Diagnosis and Treatment of Voice Disorders

Third Edition

Diagnosis and Treatment of Voice Disorders

Third Edition

Edited by
John S. Rubin, MD, FACS, FRCS
Robert T. Sataloff, MD, DMA, FACS
Gwen S. Korovin, MD, FACS

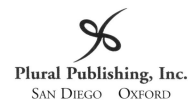

Plural Publishing, Inc.
SAN DIEGO OXFORD

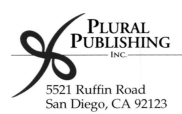

PLURAL
PUBLISHING
INC.

5521 Ruffin Road
San Diego, CA 92123

e-mail: info@pluralpublishing.com
Web site: http://www.pluralpublishing.com

49 Bath Street
Abingdon, Oxfordshire OX14 1EA
United Kingdom

Typeset in 10/12 Palatino by So Cal Graphics Printed by Sheridan Press

ISBN-13: 978-1-59756-007-8
ISBN-10: 1-59756-007-3
Library of Congress Cataloging-in-Publication Data:

Diagnosis and treatment of voice disorders / [edited by] John S. Rubin, Robert T.
    Sataloff, Gwen S. Korovin.— 3rd ed.
      p. ; cm.
    Includes bibliographical references and index.
    ISBN-13: 978-1-59756-007-8 (hardcover)
    ISBN-10: 1-59756-007-3 (hardcover)
    1. Voice disorders—Diagnosis. 2. Voice disorders—Treatment.
[DNLM: 1. Laryngeal Diseases—diagnosis. 2. Voice Disorders—therapy. 3. Laryngeal
Diseases—surgery. 4. Larynx. 5. Voice. WV 500 D536 2006] I. Rubin, John S. (John
Stephen) II. Sataloff, Robert Thayer. III. Korovin, Gwen S.
RF510.D53 2006
616.85′5—dc22

                          2006003332

Contents

Preface

In the age of information, science is advancing at an unprecedented rate. At the very heart of information lies communication, and at the center of communication, the voice. It has only been 3 years since the second edition of *Diagnosis and Treatment of Voice Disorders,* but in that short time there has been an outpouring of new information on Voice disorders such that the authors felt that it was appropriate to write a third edition. We once again dedicate this book to the memory of Wilbur James Gould, a true giant in the field of voice disorders, a tremendous advocate both for the field as well as for his patients, and a great friend and mentor.

In preparing the third edition, we have attempted to retain the format of previous editions but amplify the information with later concepts, discoveries and protocols. To this end, some chapters have few or no additions, others have been revised substantially; and several new chapters have been added. The book is subdivided into three units; basic sciences, clinical assessment, and management. The Basic Sciences and Clinical Assessment units account for approximately half of the book; the management section accounts for the remainder.

There are 11 chapters in the Basic Sciences Unit. The chapter by Laitman et al on *Formation of the Larynx: From Hox Genes to Critical Periods* has undergone an extensive rewrite commensurate with the continuous increase in information. It is an excellent complement to *Henick's Laryngeal Development* chapter, which we feel is now a classic in the literature.

Sato's *Functional Fine Structures of the Human Vocal Fold Mucosa* presents the latest insights on the fine structures of the larynx. Together with Sasaki and Kim's *Anatomy of the Human Larynx ,* and Sanders' *Microanatomy of the Vocal Fold Musculature,* the reader is presented with a truly comprehensive and in-depth survey of current anatomical perspectives. These chapters prepare the reader to explore fully Rubin and Yanagisawa's chapter *Benign Vocal Fold pathology Through the Eyes of the Laryngologist.*

We have added an entire new chapter by Spain, Mandel, and Sataloff, *The Neurology of Stuttering,* as we felt that it integrates much new information on what was previously felt to be an old subject . Newer in-

sights provided by functional brain imaging are adding tremendous information not only on stuttering but on movement disorders in general. It is an excellent companion chapter to Scherer's *Laryngeal Function During Phonation* and Benninger et al's erudite chapter, *Laryngeal Neurophysiology,* both of which have also been updated.

Baken's chapter, *Dynamic Disorders of the Voice: A Chaotic Perspective on Vocal Irregularities,* was an instant classic when it was presented in the second edition. It has been subtly updated while still offering the reader a surprisingly accessible window into the world of nonlinear dynamics and its potential benefit in the understanding of voice disturbances. The section ends with Woodson's chapter, *Research in Laryngology,* which has been thoroughly revised since the last edition and suggests directions the field is likely to follow in the near future.

Unit 2, Clinical Assessment, consists of an additional 11 chapters. It begins with two chapters, both by the Sataloff team, *History of Patients with Voice Disorders* and *Physical Examination of Patients with Voice Disorders.* These are the cornerstones of assessment and are presented in a clear, patient-oriented fashion. The following two chapters focus on flexible endoscopic evaluation. *Evaluation of Laryngeal Biomechanics by Fiberoptic Laryngoscopy* by Koufman has been substantially updated. It lays the framework for the theme of the musculoskeletal system in voice disorders, which is picked up and expanded on in later chapters by Lieberman et al and Rubin et al, which are discussed in greater detail further on. Sarpano and Mirsa's chapter, *Transnasal Esophagoscopy,* is new to this edition and expounds on the natural expansion of the office assessment further down the gullet.

Korovin and Rubin's chapter, *Introduction to the Laboratory Diagnosis of Vocal Disorders,* prepares the way for the following .four chapters. These include updated chapters by Colton and Woo on *Measuring Vocal Fold Function,* Sulica et al on *Laryngeal Electromyography,* Yanagisawa et al on *Laryngeal Photography and Videography,* and Abitbol and Castro on *3D Laryngeal CT Scan for Voice Disorders: Virtual Endoscopy—Virtual Dissection.* These chapters provide readers with insights into nonsurgical diagnostic evaluation techniques of the larynx and voice, that, taken as a group, should allow for pinpoint accuracy in diagnosis. Abitbol and Castro's chapter, when introduced into the second edition was an instant classic, and it continues to be as presented herein. The final two chapters in this section, Benninger and Gardner's *The Evaluation of Voice Outcomes and Quality of Life* and Sataloff's *Voice Impairment, Disability, Handicap and Medical/Legal Evaluation,* take the assessment of voice that one step further to the critical issue of the patient's own perception. This is, at the end of the day, the crucial outcome measure.

The remaining 26 chapters comprise the Unit 3: Managemment. A framework is given by Sataloff and Hawkshaw's *Common Medical Diagnoses and Treatment in Patients with Voice Disorders.* This is followed by three chapters on infant and pediatric voice disorders, from three different, hugely experienced teams. Tewfik and colleagues present insights on *Congenital Anomalies of the Larynx* and Rahbar and *Healy on Voice Disorders in the Pediatric Population.* A additional new chapter for this edition by Hartnick, *Diagnosis and Treatment of Pediatric Voice Disorders,* emphasizesthe office approach and management.

The following chapter by the Abitbols, *The Larynx: A Homonal Target,* stands on its own, with useful information on the effects of the endocrine system on the voice, and with particular emphasis on the sex hormones and their effects on women's voices. The later chapter by Harris and Rubin, *Medications and the Voice,* and the chapter by Spector and Rosen, *Corticosteroid Use in Otolaryngology* (new to this edition), help flesh this out as well as supply extremely important information on drug effects, interactions and complications which is essential to all workers in the field.

There are two chapters on irritants and infections of the larynx, Koufman and Watkin's heavily revised and updated chapter, *Laryngopharyngeal Reflux and Voice Disorders,* and Lebovics and Neel's classic chapter, *Infectious and Inflammatory Disorders of the Larynx.* Both provide up-to-the-moment insights. Three chapters on neurologic disorders follow. Smith and Ramig provide a broad overview in *Neurologic Disorders and the Voice.* *Vocal Fold Paralysis* is then presented by Gardner and Benninger, looking particularly at peripheral disorders and treatment. Kearney and her team give an elegant update in *Management of Spasmodic Dysphonias.*

Rosen and her team present their insights into *Psychologic Aspects of Voice Disorders.* This includes newer information on psychotropic drugs. The medication chapters have already been alluded to. Then follow two critical chapters on nonsurgical management, *The Role of the Speech-Language Pathologist in the Treatment of Voice Disorders* by Murry and Rosen and *The Role of the Voice Specialist in the Nonmedical Management of Benign Voice Disorders* by Carroll These two practical and detailed

chapters crystallize the most modern therapies available.

As noted, the entire subfield of musculoskeletal abnormalities and voice is growing. Two authoritative chapters follow in this area. Lieberman and his team present their management protocols in *Laryngeal Manipulation.* Rubin and his team then submit a chapter new to this edition, *The Effects of Posture on Voice.* Although still slightly speculative, these two chapters broadly and boldly expand this crucial area of our armamentarium and knowledge. These are followed by Rubin et al's update on *Special Considerations for the Professsional Voice User.* Of particular interest are the clinical vignettes in this chapter and the update on the role of complementary medicine.

The following several chapters are surgical in focus. Heman-Ackah et al update their experience on *Laryngotracheal Trauma* in a clear and beautifully illustrated chapter. This is followed by Courey and Ossoff's classic, *Surgical Management of Benign Voice Disorders.* Sandhu and Howard's chapter, *Management of Adult Onset Subglottic and Tracheal Stenosis* is new to this edition, and it presents the largest personal experience in Europe and possibly in the world on this complex area. Zeitels' *Vocal Fold Medialization: Injection and Laryngeal Framework Surgery,* is greatly revised and beautifully written. It is followed by Tucker's elegant and clearly illustrated chapter Laryngeal Reinervation. Dean and Sataloff's chapter *Premalignant Lesions of the Larynx* follows, setting the stage for perhaps the most innovative chapter in the book, Zeitels' *Surgery for Laryngeal Cancer.* This chapter, extensively revised, is a beacon into the future of oncologic surgery for the larynx. The book ends with the classic chapter by Woo, *Diagnosis and Management of Postoperative Dysphonia.*

In summary, the third edition of Diagnosis and Treatment of Voice Disorders provides an up-to-date, accessible, and clear reference for the various professionals entrusted with the care of patients with voice disorders, be they laryngologists or phoniatricians, speech-language pathologists or logopeds, physical therapists, osteopaths or other practitioners of complementary medicine, singing or acting voice specialists, acoustic and voice scientists, psychiatrists or psychologists, gastroenterologists or pulmonary physicians, nurses, and other allied medical specialists. It is written in language intended to be accessible to an interdisciplinary readership; and we hope that the information presented will prove not only useful, but also inspirational to all voice care professionals since each of us has the opportunity to add new knowledge to this exciting and rapidly advancing field.

JSR
RTS
GK

Contributors

Jean Abitol, MD
Ancien Chef de Clinique
Faculty of Medicine of Paris
Oto-Rhino-Laryngolotiste
Phoniatrie—Chirurgie
Paris, France
Chapters 20 and 27

Patrick Abitol, MD
Faculty of Medicine
Oto-Rhino-Laryngolofiarw
Paris, France
Chapter 20 and 27

Khalil Al Macki, MD
Resident Physician
Department of Otolaryngology
McGill University Health Center
Montreal, Canada
Chapter 24

Joseph Anticaglia, MD
Ear, Nose, and Throat Associates of New York
Flushing, New York
Chapter 12

Ronald J. Baken, PhD
Professor and Director of Laryngology Research
New York Eye and Ear Infirmary
New York, New York
Chapter 10

Michael S. Benninger, MD
Chair, Department of Otolaryngology-Head and
Neck Surgery
Henry Ford Hospital and Medical Centers
Detroit, Michigan
Chapters 8, 21, and 31

Ed Blake, MSc (Phty), MCST, SRP
Physiatrist
Specialist in Dance and Vocal Medicine
Physio-Ed Medical
London, England

Andrew Blitzer, MD, DDS
Professor of Clinical Otolaryngology
College of Physicians and Surgeons
Columbia University
Director
New York Center for Voice and Swallowing
Disorders
Medical Director
New York Center for Clinical Research
Chapter 18

Tanya Meyer, MD
Assistant Professor of Otorhinolaryngology-Head
and Neck Surgery
University of Maryland
Baltimore, Maryland

Linda M. Carroll, MS
Speech-Language Pathologist and Singing Voice
Specialist
Doctoral Student, Teachers College
Columbia University
New York, New York
Voice Consultant, Department of Otolaryngology
Lenox Hill Hospital
New York, NY 10024
Chapter 37

Albert Castro, MD
Radiologue
Directeur Centre d'Imagerie Médicale Numérisér
Monceau
Paris, France
Chapter 20

Raymond H. Colton, PhD
Professor and Chair, Department of Communication
Sciences and Disorders
Syracuse University
Syracuse, New York
Chapter 17

Mark S. Courey, MD
Professor, Otolaryngology-Head and Neck Surgery
Director, Division of Laryngology
University of California-San Francisco
San Francisco, California
Chapter 42

Carole M. Dean, MD, FRCS)
Otolaryngologist
Northside Hospital
Atlanta, Georgia

Venu Divi, MD
Department of Otolaryngology-Head and Neck
Surgery
Henry Ford Hospital and Medical Centers
Detroit, Michigan
Chapter 8

Brian P. Driscoll, MD
Ear, Nose, Throat, and Plastic Surgery Associates
Attending Otolaryngologist
Florida Hospital
Orlando, Florida
Chapter 19

Ruth Epstein, PhD, MCRCSLT
Lead Principal Speech Unit
Language Therapist
Royal National Throat, Nose, and Ear Hospital
Royal Free HNS Trust
London, England
Chapter 40

Adrian J. Fourcin, Ph.S.
Emeritus Professor of Experimental Phonetics,
Phonetics, and Linguistics
University College London
London, United Kingdom
Chapter 38

Glendon M. Gardner, MD
Department of Otolaryngology-Head and Neck
Surgery
Department of Neurology
Henry Ford Hospital
Detroit, Michigan
Chapters 8, 21, and 31

Georg S. Godding, Jr., MD
Associate Professor
Department of Otolaryngology
University of Minnesota School of Medicine
and
Department of Otolaryngology
Hennepin County Medical Center
Minneapolis, Minnesota
Chapter 41

Rodolphe Gombergh, MD
Radiologue, Directeur du Centre d'Imagerie
Médicale Numérisér Monceau
Paris, France
Chapter 20

Thomas M. Harris, MA, FRCS
Consultant ENT Surgeon
University Hospital Lewisham
Director, The Voice Clinic
Queen Mary's Hospital
Honorary Senior Lecturer, Guy's King's St. Thomas'
Medical Schools
London, United Kingdom
Chapter 34

Christopher J. Hartnick, MD, MS Epi
Assistant Professor
Harvard Medical School
Massachusetts Eye and Ear Infirmary
Boston, Massachusetts
Chapter 26

Mary J. Hawkshaw, RN, BS
Otolaryngologic Nurse Clinician
Executive Director
American Institute for Voice and Ear Research
Philadelphia, Pennsylvania
Chapters 12, 13, and 23

Gerald B. Healy, MD
Professor of Otology and Laryngology
Harvard Medical School
and
Otolaryngologist-in-Chief
Children's Hospital
Boston, Massachusetts
Chapter 25

Yolanda D. Heman-Ackah, MD
Assistant Professor
Department of Otolaryngology–Head and Neck
Surgery
Jefferson Medical College
Thomas Jefferson University
Philadelphia, Pennsylvania
Chapter 41

David H. Henick, MD
Clinical Assistant Professor
Albert Einstein College of Medicine
New York, New York
Chapter 2

Reinhardt J. Heuer, PhD
Professor, Department of Communication Sciences
and Disorders
College of Allied Health Professionals
Temple University
Philadelphia, Pennsylvania
Chapter 33

David J. Howard, PhD
The Royal National Throat, Nose, and Ear Hospital
University College
London, England
Chapter 43

Jagdeep Hundal, MD
Section of Otolaryngology
Department of Surgery
Yale University School of Medicine
New Haven, Connecticut
Chapter 3

Pamela R. Kearney, MD
Assistant Professor
Otolaryngology-Head and Neck Surgery
George Washington University
Washington, DC
Chapter 32

Gwen S. Korovin, MD, FACS
Clinical Assistant Professor
Department of Otolaryngology
New York School of Medicine
And
Consulting Otolaryngologist
Ames Vocal Dynamics Laboratory
Lenox Hill Hospital
And
Attending Physician
Department of Otolaryngology
Manhattan Eye, Ear, and Throat Hospital
And
Attending Physician
Department of Otolaryngology
Lenox Hill Hospital
New York, New York
Chapters 16 and 40

Jamie A. Koufman, MD
Director, Center for Voice Disorders
Professor of Otolaryngology
Wake Forest University School of Medicine
Winston-Salem, North Carolina
Chapter 14

Christy L. Ludlow, PhD, CCC-SLP
Chief, Laryngeal and Speech Section
National Institute of Neurological Disorders and
Stroke
National Institutes of Health
Bethesda, Maryland
Chapter 32

Jeffrey T. Laitman, PhD
Professor of Cell Biology and Anatomy
Department of Otolaryngology
Director of Anatomy and Functional Morphology
Professor of Otolaryngology
Mt. Sinai School of Medicine
and
Research Associate
Department of Anthropology
American Museum of Natural History
New York, New York
Chapter 1

Robert S. Lebovics, MD
Surgical Consultant
National Institutes of Health
Bethesda, Maryland
Chapter 29

Steven L. Levy, MD, PhD
Medical Director
Psych Arts Center
Research Associate, American Institute for Voice
and Ear Research
Philadelphia, Pennsylvania
Chapter 33

Jacob Lieberman, DO, MA
Osteopathic Physician and Psychotherapist
and
Team Member
The Voice Research Laboratory
Queen Mary's Hospital
Sidcup, Kent, England
Chapter 38

Steven Mandel, MD
Clinical Professor of Neurology
Thomas Jefferson University
Philadelphia, Pennsylvania
Chapter 9

Eric A. Mann MD, PHD
Staff Otolaryngologist
Laryngeal and Speech Section
National Institute of Neurological Disorders and
Stroke

National Institutes of Health
Bethesda, Maryland
Chapter 32

Leslie Mathieson, DipCST, FRCSLT
Visiting Lecturer in Voice Pathology
The University of Reading
Reading, United Kingdom
Chapter 39

Natasha Mirza, MD, FACS
Associate Professor Otolaryngology, Head and Neck
Surgery Hospital of the University of Pennsylvania
Philadelphia, Pennsylvania
Chapter 15

Thomas Murry, Ph.D.
Professor of Speech Pathology
College of Physicians and Surgeons
Clinical Director of the Voice and Swallowing
Center
Columbia University
New York, New York
Chapter 36

H. Bryan Neel, III, MD, PhD
Professor
Department of Otolaryngology—Head and Neck
Surgery
Mayo Clinic Medical School
Rochester, Minnesota
Chapter 29

Drew M. Noden, PhD
Professor
Department of Biomedical Sciences
New York State College of Veterinary Sciences
Cornell University,
Ithaca, New York
Chapter 1

Lorraine Olson Ramig, PhD
Professor
Department of Speech, Language and Hearing
Sciences
University of Colorado-Boulder
and
Research Associate
Wilbur James Gould Voice Center
The Denver Center for the Performing Arts
Denver, Colorado
Chapter 30

Robert H. Ossoff, DMD, MD
Associate Vice Chancellor for Health Affairs
Director

Vanderbilt Bill Wilkerson Center for Otolaryngology
and Communication Sciences

Guy M. Maness Professor and Chairman
Department of Otolaryngology
Vanterbilt University Medical Center
Nashville, TN
Chapter 42

Reza Rahbar, DMD, MD, FACS
Department of Otolaryngology
Children's Hospital
and
Assistant Professor of Otology and Laryngology
Department of Otology and Laryngology
Harvard Medical School
Boston, Massachusetts
Chapter 25

Vijay Rao, MD
Professor
Department of Radiology
Jefferson Medical College
Thomas Jefferson University
Philadelphia, Pennsylvania
Chapter 41

Clark A. Rosen, MD
Director, University of Pittsburgh Voice Center
Associate Professor, Department of Otolaryngology
University of Pittsburgh School of Medicine
Pittsburgh, Pennsylvania
Chapter 35

Deborah Caputo Rosen, RN, PhD
Medical Psychologist and Director of Health
Outreach
External Affairs and Communications
Temple University Health System
Philadelphia, Pennsylvania
Adjunct Professor
Department of Counseling and Human Relations
College of Education
Villanova University
Villanova, Pennsylvania
Chapter 33

Marc Rosen, MD
Associate Professor
Department of Psychiatry
Yale University Medical School
New Haven, Connecticut
Chapter 35

John S. Rubin, MD, FACS, FRCS
Consultant Otolaryngologist
Royal National Throat, Nose, and Ear Hospital
and
Honorary Consultant Otolaryngologist
St. Bartholomew's Hospital
London, England
and
Honorary Senior Lecturer
Institute of Laryngology and Otology
University College of London
and
Visiting Associate Professor
Department of Otolaryngology
Albert Einstein College of Medicine
Bronx, New York
Chapters 6, 16, 38, 39, and 40

Ira Sanders, MD
Associate Clinical Professor
Department of Otolaryngology
Director of Research, Grabscheid Voice Center
Mount Sinai School of Medicine
New York, New York
Chapter 5

Guri S. Sandhu, MD, FRCS
The Royal National Throat, Nose and Ear Hospital
University College
London, England
Chapter 43

Marshall E. Smith, MD
Associate Professor
Division of Otolaryngology-Head and Neck Surgery
University of Utah Medical Center
Salt Lake City, Utah
And
Research Associate
Wilbur James Gould Voice Center
The Denver Center for the Performing Arts
Denver, Colorado
Chapter 30

Clarence T. Sasaki, MD
Ohse Professor of Surgery and Chief
Department of Surgery, Section of Otolaryngology
Yale University School of Medicine
New Haven, Connecticut
Chapter 3

Robert T. Sataloff, MD, DMA, FACS
Professor and Chairman
Department of Otolaryngology-HNS
Associate Dean for Clinical Academic Specialties
Drexel University College of MedicineProfessor of

Otolaryngology
Jefferson Medical College
Thomas Jefferson University
and
Chairman
Department of Otolaryngology-Head and Neck
Surgery
The Graduate Hospital
and
Adjunct Professor of Otorhinolaryngology-Head
and Neck Surgery
University of Pennsylvania
and
Chairman of the Boards of Directors
The Voice Foundation
American Institute for Voice and Ear Research
Chapters 12, 13, 22, 23, 33, 46

Kiminori Sato, MD, PhD
Clinical Professor
Department of Otolaryngology-Head and Neck
Surgery
Kurume University School of Medicine
Kurume, Japan
Chapter 4

Ronald C. Scherer, PhD
Professor, Department of Communication Disorders
Bowling Green State University
Bowling Green, Ohio
Chapter 7

Craig Schwirmer, MD
Private Practice
Dallas, Texas
Chapter 8

H. Steven Sims, MD
Clinical Fellow in Laryngology and Care of the
Professional Voice
Department of Otolaryngology
Vanderbilt University Medical Center
Nashville, Tennessee
Chapter 19

Steven E. Sobol, MD, FRCSC
Assistant Professor
Department of Otolaryngology
Emory University School of Medicine
Atlanta, Georgia
Chapter 24

Rebecca Spain, MD
Assistant Professor
Department of Neurology
Jefferson Medical College

Thomas Jefferson University
Philadelphia, Pennsylvania
Chapter 9

Anthony M. Sparano, MD
Department of Otolaryngology-Head and Neck
Surgery
University of Pennsylvania Medical Center
Philadelphia, Pennsylvania
Chapter 15

Andrew Spector, MD
Chapter 35

Lucian Sulica, MD
Director
Center for Voice Disorders
Department of Otolaryngology
New York Eye and Ear Infirmary
Beth Israel Medical Center
New York, NY
and
Assistant Professor
Department of Otolaryngology
New York Medical College
and
Assistant Professor
Deparment of Otolaryngology
Albert Einstein College of Medicine
Bronx, New York
Ted L. Tewfik, MD, FRCSC
Professor and Director of Continuing Medical
Education (CME)
Department of Otolaryngology
Montreal Children's Hospital and McGill University
Health Center
Montreal, Canada
Chapter 24

Harvey M. Tucker, MD, FACS
Professor of Otolaryngology-Head and Neck
Surgery
Case Western Reserve School of Medicine
Cleveland, Ohio
Chapter 45

Peak Woo, MD
Director of Clinical Services
Eugene Grabscheid, MD, Voice Center
The Mount Sinai Medical Center

Professor
Department of Otolaryngology
Mount Sinai School of Medicine
New York, New York
Chapters 17 and 48

Gayle E. Woodson, MD
Professor, Department of Otolaryngology
Southern Illinois University School of Medicine
Springfield, Illinois
S. Carter Wright, Jr., MD
Wake Forest University School of Medicine
Winston-Salem, North Carolina
Chapter 28

Eiji Yanagisawa, MD, FACS
Clinical Professor of Otolaryngology
Yale University School of Medicine
Attending Otolaryngologist, Yale-New Haven
Hospital
Attending Otolaryngologist, Hospital of Saint
Raphael
New Haven, Connecticut
Chapter 8 and 19

Young-Ho Kim, MS, PhD
Section of Otolaryngology
Department of Surgery
Yale University School of Medicine
New Haven, Connecticut
Chapter 3

Thomas R. Van De Water, PhD
Director
Cochlear Implant Research Program
Professor
University of Miami Ear Institute
Department of Otolaryngology
Miami, Florida
Chapter 1

Steven M. Zeitels, MD, FACS
Eugene B. Casey Chair of Laryngeal Surgery
Harvard Medical School
Director, Center for Laryngeal Surgery and Voice
Rehabiltation
Massachusetts General Hospital
Boston, Massachusetts
Chapter 44 and 47

Dedication

It has been 10 years since the untimely death of Wilbur James Gould. We wish to again dedicate this book to his memory. Dr. Gould was a true master of laryngology, a giant in the field of voice disorders, and a personal mentor to all the authors.

One of the authors (JSR) wrote a brief poem about Jim, shortly following his death, which is included below and which we feel at the distance of the intervening years still encompasses our feelings about this remarkable man.

The authors

to Wilbur James Gould
in memoriam

We are a special club,
those of us whose lives he changed.
We are select
but not so few,
for he threw his net widely
and he chose wisely.

We are a special club—
we had the audacious luck
to learn from him,
to be taught by him,
to be with him
as his brain hatched up
idea after idea,
project after project.

He pushed us,
or he cajoled us,
or he talked us
into the lab,
into learning voice,
into loving laryngology.
He did whatever he felt it took—

and he did it time and again,
until it worked.

And then there are his patients,
for almost 50 years
the tens of thousands whom he touched,
whom he was always willing to see,
whom he healed
as much by caring
as by treating.

He is Wilbur James Gould
I doubt that there will ever be another
such as he.
We are his legacy,
and now we must, each of us,
fufill it.

Unit 1
BASIC SCIENCE

1

Formation of the Larynx: From Hox Genes to Critical Periods

Jeffrey T. Laitman, PhD
Drew M. Noden, PhD
Thomas R. Van De Water, PhD

The human larynx is a compact and complex structure that must serve respiratory, protective, and vocalization functions. Although there have been several descriptions of the major histogenic and morphogenic events during laryngeal development in humans[1] and other mammals,[2] only recently have accurate fate mapping and molecular expression data become available.

The larynx arises at the interface of "head" and "trunk" regions of the embryo and cells from both sides of this interface move to the site of laryngeal development. Also, it is the only musculoskeletal assembly intimately associated with the endodermal gut tube. These unique attributes make dissecting the cellular and molecular basis of laryngeal development especially difficult and, to date, neglected.

This chapter addresses two aspects of laryngeal development that are especially critical to understanding the structure-function relations both within this complex and between it and adjacent structures. First, we review early embryologic events and processes, including the genesis of laryngeal tissues and interactions, both cellular and genetic, which are essential for the normal histogenesis and morphogenesis of the larynx. Second, we identify and discuss significant critical periods in prenatal and postnatal laryngeal development in humans.

ESTABLISHING LARYNGEAL PRIMORDIA

Common Developmental Themes

Laryngeal development requires the determination and integrated movements of several cell lineages that converge beside the caudal aspect of the pharynx. These epithelial and mesenchymal precursors of mucosa, loose and dense connective tissues, voluntary and smooth muscles, blood vessels, and nerves have greatly varied embryonic histories, and each cell lineage undergoes developmental programming that prepares its members to participate as chondrocytes, myocytes, and other components of laryngeal morphogenesis.

Achieving this programming is an epigenetic process for each precursor population. This means that cells engage in a progressive series of interactions involving other cells and the extracellular milieu that alter the function of specific genes, which in turn changes the response characteristics of cells to subsequent interactions. These interactions affect rates of cell proliferation, pathways and speeds of cell migration, and both the commitment to and the expression of specific cell phenotypes. Clearly, such processes must be temporally and spatially coordinated in order for so many disparate progenitors to achieve an integrated outcome.

A multicomponent musculoskeletal laryngeal apparatus is absent in anamniotes, although some terrestrial amphibians do have cartilaginous rods that partially circumscribe an elongated glottis. This single skeletal element is often cited as being derived aa antecedent to at least one of the laryngeal skeletal elements and is thought to have evolved from gill-associated cartilages. However, there is little direct evidence for either of these claims. Among amniotes many laryngeal precursor populations have sites of origin that are evolutionarily conserved. A key feature of this conserved plan is the presence in all vertebrate embryos of a *segmental organization* within many tissues that are developmentally related to the larynx. This is manifest especially in hindbrain, branchial arch, and trunk axial regions. While the larynx is not generally viewed as a segmentally organized set of structures, tissues developing nearby, many formed from common progenitors, do exhibit a metameric organization during their development.

The expression patterns of several members of gene families that are involved in lineage delineation and spatial programming of head and neck tissues similarly show a segmental organization. Abnormal expression of some of these genes, either as a result of germ line mutations in humans or experimental gene manipulation in transgenic mice, also results in disruptions of hindbrain, branchial, otic, and laryngeal morphogenesis.

The first objective of this section is to identify the origins of laryngeal precursors and document their movements to the site of laryngeal morphogenesis. The second goal is to identify when and where each of these populations become programmed to form tissues of the types and shapes appropriate to their final location, including the genetic bases for their decisions. The reader should be warned that laryngeal development has received little attention by experimental biologists. Thus, many of the hypotheses regarding laryngeal development presented here are by inference, based on properties of neighboring structures and experimental analyses in only a few model systems.

Origins of Laryngeal Precursors

Overview

The epithelial lining of the larynx forms close to the cauda of the pharynx, although this site is otherwise indistinct from the adjacent parts of the primitive endodermal tube. Rostral to this site the pharynx forms a set of segmentally arranged endodermal outpocketings, the *pharyngeal pouches*, between which are located the *branchial arches* (also referred to as pharyngeal or visceral arches). Present within each branchial arch are precursor populations for connective tissues, skeletal muscle, blood vessels, and peripheral neurons. These may be segregated from their neighbors (eg, skeletal myoblasts) or fully interspersed (eg., endothelial precursors). Some vertebrates establish a large number of branchial arches, retaining many as gills, but amniotes (reptiles, birds, and mammals) form only three or four recognizable branchial arch swellings on each side of the head (Figure 1–1). True fifth and sixth branchial arches do not form in amniotes.

During the neurula stage, embryos establish sets of structures common to all developing vertebrates. The *neural tube* is located dorsally (posteriorly) and is flanked on each side by *paraxial mesoderm*. Along most of the body length, this mesoderm forms cuboidal epithelial blocks called *somites*. In the head, however, paraxial mesoderm fails to epithelialize and does not display any overt segmental organization. Ventrally, the endodermal sheet folds to form a gut tube, consisting of the pharynx, rostrally, that is continuous with the future fore-, mid-, and hind-gut passageways. When first formed, this endodermal tube is enveloped by *lateral mesoderm*, which will form the smooth muscles and associated loose connective tissues of the digestive tract. Beside the lateral walls and floor of much the pharynx located rostral to the larynx, this sparse mesoderm becomes fully displaced by a secondary population of mesenchymal cells, the *neural crest*.

The neural crest brings a new population of connective tissue precursors to parts of the head in all vertebrates. Crest cells arise from the roof of the brain or

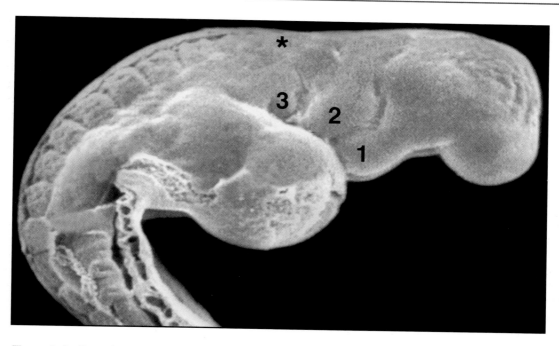

Figure 1–1. Scanning electron micrograph showing the swellings of the first (1), second (2), and third (3) branchial (pharyngeal) arches, which have formed by the movement of neural crest cells from dorsal, neural to ventral, pharyngeal regions. The grooves between each arch represent the sites of apposition between surface ectoderm and underlying pharyngeal pouches. Note the location of the prominent heart primordium, which at this stage has already begun to loop. The heart will subsequently shift its position caudally as the branchial arches and caudal pharyngeal region remodel. About 14 somites are visible; * indicates somite number 1. The specimen is a 16-day, 22-somite domestic cat embryo, which corresponds to a stage 12 (30-day) human embryo.

neural folds and move en masse to fill the areas between each pharyngeal pouch and also circumscribe the prosencephalon (Figure 1–2). The hindbrain, from which the majority of branchial arch crest cells originate, is a segmentally organized tubular structure, and the crest cells that enter each branchial arch can be traced to specific segments.

The larynx develops near the caudal boundary of connective tissues derived from the neural crest. Caudal (posterior) to this, all connective tissues associated with the endodermal tube—including most of those associated with the larynx—are of lateral mesoderm origin. Later, after the *respiratory diverticulum* buds off from the pharynx, some of these mesodermal cells will aggregate to form laryngeal cartilages and the highly ordered tracheal rings. The molecular basis for these patterned assemblies is not known.

The preceding overview highlights the complexity of laryngeal embryology owing in large part to its association with the ventral endodermal tube and location at the head-trunk interface. The following sections provide detailed accounts of each component of the developing larynx.

The Respiratory Diverticulum

The epithelial lining of the pharynx, from which the respiratory diverticulum arises, is formed along with the endodermal lining of the pharynx and gut during early gastrulation stages. Cells within the epiblast, which is the superficial layer of the embryonic disk (inner cell mass), move internally beginning at the junction of the epiblast and early primitive streak: these establish a new, internal epithelial layer, the endoderm.[3] Once internalized, the endodermal sheet expands rapidly and forms the entire extraembryonic endodermal primordium. Shortly thereafter, the positional identities of most endodermal structures (eg, thyroid, thymus, stomach, pancreas) become specified.

Endodermal cells that will give rise to laryngeal mucosa are initially located beneath (ventral to) the future post-otic hindbrain region. Analyses of dicephalic (two-headed) neonates reveal that only when the site of skull duplication occurs as far caudally as the occipito-atlanto-axial region, which flanks the caudal hindbrain, will there also be paired larynges. Duplications that extend only to the spheno-occipital (mid-hindbrain) level will have a single laryngeal apparatus.

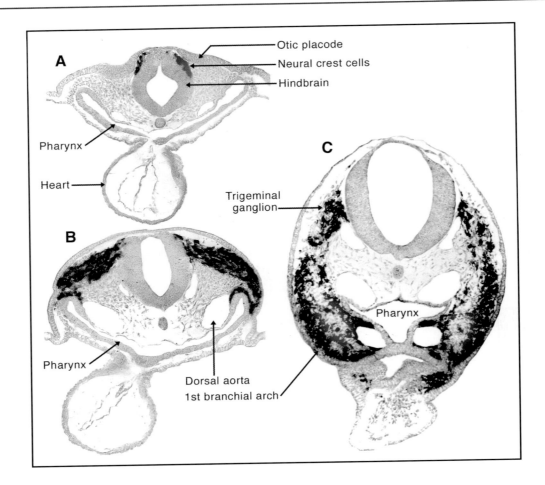

Figure 1–2. Transverse sections of chick embryos stained with an antibody to neural crest cells. **A** shows a 12-somite embryo at the level of the otic placode (inner ear primordium). Crest cells have recently emerged from the roof of the hindbrain. **B** is at the pre-otic (rhombomere 4), first pharyngeal pouch region of a 16-somite chick embryo; note the sharp boundary between crest and underlying paraxial mesoderm. **C** is a 25-somite embryo. By this stage crest cells have completed their ventral movements and, after the outflow tract of the heart (O.T.) shifts caudally, will join in the midline to complete the formation of the lower jaw region. Unlabeled cells within the branchial arch are mesodermal cells that will form the jaw musculature.

The *respiratory diverticulum* (laryngotrachial groove, tracheal diverticulum) is first evident as a ventrally expanded trough projecting from the floor of the pharynx beginning at the level of the fourth (most caudal) pharyngeal pouch.[1] Shortly after this evagination forms, distinct lateral outpocketings emerge bilaterally from the caudal margin of this trough; these demarcate the future bronchial-pulmonary structures. Partial separation of the ventral (respiratory) from dorsal (esophageal) regions of the caudal pharynx occurs by a caudal-to-cranial dying off of intermediate endodermal epithelial cells.[4-6] This is followed by a rapid caudal elongation of both the respiratory diverticulum and the esophagus.[7,8] Subsequent stages in the devel-

opment of the respiratory diverticulum are presented in greater detail in Chapter 2.

It is not known how the precise site at which the respiratory diverticulum forms is specified. Similar to several other endoderm-derived structures (eg, the thyroid and pancreas), the early histogenic remodeling of the respiratory diverticulum requires the presence of a cholesterol-associated growth factor called sonic *hedgehog*.[9] Reducing the level of sonic hedgehog biosynthesis by cells of the respiratory diverticulum, or disabling the ability of adjacent mesoderm cells to properly respond, results in defects of tracheo-esophageal separation and tracheal chondrogenesis.[10] These dysmorphologies can be isolated, but in humans are more commonly syndromic (eg, Pallister-Hall, Smith-Lemli-Opitz, and VACTERL syndromes).[11,12]

Lateral Mesoderm

The onset of intraembryonic mesoderm formation follows the appearance of endoderm, but this mesenchymal population rapidly expands to fully overlie the endodermal sheet. In human embryos this process is complete by the end of the second week of gestation, and spatial relations established at these early stages remain constant throughout subsequent stages.

Fate-mapping studies in avian embryos have identified lateral mesoderm located beside the first and second somites as the source of laryngeal connective tissues, including the arytenoid and cricoid cartilages (Figure 1–3).[7] These data contradict previous assertions based on descriptive studies, which postulated that all skeletal elements associated with the larynx are homologous to gill-associated skeletal structures in anamniotes and as such would be derived from branchial arch neural crest cells. Birds do not have a structure homologous to the thyroid cartilage, and thus the embryonic origin of this element has not been positively identified. However, based on its relation to other structures, an origin from the neural crest is most likely.

Lateral mesoderm located caudal to the laryngeal primordium forms the tracheal cartilages and associated connective tissues. Analyses of expression pat-

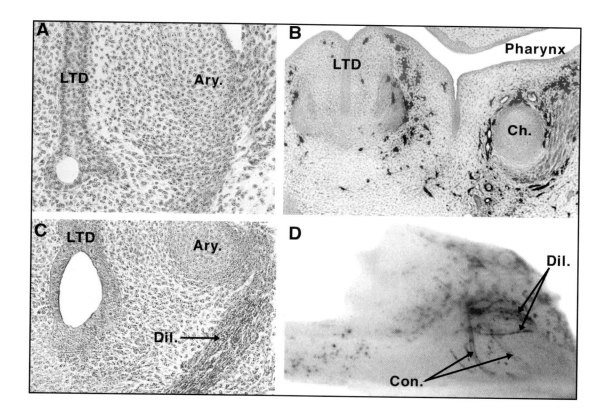

Figure 1–3. Origins of laryngeal cartilages and blood vessels. **A** shows the larynx from a chick embryo that received a transplant of quail lateral mesoderm at an earlier stage. Quail cells are identified in the arytenoid (*Ary*) cartilage by their prominent dense nuclear marker, which is not present in other tissues. **B** is from a similar embryo, but this section was stained to reveal only the endothelial cells derived from the transplant. Note the extensive spreading that resulted from invasive movements of grafted angioblasts. In **C**, quail somites 1 to 2 were grafted into a chick host. In this case a laryngeal muscle (*Dil.*, dilator glottides) but not associated connective tissues are derived from the transplant. **D** confirms the somitic origin of laryngeal muscles, but in this case a reporter gene was introduced into somite 2 using a retroviral vector. In addition to both avian laryngeal muscles (*Con*, constrictor glottides), many surrounding endothelial cells are evident by their labeling. *LTD*, laryngotracheal diverticulum. Sources, **A**,[18] **C**.[19]

terns of early chondrogenic genes such as *sox9* and *collagen 2A1* reveal that tracheal cartilage precursors are initially specified as a continuous longitudinal band within mesoderm located dorsolateral to the proximal (cranial) half of the respiratory diverticulum.[10] Later, this band becomes subdivided into discrete, regularly spaced chondrogenic foci, each of which subsequently expands ventrally.

A detailed molecular biography of laryngeal chondrogenesis is not yet available. Human patients and transgenic mice with haplo-insufficiency of *sox9* expression have, among other skeletal defects, upper airway defects secondary to hypoplasia of laryngeal and tracheal cartilages.[13]

Lateral mesoderm located rostral to the laryngeal primordium is exclusively angiogenic and cardiogenic. Embryonic angioblasts are one of the earliest progenitor populations to be delineated and constitute over one-third of the early mesodermal population.[14] These endothelial precursors are a unique and poorly understood population. Most early intraembryonic angioblasts undergo extensive, highly invasive movements that are unrivaled by any other migratory population in the embryo.[15] Thus, many endothelial cells associated with the larynx will have arisen elsewhere in head mesoderm, and some angioblasts originally located adjacent to the caudal pharynx will have participated in the formation of outflow tract endocardial formation.[16]

Paraxial Mesoderm

Despite the pronounced differences in appearance between trunk (somitic, epithelial) and head (unsegmented, mesenchymal) paraxial mesoderm populations, they are similar in the lineages to which they give rise. All striated voluntary muscles in the body arise within paraxial mesoderm. These may differentiate in situ, forming, for example, muscles associated with the vertebral column. Many myogenic populations move peripherally. In the trunk these include hypaxial (e.g., thoracic and abdominal body wall) and appendicular muscle precursors.[17]

All voluntary muscles in the head undergo extensive morphogenetic movements prior to their terminal differentiation. Myogenic cells originating within the first two somites join with myoblasts from somites 2 to 5 to form the *hypoglossal cord*, which rapidly expands ventrally (Figure 1–4). As this column approaches the level of the pharynx, myoblasts from somites 1 to 2 break away from the cord and move beside the rostral margin of the respiratory diverticulum.[18,19] The remaining myoblasts continue moving ventrally then rostrally to seed the primordium of the tongue. These cells are committed to the myogenic lineage prior to leaving the somites, as evidenced by their expression of the skeletal muscle specific gene *myf5* and other muscle-specific genes.[20]

These movements bring muscle primordia out of the paraxial mesoderm domain. Upon leaving the hypoglossal cord, laryngeal muscles become surrounded by lateral mesoderm cells, which will form the connective tissues associated with these muscles. In contrast, the tongue muscle primordia cross into the neural crest-populated branchial arch region. Unlike most nearby branchial muscles, the intrinsic laryngeal musculature does not show overt signs of muscle organization, such as alignment of primary myocytes, until after adjacent cartilaginous structures have begun to condense.[21] These sites of origin of laryngeal and glossal muscles are reflected in their innervation by cranial nerves X and XII, respectively. Myoblasts arising more rostrally, in unsegmented paraxial mesoderm, form branchial muscles that are innervated by somatic components of cranial motor nerves V, VII, and IX and extraocular muscles innervated by cranial nerves III, IV, and VI.[19,22,23]

Paraxial mesoderm is also the primary source of skeletal elements that constitute the neurocranium (Figure 1–5).[17,24,25] Cells originating in unsegmented paraxial mesoderm surround the midbrain and much of the hindbrain and otic (inner ear) vesicle, and will form the parietal, petrosal, and basisphenoid bones. The occipital skeletal array is derived from somites 1 to 5.

Hindbrain and Neural Crest Cells

Shortly after the cranial region of the neural tube closes, a series of transverse indentations in the walls and floor of the tube reveals the metameric organization of the brain. Within the hindbrain, these indentations delineate compartments called *rhombomeres* that presage the sites where specific motor nuclei and specialized sensory processing centers will subsequently arise (Figure 1–6). For example, histogenesis of motor neurons that will project to the first (cranial nerve V), second (VII) and third (IX) branchial arches begins in rhombomeres 2, 4, and 6, respectively, a pattern that has been highly conserved during vertebrate evolution. Somatic motor neurons associated with cranial X (including the so-called "cranial root" of cranial nerve XI) arise over an extended length of the hindbrain that includes several rhombomeres. This region spans both unsegmented and somitic regions of paraxial mesoderm.

Neural crest cells form within neural folds or the roof of the neural tube beginning near the prosen-

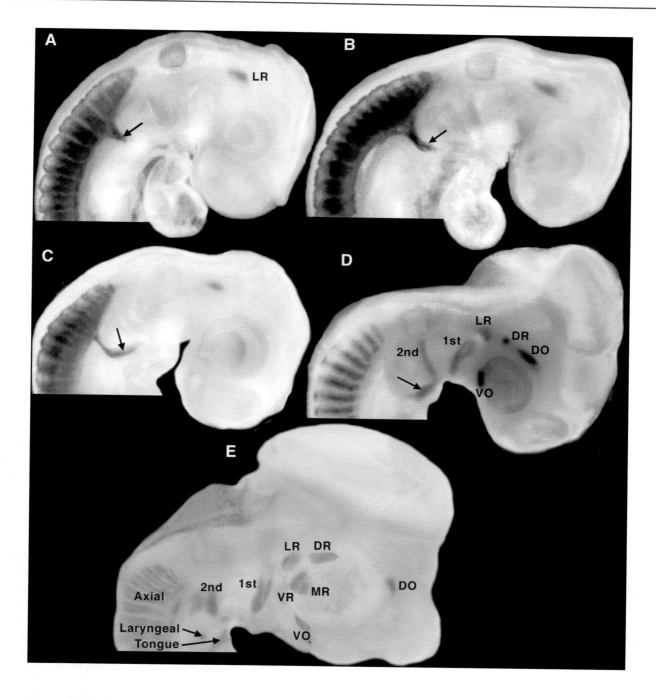

Figure 1–4. The development of tongue and laryngeal muscle precursors, shown in chick embryos at 2 to 5 days of incubation (equivalent to stages 12–18 [weeks 5–6] of human development). Arrows in **A–D** show the hypoglossal cord. This contains myoblasts that originate in the lateral margin of somites 1 to 5 then migrate ventrally to the level of the pharynx. **A–C** are *in situ* hybridizations for expression of *Paraxis*, a transcription factor expressed in all somite-derived muscle progenitors and also in the lateral rectus (*LR*) primordium. **D** is probed for *myf5*, which is expressed in all skeletal myoblasts. **E** is stained with an antibody to a myosin heavy chain. By this stage the laryngeal and glossal muscle precursors have separated from one another; the former are beside the caudal pharynx immediately behind the 4th pharyngeal pouches, but have not separated into individual muscles. The glossal muscles have not penetrated the tongue primordium. *1st, 2nd* are muscle condensations in the corresponding branchial arches. *DR, MR, VR,* dorsal (superior), medial, and ventral rectus muscles; *DO, VO,* dorsal and ventral oblique muscles.

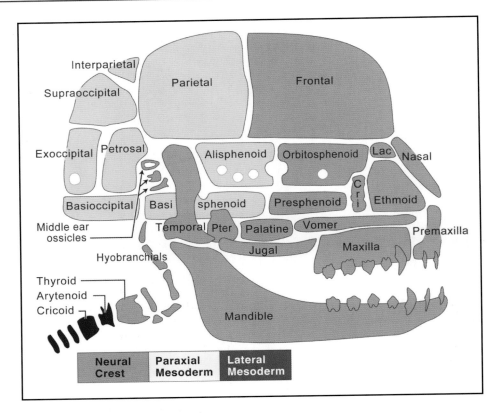

Figure 1–5. Schematic skull showing the embryonic origins of each bone. The larynx forms at the interface between connective tissues derived from neural crest and paraxial and lateral mesoderms.

cephalic-mesencephalic junction and extending caudally along the entire length of the spinal cord. There are two sites—rhombomeres 3 and 5—at which few crest cells are formed. This punctuation in the large head crest population allows for an early separation of crest cells destined to occupy each of the first three branchial arches.[26,27] Neural crest cells generated at mid- and hindbrain levels fully emigrate from the neural tube. Some will later re-establish contact as they form the cranial sensory ganglia, but most will disperse peripherally within branchial arches, the integument (eg, melanocytes), the gut tube (eg, enteric neurons and glia), peripheral nerves (eg, Schwann cells), and parts of the cardiac outflow tract (eg, distal aorticopulmonary septum).

Within each branchial arch, all the connective tissues and smooth muscle cells are derived from these crest populations. This includes tendons associated with all muscles that attach to jaw or branchial skeletal structures, such as suprahyoid and some infrahyoid (eg, thyrohyoid) muscles, and muscles that span from laryngeal or hyoid elements to the tongue.[24,28] In contrast, muscles that are fully intrinsic to the larynx

or that extend caudally from its cartilages derive their connective tissues from lateral mesoderm.

Neural crest cells generated more rostrally envelop the prosencephalon and optic vesicles, and as such constitute the sole source of connective tissues in the midfacial and upper jaw regions.[29] This includes precursors of the frontal, most orbital, and facial bones and meningeal layers associated with the diencephalon and telencephalon (Figure 1–7). Also, crest cells are present at the sites where sutures form between frontal, parietal, and interparietal bones, and are necessary for maintenance of these growth zones.[25]

Analyses of Spatial Organization

Cellular Interactions

Early in its development, each cell lineage undergoes a series of progressive restrictions or commitments that result in the expression of phenotypic properties unique to its history and appropriate to its locations. For example, only those myotome epithelial cells lo-

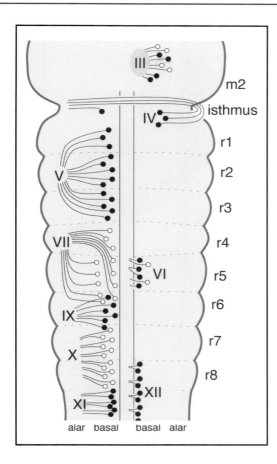

Figure 1–6. Schematic representation of the distribution of primary motor neurons in a mammalian embryo. Note the clear segregation of most, but not all, motor nuclei; there is greater overlap in the more caudal parts of the hindbrain, probably reflecting the enhanced functional domains serves by cranial nerves IX and X. Some neurons in nuclei III and VI will later undergo transmedian migrations.

cated at the ventrolateral margins of somites 1 through 5 will become migration-competent myoblasts. Comparably positioned cells in adjacent somites do not express the genes characteristic of migration myoblasts (eg, *c-met*), and neighboring cells in these occipital somites either do not commit to the myogenic lineage or, if they do, are not migratory.[30]

Similarly, neural crest cells emigrating from the roof are heterogeneous. In vivo and in vitro clonal analyses indicate that a small number of newly formed crest cells are committed to neuronal and melanogenic lineages. However, most remain multipotential during the early stages of dispersal, and become committed to specific fates in response to signals emanating either from tissues adjacent to their migratory routes or from other neural crest cells. [31,32]

In the embryo, *lineage commitment* must be fully integrated with *spatial organization*. For over a century developmental biologists have searched for the mechanisms underlying each of these processes and their integration. Although much is known about the induction of myoblasts within paraxial mesoderm[18] or chondroblasts within branchial neural crest,[33] understanding the basis for the spatial determination of, for example, the cricothyroid muscle or the arytenoid cartilage has been more elusive. Establishing spatial organization within embryonic tissues is an obligate multicellular activity. The structures formed by each cell population must have the three-dimensional shape and size appropriate for their location and functions. Extensive cellular and genetic analyses have shown that *the processes of lineage commitment and spatial organization involve different and distinct mechanisms.*

Clues regarding spatial organization within neural crest and paraxial mesodermal populations came initially from mapping data that defined the relations between them during their movements into each branchial arch (Figure 1–7). Shortly after leaving the neural tube, crest cells that subsequently will occupy each branchial arch overlie regions of paraxial mesoderm from which muscles associated with the same branchial arches will develop, and *both populations move in concert into the appropriate arches.* Furthermore, they subsequently become innervated by motor and sensory neurons that arise at the identical axial levels. Thus, all branchial arch constituents (except angioblasts) arise and maintain a strict registration from their time of origin through their terminal differentiation.[34]

Of course, this close registration only shows that opportunities for integrated spatial organization are available. To investigate whether this relationship is in fact a necessary prerequisite to the integrated morphogenesis of branchial skeletal and muscular tissues, experiments in which these spatial relations are disrupted have been performed. Taking advantage of the accessibility of avian embryos for microsurgical manipulations, precursors of trunk muscles (ie, somites) have been grafted in the place of head mesoderm. The results of these experiments, and comparable analyses of limb muscles, are consistent: grafted muscle precursors from any part of the body are able to form muscles that are structurally normal in their new location.[35-37] Thus, despite having a different ancestry and place of "birth," grafted trunk muscle precursors receive and are able to recognize both histogenic and morphogenic cues from surrounding cephalic tissues.

The implication of defining myoblasts as a subordinate, responsive population is that there must be one or more ordinate tissues responsible for initiating and sustaining myocyte differentiation and for orchestrat-

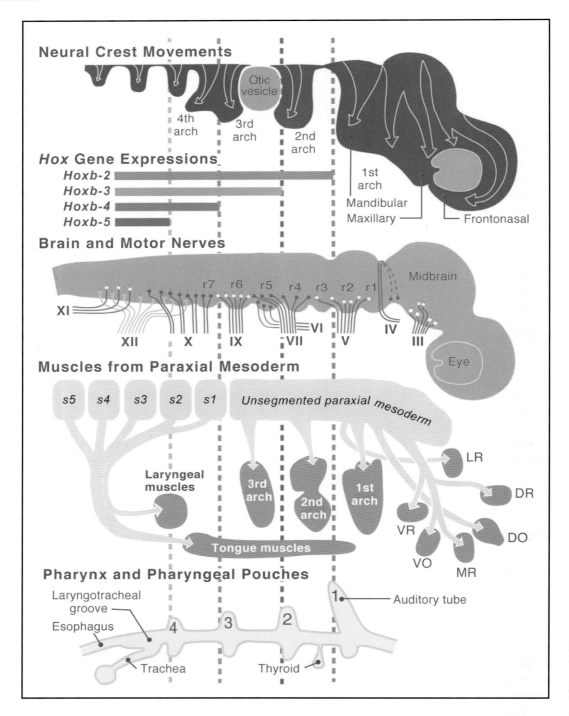

Figure 1–7. Schematic staggered view showing the spatial relations among progenitor populations of different embryonic origins. Sites of origin and patterns of movements for neural crest and myogenic mesodermal cells are shown, as are locations of cranial motor nerves and pharyngeal pouches. Note that the progenitors of all branchial arch tissues trace their origins to a common axial level, whereas musculoskeletal and neural progenitors for frontonasal and periocular regions have widely disparate origins. *Hox* genes have extensive longitudinal zones of expression, but it is the boundary of each that is critical in establishing spatial identity within rhombomeres and neural crest cells. Only one of the multiple sets of *Hox* genes that are active in the hindbrain and neural crest cells is shown. Note that these expression boundaries correspond to the gaps between crest cells destined to occupy each branchial arch. *r1, r2,* etc. identify rhombomeres in the hindbrain; *1, 2,* etc. identify pharyngeal pouches. *III, IV, V,* etc. label cranial motor nerves.

ing muscle morphogenesis. Early differentiation of somitic muscles occurs in response to a consortium of signals from surrounding tissues, such as overlying ectoderm, lateral mesoderm, the notochord, and the neural tube.[18] Acquisition of migratory competence in hypoglossal and appendicular myoblasts requires signals, including hepatocyte growth factor, from lateral mesoderm.[30] However, the basis for subsequent segregation of laryngeal from glossal progenitors is not known.

Morphogenesis of branchial and extraocular muscles has been experimentally examined, and a key role for neural crest cells established. Transplanting presumptive first branchial arch (jaw) neural crest cells in the place of prospective second arch (hyoid) crest cells results in the formation of a complete jaw skeleton in the second arch location.[38] Thus, key aspects of spatial organization in each branchial arch reside within the neural crest population that fills it, and is predicated upon the original axial site of origin of the crest cells. The myogenic cells in paraxial mesoderm that were contacted by these grafted crest cells formed muscles that, while located in the second branchial arch region, were anatomically appropriate for the first branchial arch. The morphogenesis of endothelial cells and overlying surface ectoderm was similarly respecified in accordance with the origin of the grafted neural crest cells. These data establish a hierarchy of spatial organizing influences in which connective tissue precursors (eg, neural crest cells in the head and lateral mesoderm cells in the limbs) are pattern-generating populations.

Molecular Analyses: Signals and Hox Genes

The phenomenologic data presented above focused attention on the problems of how neural crest cells acquire then manifest their spatial organization. Prospective first branchial arch crest cells are generated at or immediately caudal to the midbrain-hindbrain boundary, which coincidentally is a prominent signaling center in the brain. Signals, including *fgf8* and many downstream genes it activates, are activated at the boundary and establish the positional identities within adjacent metencephalic and mesencephalic regions of the neural tube. This results in the differentiation of the cerebellum, colliculi, and motor nuclei III and IV.[39,40] The first arch crest transplants described above were repeated but with the inclusion or exclusion of this signaling center. The results demonstrated that the ability of prospective first branchial arch neural crest cells to acquire their positional specification requires signals from this midbrain-hindbrain center.[41]

No comparable signaling centers have been found elsewhere in the hindbrain. Rather, this region and the neural crest cells that emigrate from it acquire their positional identities based on the expression of members of a large family of transcription factors encoded by *Hox* genes. Members of this family were first identified in *Drosophila* larvae and adults that, following exposure to known mutagens, developed with extra body parts located on inappropriate body segments. Often, an entire body segment would develop with all the anatomic features of a different segment. When all members of the family were identified in the fruit fly, investigators were surprised to discover that all were arranged on a single chromosome in the same relative positions as they were expressed in the body; their 3′ to 5′ order corresponds to head-to-tail expression sites (Figure 1–8).[42]

Early in chordate evolution a series of partial chromosomal duplications produced four nearly complete copies of the *Hox* gene cluster. The significance of these duplications is that for each *Hox* gene in mammals there are one, two, or even three very similar genes (eg, b1, b2, b3, b4 in Figure 1–8). This redundancy is a key feature of genetic evolution in that it allows essential functions to be maintained (by the original member) while base pair changes in the duplicates allow for variation of phenotypic expression that is unlikely to occur if only one member were present.[43]

Select members of the *Hox* gene family are expressed during the early stages of most organ systems, including the central nervous system, axial skeleton, limbs, gut, and reproductive tract. [43,44] The locations of expression boundaries in the brainstem (and corresponding neural crest) and in somites (vertebral precursors) are illustrated in Figures 1–7 and 1–8. Through the application of transgenic methods in mice, it is possible to delete or spatially misdirect the expression of specific *Hox* genes. For example, the loss of a functional *Hox d-3*, whose expression boundary in somites corresponds to the occipital-cervical junction, results in a frame shift such that the first cervical vertebra develops with characteristics of the occipital bone (Figure 1–8).[45] While these skeletal tissues have an altered spatial organization, tongue and laryngeal muscles derived from the same somites are normal, as would be expected if the spatial organization of myoblasts is imposed by connective tissue elements surrounding the respiratory diverticulum.

Transgenic mice with loss of *Hox a-2* function develop with rhombomeres 4 and 5 having no *Hox* genes of the "a" cluster expressed, which renders them genetically similar to rhombomeres 2 and 3 in this respect. In these animals, neural crest cells migrating from rhombomere 4 enter the second branchial

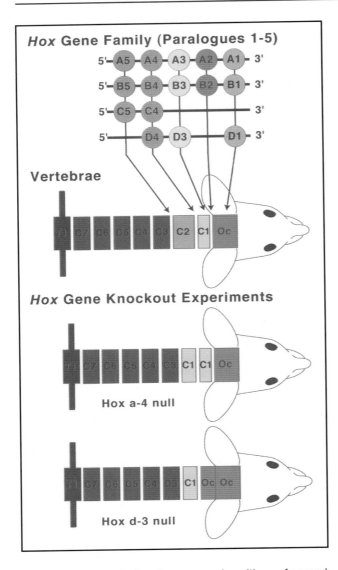

Figure 1–8. The relative chromosomal positions of several *Hox* family genes and their boundaries of expression in somites (which give rise to vertebrae) are shown. In most cases closely related genes (eg, *Hox a-4, b-4, c-4, and d-4*) have similar sites and times of expression. Note that the anatomic location of expression boundaries matches the 3' to 5' location of each gene along a chromosome. In somites, *Hox* gene expression boundaries tend to be clustered around sites of anatomic transition, such as occurs within and between occipital C1-C2 vertebrae. The effects of losing expression of specific *Hox* genes are illustrated in the lower two sketches. In the absence of *Hox a-4*, the primordium of the axis (2nd cervical vertebra) acquires the shape of the atlas (1st cervical vertebra); in *Hox d-3* nulls the atlas becomes occipitalized.

arch, but therein form a first branchial arch skeleton.[46,47] This genetic lesion produces the same results as neural crest transplantations.

Analyses of *Hox* gene loss of function transgenic mice have identified two that are involved in laryngeal and tracheal cartilage development. Loss of *Hox a-3* expression results in multiple skeletal defects, including dysmorphogenesis of the cricoid and thyroid cartilages, which are shortened with thick pedicles.[48] This gene is normally expressed in caudal pharyngeal endoderm. Analyses of mutations involving *Hox a-5*, which is normally expressed throughout mesenchyme surrounding the respiratory diverticulum, reveal a hyperplastic cricoid, disorganization of the tracheal rings and resultant tracheal occlusion, and hypoplasia of the pulmonary tree.[49]

These studies reveal that many strategies are invoked to provide connective tissue progenitors with the spatial information necessary to execute their own skeletal morphogenesis and also to orchestrate the morphogenesis of nearby muscles, blood vessels, and peripheral nerves. Given the unique location of the laryngeal connective tissue progenitors at the interface between head (ie, neural crest-dominated) and trunk (lateral mesoderm-derived) regions, and the juxtaposition of these to the respiratory diverticulum derived from pharyngeal endoderm, it is not surprising that simple, single *Hox* gene ablations produce defects in these structures that are less severe than found elsewhere.

CRITICAL PERIODS IN THE DEVELOPMENT OF THE FETAL AND POSTNATAL LARYNX

Although the foundations for laryngeal morphology are established during the period of organogenesis, recent studies have shown that significant aspects of maturation also occur in critical periods of both fetal (8 weeks to birth) and postnatal development. Of particular importance during this time are maturational events concerning changes in laryngeal position relative to contiguous aerodigestive tract structures.

Basic Mammalian Pattern of Laryngeal Position

In order to appreciate fully the development of the fetal larynx, it is necessary to review briefly the nature of laryngeal position in mammals. In most mammals, at all stages of postnatal development, the larynx during normal respiration is situated relatively "high" in the neck.[50] Its position, measured from the cranial aspect of the epiglottis to the caudal border of the cricoid cartilage, corresponds to the level of the basiocciput or first cervical vertebra (C1) to the third or fourth cervical vertebra (C3 or C4) in most terrestrial mammals.

This laryngeal position corresponds to high positions for the hyoid bone, tongue, and pharyngeal constrictors. For example, the tongue at rest lies almost entirely within the oral cavity, with no portion of it forming part of the anterior pharyngeal wall. Accordingly, the supralaryngeal region of the pharynx is noticeably small, with little or no oral portion.

A major corollary of high laryngeal position is that the epiglottis abuts, or direct overlaps, the soft palate. The epiglottis can thus pass up behind the soft palate and allow the larynx to open directly into the nasopharynx, creating what is often called the *intranarial* larynx. This configuration provides a direct air channel from the external nares through the nasal cavities, nasopharynx, larynx, and trachea to the lungs. Liquids, and in some species even chewed or solid material, can pass on either side of the interlocked larynx and nasopharynx via the isthmus faucium, through the piriform sinuses to the esophagus, following the so-called lateral food channels. This anatomic configuration may permit the patency of the laryngeal airway in some species while streams of liquid or semisolid food are transmitted around each side of the larynx during swallowing. In essence, two largely separate pathways are created: a respiratory tract from the nose to the lungs, and a digestive tract from the oral cavity to the esophagus (see References 50–55). The importance of this dual pathway system for many mammals has often been noted (see particularly References 51–53).

Development of Laryngeal Position in the Human Fetus

The position of the larynx relative to contiguous structures in human newborns and young infants closely resembles the basic mammalian pattern described above. While the high position of the infant larynx has been noted in many studies (eg, Crelin[51] and Laitman[52]), only recently have investigations begun to pinpoint the late fetal period as the crucial time for the establishment of laryngeal position sufficient to allow epiglottic-soft palate overlapping.[56,57] Indeed, recent studies have shown that fetal life is a critical period for the development of *both* structure and future functions of the upper respiratory and digestive pathways.[56-58]

The second trimester (13 to 26 weeks of gestation), in particular, has been shown to be a period of intense developmental activity. Studies have shown that by week 15 of development, earlier than previously reported, the epiglottis is already present, indicating that the epiglottic primordium may appear earlier in development than classically believed (Figure 1–9A).[56]

Throughout this period the larynx is found high in the neck, generally corresponding (from epiglottic tip to inferior border of the cricoid) to the level of the basioccipital bone to the third cervical vertebra. By week 21 the epiglottis is found to be almost in apposition to the uvula of the soft palate. Between weeks 23 and 25 the epiglottis and soft palate are found to overlap for the first time, thus providing the anatomic "interlocking" of the larynx into the nasopharynx characteristic of most mammals (Figure 1–9B).

A major maturational horizon in the aerodigestive region is accomplished with the attainment of larynx-nasopharynx interlocking. Establishment of this anatomic relationship allows the creation of essentially separate respiratory and digestive routes that will function as such in the newborn infant. Recent ultrasound investigations have shown upper respiratory activity patterns strongly suggestive of an operational "two-tube" system beginning to function even prenatally, that is, the larynx remains highly positioned and intranarial during fetal swallowing movements.[57]

A developmental Rubicon may thus be achieved between weeks 23 and 25. Indeed, this period may reflect a critical time in the development of the entire upper respiratory region. Not only is the larynx attaining a position that for the first time can accomplish an intranarial larynx, but contiguous portions of the skull base, the de facto roof of the upper respiratory tract, also appear to be undergoing considerable remodeling.[56,59] This may be quite significant, as the shape of the basicranium has been shown both comparatively and experimentally to bear a direct relationship to the location of the larynx in the neck.[60,61] What may be beginning at this time is a remodeling and refinement of the positional anatomy of the entire upper respiratory region in order to provide the anatomic framework for the newborn upper respiratory and digestive tracts. Aspects of soft tissue structures such as the larynx, and skeletal framework such as the skull base, are assuming both the morphology and positional relationships that will be required to sustain life postnatally.

The upper respiratory region is thus an area undergoing intense developmental activity at this time. While laryngeal and basicranial modifications are occurring during this stage of fetal life in the *upper* respiratory region, concomitant changes are also occurring in the *lower* respiratory tract. For example, the period of 23 to 25 weeks corresponds to the maturation of the pulmonary glandular epithelium.[51,62] This alveolar epithelium is responsible for the production of surfactant in the fetal lung, a substance that has been shown to be essential for independent respiratory function. The contemporaneous occurrence of the anatomic de-

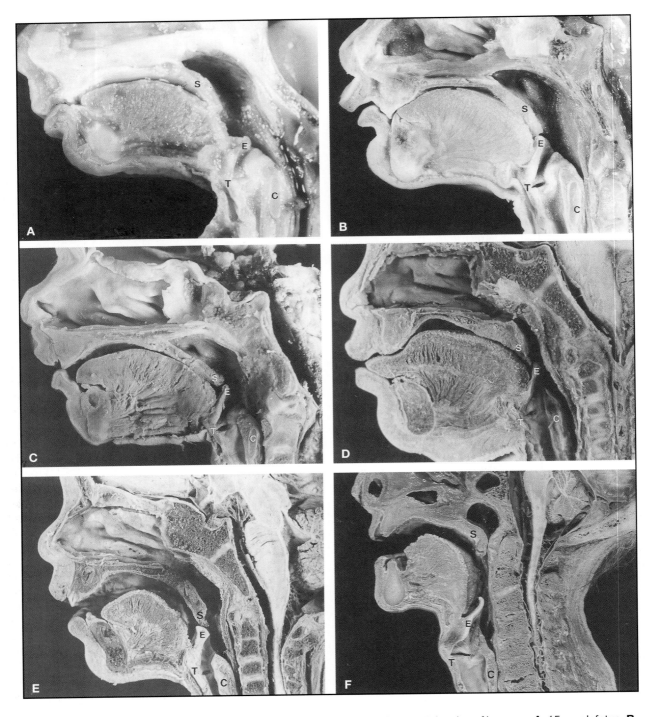

Figure 1–9. Midsaggital sections through the head and neck of a developmental series of humans. **A.** 15-week fetus. **B.** 24-week fetus. **C.** Newborn. **D.** 7 months. **E.** 15 months. **F.** Adult. (*C* = cricoid cartilage; *E* = epiglottic cartilage; *S* = soft palate; *T* = thyroid cartilage.) The larynx is not fully developed at 15 weeks, and the epiglottis is not able to approximate the soft palate. By 24 weeks, the epiglottis is able to overlap the soft palate. Notice the high position of the larynx in all except the adult. (From Laitman and Reidenberg.[72])

velopment of the fetal larynx to permit soft palate-epiglottic overlap with increasing levels of lung surfactant suggests that the timing of upper and the timing of lower respiratory tract maturation are closely related. Indeed, it appears that proper fetal maturation of the larynx may well be a major factor in determining the beginnings of respiratory independence in particular, and fetal viability overall. Understanding with increasing precision the attainment of these horizons, or factors that may alter them, can be of considerable importance in planning measures for the intervention and treatment of premature births.

Postnatal Changes in the Human Larynx

The newborn and young infant period is more accurately seen as an extension of the pattern established during the late second and early third trimester in upper respiratory and digestive tract anatomy rather than as a distinct stage. Indeed, newborns and young infants until approximately 1½ to 2 years of age continue to maintain a larynx situated high in the neck (Figure 1–9C to 1–9E). The larynx corresponds to the basiocciput-C1 and extends to the superior border of C4 in newborn infants, and descends slightly to the level between C2 and C5 by about 2 years of age. As exhibited in the late fetal period, the tongue at rest is found entirely within the oral cavity, with no portion of it forming the upper anterior wall of the pharynx.

The maintenance of high laryngeal position in newborns and young infants enables the existence of largely separate respiratory and digestive pathways similar to those described in other terrestrial mammals. These essentially separate pathways prevent the mixing of most ingested food and inhaled air. These routes may also enable the baby to breathe and swallow some liquids almost simultaneously in a manner similar to that shown in nonhuman primates.[51,52,54,55,63–65] Because of this high laryngeal position, newborns appear to be essentially, if not as classically believed obligatory,[66] nose breathers. As with nonhuman primates, the connection between the epiglottis and the soft palate is constant except for interruptions that may occur during the swallowing of a particularly large or dense bolus of food or liquid, during vocalization, during crying, or when disease is present. Indeed, developmental abnormalities that cause the epiglottis to be dislodged from its normal position have been shown to relate directly to concomitant feeding disorders.[67]

From a linguistic point of view, the high position of the larynx in a human newborn or young infant strongly affects the ability to modify sounds. Although high laryngeal position effectuates the dual pathway system, it severely limits the array of sounds babies produce. Many studies (eg, Laitman[68] and Lieberman[69]) have shown that the high position of the larynx greatly restricts the supralaryngeal portion of the pharynx available to modify the initial, or fundamental, sounds produced at the vocal folds. Thus, an individual with a larynx situated high in the neck, such as is found in a newborn human or monkey, would have a more restricted range of vocalizations available than would individuals with larynges placed lower in the neck. The linguistic analyses by Lieberman,[69,70] in particular, have identified the quantal vowels [i], [u], and [a] as sounds that human infants or nonhuman primates cannot produce. As these vowels are the limiting articulations of a vowel triangle that is language-universal, their absence considerably restricts an individual's speech capabilities.

While the larynx remains high in the neck until around the second year, functional changes, such as the first occasional instances of oral respiration, have been noted to occur considerably earlier, indeed within the first half year of life.[63] The period between 4 and 6 months, in particular, may represent a crucial stage in aerodigestive tract activity. At this time, neuromuscular control mechanisms of the larynx and pharynx are beginning to change even before true structural "descent" of the larynx has occurred. This changeover period may also indicate a time of potential respiratory instability owing to the transition from one respiratory pattern to another. It should be remembered that this is also a time of considerable maturational change within the central nervous system itself. The combination of nervous system maturation and developmental change in respiratory patterns may predispose the infant to a number of developmentally related problems. The occurrence of the sudden infant death syndrome (SIDS or crib death), for example, may be related to these first upper respiratory changes and to the subtle changes in laryngeal position or central and peripheral neuromotor control of the larynx.[71] The precise time of shifts that occur in breathing patterns, concomitant changes in digestive tract coordination, or the neurophysiologic mechanisms that would accompany them, remain poorly understood and warrant detailed study.

While the focus of this chapter has been on the prenatal development of the larynx, it is important to note that major maturational shifts in laryngeal position and function continue as development continues during the postnatal period.[72,73] The path of human laryngeal development is as much one of postnatal change as it is of prenatal formation and modification. Humans undergo a substantial postnatal reorganization of both laryngeal position and associated functions, dramatically more so than that found in other mammals.

The postnatal descent of the larynx into the neck is one of the most distinctive aspects of human ontogeny.[50,72,74] Whereas the purpose of the fetal period appears to be to establish those positional arrangements commensurate with the requirements of the infantile (ie, mammalian) pattern of laryngeal interlocking, the postnatal descent of the human larynx appears as a uniquely human occurrence. Permanent laryngeal descent, which seems to commence during the second year, eventually results in a larynx with a position corresponding to the level between the upper border of C3 and the lower border of C5 in a 7-year-old child, and lying opposite the lower border of C3 and the upper part of C4 to the upper border of C7 by adulthood (Figure 1–9F).[71] This positional change of the larynx dramatically alters our patterns of breathing and swallowing, as by necessity these routes must now intersect. The permanently lowered larynx also produces an enlarged supralaryngeal aspect of the pharynx. This resultant pharyngeal expansion, in turn, allows greater modification of sounds produced at the vocal folds than that possible for infant humans or other mammals. The descent of the larynx has thus provided the anatomic ability to produce fully articulate speech.

REFERENCES

1. Zaw-Tun HA, Burdi AR. Re-examination of the origin and early development of the human larynx. *Acta Anat (Basel)*. 1985; 122:163–184.
2. Henick DH. Three-dimensional analysis of murine laryngeal development. *Ann Otol Rhinol Laryngol*. 1993; 102(suppl 159):1–24.
3. Garcia-Martinez V, Alvarez IS, Schoenwolf GC. Locations of the ectodermal and nonectodermal subdivisions of the epiblast at stages 3 and 4 of avian gastrulation and neurulation. *J Exp Zool*. 1993;267:431–46.
4. Sutliff KS, Hutchins GM. Separation of the respiratory and digestive tracts in the human embryo: crucial role of the tracheoesophageal sulcus. *Anat Rec*. 1994;238:237–247.
5. Henick DH. Three-dimensional analysis of murine laryngeal development. *Ann Otol Rhinol Laryngol Suppl*. 1993;159:3–24.
6. Williams AK, Quan QB, Beasley SW. Three-dimensional imaging clarifies the process of tracheoesophageal separation in the rat. *J Ped Surg*. 2003;38:173–177.
7. Huang R, Zhi Q, Ordahl CP, Christ B. The fate of the first avian somite. *Anat Embryol (Berl)*. 1997;195:435–49.
8. Hilfer SR, Marrero L, Sheffield JB. Patterns of cell movement in early organ primordia of the chick embryo. *Anat Rec*. 1990;227:508–517.
9. Arsic D, Keenan J, Quan QB, Beasley S. Differences in the levels of sonic hedgehog protein during early foregut development caused by exposure to Adriamycin give clues to the role of the Shh gene in oesophageal atresia. *Pediatr Surg Int*. 2003;19:463–466.
10. Miller L-AD, Wert SE, Clark JC, et al. Role of sonic hedgehog in patterning of tracheal-bronchial cartilage and the peripheral lung. *Dev Dyn*. 2004;231:57–71.
11. Kim J, Kim P, Hui CC. The VACTERL association: lessons from the sonic hedgehog pathway. *Clin Genet*. 2001;59:306–315.
12. Oldak M, Grzela T, Lazarczyk M, et al. Clinical aspects of disrupted hedgehog signaling. *Int J Mol Med*. 2001; 8:445–452.
13. Elluru RG, Whitsett JA. Potential role of Sox9 in patterning tracheal cartilage ring formation in an embryonic mouse model. *Arch Otolaryngol Head Neck Surg*. 2004; 130:732–736.
14. von Kirschhofer K, Grim M, Christ B, et al. Emergence of myogenic and endothelial cell lineages in avian embryos. *Dev Biol*. 1994;163:270–278.
15. Noden DM. Embryonic origins and assembly of blood vessels. *Am Rev Respir Dis*. 1989;140, 1097–1103.
16. Noden DM. Mesenchymal cell movements and tissue assembly during craniofacial development. *J Craniofac Genetics Dev Biol*. 1991;11:192–213.
17. Borycki AG, Emerson CP Jr. Multiple tissue interactions and signal transduction pathways control somite myogenesis. *Curr Top Dev Biol*. 2000; 48:165–224.
18. Noden DM. The use of chimeras in analyses of craniofacial development. In: Le Dourarin N, McLaren A, eds. *Changes in Developmental Biology*. London, England: Academic; 1984:241–280.
19. Noden DM. The embryonic origins of avian cephalic and cervical muscles and associated connective tissues. *Am J Anat*. 1983;168: 257–276.
20. Noden DM, Marcucio RM, Borycki A-G, Emerson CP. Differentiation of avian craniofacial muscles. I. Patterns of early regulatory gene expression and myosin heavy chain synthesis. *Dev Dyn*. 1999; 216: 96–112.
21. McClearn D, Noden, DM. Ontogeny of architectural complexity in embryonic quail visceral arch muscles. *Amer J Anat*. 1988; 183:277–293.
22. Wahl CM, Noden DM, Baker R. Developmental relations between sixth nerve motor neurons and their targets in the chick embryo. *Dev Dyn*. 1994;201:191–202.
23. Trainor PA, Tan SS, Tam PP. Cranial paraxial mesoderm: regionalization of cell fate and impact on craniofacial development in mouse embryos. *Development*. 1994;120: 2397–2408.
24. Noden DM. Interactions and fates of avian craniofacial mesenchyme. *Development*. 1988;103:121–40.
25. Jiang X, Iseki S, Maxson RE, Sucov HM, Morriss-Kay GM. Tissue origins and interactions in the mammalian skull vault. *Dev Biol*. 2002;241:106–16.
26. Santagati F, Rijli FM. Cranial neural crest and the building of the vertebrate head. *Nat Rev Neurosci*. 2003;4: 806–818.
27. Francis-West PH, Robson L, Evans DJ. Craniofacial development: the tissue and molecular interactions that control development of the head. *Adv Anat Embryol Cell Biol*. 2003;169:1–138.
28. Koentges G, Lumsden A. Rhombencephalic neural crest segmentation is preserved throughout craniofacial ontogeny. *Development*. 1996; 122:3229–3242.

29. Helms J, Schnieder RA. Cranial skeletal biology. *Nature.* 2003;423:326–331.

30. Buckingham M, Bajard L, Chang T, Daubas P, Hadchouel J, Meilhac S, Montarras D, Rocancourt D, Relaix F. The formation of skeletal muscle: from somite to limb. *J Anat.* 2003;202:59–68.

31. Fraser SE, Bronner-Fraser M. Migrating neural crest cells in the trunk of the avian embryo are multipotent. *Development.* 1991;112:913–920.

32. Sieber-Blum M. Factors controlling lineage specification in the neural crest. *Int Rev Cytol.* 2000;197:1–33.

33. Thorogood P. Differentiation and morphogenesis of cranial skeletal tissues. In: Hanken J, Hall BK, eds. *The Skull, Vol. 1: Development.* Chicago, IL: University of Chicago Press; 1993:112–152.

34. Noden DM. Spatial integration among cells forming the cranial peripheral nervous system. *J Neurobiol.* 1993;24: 248–261.

35. Noden DM. Patterning of avian craniofacial muscles. *Dev Biol.* 1986;116:347–356.

36. Hacker A, Guthrie S. A distinct developmental programme for the cranial paraxial mesoderm in the chick embryo. *Development.* 1998;125:3461–3472.

37. Borue X, Noden DM. Normal and aberrant craniofacial myogenesis by grafted trunk somitic and segmental plate mesoderm. *Development.* 2004;131:3967–3980.

38. Noden DM. The role of the neural crest in patterning of avian cranial skeletal, connective, and muscle tissues. *Dev Biol.* 1983;96:144–165.

39. Rhinn M, Brand M. The midbrain-hindbrain boundary organizer. *Curr Opin Neurobiol.* 2001;11:34–42.

40. Joyner AL, Liu A, Millet S. Otx2, Gbx2 and Fgf8 interact to position and maintain a mid-hindbrain organizer. *Curr Opin Cell Biol.* 2000;12:736–744.

41. Trainor PA, Ariza-McNaughton L, Krumlauf R. Role of the isthmus and FGFs in resolving the paradox of neural crest plasticity and prepatterning. *Science.* 2002;295: 1288–1291.

42. Trainor PA, Krumlauf R. *Hox* genes, neural crest cells and branchial arch patterning. *Curr Opin Cell Biol.* 2001; 13:698–705.

43. Schilling TF, Knight RD. Origins of anteroposterior patterning and *Hox* gene regulation during chordate evolution. *Philos Trans R Soc Lond B Biol Sci.* 2001;356:1599–1613.

44. Trainor PA. Making headway: the roles of *Hox* genes and neural crest cells in craniofacial development. *Scientific World J.* 2003;3:240–264.

45. Condie BG, Capecchi MR. Mice homozygous for a targeted disruption of *Hox*d-3 (*Hox-4.1*) exhibit anterior transformations of the first and second cervical vertebrae, the atlas and the axis. *Development.* 1993;75:1317–1331.

46. Gendron-Maguire M, Mallo M, Zhang M, Gridley T. *Hox*a-2 mutant mice exhibit homeotic transformation of skeletal elements derived from cranial neural crest. *Cell.* 1993;75:1317–1331.

47. Rijli FM, Mark M, Lakkaraju S, Dierich A, Dolle P, Chambon P. A homeotic transformation is generated in the rostral branchial region of the head by disruption of Hoxa-2, which acts as a selector gene. *Cell.* 1993;75:1333–1349.

48. Manley NR, Capecchi MR. Hox group 3 paralogous genes act synergistically in the formation of somitic and neural crest-derived structures. *Dev Biol.* 1997;192:274–288.

49. Aubin J, Lemieux M, Tremblay M, et al. Early postnatal lethality in *Hoxa-5* mutant mice is attributable to respiratory tract defects. *Dev Biol.* 1997;192:432–445.

50. Laitman JT, Reidenberg JS. Specializations of the human upper respiratory and upper digestive systems as seen through comparative and developmental anatomy. *Dysphagia.* 1993;8:318–325.

51. Crelin ES. Development of the upper respiratory system. *Ciba Clin Symp.* 1976;28(3):3–26.

52. Laitman JT. *The Ontogenetic and Phylogenetic Development of the Upper Respiratory System and Basicranium in Man.* (Ph.D. dissertation. Yale University). Ann Arbor, MI: University Microfilms; 1977.

53. Negus VE. *The Comparative Anatomy and Physiology of the Larynx.* New York, NY: Grune & Stratton; 1949.

54. Laitman JT, Crelin ES, Conlogue GJ. The function of the epiglottis in monkey and man. *Yale J Biol Med.* 1977; 50:43–49.

55. German RZ, Crompton AW. Integration of swallowing and respiration in infant macaques (*Macaca fascicularis*). *Am J Phys Anthropol.* 1993;16(suppl):94.

56. Magriples U, Laitman JT. Developmental change in the position of the fetal human larynx. *Am J Phys Anthropol.* 1987;72:463–472.

57. Wolfson VP, Laitman JT. Ultrasound investigation of fetal human upper respiratory anatomy. *Anat Rec.* 1990; 227:363–372.

58. Isaacson G, Birnholz JC. Human fetal upper respiratory tract function as revealed by ultrasonography. *Ann Otol Rhinol Laryngol.* 1991;100:743–747.

59. Moore SL, Laitman JT. A critical period in fetal human cranial base development. *Anat Rec.* 1991;229:61A.

60. Laitman JT, Heimbuch RC, Crelin ES. Developmental change in a basicranial line and its relationship to the upper respiratory system in living primates. *Am J Anat.* 1978;152:467–483.

61. Reidenberg JS, Laitman JT. Effect of basicranial flexion on larynx and hyoid position in rats: an experimental study of skull and soft tissue interactions. *Anat Rec.* 1991;220:557–569.

62. Liggins GC, Schellenberg JL. Aspects of fetal lung development. In: Jones CT, Nathanielsz PW, eds. *The Physiological Development of the Fetus and Newborn.* London, England: Academic Press; 1985:178–189.

63. Sasaki CT, Levine PA, Laitman JT, et al. Postnatal descent of the epiglottis in man: a preliminary report. *Arch Otolaryngol.* 1977;103:169–171.

64. Polgar G, Weng TR. The functional development of the respiratory system: from the period of gestation to adulthood. *Am Rev Respir Dis.* 1979;120:625–695.

65. Harding R. Function of the larynx in the fetus and newborn. *Ann Rev Physiol.* 1984;46:645–659.

66. Moss ML. The veloepiglottic sphincter and obligate nose breathing in the neonate. *J Pediatr.* 1965;67:330–331.

67. Mukai S, Mukai C, Asaoka K. Ankyloglossia with deviation of the epiglottis and larynx. *Ann Otol Rhinol Laryngol.* 1991;100:3–20.

68. Laitman JT. The evolution of the hominid upper respiratory system and implications for the origins of speech. In: de Grolier E, ed. *Glossogenetics: The Origin and Evolution of Language.* Paris, France: Harwood Academic; 1983: 63–90.

69. Lieberman P. *The Biology and Evolution of Language.* Cambridge, MA: Harvard University Press; 1984.

70. Lieberman P, Laitman JT, Reidenberg JS, et al. The anatomy, physiology, acoustics and perception of speech: essential elements in analysis of the evolution of human speech. *J Hum Evol.* 1992;23:447–467.

71. Laitman JT, Crelin ES. Developmental change in the upper respiratory system of human infants. *Perinatol Neonatol.* 1980;4:15–22.

72. Laitman JT, Reidenberg JS. Comparative and developmental anatomy of laryngeal position. In: Bailey B, ed. *Head and Neck Surgery-Otolaryngology.* Philadelphia, PA: Lippincott; 1993:36–43.

73. Roche AF, Barkla DH. The level of the larynx during childhood. *Ann Otol Rhinol Laryngol.* 1965;74:645–654.

74. Laitman JT, Crelin ES. Postnatal development of the basicranium and vocal tract region in man. In: Bosma JF, ed. *Symposium on Development of the Basicranium.* Washington, DC. US Government Printing Office; 1976:206–220.

2

Laryngeal Development

David H. Henick, MD

The critical stages in the prenatal development of the human larynx provide valuable insight into the anatomy and clinical malformations of the mature larynx. Earlier theories of laryngeal development espoused the concept of a tracheoesophageal septum. Observations of laryngeal development over the past decade challenge the validity of these earlier theories. Computer-generated solid-model three-dimensional reconstructions have allowed for a more precise analysis of embryologic events than the wax-model reconstructions used over the past century. Furthermore, the computer image has allowed the observer to understand complex anatomic changes over both space and time. The development of clinical laryngeal malformations presented in this chapter can be correlated with arrested stages of normal laryngeal development.

DEVELOPMENT OF THE LARYNGOPHARYNGEAL REGION

Before discussing the history of laryngeal development, it is helpful to consider Figure 2–1, a dorsal view of the developing laryngopharyngeal region taken from a popular embryology textbook. It provides a perspective of the developing larynx as one would view a larynx endoscopically. Imagine if the dorsal

wall of the foregut were removed, and one was now viewing the epithelium of the ventral foregut floor. The limitation of this illustration, however, is that it provides only one perspective of laryngeal development. It fails to portray the complex anatomic changes occurring in both the sagittal and the coronal planes of the developing larynx.

As a reference point, this illustration views the level of the pharyngeal floor *(PhF)*, which is equivalent to the level of the fourth pharyngeal pouch *(4PP)*. The sagittal slit seen in the pharyngeal floor (labeled as *Laryngeal orifice*) has been interpreted by many authors as meaning different anatomic locations. For example, some authors believe that it represents the opening to the infraglottic region,[1] or the glottic region,[2,3] and finally, more recent observations support evidence that it represents the opening to the supraglottic region.[4]

This confusion in the literature can be attributed to several factors. (1) Previous authors have labeled various anatomic sites inconsistently. (2) Wax models, which are created from postmortem human fetal histologic sections, have been the mainstay of our current understanding of laryngeal development. Observations that are made on these models are subject to individual interpretation. (3) Prior to the existence of the Carnegie collection, there was no centralization of the specimens and wax-model reconstructions. This has

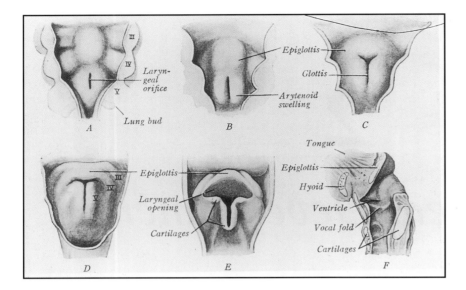

Figure 2–1. Development of the human larynx, as seen by unroofing the embryo to show floor of the pharyngeal cavity. **A.** At 5 mm; **B.** at 9 mm; **C.** at 12 mm; **D.** at 16 mm; **E.** at 40 mm (x7); **F.** sagittal hemisection, at birth (x1.5). In A-E, His[2] assumed the "ascending notch" reached the level of the pharyngeal floor, and the tracheoesophageal separation would be at the level shown. Hence, according to His, figures A-E would represent the cephalic end of the trachea. According to Zaw-Tun, figures A-E represent the entrance to the primitive laryngopharynx, which eventually becomes the supraglottis. (From Arey LB. *Developmental Anatomy*, 7th ed. Philadelphia, PA: WB Saunders; 1954. Used by permission.)

presented each subsequent scientist with the need to analyze and compare new findings and updated information from earlier studies.

RESEARCH STUDIES

There have been several landmark studies on the origin and development of the larynx. Probably the most influential work, performed in the late 19th century, was contributed by His.[2] In his description of the developing gastrointestinal tract and pharyngeal arches, His[2] proposed that the respiratory primordium *(RP)* appears as an outpouching from the cephalic portion of the pharynx by the third week of gestation. His[2] described an ascending tracheoesophageal septum, identified as a groove behind the respiratory primordium, which would ascend to the level of the fourth pharyngeal pouch. This would divide the foregut into a ventral trachea and a dorsal esophagus. This theory implied that the distance between the fourth pharyngeal pouch, or pharyngeal floor, and the separation of the trachea and esophagus would gradually decrease over time.

Several investigators subsequently accepted His's[2] theory of an ascending tracheoesophageal septum, and added their own novel interpretations. In Figure 2–2, schematic drawings represent developmental theories of the larynx according to Kallius, Frazer, and Walander. Each author demonstrated the presence of the ascending tracheoesophageal septum (the striped line,) which separates the trachea and esophagus up to the level of the fourth pharyngeal pouch or pharyngeal floor. Although these authors agreed that the trachea and the esophagus are separated by an ascending tracheo-esophageal septum, they disagreed about the site of the obliteration of the pharynx, otherwise

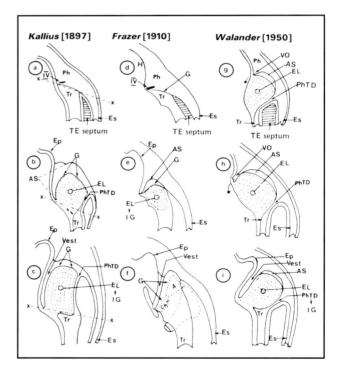

Figure 2–2. Historical concepts of development of laryngeal cavity. Kallius (**A-C**), Frazer (**D-F**), and Walander (**G-I**) accepted concept of tracheoesophageal septum originally proposed by His, Zaw-Tun, and Burdi (Figs. 2-2 to 2-6, 2-9 to 2-11 from Henick DH. Three-dimensional analysis of murine laryngeal development. In *Annals of Otology, Rhinology and Laryngology*. 102:(suppl 159), 1993. Reproduced with permission.)

known as the epithelial lamina *(EL)*. Kallius thought it occurred above the pharyngeal floor, Frazer thought it occurred below the pharyngeal floor, and Walander thought it occurred precisely at the level of the pharyngeal floor.[1,3,5]

In contrast to the foregoing hypothesis, Zaw-Tun[4] demonstrated that no such tracheoesophageal septum exists, even as a transitory structure during normal laryngeal development. To review, His demonstrated an ascending tracheoesophageal septum, which begins at the level of the respiratory primordium, dividing the foregut to form the trachea ventrally and the esophagus dorsally. This theory suggests that the distance between the tracheoesophageal separation point and the level of the fourth pharyngeal pouch would decrease over time, as indicated by the stippled box.[2] Zaw-Tun, however, found that the respiratory primordium continues as a ventrocaudal outgrowth of the foregut lumen, which ultimately gives rise to the entire upper and lower respiratory system. Zaw-Tun demonstrated that the separation of the esophagus and trachea was not the result of an ascending tracheoesophageal septum, but was caused by the descending outgrowth of the respiratory primordium.

In contrast to His, Zaw-Tun found that the foregut segment which separates the original site of the respiratory primordium from the pharyngeal floor does not change over time. Zaw-Tun classified this foregut segment as the primitive laryngopharynx (PLPh). The primitive laryngopharynx would eventually give rise to the supraglottic larynx.[4,6]

SCIENTIFIC ANALYSIS

The computer has enabled the scientist to analyze complex anatomic relationships as they change over space and time. A recent study[7] utilized computer-generated three-dimensional solid-model reconstructions to portray the critical stages in the development of the murine larynx. The mouse was chosen as an animal model because (1) laryngeal development is essentially uniform in all mammals, (2) the genetic analysis of murine development is well defined, and (3) embryos of a predetermined age can be easily and accurately staged. The results of this developmental study were in close correlation with the findings of Zaw-Tun and will be described in further detail.

Serial histologic sections of the laryngopharyngeal region of mice embryos were obtained from day 9 of gestation to day 18. STERECON, a computer graphics system designed to allow three-dimensional tracings of structural contours from two-dimensional images, was used to generate the three-dimensional models.[8,9] Photographic transparencies of each histologic section were then projected onto a screen that was the same size as a high-resolution computer monitor. By means of a digitizing tablet, color-coded lines were drawn on

the monitor, outlining the structures of interest, for example, the epithelial lining of the foregut, foregut lumen, muscles, cartilages, and arteries. The resulting contours were stored in a database and used to form wire-frame models. Wire-frame models were then transferred to a Silicon Graphics workstation and rendered as solid, shaded reconstructions with Wavefront Technologies software. This allowed anatomic structures to be viewed in continuity, in any desired orientation, and in relation to any other given structure. In addition, internal structures could be visualized by sectioning the models in various planes.

HUMAN DEVELOPMENT

Human development is divided into an embryonic period, or the first 8 weeks of human gestation, and the subsequent fetal period.[10] The embryonic period has a total of 23 stages of development according to the Carnegie staging system. Each stage has a characteristic feature not seen in a previous stage. Laryngeal development is first seen at stage 11 (approximately 4 weeks of human gestation, and 9 days of murine gestation).

Figure 2–3 is a lateral view of a three-dimensional reconstruction of the epithelial lining of the developing laryngopharyngeal region. The first sign of the respiratory system is seen as an epithelial thickening along the ventral aspect of the foregut known as the respiratory primordium (RP). The respiratory primordium is separated from the hepatic primordium (HP) by the septum transversum (ST), a structure that will eventually develop into the central tendon of the diaphragm.

Figure 2–4 is a schematic representation of the laryngopharyngeal regions of a stage 12 embryo in comparison with the mature fetal larynx in a midsagittal plane. The respiratory diverticulum (RD) is a ventral outpocketing of foregut lumen that extends into the respiratory primordium. The site of origin of the respiratory diverticulum is called the primitive pharyngeal floor (PPhF) and eventually develops into the glottic region of the adult larynx. The cephalic portion of the respiratory diverticulum eventually develops into the infraglottic (IG) region of adult larynx. The primate pharyngeal floor is separated from the pharyngeal floor (PhF), or the level of the fourth pharyngeal pouch (4PP), by a segment of foregut originally classified by Zaw-Tun as the primitive laryngopharynx (PLPh);[4-6] this will eventually become the adult supraglottic larynx.

Figure 2–4B is a ventral view of a three-dimensional reconstruction of the epithelial lining of the laryngopharyngeal region of a stage 12 embryo. The respiratory diverticulum has given rise to bilateral pro-

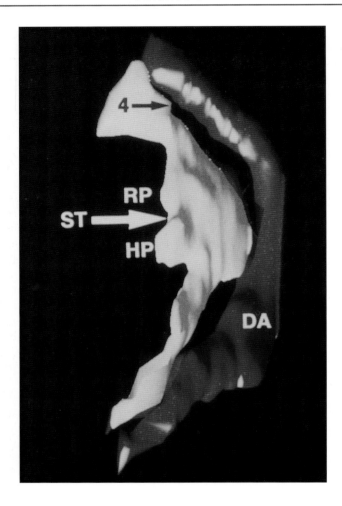

Figure 2–3. Stage 11 (17-somite mouse embryo, E9.5). Lateral view of 3-D reconstruction of epithelial lining of foregut. First evidence of respiratory system is indicated by epithelial thickening along ventral aspect of foregut called respiratory primordium (*RP*). Respiratory primordium is separated from hepatic primordium (*HP*) by septum transversum (*ST*), which is indicated by solid white arrow. Septum transversum will eventually develop into central tendon of developing diaphragm. 4—site of developing fourth pharyngeal pouch, *DA*—dorsal aorta.

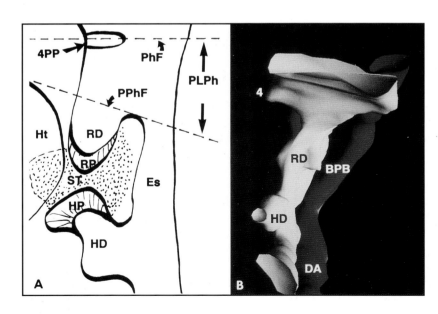

Figure 2–4. Stage 12 (22-somite mouse embryo, E10). **A.** Schematic representation of midsagittal section through laryngopharyngeal region. Respiratory diverticulum (*RD*) is ventral outpocketing of foregut lumen that extends into respiratory primordium (*RP*). Similarly, hepatic diverticulum (*HD*) results from extension of foregut lumen into hepatic primordium (HP). Cephalic portion of RD will eventually develop into infraglottic region of adult larynx. Site of origin of RD is called primitive pharyngeal floor (*PPhF*); it will eventually develop into glottic region of adult larynx. Esophagus (*Es*) separates from RD at level of PPhF. Primitive pharyngeal floor is separated from fourth pharyngeal pouch (4PP) by segment of foregut called primitive laryngopharynx (*PLPh*). Pharyngeal floor (PhF) is at same level as 4PP. Primitive laryngopharynx will eventually develop into supraglottic region of adult larynx. *Ht*—heart, *ST*—septum transversum. **B.** Ventral view of 3-D reconstruction of epithelial lining of laryngopharyngeal region. Respiratory diverticulum has given rise to bilateral projections called bronchopulmonary buds (*BPB*); they will eventually develop into lung parenchyma. *DA*—dorsal aorta, *4*—fourth pharyngeal pouch.

jections called bronchopulmonary buds (BPB); these will eventually develop into the lower respiratory tract. The bronchopulmonary buds are tethered to the superior aspect of the septum transversum.

Dynamic changes to the developing foregut region are occurring at this and subsequent stages. For example, the heart (*Ht*) and the hepatic primordium are proliferating at a rapid rate on opposing surfaces of the septum transversum. These differential forces are exerted upon the adjacent foregut region, which leads to a dramatic lengthening of the foregut in a cephalo-caudal plane. The result can be seen as the distance between the respiratory primordium and the hepatic primordium increases over time.

In stage 13 (Figure 2–5), the bronchopulmonary buds are drawn caudally and inferiorly because they are tethered to the septum transversum and the

cephalic aspect of the foregut, and the respiratory diverticulum migrates superiorly. As a result, (1) two primary main-stem bronchi develop and (2) the carina is seen as a distinct region that develops from the caudal aspect of the respiratory diverticulum, and it is the site of origin of the two primary bronchi.

Figure 2–6 shows the distance between the carina and the respiratory diverticulum by two white solid arrows in a stage 14 embryo. The lengthening of this foregut segment will eventually give rise to the developing trachea. At this point in development, dramatic lengthening of the trachea and esophagus occurs. Anatomically, the esophagus is in close proximity to the region of the carina. Vascular compromise to the developing esophagus may give rise to esophageal atresia, or the spectrum of tracheoesophageal anomalies seen in Figure 2–7.

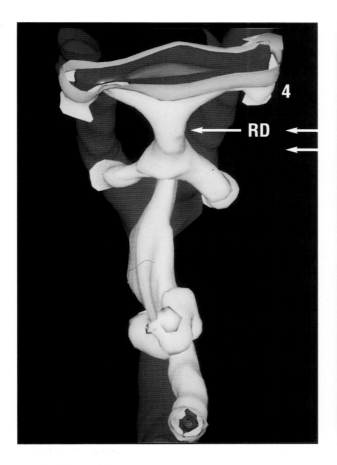

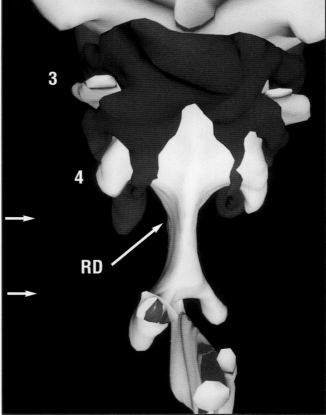

Figure 2–5. Stage 13 (28-somite mouse embryo, E10.5). Ventral view of epithelial lining of foregut. Bronchopulmonary buds have continued to be drawn dorsocaudally from carina (*Ca*) because of cephalic rotation of embryo and because bronchopulmonary buds are tethered to septum transversum. Carina (*Ca*) develops from caudal aspect of respiratory diverticulum (*RD*). Two white solid arrows indicate distance between RD and Ca. *HD*—hepatic diverticulum.

Figure 2–6. Stage 14 (35-somite mouse embryo, E11). Ventral view of 3-D reconstruction of epithelial lining of laryngopharyngeal region. Compared with Figure 2–5, lengthening of Ca from RD is demonstrated with two white solid arrows. Lengthening of this foregut segment will eventually give rise, in part, to developing trachea. Carina (*Ca*) continues to descend from site of respiratory diverticulum (*RD*). Numerals 3 and 4—third and fourth pharyngeal pouches, respectively.

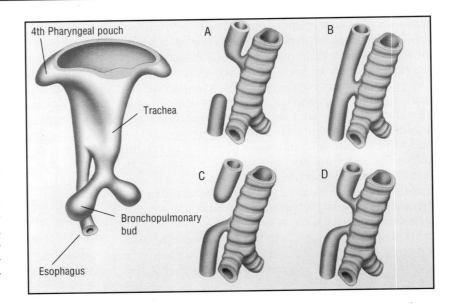

Figure 2–7. Esophageal atresia and spectrum of tracheoesophageal fistulae. **A.** Esophageal atresia, proximal tracheoesophageal fistula (<1%). **B.** Tracheoesophageal H-Fistula, no atresia (4%). **C.** Esophageal atresia, distal tracheoesophageal fistulae (87%). **D.** Esophageal atresia, proximal and distal tracheoesophageal fistulae (<1%).

Esophageal atresia in a newborn infant usually presents clinically with increased salivation requiring frequent suctioning, with the pulmonary triad of coughing, choking, and cyanosis. These symptoms are the result of saliva pooling in the blind proximal esophageal pouch with the subsequent overflow into the infant's airway. Aspiration is greater in infants who have a direct airway connection because of an associated tracheoesophageal fistula.

Tracheoesophageal fistula with a proximal esophageal pouch and distal tracheoesophageal fistula occurs in 80% to 85% of affected patients and results in gastric distention caused by air ingested with each breath. The stomach distention associated with increased gastric acid production results in respiratory symptoms caused by (1) direct tracheal aspiration of the mixture of refluxed air or gastric acid and (2) decreased diaphragmatic excursion. If the diagnosis is delayed or missed and feeding is begun, choking episodes occur, with the potential for further airway soilage.

Vascular compromise to the developing trachea at this stage of development may give rise to complete tracheal agenesis, or tracheal stenosis with complete tracheal rings (Figure 2–8). Classically, both these anomalies are associated with normal laryngeal and pulmonary development as the insult is limited to the region of the developing trachea.

Figure 2–9 demonstrates a coronal reconstruction of a late stage 14 embryo. The infraglottis *(IG)*, which is the most cephalic portion of the respiratory diverticulum, has the characteristic shape of an upright triangle when sectioned in coronal plane; this is characteristic of the adult conus elasticus. The primitive laryn-

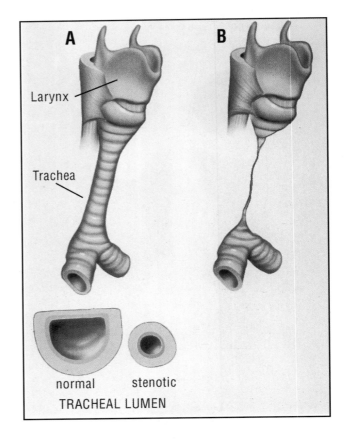

Figure 2–8. Tracheal anomalies. **A.** Tracheal stenosis. Axial sections demonstrate the concentric circular tracheal cartilage with the loss of the membranous trachea posteriorly. **B.** Tracheal atresia. Relatively normal laryngeal and pulmonary development is seen in both of these anomalies.

gopharynx, which extends from the infraglottis to the level of the fourth pharyngeal pouch, has become compressed bilaterally along its ventral aspect, called the epithelial lamina *(EL)*. This compression is caused by forces exerted by the proliferating triangular-shaped, laryngeal mesodermal anlage *(LMA)* and branchial arch arteries. The laryngeal mesodermal anlage eventually develops into the laryngeal cartilages and muscles. An elevation of the median pharyngeal floor gives rise to the arytenoid swellings. This occurs at the same level as the fourth pharyngeal pouch. The trachea *(Tr)* is seen as the uniformly circular lumen separating the infraglottis from the carina *(Ca)*.

In stage 15, the epithelial lamina continues to obliterate the primitive laryngopharynx from a ventral to dorsal direction until obliteration is essentially complete by stage 16. Figure 2–10 is a lateral view of a three-dimensional reconstruction of the laryngopharyngeal region of a stage 16 embryo. A glass simulation is used to represent the epithelial lining of the foregut so that the internal changes to the lumen *(blue)* can be seen. The primitive laryngopharynx is seen as the segment of the foregut between the infraglottis, which was a characteristic shape of an inverted triangle when sectioned in the sagittal plane, and the arytenoid swellings *(yellow)*. Complete obliteration of the primitive laryngopharynx is seen except for a ventral laryngeal cecum *(LC)*, and a dorsal pharyngoglottic duct *(PhGD)*. The dorsal pharyngoglottis is the last remnant of patent communication between the hypopharynx and the infraglottis.

The laryngeal cecum originates as a triangular-shaped lumen along the ventral aspect of the arytenoid swellings and progresses caudally along the ventral aspect of the primitive laryngopharynx until it reaches the level of the glottis in stage 18 (Figure 2–11). In stage 19, the epithelial lamina begins to recanalize from a dorsocephalad to a ventrocaudal direction. In

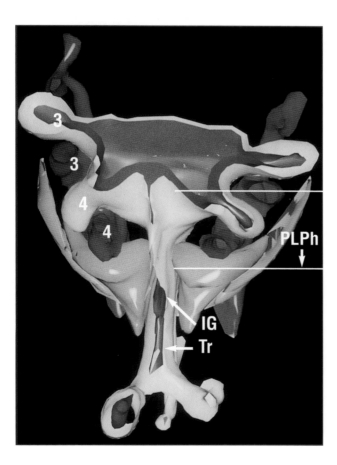

Figure 2–9. Stage 14 (36-somite mouse embryo, E11.5). Coronal section of a 3-D reconstructed embryo. Region of primitive laryngopharynx *(PLPh)* has become compressed bilaterally, likely because of forces exerted by the (purple) laryngeal mesodermal anlage and fourth branchial artery (4, red). Infraglottis *(IG)* has the characteristic shape of an upright triangle when sectioned in this coronal plane. Infraglottis is separated from the carina by the ovoid-circular the lumen of trachea (Tr). Also, at level of fourth pharyngeal pouch (4), elevation of median pharyngeal floor will give rise to developing arytenoid swellings.

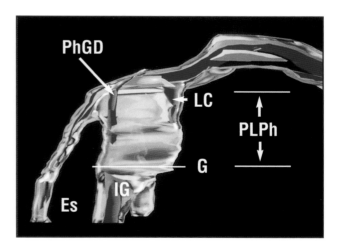

Figure 2–10. Stage 16 (50-somite mouse embryo E12 to E12.5) Lateral view of 3-D reconstruction of foregut epithelial lining. Glass simulation was used so that internal *(blue)* luminal anatomy could be visualized. Primitive laryngopharynx *(PLPh)* extends from floor of pharynx *(level of AS; yellow)* to infraglottic region below *(IG;* previously cephalic end of respiratory diverticulum). Glottis *(G)* is just cephalic to IG. Primitive laryngopharynx is completely obliterated except for narrow pharyngoglottic duct *(PhGD)* dorsally and developing laryngeal cecum *(LC)* ventrally.

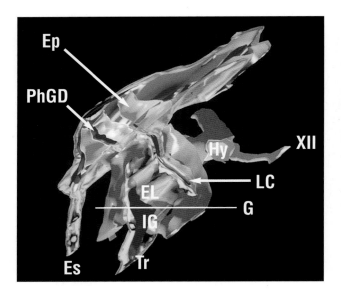

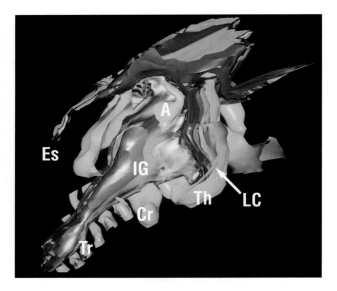

Figure 2–11. Stages 17 and 18 (62-somite mouse embryo, E14). Lateral view of 3-D reconstruction of foregut epithelial lining of laryngopharyngeal region with its surrounding laryngeal mesodermal anlagen (*purple*). Glass simulation was used to enhance visualization of internal luminal anatomy (*blue*). Compared to Figure 2–10 (stage 16), primitive laryngopharynx is still obliterated except for pharyngoglottic duct (*PhGD*) dorsally and laryngeal cecum (*LC*) ventrally, which has, at this stage, descended to glottic (*G*) region (white line). Eventually, recanalization of epithelial lamina (*EL*) will bring dorsal PhGD into communication with ventral LC to give rise to laryngeal vestibule, or supraglottic larynx. *Ep*—epiglottis anlage, *Hy*—hyoid anlage, XII—12th cranial nerve, *Tr*—trachea, *Es*—esophagus.

Figure 2–12. Stages 19 through 23 (E16 mouse embryo). 3-D reconstruction of laryngopharyngeal region, sectioned in midsagittal plane exposing right medial aspect of embryo. Glass simulation is used to view luminal (*dark blue*) anatomy. White broken lines indicate area in which epithelial lamina has not completely recanalized. It has been suggested that incomplete recanalization of epithelial lamina can give rise to full spectrum of supraglottic stenosis and glottic webs seen clinically. *Es*—esophagus, *A*—arytenoid cartilage, *Th*—thyroid cartilage, *Cr*—cricoid cartilage, *Tr*—trachea, *IG*—infraglottis, *LC*—laryngeal cecum.

the process, communication is reestablished between the ventral laryngeal cecum and the dorsal pharyngoglottis. The last portion of the primitive laryngopharynx to recanalize is at the glottic level, as indicated by the white broken line in Figure 2–12. It is the incomplete recanalization of the epithelial lamina that can give rise to the full spectrum of supraglottic and glottic atresias seen clinically. In stage 21, the laryngeal cecum gives rise bilaterally to the laryngeal ventricles.

Figure 2–13 is a schematic representation of a stage 18 embryo prior to the recanalization of the epithelial lamina. Complete failure of the epithelial lamina to recanalize would give rise to a type 1 atresia (Figure 2–13D). Complete recanalization of the epithelial lamina except at the glottic level would give rise to a type 3 atresia, or a glottic web (Figure 2–13F). Partial recanalization of the epithelial lamina would give rise to a type 2 atresia (Figure 2–13E). In types 1 and 2 atresia, there is an associated subglottic stenosis as the insult

in development occurred at an earlier point in development, preventing the complete development of the infraglottic region. In addition, there are no signs of laryngeal ventricles, as this is one of the last structures to normally develop.

Development of the laryngeal cartilages and muscles is first seen in a stage 14 embryo, seen initially as the triangular-shaped laryngeal mesodermal anlage adjacent to the primitive laryngopharynx (Figure 2–9). Eventually, the laryngeal mesodermal anlage consolidates into two distinct regions, a hyoid and a thyrocricoid anlage. Fusion of the laryngeal mesodermal anlage occurs dorsally in the cricoid region by stage 18. Chondrification begins along the ventral aspect of the cricoid in stage 17 and progresses dorsally until fusion occurs along the posterior cricoid lamina by stage 20. It is the incomplete fusion dorsally of the laryngeal mesodermal anlage or the chondrification process that can give rise to the full spectrum of laryngotracheal clefts seen clinically.

Four types of clefts have been described in a classification system proposed by Benjamin[11]: type 1, interarytenoid area; type 2, partial cricoid; type 3, total

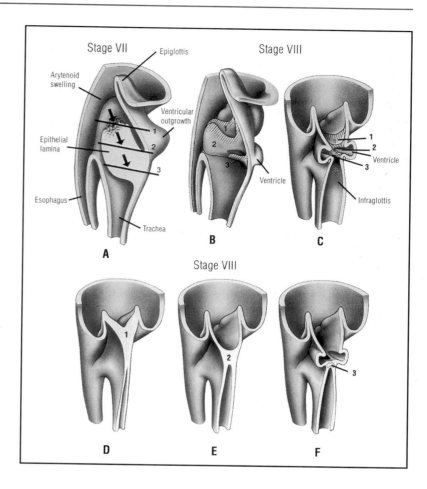

Figure 2–13. Stage 18 embryo prior to the recanalization of the epithelial lamina. **A-C** Normal development. **D.** Type I atresia results in a complete supraglottic stenosis. **E.** Type II atresia results in partial supraglottic stenosis. Communication between supraglottis and infraglottis is usually maintained through a patent pharyngoglottic duct. **F.** Type III atresia corresponds to formation of a glottic web.

cricoid: remains above the thoracic inlet; type 4, laryngotracheoesophageal cleft. Chapter 24 will review these anomalies in greater detail.

REFERENCES

1. Frazer JE. The development of the larynx. *J Anat Physiol.* 1910;44:156–191.
2. His W. *Anatomic Menschlicher Embryonen. III: Zur Geschichte der Organe. Leipzig*: Vogel; 1885:12–19.
3. Kallius E. Beitrage zur Entwicklungsgeschichte des Kehlkopfes. *Anat Hefte Wiesbadan.* 1897;9:303–363.
4. Zaw-Tun HA. The tracheo-esophageal septum—Fact or fantasy? Origin and development of the respiratory primordium and esophagus. *Acta Anat (Basel).* 1982;114:1–21.
5. Walander A. Prenatal development of the epithelial primordium of the larynx in the rat. *Acta Anat (Basel).* 1950; 10(suppl 13).
6. Zaw-Tun HA, Burdi AR. Re-examination of the origin and early development of the human larynx. *Acta Anat (Basel).* 1985;122:163–184.
7. Henick DH. Three-dimensional analysis of murine laryngeal development. *Ann Otol Rhinol Laryngol.* 1993; 102(suppl 159):1–24.
8. Marko M, Leith A, Parsons D. 3-Dimensional reconstructions of cells from serial sections and whole cell mounts using multi-level contouring of stereomicrographs. *J Electron Microsc Tech.* 1988;9:395–411.
9. Leith A, Marko M, Parsons D. Computer graphics for cellular reconstructions. *IEEE Comput Graphics Applicat.* 1989;9:16–23.
10. O'Rahilly R, Muller F. Respiratory and alimentary relations in staged human embryos. New embryological data and congenital anomalies. *Ann Otol Rhinol Laryngol.* 1984;93:421–429.
11. Benjamin B, Inglis A. Minor congenital laryngeal clefts: Diagnosis and classification. *Ann Otol Rhinol Laryngol.* 1989;98:417–420.

3

Anatomy of the Human Larynx

Clarence T. Sasaki, MD
Young-Ho Kim, MD, PhD
Jagdeep Hundal, MD

The human larynx functions as a complex sphincter that directs both airflow and bolus transport at the junction of the digestive and lower respiratory tracts. The larynx has evolved to fulfill three obligations.[1] First, the larynx protects the airway during swallowing. Second, the phasic contraction and relaxation of laryngeal muscles during inspiration and expiration modulate airflow to the lungs. Last, the larynx plays a central role in phonation. Laryngeal anatomy reflects the specialization required by these multiple roles.

INTRODUCTION

Conceptually, the larynx consists of a cartilaginous, bony, and membranous framework, over which a mucosal lining is draped.[2] The laryngeal muscles control the relative positions of individual components of the framework during the various laryngeal actions of swallowing, respiration, and phonation.

Laryngeal Framework

The thyroid, the cricoid, the epiglottic, and the paired arytenoid cartilages constitute the major framework of the larynx (Figures 3–1 through 3–3). The corniculate and cuneiform cartilages, which are also both paired structures, are of considerably less importance. The quadrangular and the triangular membranes are connected to the laryngeal cartilages and comprise the underlying structure for the vocal folds.

Hyoid Bone

Because the hyoglossus, geniohyoid, and mylohyoid muscles attach to the hyoid bone, this bone has been called a lingual bone. Nonetheless, the hyoid serves as an important place of attachment for the larynx; consequently, this bone also can be considered to be a part of the larynx. The hyoid bone is a U-shaped bone that consists of a body centrally and the greater and lesser cornua laterally (Figure 3–1). On each side, the greater

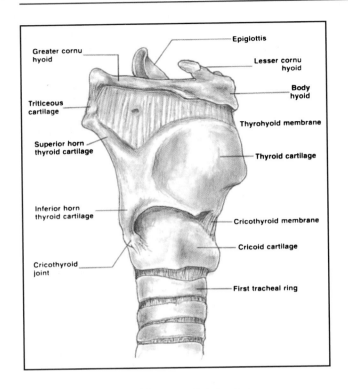

Figure 3–1. Laryngeal framework, lateral view.

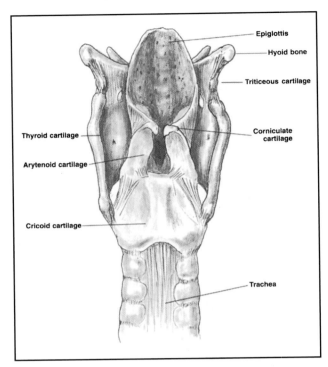

Figure 3–2. Laryngeal framework, posterior view.

cornu is inferior to the lesser cornu. The thyrohyoid membrane connects the thyroid cartilage with the hyoid bone.

The hyoid bone is only partially ossified at birth. Its ossification is usually complete by the age of 2 years.

Thyroid Cartilage

The thyroid cartilage consists of two pentagonal plates, or laminae, that meet anteriorly in the midline. The angle between the plates in the male larynx is 90°, while in the female larynx, this angle is 120°. This angle is more prominent in men than women and is colloquially known as the Adam's apple. The overall shape and positioning of the laminae also differ between men and women; that is, the thyroid cartilage assumes a funnel-type configuration in the male larynx, while the female thyroid cartilage has a more cylindrical shape. Anteriorly, the superior edges of the laminae meet to form the V-shaped thyroid notch. Extending superiorly and inferiorly from the posterior edge of the laminae are the superior and inferior horns. The lateral thyrohyoid ligament connects the superior horn to the hyoid bone. The inferior horn articulates with the cricoid cartilage in the cricothyroid joint, a true synovial joint.

The thyroid cartilage is composed of hyaline-type cartilage, which can undergo calcification and even

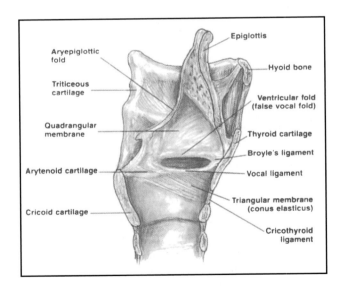

Figure 3–3. Laryngeal framework, sagittal section.

ossification with aging.[3,4] In general, this ossification, which commences at approximately 20 years of age, starts in the posterior laminae and the inferior horns. The central portions of the laminae tend not to undergo these changes, and usually remain relatively radiolucent until well into old age. These changes occur earlier in men, and the extent of the changes is also greater in men. Because the ossified cartilage is radiodense, these areas can be mistaken for intraluminal foreign bodies on plain radiographs.

The thyroid cartilage is covered by a thick perichondrium on its external surfaces, and its perichondrium is thinner on its internal surface. A small prominence on the internal surface lacks a perichondrial cover; this area corresponds to the attachment point for the anterior commissure of the vocal folds.

Cricoid Cartilage

The cricoid cartilage is classically described as a signet ring, with a thin anterior arch and a broader posterior lamina about 20 to 30 mm in height (Figures 3–1 and 3–2). The cricothyroid membrane connects the thyroid and cricoid cartilages anteriorly. In the midline, this membrane is thickened and forms the cricothyroid ligament. The inferior cornua of the thyroid cartilage articulate posterolaterally with the cricoid cartilage. The inferior edge of the cricoid cartilage is firmly attached to the first tracheal ring. Along the superior aspect of the cricoid lamina, facets for the articulation with the arytenoid cartilages are present.

Like the thyroid cartilage, the cricoid cartilage is composed of hyaline cartilage. The cricoid ossifies first posteriorly in the cricoid lamina, and the cricoid arch undergoes these changes later as the process sweeps anteriorly. Ossification of the cricoid cartilage starts slightly after this process begins in the thyroid cartilage. Similar in appearance to ossified thyroid cartilage, these radiodense areas can mimic intraluminal foreign bodies on soft tissue radiographs.[3,4]

Epiglottic Cartilage

The epiglottic cartilage is shaped as a leaf and defines the anterior border of the laryngeal inlet (Figures 3–2 and 3–3). Its anterior surface projects above the thyroid cartilage and faces the base of tongue and lingual tonsils. The epiglottic cartilage's inferior portion is considerably narrower than its broader, rounder superior part. The petiole, or the stemlike inferior extension of the epiglottic cartilage, is connected to the thyroid cartilage just below the thyroid notch by the thyroepiglottic ligament. The hyoepiglottic ligament runs from the lingual surface of the epiglottic cartilage to the posterior surface of the hyoid. Along the inferior aspect of the laryngeal surface of the petiole, the epiglottic tubercle partially overhangs the anterior commissure.

This cartilage consists of fibroelastic cartilage and does not calcify or ossify. It is considerably thinner than the cricoid and thyroid cartilages. The epiglottic perichondrium is more tightly bound to the underlying cartilage on the laryngeal surface of the epiglottis than on its lingual surface. Consequently, acute inflammatory processes often produce more marked mucosal edema on the lingual surface of the epiglottis, rather than on its laryngeal surface. This distribution of edema results in posterior displacement of the epiglottis into the laryngeal airway during acute epiglottitis. Mucous glands extend into tiny indentations within the cartilage on both surfaces, although more glands are present on the laryngeal surface.

Arytenoid Cartilages

The arytenoid cartilages are paired pyramidal-shaped cartilages that rest upon the superior edge of the cricoid lamina (Figures 3–2 and 3–3). Each arytenoid consists of two processes, an apex and a base. The vocal ligament attaches to the vocal process, and the intrinsic laryngeal muscles insert upon the muscular process and elsewhere. The base has a concave contour, and it articulates with the cricoid cartilage in a synovial joint. The motion of this joint is very complex and involves more than just simple rotation of the arytenoid around its vertical axis.

The apices of these cartilages and the vocal process are composed of elastic cartilage, while the remainder is mainly hyaline cartilage. The arytenoid cartilages also ossify, beginning at approximately age 30 years.[3,4]

Minor Cartilages

The corniculate cartilages, also known as the cartilages of Santorini, are located just above the arytenoid apices (Figure 3–2). They consist of fibroelastic cartilage. The cuneiform cartilages, also known as the cartilages of Wrisberg, are found within the superior aspect of the aryepiglottic folds, just lateral to the corniculate cartilages. Even though the cuneiform cartilages are composed of hyaline cartilage, they do not appear to ossify.[3,4] These cartilages provide rigidity to the aryepiglottic folds (described below), which function as ramparts that guide the food bolus away from the laryngeal inlet posterolaterally toward the piriform sinuses.

The triticeal cartilages are embedded in the lateral thyrohyoid ligaments. These cartilages are composed of hyaline cartilage, and they also may be absent in the human larynx. The triticeal cartilages commonly calcify and should not be mistaken for a foreign body on cervical radiographs.[3,4] The adjacent lateral thyrohyoid ligaments also ossify, but less frequently.

Thyrohyoid Membrane

The thyrohyoid membrane connects the posterosuperior edge of the hyoid bone and the superior edge of the thyroid cartilage (Figure 3–1). It is thickened medially and laterally, giving rise to the medial thyrohyoid ligament and the paired lateral thyrohyoid ligaments. Posterior to the lateral thyrohyoid ligaments, the internal branch of the superior laryngeal nerve and vessels pierce the thyrohyoid membrane to enter the larynx.

Quadrangular Membrane

On each side of the larynx, the quadrangular membrane extends from the lateral edge of the epiglottis to arytenoid cartilage posteriorly (Figure 3–3). The superior border of each quadrangular membrane is a free edge that extends posteroinferiorly from the epiglottis to the corniculate cartilages. The aryepiglottic fold corresponds to this free border. Each quadrangular membrane's inferior edge is also free; it extends from the inferior epiglottis to the vocal process of the arytenoid. This portion of the quadrangular membrane corresponds to the false vocal folds, also known as the ventricular or vestibular folds. Because of this arrangement, the anterior vertical height of this membrane is considerably greater than its corresponding posterior vertical dimension. The superior and inferior edges of this membrane are thickened, giving rise to the aryepiglottic ligament and the vestibular ligament, respectively.

Triangular Membrane

The triangular membrane is a paired fibroelastic structure (Figure 3–3). Its inferior edge is firmly attached to the cricoid cartilage. Its base is located anteriorly, at attachments to both the cricoid and thyroid cartilages. Each triangular membrane's apex inserts upon the vocal process of the arytenoid cartilage. The free superior edge of this membrane is thickened and forms the vocal ligament. The attachment of the vocal ligament to the thyroid cartilage is known as Broyle's ligament. Both triangular membranes together constitute the conus elasticus. Anteriorly, the thick part of the anterior conus elasticus forms the cricothyroid ligament.

LARYNGEAL MUCOSA

The laryngeal mucosa is draped over the laryngeal skeleton. The resulting relationships are best appreciated in a coronal section of the larynx (Figure 3–4). Fol-

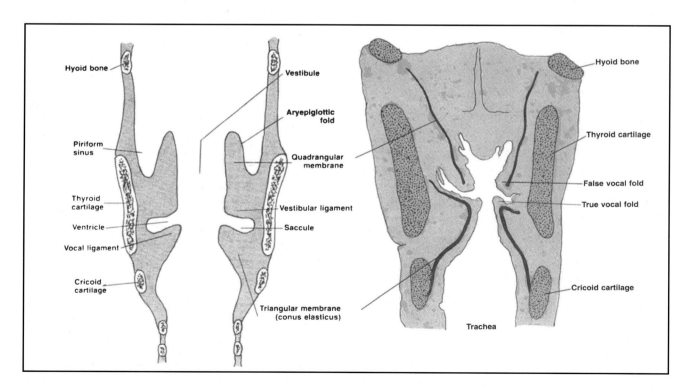

Figure 3–4. Human larynx, coronal view.

lowing the internal contour of the larynx in a superior to inferior direction, the mucosa lines the thyrohyoid membrane and a portion of the thyroid cartilage. The mucosa then extends superiorly covering the lateral aspect of the quadrangular membrane. The space between the quadrangular membrane and thyroid cartilage is the piriform sinus or recess, which has a pear shape. The lining comes over the superior edge of the quadrangular membrane, creating the aryepiglottic fold, and descends along the medial aspect of this membrane, creating the false vocal fold. That portion of the airway that is located between the aryepiglottic folds is known as the laryngeal vestibule. The mucosa then proceeds laterally forming a pouch, known as the laryngeal ventricle, or the ventricle of Morgagni. The superior aspect of the ventricle is called the laryngeal saccule, or the saccule of Hilton. Along the floor of the ventricle, the mucosa continues medially to the triangular membrane and vocal ligament. The mucosa covers the vocal ligament and the inferior aspect of the triangular membrane, and is continuous with the tracheal mucosa.

The mucosa is also reflected over the lingual surface of the epiglottis. This arrangement creates two pouches between the base of the tongue and the epiglottis. These valleculae are bounded laterally by the glossoepiglottic folds. The median glossoepiglottic fold corresponds to the hyoepiglottic ligament and separates the two valleculae.

Both pseudostratified ciliated columnar epithelium (also known as respiratory epithelium) and stratified squamous epithelium comprise the laryngeal mucosa. Stratified squamous epithelium covers the piriform sinus, the lingual surface of the epiglottis, the superior half of the laryngeal surface of the epiglottis, the superior surface of the false vocal folds, true vocal folds, and the undersurface of the true vocal folds. Respiratory epithelium lines the subglottic area, the laryngeal ventricle, the laryngeal vestibule, and the inferior half of the laryngeal surface of the epiglottis. Mucus-secreting goblet cells are found within this respiratory epithelium and are prominent within the mucosa of the false vocal folds. Beneath the respiratory epithelium, numerous seromucous tubuloalveolar glands are present, especially in the medial part of the aryepiglottic fold, the laryngeal saccule, and the posterior surface of the epiglottis. These glands and goblet cells help lubricate the surface of the larynx; such secretions are essential for normal laryngeal function, particularly vocal fold vibration. In addition, lysozyme and other antibacterial proteins and glycoproteins in the secretions of these glands and goblet cells serve to protect the larynx against bacterial infections. Inflammatory cells are also located within the stroma deep to the ep-

ithelium. These cells may be organized into germinal centers. The squamous epithelium is nonkeratinizing, although it may keratinize in certain pathologic conditions. Furthermore, the respiratory epithelium may undergo metaplastic changes with chronic irritation and become a keratinizing or nonkeratinizing stratified squamous epithelium.

This arrangement of the true vocal folds inferiorly and the ventricular folds superiorly enhances the ability of the larynx to act as a valve for airflow into and from the lungs. In the absence of active muscular contraction, the adducted true vocal folds block the flow of air into the lungs at a pressure head greater than 140 mm Hg.[1] Yet, they offer minimal resistance to flow in the opposite direction. Thus, it is essential that the glottis be actively opened for airflow to pass through the larynx and into the lung during each inspiration. Similarly, the ventricular folds passively resist egress of air at subglottic pressure of up to 30 mm Hg, but they do not significantly impede the entry of air into the lungs. It is believed that the ventricular folds are involved in the production of an adequate cough.

LARYNGEAL MUSCLES

The laryngeal muscles can be divided into three groups: intrinsic, extrinsic, and accessory. The intrinsic muscles directly act upon the arytenoids. The only extrinsic muscle is the cricothyroid muscle. The accessory muscles either elevate or depress the larynx.

Other classifications of the laryngeal muscles have been proposed. A common alternative approach places the cricothyroid muscle with the intrinsic muscles and considers all the remaining elevators and depressors of the larynx as extrinsic laryngeal muscles.

This discussion will describe intrinsic, extrinsic, and accessory laryngeal muscles, as outlined above.

Intrinsic Muscles

The articulation between the cricoid and arytenoid cartilages is a complex one, involving a sliding of the arytenoid across the cricoid cartilage, not just a rotation of the arytenoid about its vertical axis. This motion reflects the saddle-shaped contour of each surface of the cricoarytenoid joint. During adduction of the vocal processes of the arytenoid cartilages, each vocal process moves medially, inferiorly, and posteriorly, while during abduction, each vocal process moves laterally, superiorly, and posteriorly.[5] This pattern of movement occurs as each arytenoid cartilage rocks around the long axis of the cricoarytenoid joint facets. Discussion of the intrinsic muscles of the larynx often oversimplifies this joint in two ways. First, the joint is assumed to purely permit rotation of the arytenoid on the cricoid. Second, each intrinsic laryngeal muscle is assumed to act alone. In reality, arytenoid movement is the composite of all the actions of the intrinsic muscles acting together. Nonetheless, consideration of the actions of the intrinsic muscles is traditionally facilitated by making these two assumptions.

The intrinsic laryngeal muscles consist of the muscles of the quadrangular membrane and the muscles of the arytenoid cartilage.[2] The first group includes the thyroepiglottic, thyroarytenoid, and aryepiglottic muscles (Figure 3–5). The second set is composed of the interarytenoid, posterior cricoarytenoid, and lateral cricoarytenoid muscles (Figures 3–5 through 3–7).

The muscles of the quadrangular membranes consist of a nearly continuous sheet of muscles that originate from the posterior midportion of the thyroid cartilage. The thyroarytenoid muscle is made up of both horizontal and more vertically oriented fibers. The thyroarytenoid muscle inserts upon the vocal process of the arytenoid. Its deep portion constitutes the vocalis muscle. The aryepiglottic muscles run along each quadrangular membrane parallel to its free edge from the epiglottis to the arytenoid cartilages. These mus-

cles extend posteriorly and are at least partially continuous with the oblique arytenoid muscles.

The origins of the posterior and lateral cricoarytenoid muscles are the posterior and lateral aspects of the cricoid cartilage, respectively. The posterior cricoarytenoid muscle inserts upon the posteromedial surface of the muscular process of the arytenoid cartilage, while the lateral cricoarytenoid muscle inserts upon the anterolateral surface of the muscular process of the arytenoid cartilage. The interarytenoid muscle, also

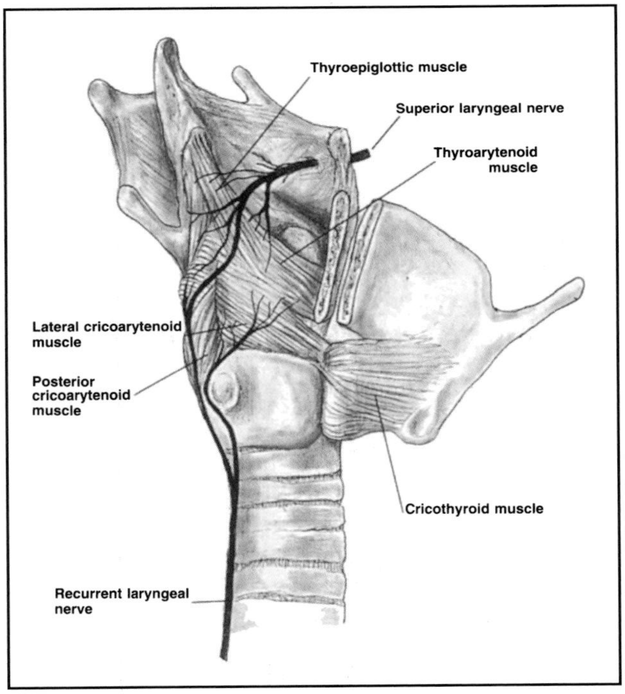

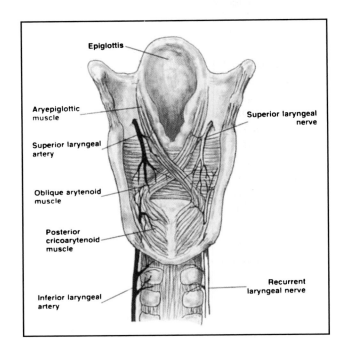

Figure 3–6. Laryngeal intrinsic muscles, posterior view. Innervation and blood supply are also depicted.

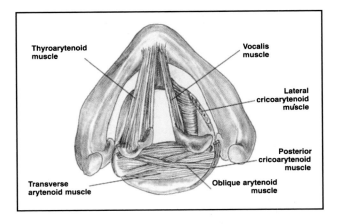

Figure 3–7. Laryngeal intrinsic muscles, arytenoid group, superior view.

Figure 3–5. Laryngeal intrinsic muscles, lateral view. Innervation is also depicted.

known as the transverse arytenoid muscle, connects the posterior parts of the arytenoid cartilages. The oblique arytenoid muscles run superficially across the interarytenoid muscles and the arytenoid cartilages. Each oblique arytenoid muscle diagonally crosses its contralateral counterpart.

The intrinsic laryngeal muscles are not merely abductors and adductors of the vocal folds. While vocal fold abduction and adduction are essential functions of these muscles, the intrinsic laryngeal muscles also determine the vibratory characteristics (ie, tension, mass per unit length) and cross-sectional contour of the vocal folds. The primary abductors of the vocal folds are the posterior cricoarytenoid muscles, which rotate the vocal process of the arytenoid laterally by pulling its muscular process medially (Figure 3–8A). Contraction of the posterior cricoarytenoid muscles expands the glottis in the horizontal dimension during forced inspiratory efforts. The posterior cricoarytenoid muscles lengthen and stiffen the vocal folds. As this happens, the vocal folds become thinner and their edges become rounder. These muscles are found to contain three distinct neuromuscular compartments: vertical, oblique, and horizontal bellies. The vertical and oblique bellies rock the arytenoid backward while

sliding it laterally, thus causing a maximal dilation of the airway. The horizontal belly causes a swiveling motion of the arytenoid. It is proposed that the vertical and oblique bellies normally cause vocal fold abduction during respiration, while the horizontal belly primarily is used to adjust the position of the vocal process during phonation.[6,7] The lateral cricoarytenoid muscles draw the muscular processes of the arytenoid cartilages laterally, thereby adducting the vocal folds and narrowing the glottic opening (Figure 3–8B). This movement of the arytenoid cartilages lowers the position of the vocal folds. The lateral cricoarytenoid muscles also thin the free edge of each vocal fold by increasing its length. The interarytenoid and oblique arytenoid muscles directly pull the arytenoid cartilages together, also adducting the vocal folds (Figure 3–8C). Because of the complexity of the cricoarytenoid joint, these muscles act primarily to stabilize the arytenoid cartilages on the cricoid cartilage during vocal fold adduction. The interarytenoid and oblique arytenoid muscles do not alter the vibratory characteristics of the vocal folds significantly.

The thyroarytenoid muscles are adductors of the vocal folds (Figure 3–8D). These muscles also shorten and tense the true vocal folds. In addition, contraction

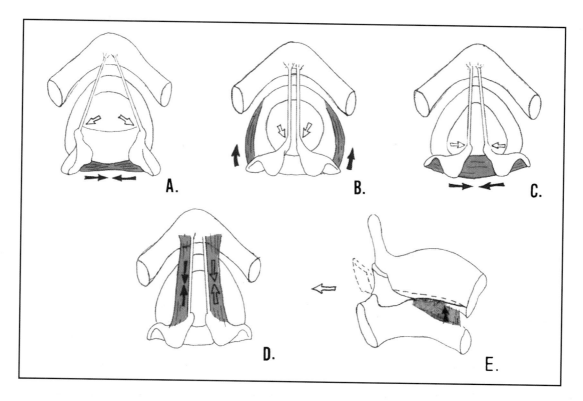

Figure 3–8. Actions of the intrinsic and extrinsic laryngeal muscles. **A** to **D.** Superior view; **E.** lateral view.

and relaxation of the vocalis muscles change the vibratory characteristics of the vocal folds by altering their mass and the tension of the vocal ligament. The vocalis muscles act to shorten and thicken the vocal folds. The aryepiglottic muscles help close the laryngeal inlet by folding the epiglottis posteriorly.

The intrinsic laryngeal muscles function to shut the larynx at three levels. Most inferiorly, forced adduction of the vocal folds by contraction of the thyroarytenoid, lateral cricothyroid, interarytenoid, and oblique arytenoid muscles closes the glottis tightly. Medial rotation of the vocal processes of the arytenoid cartilages also tightly closes the false vocal folds. Most superiorly, the epiglottis is drawn posteriorly by the aryepiglottic muscles. These three tiers of closure represent a most effective mechanism of protection of the airway against aspiration.[1]

Extrinsic Muscles

The only extrinsic muscles of the larynx are the paired cricothyroid muscles. These muscles, which are located on the exterior surface of the larynx, each consist of two parts. Their anterior portion arises from the superior edge of the cricoid arch and inserts upon the posterolateral border of the thyroid cartilage, while the oblique portion extends from the lateral surface of the cricoid cartilage to the inferior edge of the thyroid cartilage. In canine cricothyroid muscles, three distinct muscle bellies (rectus, oblique, and horizontal) have been identified, each separated by distinct connective tissue planes. Differences in their electrical activity patterns suggest these three bellies probably play separate roles in the complex function of this muscle.[8]

The cricothyroid muscle tilts the larynx by approximating the cricoid and thyroid anteriorly utilizing the cricothyroid joint (Figure 3–8E). By doing so, the cricothyroid muscle lengthens the vocal fold by up to one-third of its original length and lowers the relative position of the vocal fold within the larynx. This action effectively expands the glottis in its anteroposterior dimension during expiration and inspiration. The cricothyroid muscle also is a weak adductor of the true vocal folds. At the same time, contraction of the cricothyroid muscle augments the tension of the vocal fold while decreasing its mass per unit length during pitch elevation. Because the cricothyroid muscle stretches the vocal fold, this muscle thins the vocal fold and sharpens its edge. These characteristic changes produced by the cricothyroid muscles in the vocal folds indicate that the cricothyroid muscles are an important determinant of the pitch of the acoustic signal of the vibrating vocal folds.

Accessory Muscles

The accessory muscles can be divided into elevator and depressor groups (Figure 3–9). The first group includes the digastric (both bellies), the stylohyoid, the geniohyoid, and the mylohyoid muscles, all of which act to pull the larynx superiorly. Additionally, contraction of the hyoglossus muscle elevates the larynx if the remainder of the tongue musculature remains fixed. The anterior belly of the digastric, the geniohyoid, and the mylohyoid muscles also move the larynx under the base of tongue, an important maneuver in the prevention of aspiration during deglutition. Such action plays a vital role in deglutition by expanding the hypopharynx and thus easing the passage of the bolus inferiorly. This movement also serves to protect the airway against aspiration as the anterosuperior displacement of the tongue pulls the laryngohyoid complex away from the bolus path. The depressor muscles include the sternohyoid, sternothyroid, and omohyoid muscles, which all pull the larynx inferiorly. The thyrohyoid muscle pulls the hyoid bone and thyroid cartilage together.

The pharyngeal constrictor muscles are also closely related to the larynx. The middle and inferior constrictor muscles insert upon the greater cornua of the hyoid and the thyroid lamina, respectively. Their contraction draws the larynx posterosuperiorly. The cricopharyngeus muscle, located inferior to the inferior constrictors, arises from the cricoid cartilage and encircles the esophageal inlet. This muscle functions as an upper esophageal sphincter by maintaining a tonic state of contraction. During swallowing, the con-

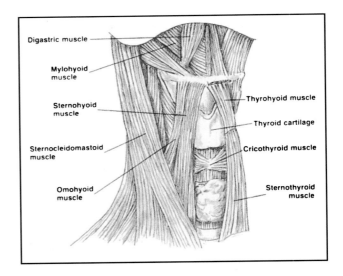

Figure 3–9. Laryngeal accessory muscles, anterior view.

stricter muscles propel the bolus into the esophagus, while the cricopharyngeus muscle relaxes as the bolus enters the esophagus.

LARYNGEAL INNERVATION

The main somatic innervation to the larynx is from the vagus nerve through the superior and recurrent laryngeal nerves (Figure 3–10). The superior laryngeal nerve passes between the external and internal carotid arteries at about the level of the crossing of the hypoglossal nerve. This nerve then travels inferiorly to the tip of the hyoid, where it divides into external and internal branches. The external branch descends with superior thyroid vessels on the surface of the inferior constrictor muscle. The internal branch pierces the thyrohyoid membrane to enter the interior larynx. The recurrent laryngeal nerves, also known as the inferior laryngeal nerves, take a longer route to the larynx. On the right side, the recurrent laryngeal nerve branches from the vagus at the subclavian artery. This recurrent laryngeal nerve then loops around the subclavian

artery and proceeds superiorly in the tracheoesophageal groove to enter the larynx between the cricopharyngeus and the esophagus. On the left side, the route of the recurrent laryngeal nerve is similar, except that the nerve passes around the aortic arch distal to the ligamentum arteriosum.

The course of the recurrent laryngeal nerve reflects the embryologic branchial arch system, whose further development and partial involution influence the positioning of the recurrent laryngeal nerve. In a small percentage of individuals, the right inferior laryngeal nerve does not pass around the subclavian artery.[9] This nonrecurrent laryngeal nerve descends directly to the larynx. Invariably associated with this anomaly is a right retroesophageal subclavian artery that arises from the aorta distal to the ligamentum arteriosum.

All the intrinsic muscles of the larynx are innervated by the corresponding ipsilateral recurrent laryngeal nerve (Figures 3–5 and 3–6). Only the interarytenoid muscle receives bilateral innervation. Sensory information from the muscle spindles of the intrinsic muscles is conveyed by the recurrent laryngeal nerve. The cricothyroid muscle is supplied by the external branch of the superior laryngeal nerve. The somatic motor nucleus for the recurrent laryngeal nerve and the external branch of the superior laryngeal nerve is the nucleus ambiguus.

Somatic sensory innervation for the mucosa above the glottis is carried by the internal branch of the ipsilateral superior laryngeal nerve, which is divided into three divisions. The superior division mainly supplies the mucosa of the laryngeal surface of the epiglottis; the middle division supplies the mucosa of the true and false vocal folds and the aryepiglottic fold; and the inferior division supplies the mucosa of the arytenoid, subglottis, anterior wall of hypopharynx, and upper esophageal sphincter.[10] The corresponding innervation for the remaining major portions of the subglottis is from the ipsilateral recurrent laryngeal nerve (Figures 3–5 and 3–6). The thyroepiglottic joint and the cricothyroid joint are both innervated by the internal branch of the ipsilateral superior laryngeal nerve. The cricothyroid joint also receives sensory innervation from the external branch of the ipsilateral superior laryngeal nerve. The external branch of the superior laryngeal nerve also conveys sensory information from the anterior midline portion of the subglottis, as demonstrated in a cat model[11]; a similar pattern of innervation is probably true in the human larynx as well. These sensory nerves project to the ipsilateral nucleus solitarius, and their corresponding sensory ganglion is the nodose ganglion.

The afferent impulses of the protective glottic closure reflex (GCR) project centrally via the internal

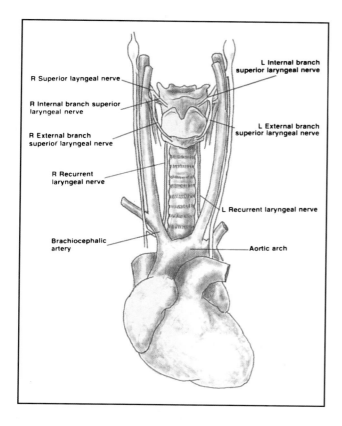

Figure 3–10. Paths of the recurrent and superior laryngeal nerves.

R Superior layngeal nerve

R Internal branch superior laryngeal nerve

R External branch superior laryngeal nerve

R Recurrent laryngeal nerve

Brachiocephalic artery

L Internal branch superior laryngeal nerve

L External branch superior laryngeal nerve

L Recurrent laryngeal nerve

Aortic arch

branch of the superior laryngeal nerve to the ipsilateral nucleus ambiguus with synapse at the level of the nucleus tractus solitarius. The motor neurons within the nucleus ambiguus then project through the recurrent laryngeal nerve to the ipsilateral adductor muscles, completing the efferent arc. The existence of a crossed GCR pathway (Figure 3–11) has also been demonstrated to exist in humans. This crossed GCR is centrally mediated and is suppressed with increasing depths of anesthesia (Figure 3–12), thereby weakening the glottic closing force and predisposing to aspiration under sedation or deep sleep.[12]

The somatic sensory receptors of the larynx are distributed in a well-characterized pattern. The true vocal folds have fewer mucosal surface receptors than the laryngeal surface of the epiglottis, which has the great-

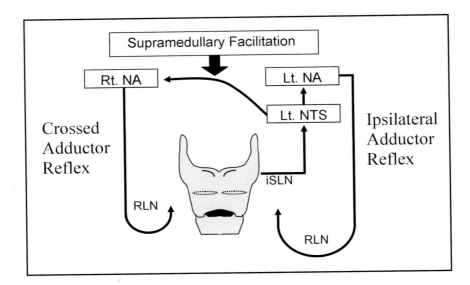

Figure 3–11. Organizational Model of the Crossed adductor reflex under light anesthesia. (*NA* = nucleus ambiguus; *NTS* = nucleus tractus solitarius; *RLN* = recurrent laryngeal nerve; *iSLN* = internal branch superior laryngeal nerve.)

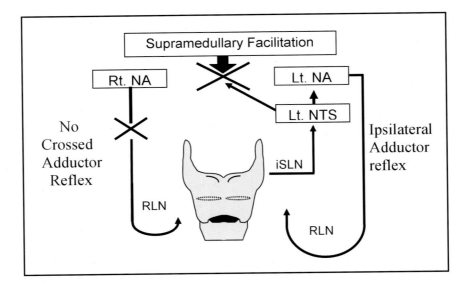

Figure 3–12. Organizational Model demonstrating the loss of crossed adductor reflex under deep anesthesia (*NA* = nucleus ambiguus; *NTS* = nucleus tractus solitarius; *RLN* = recurrent laryngeal nerve; *iSLN* = internal branch superior laryngeal nerve.

est density of receptors in the larynx.[12] In addition, the distribution of chemoreceptors is limited to the supraglottic mucosa.

Histologic examination has revealed the presence of free nerve endings, Merkel's cells, Meissner's corpuscles, and taste buds scattered in the larynx. Mechanoreceptors are located either in the superficial mucosa or in the muscles and laryngeal joints. Some of them are spontaneously active whereas others are silent until stimulated. A large number of taste buds populate the laryngeal surface of the epiglottis and extend caudally along the aryepiglottic folds, reaching peak density at the caudal extreme of the folds. These respond to a number of chemical stimuli and to water. Taste buds of the larynx tend to be stimulated by the pH and tonicity of the stimulating solution. Chemoreceptors of the larynx are adapted to detect chemicals that are not salinelike in composition and can play an important role in modifying reflexes involved in the maintenance of upper airway patency.[13,14]

The recurrent laryngeal and internal branch of the superior laryngeal nerves carry parasympathetic innervation from the dorsal motor nucleus to the subglottic and supraglottic regions, respectively. The sympathetic innervation is from the superior cervical ganglion.

The nerve of Galen, which is also known as the ramus communicans, connects the superior laryngeal nerve and the recurrent laryngeal nerve. It provides visceral motor input to the tracheal and esophageal mucosa as well as to the tracheal smooth muscle. The baroreceptors and chemoreceptors of the aortic arch are also innervated by the nerve of Galen, which relays this sensory information to the solitary nucleus.

LARYNGEAL BLOOD SUPPLY

Each side of the larynx has a dual blood supply from the inferior and superior laryngeal arteries. The inferior laryngeal artery is a branch of the inferior thyroid artery, which travels from the thyrocervical trunk superiorly to the inferior pole of the thyroid gland. Of note, the thyrocervical trunk is a constant feature on the right side, but on the left, the trunk may be so short that its branches, the inferior thyroid artery, the suprascapular artery, and the transverse cervical artery, arise directly from the subclavian artery. The inferior laryngeal artery enters the larynx with the recurrent laryngeal nerve and supplies the arytenoids, the false folds, and the laryngeal ventricle (Figure 3–6). The superior laryngeal artery is a branch from the superior thyroid artery, itself a branch of the external carotid artery. The superior laryngeal artery travels with the superior la-

ryngeal nerve and enters the larynx with this nerve's internal branch to supply the piriform sinus and the quadrangular membrane (Figure 3–6).

The venous drainage parallels the larynx's arterial supply. The superior laryngeal vein empties into the internal jugular vein, while the inferior laryngeal vein empties into the thyrocervical trunk, a tributary of the subclavian vein.

LARYNGEAL LYMPHATIC DRAINAGE

Two systems of lymphatics drain the larynx. The superficial system is intramucosal only, and there is free communication between the left and right sides. Its contribution is relatively minor. The deep system drains the ipsilateral tissues only and is located submucosally.

The lymphatic flow from the larynx travels inferiorly and superiorly. The subglottic lymphatics drain via the middle pedicle and the paired posterolateral pedicles. The middle pedicle pierces the cricothyroid membrane and travels to the pretracheal and Delphian lymph nodes, which in turn, drain to the deep cervical lymph nodes. The posterolateral pedicle follows the inferior thyroid artery to ultimately reach the inferior deep lateral cervical, the subclavian, the paratracheal, and the tracheoesophageal lymph nodes. The supraglottic lymphatic vessels form a pedicle that exits the larynx with the superior laryngeal and superior thyroid vessels. This lymph drainage travels to the superior deep cervical lymph nodes associated with the internal jugular vein. In addition, lymph from the laryngeal ventricle flows through the cricothyroid membrane and ipsilateral thyroid gland to reach the prelaryngeal, paratracheal, prethyroid, supraclavicular, and pretracheal lymph nodes. The true vocal folds themselves lack significant lymphatic drainage.

CLINICAL SUBDIVISIONS

For clinical assessments, the larynx is divided into the supraglottis, glottis, and subglottis. The supraglottis, which surrounds the laryngeal vestibule, extends from the tip of the epiglottis to the junction between respiratory and squamous epithelium in the floor of the laryngeal ventricle. From a practical viewpoint, however, this inferior boundary is considered to be at the junction of the floor and lateral wall of the ventricle, so that the entire floor of the ventricle is considered to be part of the glottic larynx. Strictly speaking, the glottic larynx consists of the true vocal folds, the anterior commissure and the so-called posterior commissure. Because the vocal folds do not join posteriorly, there is no true posterior commissure. Instead, it is more appropriate to describe a posterior part of the glottic larynx, consisting of the arytenoid cartilages and the superior edge of the cricoid lamina.[15] The subglottis extends inferiorly from the area on the undersurface of the vocal folds where the squamous epithelium becomes a respiratory epithelium. Operationally, this margin is defined as occurring 5 millimeters below the free edge of the vocal folds. The inferior edge of the subglottis is the inferior border of the cricoid cartilage.

The term *epilarynx* describes the epiglottis and aryepiglottic folds above the hyoid bone. Here, malignant disease more closely resembles hypopharyngeal carcinomas, but this region is considered to be part of the anatomic larynx.

The valleculae, piriform sinuses, and the posterior cricoid esophageal inlet regions are all extralaryngeal. They are parts of the oropharynx and hypopharynx.

LARYNGEAL SPACES

A variety of compartments in the larynx are created by the arrangement of the various laryngeal membranes and mucosal reflections. The paraglottic space is found lateral to the laryngeal ventricle. This area is bounded by the thyroid lamina, the conus elasticus, and the quadrangular membrane. The paraglottic space communicates with the gap between the cricoid and thyroid cartilages, creating an important passageway for the spread of carcinoma arising in the ventri-

cle. The pre-epiglottic space is bounded by the vallecular mucosa superiorly, the thyrohyoid membrane and thyroid cartilage anteriorly, and the epiglottis posteriorly and inferiorly. This space contains areolar tissue, lymphatic channels, and blood vessels.

VOCAL FOLD HISTOLOGY

The glottis consists of an anterior, or intermembranous, part and a posterior, or intercartilaginous, part. The true vocal fold extends from the tip of the vocal process of the arytenoid cartilage anteriorly to the anterior commissure. The cartilage of the vocal process does not participate in the vibratory actions of the true vocal fold and is not considered to be a part of the vocal fold.

The true vocal fold is a laminated structure composed of mucosa and muscle (Figure 3–13).[16-18] The overlying epithelium, as previously described, is of a nonkeratinizing, stratified squamous type. The lamina propria beneath this epithelium contains three layers: the superficial, intermediate, and deep layers. The superficial layer corresponds to Reinke's space and is made of mostly amorphous material. Elastic and collagenous fibers comprise the intermediate and deep layers, which together form the vocal ligament. The vocalis muscle is deep to the vocal ligament. The anterior macula flava is a thickening of the intermediate layer of the anterior vocal fold. The collagenous anterior commissure tendon extends from the anterior macula flava and the vocal fold deep lay-

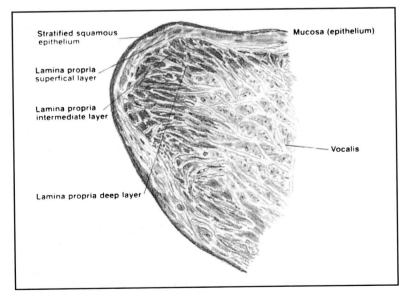

Figure 3–13. Schematic illustration of vocal histologic structure.

Stratified squamous epithelium

Lamina propria superfical layer

Lamina propria intermediate layer

Lamina propria deep layer

Mucosa (epithelium)

Vocalis

er to the thyroid cartilage. The posterior macula flava resembles the anterior macula flava. A transitional area of chondrocytes and fibroblasts lies between the posterior macula flava and the arytenoid vocal process, which is composed of elastic cartilage.

From a mechanical viewpoint, this histologic arrangement is actually three layers. The squamous epithelium and the superficial layer of the lamina propria form the cover, the intermediate and deep layers of the lamina propria form the transitional zone, and the vocalis muscle forms the body. This simplification is known as the cover-body concept and helps describe the vibratory characteristics of the vocal folds in health and disease.

THE PEDIATRIC LARYNX

The adult and pediatric larynges are not identical. Major differences include the position of the larynx, as well as the configuration and relative sizes of the laryngeal cartilages. Lastly, the histologic structure of the vocal fold differs in the pediatric population.

Position

At birth, the cricoid is approximately at the level of the fourth cervical vertebra, and the epiglottis may be visualized over the dorsum of the tongue. The larynx descends slightly so that the cricoid is at the level of the fourth and/or fifth vertebra by age 2 years. During puberty, there is a rapid descent of the larynx so that it acquires its adult position in the neck. The cricoid cartilage is anterior to the seventh and sixth cervical vertebrae in men and women, respectively.

In the neonate, the epiglottis is in close apposition to the uvula and soft palate. This placement probably accounts for the observation that the neonate is an obligate nasal breather. The epiglottis descends between the ages of 4 and 6 months to a more mature placement.[19]

Framework Configuration and Size

The infantile epiglottis has an omega shape that provides less support for the aryepiglottic folds. The angle between the thyroid laminae in the newborn is approximately 110 to 120°. In the fully developed larynx, the epiglottis has a leaflike appearance, and the angle between the thyroid laminae is 90° and 120° in men and women, respectively.

The infantile larynx is smaller relative to body size compared to the adult counterpart. In addition, the

subglottic region is the narrowest part of the child's larynx, while the glottis forms the narrowest point of the adult larynx. Rapid growth from birth until age 6 and again during adolescence occurs as the larynx assumes its more mature configuration.

Histology

The pediatric vocal fold is considerably different from its adult counterpart.[17] The ratio between the cartilaginous and the membranous portions of the vocal fold is 1:1 in the neonate and 2:3 in the adult. The lamina propria of the vocal fold lacks clearly defined layers and is relatively thick in the neonatal larynx. Between the ages of 1 and 4 years, the vocal ligament, which is absent in the neonate, develops. Two layers appear in the lamina propria between the ages of 6 and 12 years. The fully mature lamina propria, consisting of superficial, intermediate, and deep layers, is only apparent by the conclusion of adolescence.

THE GERIATRIC LARYNX

The vocal fold also undergoes considerable sex-specific changes with aging.[20] In the female larynx, both the mucosa and vocal fold cover thicken with aging. In addition, the superficial layer of the lamina propria loses density as it becomes more edematous. The intermediate layer of the lamina propria tends to atrophy only in men. The deep layer of the lamina propria of the male vocal fold thickens because of increased collagen deposition. The vocalis muscle atrophies in both men and women.

The aging process also alters the histologic appearance of the false vocal folds.[21] Within the submucosa of the respiratory epithelium of the larynx, the seromucous glands become less prominent with increasing age. These changes are more pronounced for the mucous components of these glands compared with their serous portions.

As these glands atrophy, fatty infiltration increases. Additionally, the connective tissues of the false vocal folds fragment and become less dense in the geriatric larynx. These observations may account for age-related changes in laryngeal function.

THE VOCAL TRACT CONCEPT

Two general theories have been proposed to explain human voice production. The neuromuscular hypothesis stated that contractions of the intrinsic laryngeal muscles encoded by neural input directly initiate the vocal fold vibrations. This idea has been disproven. Even the larynx with bilateral recurrent laryngeal nerve palsies is capable of voice production. According to the myoelastic-aerodynamic theory, the release of subglottic pressure through the medialized vocal folds opens the glottis. As this pressure is released, the intrinsic elastic tension of the vocal folds draws the glottis closed again. The Bernoulli effect, in which flow produces decreased pressure, also tends to bring the vocal folds together. This cycle is repeated many times. In this way, the vocal folds are caused to vibrate. The sound waves created by the balance between subglottic pressure and vocal fold tension and the Bernoulli effect is then further modified by the resonance chambers of the hypopharynx, oropharynx, nasopharynx, nasal cavity, and oral cavity.

The vocal tract then includes not only the larynx, but also the lower respiratory and upper aerodigestive tracts. The pulmonary system, including the trachea, bronchi, lungs, thorax, and the related muscles of respiration, functions as an activator for phonation by providing the airflow and subglottic pressure. The lar-

ynx houses the vibrator source (ie, the true vocal folds). The muscles of the upper aerodigestive tract alter the dimensions and shape of the superior vocal tract and in doing so change the resultant resonant frequencies. Components of the initial sound signal are thus enhanced. By relatively rapid changes in the configuration (ie, volume, cross-sectional area, etc) of the upper vocal tract, a wide range of speech sounds can be produced. In this way, the specific sounds of human speech result from this complex interaction.

Initial studies of the contribution of the upper aerodigestive tract to human voice production utilized two-dimensional plain radiographs to assess the positioning of soft tissues. Computed tomography (CT) scans have also been applied for this purpose. Most recently, magnetic resonance imaging (MRI), which has multiplanar imaging capacity, has provided information about the three-dimensional shape of the upper vocal tract during phonation.[22] In particular, the positioning of the tongue within the oral cavity is well visualized with this technique (Figure 3–14).

Consideration of the anatomy of the activator and resonator components of the vocal tract is beyond the scope of this discussion of laryngeal anatomy.

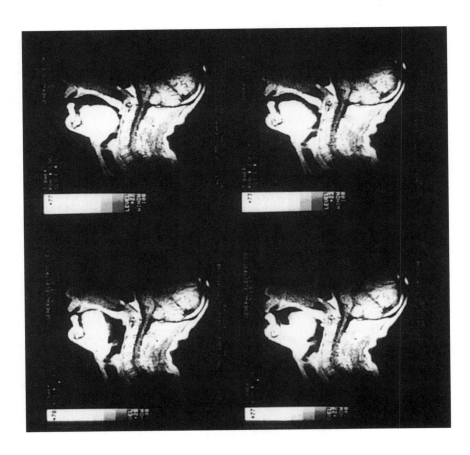

Figure 3–14. MRI of upper vocal tract, sagittal section.

REFERENCES

1. Sasaki CT, Isaacson G. Dynamic anatomy of the larynx. *Problems in Anesthesia.* 1988;2:163–174.

2. Graney DO, Flint FW. Larynx and hypopharynx: Anatomy. In: Cummings CW, Frederickson JM, Harker LA, Krause CJ, Schuller DE, eds. *Otolaryngology–Head and Neck Surgery.* 3rd ed. St. Louis, MO: Mosby Year Book; 1993:1693–1703.

3. Hately W, Evison E, Samuel E. The pattern of ossification in the laryngeal cartilages: a radiological study. *Br J Radiol.* 1965;38:585–591.

4. Chamberlain WE, Young BR. Ossification (so-called "calcification") of normal laryngeal cartilages mistaken for foreign body. *Am J Roentgenol Rad Ther.* 1935;33:441–450.

5. Hirano M, Yoshida T, Kurita S, et al. Anatomy and behavior of the vocal process. In: Baer T, Sasaki C, Harris KS, eds. *Laryngeal Function in Phonation and Respiration.* Boston, MA: Little Brown and Company; 1987:3–13.

6. Sanders I, Jacobs I, Wu BL, et al. The three bellies of the canine posterior cricoarytenoid muscle: implications for understanding laryngeal function. *Laryngoscope.* 1993; 103:171–177.

7. Sanders I, Rao F, Biller HF. Arytenoid motion evoked by regional electrical stimulation of the canine posterior cricoarytenoid muscle. *Laryngoscope.* 1994;104:456–462.

8. Zaretsky LS, Sanders I. The three bellies of the canine cricothyroid muscle. *Ann Otol Rhinol Laryngol.* 1992;156 (suppl):3–16.

9. Work WP. Unusual position of the right recurrent laryngeal nerve. *Ann Otol Rhinol Laryngol.* 1941;50:769–775.

10. Sanders I, Mu L. Anatomy of human internal superior laryngeal nerve. *Anat Rec.* 1998;252:646–656.

11. Suzuki M, Kirchner JA. Afferent nerve fibers in the external branch of the superior laryngeal nerve in cat. *Ann Otol Rhinol Laryngol.* 1968;77:1059–1070.

12. Shin T, Watanabe S, Wada S, et al. Sensory nerve endings in the mucosa of the epiglottis—morphologic investigations with silver impregnation, immunohistochemistry, and electron microscopy. *Otolaryngol Head Neck Surg.* 1987;96:55–62.

13. Anderson JW, Sant'Ambrogio FB, Mathew OP, et al. Water-responsive laryngeal receptors in the dog are not specialized endings. *Resp Physiol.* 1990;79:33–43.

14. Bradley RM. Sensory receptors of the larynx. *Am J Med.* 2000;108(suppl 4a):47–50.

15. Hirano M, Kurita S, Kiyokawa K, et al. Posterior glottis: morphological study in excised human larynges. *Ann Otol Rhinol Laryngol.* 1986;95:576–581.

16. Hirano M. Phonosurgical anatomy of the larynx. In: Ford CN, Bless DM, eds. *Phonosurgery: Assessment and Surgical Management of Voice Disorders.* New York, NY: Raven Press; 1991:25–41.

17. Hirano M, Kurita S. Histological structure of the vocal fold and its normal and pathological variations. In: Kirchner JA, ed. *Vocal Fold Histopathology—A Symposium.* San Diego, CA: College-Hill Press; 1986:17–24.

18. Hirano M, Sato K, eds. *Histological Color Atlas of the Human Larynx.* San Diego, CA: Singular Publishing Group, Inc; 1993.

19. Sasaki CT, Levine PA, Laitman JT, et al. Postnasal descent of the epiglottis in man. *Arch Otolaryngol.* 1977;103: 169–171.

20. Hirano M, Kurita S, Sakaguchi S. Aging of the vibratory tissue of human vocal folds. *Acta Otolaryngol.* 1989;107: 428–433.

21. Gracco C, Kahane JC. Age-related changes in the vestibular folds of the human larynx: a histomorphometric study. *J Voice.* 1989;3(3):204–212.

22. Baer T, Gore JC, Gracco LC, et al. Analysis of vocal tract shape and dimensions using magnetic resonance imaging: vowels. *J Acoust Soc Am.* 1991;90(2) (pt 1):799–828.

4

Functional Fine Structures of the Human Vocal Fold Mucosa

Kiminori Sato, MD, PhD

Viscoelastic properties of the lamina propria of human vocal fold mucosa determine vibratory behavior and depend on extracellular matrices, such as collagenous fibers, reticular fibers, elastic fibers, glycoproteins, and glycosaminoglycan. Three-dimensional structures of these extracellular matrices are indispensable to the viscoelastic properties of the vocal fold mucosa. Fine structures of the vocal fold mucosa influence vibrating behavior and voice quality.

This chapter discusses functional fine structures of human adult vocal fold mucosa as vibrating tissue with viscoelasticity.

HISTOANATOMY OF THE GLOTTIS

The glottis (Figure 4–1) is composed of an intermembranous portion or anterior glottis and intercartilaginous portion or posterior glottis.[1,2] Their borders are defined by a line between the tips of the bilateral vocal

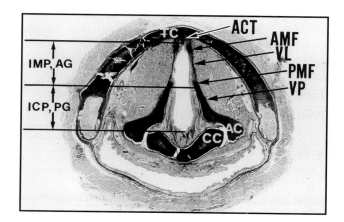

Figure 4–1. Horizontal section of human female larynx at the level of glottis (Elastica van-Gieson stain). *IMP*: intermembranous portion, *AG*: anterior glottis, *ICP*: intercartilaginous portion, *PG*: posterior glottis, *TC*: thyroid cartilage, *AC*: arytenoid cartilage, *CC*: cricoid cartilage, *ACT*: anterior commissure tendon, AMF: anterior macula flava, *VL*: vocal ligament, *PMF*: posterior macula flava, *VP*: vocal process of arytenoid cartilage.

processes.[1,2] The anterior glottis is required for phonation and the posterior glottis primarily for respiration.[2] Thus, voice disorders are usually caused by lesions of the anterior glottis.

The vibratory portion of the vocal fold is connected to the thyroid cartilage anteriorly via the intervening anterior macula flava and anterior commissure tendon. Posteriorly, this portion is joined to the vocal process of arytenoid cartilage via the intervening posterior macula flava. Thus, there are gradual changes in stiffness between the pliable vocal fold and hard cartilage.[1,3,4] The vocal processes form a firm framework of the glottis and are more pliable toward the tip.[4] Elastic cartilage is found not only at the tip of the vocal process but also at the superior portion of the arytenoid cartilage from the vocal process to the apex.[3] The vocal process bends at the elastic cartilage portion during adduction and abduction.[3,5]

Adult vocal folds have a layered structure consisting of epithelium; superficial, intermediate, and deep layers of the lamina propria; and vocalis muscle.[1,6] These layers may be grouped as three sections: a cover, consisting of the epithelium and superficial layer of the lamina propria; a transition zone, consisting of the intermediate and deep layers of the lamina propria; and a body, consisting of the vocalis muscle.[1,6] This layered structure is very important for vibration. The intermediate and deep layers of the lamina propria form the vocal ligament. Vocal ligaments run between the anterior and posterior maculae flavae.[1]

At birth, there is no structure corresponding to the vocal ligament and layered structure in adult vocal folds.[7-9] Development of the vocal ligament and layered structure of the vocal fold is complete at the end of adolescence.[7]

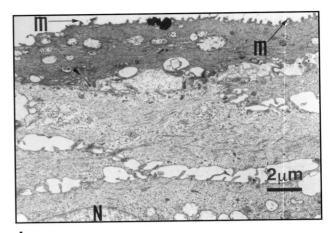

A

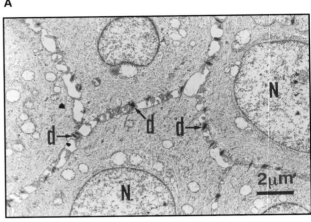

B

Figure 4–2. A. Superficial layers of stratified squamous epithelium of the vocal fold (Transmission electron micrograph [*TEM*]). *m*: microridge and microvilli, *N*: Nucleus. **B.** Intermediate layers of stratified squamous epithelium of the vocal fold (*TEM*). *d:* desmosome, *N*: Nucleus.

FINE STRUCTURES OF THE HUMAN ADULT VOCAL FOLD MUCOSA

Epithelium

The free edge of the membranous vocal fold (anterior glottis) is covered with stratified squamous epithelium. The mucosa has pseudostratified ciliated epithelium in the posterior glottis.[1,2,10]

On the surface of epithelial cells, microridges and microvilli are present (Figure 4–2A). Lubrication of the vocal folds is essential for normal phonation. Microridges and microvilli facilitate the spreading and retention of a mucous coat on the epithelium.[11]

The epithelium consist of 6 to 7 layers of squamous cells. The cells of basal layers are columnar or polyhedral. Many desmosomes at the junction of two adjacent epithelial cells make firm intercellular adhesion (Figure 4–2B). Near the surface, the number of desmosomes decreases and the cells are more flattened. The superficial layers are composed of thin squamous cells (Figure 4–2A).

Basal Lamina (Basement Membrane)

At the boundary between epithelium and underlying lamina propria, a supporting structure, the basal lamina, is present (Figure 4–3). Basal lamina of the vocal fold is composed of two zones, lamina lucida and lamina densa. The lamina lucida is a low density clear zone adjacent to the cell membrane. Lamina densa is a greater density area of filaments adjacent to the lamina propria. Lamina densa contains type IV collagen.

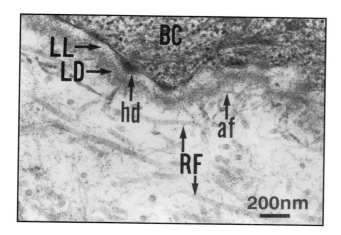

Figure 4–3. Basal lamina of the vocal fold (*TEM*). *BC*: basal cell of the stratified squamous epithelium, *LL*: lamina lucida, *LD*: lamina densa, *af*: anchoring fibril, *hd*: hemidesmosome, *RF*: reticular fiber.

Hemidesmosomes bind basal cells to the basal lamina. Anchoring fibrils tether the basal lamina to underlying connective tissue, the lamina propria of the vocal fold mucosa.[12,13]

The basal lamina mainly provides physical support to the epithelium[14] and is essential for repair of the epithelium.[15]

Superficial Layer of the Lamina Propria (SLLP)

This layer, referred to as Reinke's space, is a superficial layer that vibrates a good deal during phonation. The viscoelasticity of the lamina propria of the vocal fold mucosa, especially the superficial layer, is a major determinant of the vibratory behavior of the structure.

Supportive functions and viscoelasticity of connective tissue depend largely on extracellular matrices. The main extracellular matrices of the vocal fold mucosa are reticular, collagenous, and elastic fibers, glycoprotein, and glycosaminoglycan.[16]

Extracellular Matrices of SLLP (Reinke's Space)

As fibrillar proteins, collagenous and reticular fibers (Figure 4–4A) are required for structural maintenance. They are responsible for tensile strength and resilience and serve as stabilizing scaffolds in extracellular matrices. The predominant collagen in the superficial layer of the lamina propria of the vocal fold mucosa is type III,[12] a major constituent of slender, 50 nm or less fibers traditionally called reticular fibers.

Reticular fibers (type III collagen) have a function of structural maintenance in expansible organs.[14] Reticular fibers are present in superficial and intermediate

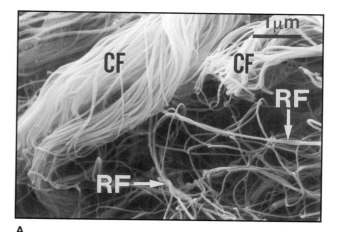

Figure 4–4. A. Reticular and collagenous fibers in SLLP of vocal fold mucosa (Scanning electron micrograph [*SEM*], NaOH maceration method). *RF*: reticular fibers, *CF*: collagenous fibers. **B.** Elastic fibers in SLLP of vocal fold mucosa (*SEM*, NaOH maceration method). *EF*: elastic fibers. **C.** Fibroblasts in SLLP of vocal fold mucosa (*TEM*). *N*: nucleus.

layers of the lamina propria of the vocal fold mucosa. They are most abundant around the vocal fold edge, then decrease in areas near the superior and inferior portions of the vocal folds. Reticular fibers are located in the portion of the vocal fold mucosa that undergoes the greatest vibration.[16] Slender fibrils of the reticular fibers do not form bundles but rather branches and anastomoses (Figure 4–4B). The delicate three-dimensional structures of reticular fibers contribute to structural maintenance of the vocal fold mucosa during vibration without disturbing vibration.[16]

Elastic fibers are also fibrillar proteins (Figure 4–4B). They stretch by small force and return to their original dimensions when the force is removed.[14] In SLLP of the vocal fold mucosa, elastic fibers are slender, run in various directions, branch, and anastomose to form loose networks (Figure 4–4B).

Ground substances of the vocal fold mucosa consist of glycosaminoglycan (acid mucopolysaccharide) and glycoprotein. One glycosaminoglycan in the vocal fold mucosa is hyaluronic acid,[16] which has very high viscosity in aqueous solution and thus is largely responsible for the consistency of ground substances.[13]

The reticular fibers which form delicate three-dimensional networks and spaces among the fibers are relatively large and there are innumerable potential spaces. The extracellular interstitial spaces are minute chambers or compartments occupied by other extracellular matrices, that is, elastic fibers and glycosaminoglycan (hyaluronic acid), which provide viscoelasticity to the tissue.[16] The three-dimensional structures of reticular fibers and other extracellular matrices are key components for structural maintenance and viscoelasticity of SLLP of vocal fold mucosa as vibrating tissue.

Fibroblasts in SLLP (Reinke's Space)

Fibroblasts are one of the interstitial cells that produce collagenous fibers and other extracellular matrices. Some fibroblasts are present throughout the human adult vocal fold mucosa (Figure 4–4C). Fibroblasts are spindle-shaped and the nuclei, elliptic. The nucleus to cytoplasm ratio is large with poorly developed rough endoplasmic reticulum and Golgi apparatus. Fibroblasts in SLLP (Reinke's space) synthesize few extracellular matrices;[18] they are inactive and at rest under normal conditions.[18]

Intermediate and Deep Layers of the Lamina Propria

The intermediate layer is primarily made up of elastic fibers, the deep layer, of collagenous fibers.[6] Both layers comprise the vocal ligament (Figures 4–1 and 4–5).

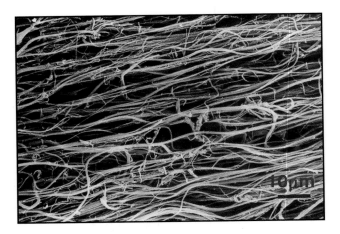

Figure 4-5. Vocal ligament of vocal fold mucosa (*SEM*, NaOH maceration method). Fibers run roughly parallel to the vocal fold edge.

FINE STRUCTURES OF MACULA FLAVA OF THE HUMAN ADULT VOCAL FOLD

Maculae flavae are located at the anterior and posterior ends of both membranous vocal folds[1,19] and make conspicuous mucosal bulges. When analyzed through the mucosa, they appear as a white-yellow mass. The macula flava is elliptical in shape, about $1.5 \times 1.5 \times 1$ mm in size, and composed of fibroblasts, elastic and collagenous fibers, and ground substance.[19]

Extracellular Matrices of the Macula Flava

The maculae flavae are dense masses of fibrous tissue (Figure 4–6A)[19,20] containing many fibrillar proteins such as collagenous, reticular and elastic fibers, and ground substances such as glycosaminoglycan (hyaluronic acid).[21]

Fibroblasts in Macula Flava

The distribution of fibroblasts differs according to the site within the vocal fold mucosa.[18] Cell density is greater in maculae flavae (Figure 4–6B) and sparse in Reinke's space.[18] In the macula flava there are numerous spindle-shaped fibroblasts and non-conventional fibroblasts stellate in shape.[21]

Stellate cells (nonconventional fibroblasts) (Figure 4–6C) are present in human adult maculae flavae but absent in Reinke's space.[21] Some morphologic and functional differences are apparent in these cells that differentiate them from conventional fibroblasts. Stel-

5

The Microanatomy of the Vocal Fold Musculature

Ira Sanders, MD

The object of this chapter is to describe the neuromuscular organization of the larynx, especially as it relates to voice production. The initial part of the chapter reviews the course of the main laryngeal nerves and the innervation and function of each muscle. The second part presents a hypothetical overview of voice production based on what is being learned about the anatomy of the laryngeal muscles. The descriptions depicted here are based on the author's review of the literature and original research in humans and animals and differ from generally described laryngeal anatomy and physiology in the following key areas:

1. In the human larynx there are a number of connections between the superior and recurrent laryngeal nerves. These connections may allow the superior laryngeal nerve to supply motor innervation to the intrinsic laryngeal muscles. The most consistent connection is present in the interarytenoid muscle. In this location both recurrent laryngeal nerves as well as both internal superior laryngeal nerves combine in a neural plexus. In about half of the population, another connection is present in the area of the

piriform sinus. This connection, which we have termed the communicating nerve, is an extension of the external superior laryngeal nerve. The communicating nerve arises from the inner surface of the cricothyroid muscle and passes across the piriform sinus to enter into the thyroarytenoid muscle. The communicating nerve is especially interesting as it appears to supply motor and sensory innervation to the area around the vocal process of the arytenoid and therefore may be of importance to phonation.

2. The thyroarytenoid muscle in both the human and the dog appears to be composed of at least two different bellies. Instead of bellies, muscle physiologists prefer the term *compartments,* and this term will be used in this chapter. The medial compartment of the thyroaytenoid muscle, the vocalis, contains a high proportion of slow-twitch muscle fibers. The lateral compartment of the thyroarytenoid, the muscularis, has a high percentage of fast-twitch muscle fibers and appears to be specialized to produce fast dynamic movements. It is hypothesized that the vocalis is responsible for controlling the tension of the vocal fold for phonation

while the muscularis is specialized for adducting the vocal cord. The histologic specializations seen in the vocalis and the muscularis are seen in other laryngeal muscles. Together these areas may function as physically separate phonatory and articulatory subsystems.

3. The vocalis itself is composed of two compartments, an inferior and a superior. It is hypothesized that these structures may correspond to the different masses in the two-mass model of vocal fold vibration. The inferior vocalis appears to control the tension in the subglottic aspect of the vocal fold. The inferior vocalis may be the area of the vocal fold responsible for determining the fundamental frequency of vocal fold vibration. In addition, it may also be responsible for controlling phonation onset. The superior vocalis is only well developed in the adult human. It is hypothesized that it has evolved to contribute to voice quality, especially the formant frequencies. In addition, the peculiar anatomy and vibratory dynamics of the superior vocalis suggest that it may operate by controlling sound production at the time of superior vocal fold closure.

LARYNGEAL NEUROMUSCULAR ANATOMY

The larynx is innervated by two main branches of the vagus nerve: the superior and recurrent laryngeal nerves (Figure 5–1).[1] The superior laryngeal nerve (SLN) branches off the vagus high in the neck at the inferior end of the nodose ganglion and bifurcates into two nerves: the internal and the external. The internal enters into the larynx at the thyrohyoid foramen and is believed to supply the sensory innervation to the entire mucosa of the larynx above the vocal folds. As will be shown below, there is reason to believe that the internal SLN also may supply some motor innervation to laryngeal muscles. The external SLN passes down the front of the larynx to supply motor innervation to the cricothyroid muscle. An extension of this nerve passes inside the larynx and may supply motor and sensory innervation to the vocal folds.

The RLNs are the main source of motor innervation to the larynx. The RLNs have an unusual course. They travel with the vagus nerve into the chest before branching. On the left the RLN usually loops under the aorta and on the right under the branchiocephalic artery. The RLNs then turn superiorly to enter into the larynx. Upon entering the larynx the RLN proceeds to supply motor innervation to the laryngeal muscles in the following sequence: posterior cricoarytenoid, interarytenoid, lateral cricoarytenoid, thyroarytenoid.

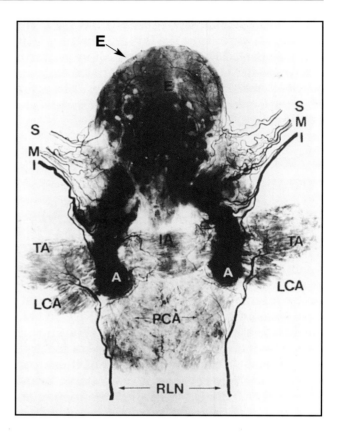

Figure 5–1. The nerve supply of the human larynx. An entire human larynx was processed with Sihler's stain, a technique that renders soft tissue translucent while counterstaining nerves. The larynx was then dissected to isolate the superior (SMI) and recurrent laryngeal nerves (RLN) as well as all laryngeal muscles and the arytenoid (A) and epiglottic (E) cartilages.

The RLNs are seen entering the larynx from the inferior direction. The first muscle to be innervated by the RLN is the posterior cricoarytenoid muscle (PCA). The second RLN branch travels beneath the PCA to innervate the interarytenoid muscle (IA). Finally, the RLN gives off a branch to innervate the lateral cricoarytenoid muscle (LCA) before terminating in the thyroarytenoid muscle (TA).

The superior laryngeal nerves enter the larynx from the superior direction. They travel down the lateral sides of the larynx and give off branches that pass medially to supply sensory innervation to the laryngeal mucosa. The superior laryngeal nerve usually divides into three main branches: a superior branch (S) innervates the epiglottis (E); a middle branch (M) innervates the false vocal fold; and an inferior branch (I) innervates the arytenoid (A) and postcricoid area.

The Posterior Cricoarytenoid Muscle

The sole abductor of the vocal folds is the posterior cricoarytenoid (PCA). This muscle originates from the back of the cricoid cartilage and inserts into the muscular process of the arytenoid cartilage. The PCA of the human is composed of at least two compartments (Figure 5–2).[2-4] On its lateral side is the vertical compartment, which inserts onto the lateral aspect of the muscular process of the arytenoid. On the medial side of the PCA is the horizontal compartment, which inserts onto the medial aspect of the muscular process of

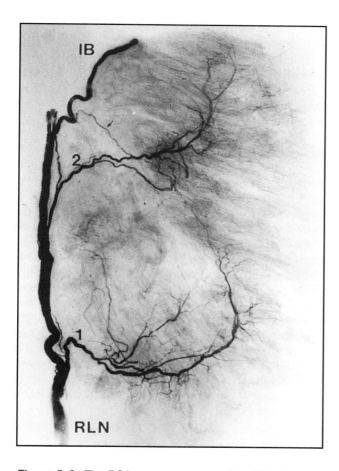

Figure 5–2. The PCA muscle processed by Sihler's stain. The initial branch of the RLN is to this muscle. Upon entering the larynx, the RLN passes superiorly along the lateral edge of the PCA muscle. In two-thirds of the specimens, two branches came off separately from the RLN to innervate two different areas of the muscle. The first branch innervates the lateral half of the muscle (the vertical) while the second branch innervates the medial half (the horizontal compartment). The clear separation of the nerve supplies to the two compartments suggests that they may be independently controlled by the nervous system. The small arrow points to one of the communicating nerve branches that connect the nerves to the PCA and interarytenoid muscles. Numerals 1 and 2 mark the two separate RLN nerve branches to the two compartments of the PCA muscle. (IB = nerve branch to interarytenoid muscle.)

the arytenoid cartilage. In the human each of these compartments usually receives its own nerve branch from the RLN. This nerve branch innervates only one compartment with little overlap between them. Anatomically, these compartments can almost be considered separate muscles. The vertical and horizontal compartments of the PCA may have different functions.

The role of the whole PCA during phonation is controversial. Speech consists of voiced and unvoiced segments in rapid succession. It is widely accepted that the PCA pulls the vocal folds apart after voicing.[5-8] In this way it can be thought of as participating in the articulation of the vocal folds that occurs during speech. However, the role of the PCA during voicing is less clear. Human electromyography shows that at high intensities and high pitches, the PCA is noticeably active. It is believed that under these conditions the PCA activity counterbalances the anterior pull of the thyroarytenoid and cricothyroid muscles.[9-11]

Although the functions of the compartments of the human PCA are unknown, a variety of experiments have been performed in the dog in an attempt to clarify the association between PCA anatomy and function.[12-14] The canine PCA is composed of three grossly distinct compartments: the vertical, oblique, and horizontal. The orientation of these compartments differs by 20° to one another so that the entire muscle spans a 60° arc. Each of these compartments has a different insertion on the muscular process of the arytenoid cartilage, and this potentially allows the compartments to move the arytenoid in different ways. Indeed the cricoarytenoid joint is believed to have three arcs of motion.[15-19] The cricoid side of this joint is shaped like a cylinder upon which sits the concave bottom of the cricoid cartilage. The arytenoid cartilage can slide laterally along the cylindrical facet of the cricoid. This motion is seen during quiet respiration when the glottic opening appears triangular. During forceful inspiration a second abducting motion occurs. This is a backward rocking of the arytenoid cartilage. This rocking causes the vocal process of the arytenoid cartilage to swing laterally. This motion maximally opens the glottis and gives it the appearance of a pentagon. The third abducting motion of the arytenoid cartilage is a swiveling motion. This motion consists of the arytenoid's rotating like a gate without any of the sliding or rocking motions. The existence and possible function of this third motion are controversial.

When electrical stimulation is applied to each of the compartments of the dog PCA, the stimuli do move the arytenoid in different ways.[13] Specifically, the vertical and oblique compartments slide the arytenoid laterally and rock it backward, the motions that can be seen during inspiration. In contrast, stimulating the horizontal compartment results in what appears to be a swiveling of the arytenoid. This causes an abduction of the vocal process with little displacement of the body of the arytenoid. When and how the swiveling action is used during vocal fold motion is obscure. It is possible that the swiveling motion is used during phonation to help position the vocal process. It is also conceivable that the horizontal compartment is not an abductor at all. Instead it may act as an adductor, just like the interarytenoid, and bring the posterior ends of the arytenoid together.

The actual role of the PCA compartments in the dog has not been tested by electromyography. However, the basic activity can be inferred by examining certain histologic indicators. Perhaps the most useful of these indicators is the distribution of fast- and slow-twitch muscle fibers. Muscle fibers can be divided into fast and slow on the basis of their reaction to myofibrillar ATPase stain.[20] Fast muscle fibers tend to contract more rapidly and develop more force than slow-twitch fibers. It has long been recognized that some whole muscles are mostly composed of either slow or fast fibers and are therefore specialized for either tonic or dynamic motions. Recently it has become clear that within the same muscle there can be regions that have differing proportions of the two fiber types. These regions, which are called compartments, have different activity patterns.[21]

Examination of the PCA of the dog shows that this muscle contains compartments with different proportions of fast- and slow-twitch muscle fibers. The proportion of slow-twitch muscle fibers in the horizontal compartment (41%) is almost twice that of the oblique compartment (23%).[12] These results suggest that the activity pattern of the horizontal compartment differs from that of the oblique. As will be shown below in the thyroarytenoid muscle, slow-twitch muscle fibers within a laryngeal muscle compartment appear to indicate that the compartment is involved with phonation. Whether this is true for the horizontal compartment of the PCA awaits confirmation through electromyography.

The Interarytenoid Muscle

The interarytenoid muscle is an unpaired muscle that originates from the back of each arytenoid cartilage. It is sometimes referred to as the transverse interarytenoid to differentiate it from the oblique interarytenoids, which are actually continuations of the aryepiglottic musculature.[21] When contracting, the interarytenoid muscle approximates the posterior ends of the arytenoid cartilages, thereby playing an

important role in both the phonatory and the sphincteric mechanisms of the larynx.

In 1882, Mandelstamm reported that the interarytenoid muscle appeared to be innervated by both RLNs.[22] This was subsequently supported by dissections of human and animal laryngeal nerves and is now the accepted view in modern anatomy texts.[23-25] A more controversial idea is that the interarytenoid muscle is also innervated by the internal SLN. Anatomic dissections and histologic studies support the possibility that the internal SLN innervates the interarytenoid muscle.[1,26,27] However, because electrical stimulation of the internal SLN does not cause vocal fold motion and sectioning of the nerve does not affect normal motion, it is generally assumed that the internal SLN branches pass through the muscle to supply sensation to the mucosa.[13,25,28]

When the interarytenoid muscle is examined in human larynges that have been processed by Sihler's stain, the four main laryngeal nerves are seen to contribute to a complicated plexus (Figure 5–3).[29] In addition, in almost every case, some axons from the internal SLN can be seen terminating among muscle fibers. It is not known whether the internal SLN axons that terminate within the muscle are contributing motor innervation to the interarytenoid muscle fibers or sensory innervation to the proprioceptive elements within the muscle. As for the internal SLN axons that join the plexus, they may pass through this plexus to travel into the RLN and then enter into the intrinsic laryngeal muscles. There is evidence that some axons travel downward from the interarytenoid muscle to innervate the PCA.[30] The interarytenoid nerve plexus has connections from side to side, and these may contain axons that travel from either the SLN or the RLN to the contralateral side of the larynx.

The Lateral Cricoarytenoid Muscle

The lateral cricoarytenoid muscle originates from the cricoid arch and inserts onto the muscular process of the arytenoid cartilage.[4] Contraction of the muscle adducts the vocal folds, and this adduction is important for phonation and reflex glottic closure.[31] A minority of investigators have also claimed an abductor function for the lateral cricoarytenoid muscle.[32] The most lateral fibers of the muscle are almost in line with the long axis of the cricoarytenoid joint so that their contraction may pull the arytenoid laterally. Zemlin has pointed out that both actions of the lateral cricoarytenoid are seen during whispering. Specifically, the tips of the arytenoids are adducted toward the midline while the bodies of the arytenoid are pulled apart. These actions result in a small triangular chink

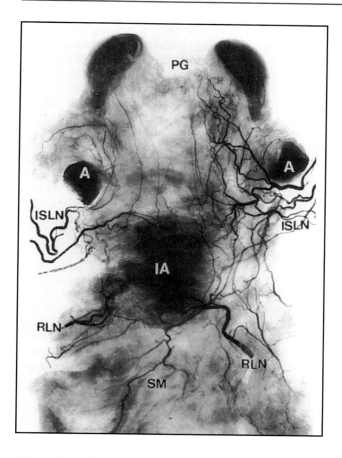

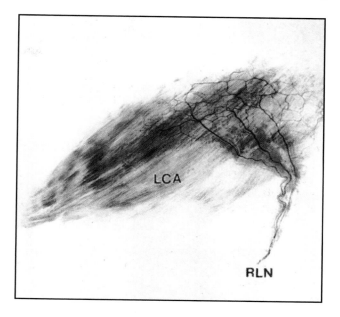

Figure 5-4. The lateral cricoarytenoid muscle processed by Sihler's stain. The innervation of the lateral cricoarytenoid muscle is fairly consistent between specimens. A single branch from the RLN enters the muscle near its insertion on the arytenoid cartilage. The intramuscular nerve pattern consists of a plexus that is limited to the superior half of the muscle. Note that the plexus appears to be organized around muscle fascicles. (*LCA* = lateral cricoarytenoid.)

The Thyroarytenoid Muscle

The thyroarytenoid muscle (TA) is clearly the most important muscle for phonation. There have been many attempts to characterize this muscle as being composed of two basic compartments: a medial part, the vocalis, which is more involved in phonation; and a lateral part, the muscularis, which is more involved with adduction.[35] Some anatomists have claimed that the organization of the muscle fibers in the vocalis is different from that of the muscularis. However, in 1960, Sonensson reviewed this topic and concluded that there is no anatomic or histologic evidence to support the idea of a separate vocalis and muscularis.[36] Since Sonensson, various new histologic methods have been developed to study muscle. The most helpful of these is the myofibrillar ATPase reaction, which, as described above, basically divides muscle fibers into a fast and slow type. Numerous studies have applied this stain to the human TA, but none has reported any local concentrations of fast- or slow-twitch fibers.[37-39] Very recently, work has been performed to show that in the human TA there are indeed histologic differences suggesting separate vocalis and muscularis compart-

Figure 5-3. The interarytenoid muscle processed by Sihler's stain. The interarytenoid muscle is innervated by nerve branches from both RLNs as well as both SLNs. The nerve branches combine within the muscle to form a complicated plexus. This arrangement allows axons to transfer between each of the main laryngeal nerves. It is possible that superior laryngeal axons transfer to the RLN to supply innervation to the intrinsic laryngeal muscles. In addition, axons from the SLN often terminate within the interarytenoid muscle and appear to be innervating muscle fibers. However, whether these axons actually control the muscle fibers is unknown. The interarytenoid innervation pattern is one of the most variable of the laryngeal muscles. (*A* = arytenoid cartilage; *ISLN* = internal *SLN;* and *SM* = subglottic mucosa.)

in the posterior glottis through which the airstream passes.[33]

The lateral cricoarytenoid muscle is innervated by a single branch from the RLN (Figure 5-4).[34] Upon entering the muscle, the nerve forms a neural plexus within the center of the muscle. There does not appear to be any difference in the neural branching pattern in the medial or lateral sides of the muscle. In general the nerve supply to the lateral cricoarytenoid muscle appears to be the simplest and most consistent of all the laryngeal muscles.

ments.[40] However, as these compartments are more clearly seen in the canine TA, it will be discussed first.

So that the compartments of the canine TA could be studied, the muscle was totally sectioned from anterior to posterior and stained for ATPase.[41] Areas within the muscle were then followed in serial sections from

their origins to insertions and the proportion of slow- and fast-twitch muscle fibers was calculated for each of these areas. It was found that the canine TA was divided into three basic compartments (Figure 5–5). Laterally is the muscularis; it originates from the muscular process of the arytenoid cartilage and inserts

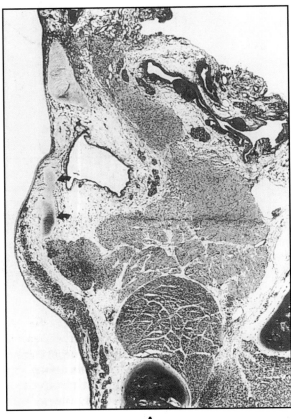
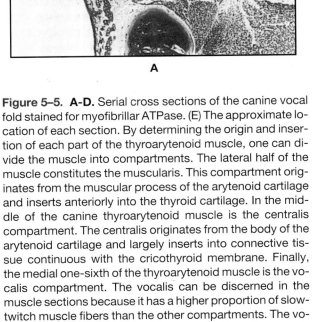

A

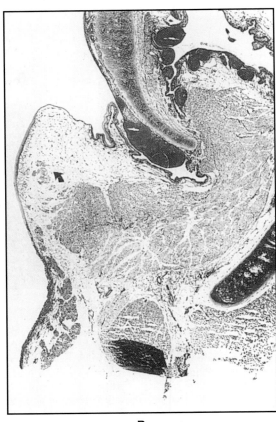

B

Figure 5–5. A-D. Serial cross sections of the canine vocal fold stained for myofibrillar ATPase. (E) The approximate location of each section. By determining the origin and insertion of each part of the thyroarytenoid muscle, one can divide the muscle into compartments. The lateral half of the muscle constitutes the muscularis. This compartment originates from the muscular process of the arytenoid cartilage and inserts anteriorly into the thyroid cartilage. In the middle of the canine thyroarytenoid muscle is the centralis compartment. The centralis originates from the body of the arytenoid cartilage and largely inserts into connective tissue continuous with the cricothyroid membrane. Finally, the medial one-sixth of the thyroarytenoid muscle is the vocalis compartment. The vocalis can be discerned in the muscle sections because it has a higher proportion of slow-twitch muscle fibers than the other compartments. The vocalis is itself composed of two identifiable subcompartments, the superior and inferior. The superior vocalis

originates from the vocal process of the arytenoid cartilage and inserts into mucosa at the mid-vocal cord. The inferior vocalis originates from the medial edge of the arytenoid cartilage and inserts anteriorly into the conus elasticus. It is hypothesized that during phonation the vocalis controls the tension along the medial edge of the vocal fold. In addition, the inferior and superior subcompartments may function independently. The inferior vocalis may control the fundamental frequency of phonation, while the superior vocalis may control the higher frequencies, which determine phonation quality.

A. This section is 2 mm posterior to the tip of the vocal process of the arytenoid cartilage. The arrows point to the vocal process. **B.** A section just in front of the vocal process. Note that where there was cartilage in the previous slide there now is a series of muscle fascicles that originated from the vocal process. These muscle fascicles constitute the superior vocalis. (*Continues*)

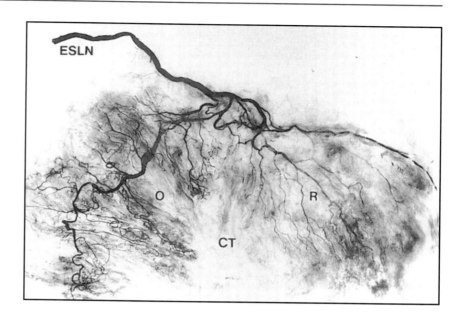

Figure 5–8. The cricothyroid muscle processed by Sihler's stain. The external SLN enters the cricothyroid muscle near the division between the rectus and the oblique compartment. After an initial rearrangement it divides into two main branches that supply the two compartments. Note that in both compartments, but especially in the oblique, the secondary nerve branches appear to extend into the origin and insertions of the muscle fibers. (*CT* = cricothyroid muscle; *ESLN* = external SLN; *O* = oblique belly of cricothyroid; *R* = rectus belly of cricothyroid.)

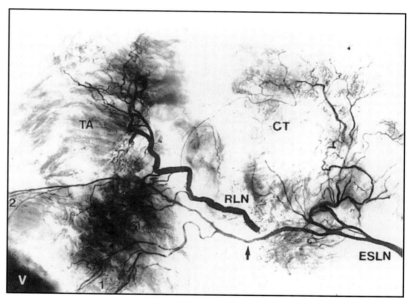

Figure 5–9. The communicating nerve branch is shown processed by Sihler's stain. A neural communication is often found between the SLN and the RLN in the region of the piriform fossa (*arrow*). The communication is a continuation of the external SLN through the cricothyroid muscle. In its most common form the communicating nerve divides into two parts. One part is presumed to be motor and either joins the RLN or terminates in the TA muscle (*1*). A second part is sensory and terminates around the vocal process of the arytenoid (*2*). The structures innervated by the communicating nerve are heavily involved in phonation; however, the exact function of this nerve has yet to be determined. (*CT* = cricothyroid muscle; *ESLN* = external SLN.)

The Lower Vocalis and the Control of Fundamental Frequency

In 1940, Farnsworth published photographs of the vocal folds of the human that were taken with an ultra-high-speed movie camera.[50] The most striking finding from this study was that the lower part of the vocal fold vibrates slightly out of phase from the upper part. During vocal fold closure the lower part can be seen as a sharp ledge while the upper part lags in a more lateral position. These observations led directly to the

two-mass model,[51] the most commonly cited theory of how the vocal folds vibrate. The presence of a ledge similar to that seen by Farnsworth has subsequently been reported in a variety of different experiments. For example, Matsushita viewed excised human and dog larynges from below and noted that a ledge was seen in the subglottic area.[52] This ledge served as the initiation line of the mucosal wave so that it was given the descriptive, albeit unwieldy, name of *the mucosal upheaval*. Berke et al have reported a similar configuration in the canine larynx when it is artificially made to phonate in vivo.[53] Finally, Hirano et al have reported the presence of the mucosal upheaval in humans when the vibrating folds are viewed from below, although the ledge is not as sharply defined as in excised larynges.[54] The existence of a line from which the mucosal wave begins has therefore been documented in vivo when human larynges are viewed from both above and below, in experimental canine larynges, and in excised human and canine larynges when artificially vibrated and viewed from below. It may be that the line seen in these different experiments is the same phenomenon and relates to a basic structure of the vocal fold.

The structure that corresponds to the mucosal upheaval is suggested by a recent experiment by Yumoto et al.[55] Excised canine larynges were viewed from below and artificially set into vibration. The mucosal upheaval was marked on the mucosa, and the larynx was then sectioned. The area of the mucosal upheaval was seen to begin at the point where the TA muscle approaches the subglottic mucosa. To be more specific, the mucosal upheaval is exactly at the juncture between what has been described earlier in this chapter as the inferior and the superior vocalis. Tying these observations together, it appears that the upper and lower masses of the two-mass model may correspond to concrete structures within the TA, the superior and the inferior vocalis.

In the human, the inferior vocalis is less well-defined than in the dog. One reason for this is that the human TA has expanded to form a large superior vocalis so that the gross appearance of the entire medial part of the TA appears to be that of a continuous muscle. However, with muscle fiber typing the inferior vocalis appears to correspond to a collection of slow-twitch fibers directly adjacent to the subglottic mucosa.

The question now arises as to the function of the inferior vocalis. It is hypothesized that the inferior vocalis is primarily responsible for the control of fundamental frequency. This area leads the rest of the vocal fold during vibration and has a much lower amplitude of vibration.[56] The appearance of this area during vibration is that it is the generator of the vocal fold oscillation and that the mucosal wave is generated from its motion. Once the mucosal wave begins, it will complete its motion upward and across the remainder of the vocal fold surface. Tension changes above the inferior area would be expected to have no effect on the frequency of vibration. The tension in the inferior vocalis may therefore be controlled separately from that of surrounding TA muscle. It is even possible that during the initiation of vibration, the actual start of oscillation is dependent on the inferior vocalis's achieving a set tension.

The Superior Vocalis and the Control of Quality

The human superior vocalis is a unique structure. In the adult human the area is packed with muscle fibers innervated by an extremely complex nerve supply. In contrast, in the dog, the chimpanzee, and even the newborn human, the area is mostly composed of soft tissue. These differences suggest that the superior vocalis has evolved to perform a key role for human speech.

Observations of vocal fold vibration suggest that the superior vocalis itself contains smaller subcompartments that can be independently controlled by the nervous system. For example, to raise pitch during falsetto, the vibrating edge of the vocal folds is progressively shortened.[57] This shortening begins posteriorly by bringing the vocal folds together to dampen vibration. At higher pitches more and more of the vocal folds are brought together until the vibrating edge is confined to a few millimeters in the very anterior aspect of the vocal fold. This phenomenon can be explained as the progressive damping of vocal fold vibration by the recruitment of small bundles of muscle fibers in the superior part of the vocalis. During modal speech the same independent control of muscle fiber groups may be occurring. Instead of dampening vibration, the nervous system could control tension in discrete areas of the superior vocalis so as to mold the vibration of the vocal fold.

Why would the shape of the superior edge of the vocal fold be important? The answer is suggested by studies that examine vocal fold shape during phonation. For example, cross-sectional radiographs of the vocal folds (tomograms) have been made of individuals phonating different vowels at the same pitch and intensity.[58,59] In these experiments the shape of the vocal folds varies dramatically. It can be speculated that one role of superior vocalis muscle groups is to mold the shape of the vocal fold during the phonation of different vowels. Vowels are characterized by their first and second formants, and because fundamental frequency was held constant during these experiments, it suggests that the superior vocalis molds the shape of the vocal fold to enhance the production of the speech formants, along with the greater effect of tongue shape. In support of this is one of the first inverse filter studies of voicing by Miller.[60] He found that individuals could vary the relative amounts of acoustic energy in different formants by more than 20-fold. This control of the higher formants appeared to be independent of the control of fundamental frequency.

A final speculation on the superior vocalis regards the mechanism by which its action produces changes in sound. Usually the actual sound produced by the vocal folds is believed to be produced in the open phase of the vibration cycle. However, there have been occasional reports that claim that the higher frequencies are actually produced during the instant of vocal fold contact at the beginning of the closure phase. These reports begin with Helmholtz, who compared his perception of the human speaking voice with that of multiple acoustic experiments.[61] Another example is that of Miller,[60] who found that the production of the higher frequencies of sound evidently occurs at vocal fold closure. Other investigators have also reported that the highest acoustic energies are produced around the instant of vocal fold closure.[62] Recent experiments that have measured the actual forces within the glottis report that peak intraglottal pressure occurs at the time of vocal fold closure, these closure pressures being much higher than at any point of the open cycle. These observations suggest that some part of the sound production occurs during vocal fold closure.

Furthermore, the unusual dynamics of the vocal fold during closure suggest a unique mechanism of sound production. As mentioned above, the movement of the vocal folds is such that the inferior and superior aspects of the vocal fold are out of phase. During closure, the inferior vocalis area contacts first, and this is rapidly followed by closure of the superior vocalis area. Therefore, the subglottic area is first sealed and then the small volume of air between the rapidly closing superior vocalis areas must be displaced superiorly at high acceleration. This acceleration may be sufficient to produce sound.

Most recently, additional information has been obtained regarding the unique nature of the human thyroarytenoid (TA) muscle, and especially the superior vocalis compartment (SV). The superior vocalis has certain microstructural and molecular characteristics which make it an unusual if not unique type of mammalian muscle (Figure 5–10). Within the human TA the SV compartment appears to contain the most specializations, including rare muscle fiber types and high concentrations of muscle spindles.[63] Histologic examination shows that the SV is also remarkable for its high proportion of extremely short muscle fibers and unusual intramuscular connection system.[64] In teased SV samples, about 70% muscle fibers could be microdissected intact. Ninety-five percent of the microdissected muscle fibers were less than 5 mm in length and more than half were less than 2 mm. As the average TA muscle is at least 2 cm in length the majority of muscle fibers within the SV must originate and insert within the muscle without directly connecting to either the thyroid or arytenoid cartilages.

The high proportion of short muscle fibers is reflected in the many types of connections seen in the SV.

Muscle fibers often are connected in series by thin tendons. In addition these tendons also merged into the endomysium of the larger diameter muscle fibers. The shapes of muscle fibers are also variable. Thin cylindrical muscle fibers with tapered ends are most common; however, short bulbous muscle fibers are also common. Variably shaped muscle fibers were often found in the same microdissected preparation, suggesting that these unusual shapes were not an artifact but did represent the in vivo condition. The SV subcompartment also contained many muscle fibers that were seen to divide into two or more smaller fibers. These branches often connected to other muscle fibers to form netlike arrays. Similar branching muscle fibers have been described in the extra-ocular muscles and a few other muscles. It is believed that the branching muscle fibers and dense connecting network reflects a special way of distributing force within the muscle.

Using antibodies to different types of the contractile protein myosin, it has been shown that the superior vocalis contains muscle fibers with very rare types of myosin, such as alpha cardiac, slow tonic, and developmental myosins. The most interesting of these is undoubtedly the slow tonic muscle fibers (STMF), as they have a different anatomy and physiology than normal twitch muscle fibers. STMF have multiple motor endplates with the characteristic *en grappe* shape.[65,66] Each motor endplate controls the contraction of the part of the muscle fiber in its area, as the STMF membrane does not propagate an action potential. Instead of contracting with a twitch, STMF exhibit slow and prolonged contractions, much like smooth muscle.

Although rare in mammals, STMF are relatively common in birds and amphibians. What is known about their physiology comes mostly from observing the function of muscles containing large amounts of STMF. In birds, shoulder muscles which connect the wings to the trunk contain a high proportion of STMF; these muscles are believed to keep the wings locked in place,[67] especially during soaring or gliding activities when the wings are relatively immobile. In contrast, the dynamic flight muscles of the wings are composed of almost entirely fast-twitch muscle fibers. One muscle that has been extensively studied is the anterior latissimus dorsi muscle. This muscle contains nearly 100% STMF and acts to stabilize the wing in the shoulder joint for extended periods, such as when a bird is soaring. As such, it serves to maintain continual tone because of its high resistance to fatigue. In other muscles they seem to be intermixed with large numbers of muscle spindles, the receptor that senses the length of a muscle. This association of STMF and muscle spindles is believed to act as a large sensory unit, the STMF

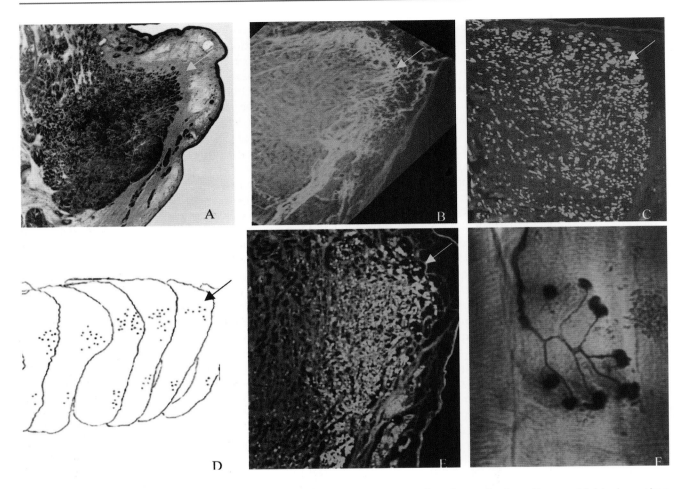

Figure 5–10. Specializations of the human vocalis compartment of the thyroarytenoid muscle. **A.** Frontal section of human mid-vocal fold. Medial (*right*) side of the thyroarytenoid muscle is the vocalis compartment; arrow points to the superior vocalis in the region of the vocal ligament. **B.** Immunoreaction for elastin, an elastic type of connective tissue that is uncommon in most muscles. A thick band of elastin is seen along the whole perimeter of the vocalis. It infiltrates into the muscle just below the vocal ligament. **C.** Immunoreaction for alpha cardiac myosin, a rare type of myosin found in the muscle fibers of the atria of the heart, the extra-ocular muscles and, now, the human vocalis. **D.** Location of slow tonic muscle fibers. Drawing of frontal section taken from intervals along the vocal fold where slow tonic muscle fibers were found and mapped from sections such as photomicrograph. Note that the largest concentration of slow tonic muscle fibers is found just next to the vocal ligament. A smaller group is present in the inferior vocalis. **E.** Immunoreaction for slow tonic myosin. Although some reaction is present throughout the vocalis, the reaction is greatest in the superior vocalis. Note that the muscularis compartment of the thyroarytenoid muscle (the lateral side) contains no slow tonic myosin reaction. **F.** An *en grappe* motor endplate from a muscle fiber in the superior vocalis. These unusual motor endplates are found only on slow tonic muscle fibers.

somehow allowing the muscle spindles to do their job better.

In mammals STMF have been found in two muscle groups. All species appear to contain the STMF in their extra-ocular muscles. In humans the stable contraction of STMF are believed to allow for gaze fixation and slow pursuit movements. The only other muscles known to contain STMF are the middle ear muscles of certain social carnivores such as the cats, but not in other species such as some nonhuman primates. Under experimental conditions it has been shown that mild contraction of the STMFs serves to stiffen the middle ear ossicles and results in the filtering of certain frequencies.[68] If this mechanism is used in vivo it may be a way that animals filter out extraneous frequencies other than those from their *con specifics* (same species).

The presence of STMF in the human vocal fold is, then, a bit of a surprise. This is only the second area in the human that is known to contain these special fibers. The area where the STMF are at highest concentrations, the superior vocalis, is just beneath the vibrating edge of the vocal fold. The highest numbers of muscle fibers were found in the center of the membranous vocal fold, and decreased both anteriorly and posteriorly. This region is the most mobile during vocal fold vibration and changes in muscle stiffness would be expected to greatly affect this vibration, and thereby change the acoustic output. Therefore, it may be that the STMF have evolved to allow some control of the vocal fold edge that is important for human speech. This is supported by the fact that the entire superior vocalis does not appear to exist in other species, including other primates such as the chimpanzee. Instead, the same area contains only soft tissue. Interestingly, neonatal human vocal folds also only contain soft tissue in this area.

If it is hypothesized that a special system has evolved to produce critical aspects of human speech, it would follow that speech disorders affect this system. Certainly there is much to learn before we can make any conclusions; however, preliminary evidence suggests that this may be true. For example, idiopathic Parkinson's disease is a neurologic disorder in which the voice is affected. Patients adopt a weak breathy speaking voice and, upon examination, the vocal folds are bowed. Comparison of vocal folds from patients with IPD with those of normals shows that the IPD have a dramatic decrease in the amount of STMF and other associated specializations normally seen in the SV area (Figure 5–11). Whether the bowing of the vocal folds seen in these cases is secondary to volume loss in the SV compartment is not known. However, the example shows how the understanding of the basic science of voice production may be relevant to the pathologic condition.

Whatever the exact mechanism may be for sound production during vocal fold closure, the superior vocalis may play a critical role. Through independent control of superior vocalis tension, the nervous system can strongly affect the amplitude and strength of vibration at the area of the vocal ligament. These changes may control the overtones produced at the vocal folds, which are interpreted perceptually as changes in quality of the voice.

The Muscularis and Centralis Compartments of the TA

The vocalis takes up only a small percentage of the TA. In the canine larynx, two other distinct compartments can be appreciated on the basis of their positions within the muscle and the course of their muscle fibers. The most lateral fibers of the TA in both the human and the dog originate from the muscular process of the arytenoid cartilage and insert into the thyroid cartilage. This compartment, which we have termed the muscularis, is composed of almost 100% fast-twitch muscle fibers. The architecture of the muscularis gives it a mechanical advantage in adducting the arytenoid cartilage. It may be inferred that this area may be a separate functional compartment that is mostly active during reflex glottic closure and adduction into the phonatory position.

A third compartment, the centralis, can be appreciated in the dog TA. The centralis originates from the flat anterior face of the body of the arytenoid cartilage and passes anteriorly to insert into connective tissue of the cricothyroid membrane. The centralis appears to have a mechanical advantage in pulling the whole arytenoid forward. An intriguing aspect of the canine centralis is that it appears to be innervated by the communicating nerve and not the RLN. As mentioned above, the communicating nerve is present about 50% of the time and is an extension of the external SLN. Glycogen depletion and degeneration experiments in the dog suggest that the centralis receives its motor innervation from the communicating nerve. The arrangement suggests that the centralis may be evolutionarily related to the cricothyroid muscle. Possibly the relationship is functional, with both the centralis and cricothyroid co-operating to control the intrinsic tension of the vocal fold. There are many unanswered questions regarding both the centralis and the communicating nerve, and this will be a fertile area for future research.

Phonatory Subsystems

In the vocalis, slow-twitch muscle fibers appear to be associated with phonation and fast-twitch muscle fibers with adduction. As concentrations of slow-twitch muscle fibers occur within other laryngeal muscles, it is possible that these areas are also directly involved in phonation. The areas of slow-twitch muscle fiber concentrations may function together as a phonatory subsystem within the larynx. The organization of a hypothetical phonatory subsystem can be summarized as follows: Once the vocal folds are adducted into position for phonation, only small parts of the laryngeal muscles are highly active. The candidates for a phonatory subsystem include the vocalis compartment of the TA, the horizontal compartment of the posterior cricoarytenoid muscle, the transverse interarytenoid muscle (but not the oblique interarytenoid), and a poorly defined part of the cricothyroid muscle. It is interesting that anatomic studies of the human larynx have demonstrated that muscle spindles, a proprioceptive element involved in fine control of muscle tension, are only found in those four locations.

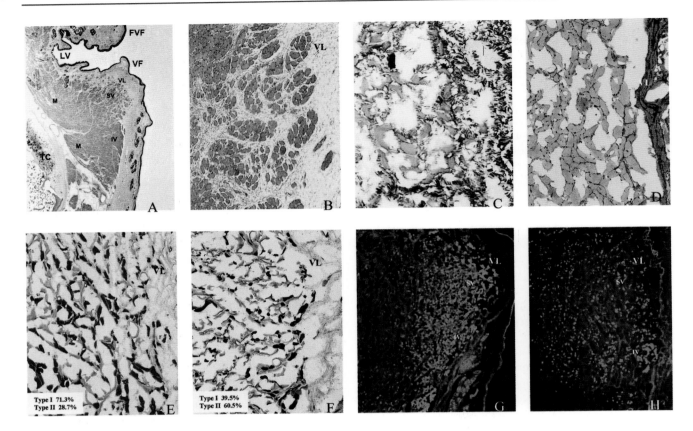

Figure 5–11. Loss of vocalis specialized structure in idiopathic Parkinson's disease (IPD). (A&B are from a normal individual without IPD; C/D, E/F, G/H are all comparisons of normal/IPD.) The specialized qualities seen in the human vocalis appear to be related to human speech, and may be preferentially affected by certain neurologic disorders. For example, preliminary results in patients with IPD suggest that these specialized characteristics are preferentially lost in this disease, a possible explanation for the bowed appearance of the vocal folds in this disease. **A.** Frontal section of normal human vocal fold showing the various compartments. **B.** High power view of normal superior vocalis compartment and its distinctive separate fascicles with muscle fibers of variable diameters (10x). **C.** Stained for elastin (*dark purple*) shows that the muscle fibers of the normal superior vocalis are surrounded by elastic fibers. **D.** A specimen from the same area of superior vocalis in an age-matched subject with IPD shows that the elastin is almost completely missing. **E.** ATPase staining of normal superior vocalis shows that a majority of muscle fibers are slow-twitch (dark). **F.** A specimen from the IPD patient shows that the ratio has shifted to one of predominantly fast muscle fibers. **G.** Immunofluorescence for slow tonic myosin in a normal patient shows reaction throughout the vocalis with most concentrated in the superior vocalis area. **H.** In the IPD patient the amount of slow tonic myosin is dramatically less and the concentration in the superior vocalis is lost.

Just as phonation is associated with slow-twitch muscle fibers, articulation of the vocal folds may be associated with fast-twitch muscle fibers. The muscle fibers of the lateral compartment of the TA (the muscularis) are almost 100% fast-twitch in both humans and dogs. It is possible that this specialization for rapid motion in the muscularis is to perform the adduction required in reflex glottic closure. High concentrations of fast-twitch muscle fibers are also found in the false vocal fold and in the lateral cricoarytenoid. Together these areas form a sheet of muscle on the outside of the larynx that cooperates to rapidly adduct the vocal folds.

REFERENCES

1. Dilworth TFM. The nerves of the human larynx. *J Anat.* 1922;56:48–52.
2. Sanders I, Wu BL, Mu L, et al. The innervation of the human posterior cricoarytenoid muscle: evidence for at least two neuromuscular compartments. *Laryngoscope.* 1994;104:880–884.
3. Zemlin WR, Davis P, Gaza C. Fine morphology of the posterior cricoarytenoid muscle. *Folia Phoniatr (Basel).* 1984;36:233–240.
4. Negus VE. *The Comparative Anatomy and Physiology of the Larynx.* New York, NY: Grune & Stratton; 1949.

5. Faaborg-Andersen K. Electromyographic investigation of intrinsic laryngeal muscles in humans. *Acta Physiol Scand.* 1957;41(suppl 140).

6. Ishizaka K, Flanagan JF. Synthesis of voice sounds from a two mass model of the vocal cords. *Bell Sys Tech J.* 1972;51:1233–1267.

7. Hirano M, Ohala J. Use of hooked wire electrodes for electromyography of the intrinsic laryngeal muscles. *J Speech Hear Res.* 1969;12:362–373.

8. Hirose H, Gay T. The activity of the intrinsic laryngeal muscles in voicing control—an electromyographic study. *Phonetica.* 1972;25:140–164.

9. Dedo HH. The paralyzed larynx: an electromyographic study in dogs and humans. *Laryngoscope.* 1970;80:1455–1517.

10. Kotby MN, Haugen LK. Critical evaluation of the action of the posterior cricoarytenoid muscle, utilizing direct EMG study. *Acta Otolaryngol (Stockh).* 1970;70:260–268.

11. Gay T, Hirose H, Strome M, et al. Electromyography of the intrinsic laryngeal muscles during phonation. *Ann Otol Rhinol Laryngol.* 1972;81:401–409.

12. Sanders I, Jacobs I, Wu BL, et al. The three bellies of the canine posterior cricoarytenoid muscle: implications for understanding laryngeal function. *Laryngoscope.* 1993;103:171–177.

13. Sanders I, Rao F, Biller HF. Arytenoid motion evoked by regional electrical stimulation of the canine posterior cricoarytenoid muscle. *Laryngoscope.* 1994;104:458–462.

14. Drake W, Li Y, Rothschild MA, et al. A technique for displaying the entire nerve branching pattern of a whole muscle: results in ten canine posterior cricoarytenoid muscles. *Laryngoscope.* 1993;103:141–148.

15. Willis R. On the mechanism of the larynx. *Trans Cambridge Philosoph Soc.* 1933;4:323–352.

16. Sonesson B. Die funktionelle Anatomie des Cricoarytenoid-gelenkes. *Z Anat Entwick Lungsgesch.* 121:292–303.

17. von Leden H, Moore P. The mechanics of the cricoarytenoid joint. *Arch Otolaryngol.* 1961;73:541–550.

18. Frable MA. Computation of motion at the cricoarytenoid joint. *Arch Otol.* 1961;73:551–555.

19. Ardran GM, Kemp FH. The mechanism of the larynx. Part I: The movements of the arytenoid and cricoid cartilages. *Br J Radiol.* 1966;39:641–654.

20. Guth L, Samaha FJ. Procedure for the histochemical demonstration of actomyosin ATPase. *Exp Neurol.* 1970;28:365–367.

21. Williams PL, Warwick R, Dyson M, et al. *Gray's Anatomy.* 37th ed. Edinburgh: Churchill Livingstone; 1989:1117,1256,1258.

22. Windhorst U, Hamm TM, Stuart DG. On the function of muscle and reflex partitioning. *Behav Brain Sci.* 1989;12:629–681.

23. Lemere F. Innervation of the larynx. I: Innervation of laryngeal muscles. *Am J Anat.* 1932;51:417–438.

24. King BT, Gregg RL. An anatomical reason for the various behaviors of paralyzed vocal cords. *Ann Otol Rhinol Laryngol.* 1948;57:925–944.

25. Rueger RS. The superior laryngeal nerve and the interarytenoid muscle in humans: an anatomical study. *Laryngoscope.* 1972; 82:2008–2031.

26. Pressman JJ. Sphincter action of the larynx. *Arch Otolaryngol.* 1941;33:351–377.

27. Vogel PH. The innervation of the larynx of man and the dog. *Am J Anat.* 1952;90:427–447.

28. Ogura JH, Lam RL. Anatomical and physiological correlations on stimulating the human superior laryngeal nerve. *Laryngoscope.* 1953;63:947–959.

29. Mu L, Sanders I, Wu BL, et al. The intramuscular innervation pattern of the human interarytenoid muscle. *Laryngoscope.* 1994;104:33–39.

30. Li Y, Sanders I, Biller HF. Axons enter the human posterior cricoarytenoid muscle from the superior direction. *Arch Otolaryngol-Head Neck Surg.* 1995;121(7):754–757.

31. Hirano M, Ohala J, Vennard W. The function of the laryngeal muscles in regulating fundamental frequency and intensity of phonation. *J Speech Hear Res.* 1969;12:616–628.

32. Stroud MH, Zwiefach E. Mechanism of the larynx and recurrent nerve palsy. *J Laryngol Otol.* 1956;70:86–96.

33. Zemlin WR. *Speech and Hearing Science: Anatomy and Physiology.* Englewood Cliffs, NJ: Prentice-Hall; 1968.

34. Sanders I, Mu L, Wu BL, et al. The intramuscular nerve supply of the human lateral cricoarytenoid muscle. *Acta Otolaryngol (Stockh).* 1993;113:679–682.

35. Wustrow F. Bau und funktion des menschlichlen Musculus vocalis. *Z Anat Entwick Lungsgesch.* 1952;116:506–552.

36. Sonesson B. On the anatomy and vibratory pattern of the human vocal folds. *Acta Otolaryngol.* 1960;(suppl 156).

37. Tieg E, Dahl HA, Thorkelson H. Actinomyosin ATPase activity of human laryngeal muscles. *Acta Otolaryngol.* 1978;85:272–281.

38. Sahgal V, Hast MH. Histochemistry of primate laryngeal muscles. *Acta Otolaryngol.* 1974;78:277–281.

39. Kersing W. *De stembandmusculatur een histologische en histochemische studie* [Thesis]. University of Utrecht, Utrecht, Holland. 1983.

40. Sanders I, Wu BL, Biller HF. Phonatory specializations of human laryngeal muscles. *Ann Otol Laryngol.* In press.

41. Sanders I, Han Y, Biller HF. *Evidence that the tension of the vocal cord mucosa is under the direct control of vocalis muscle fibers.* Presented at the 23rd Annual Symposium of The Voice Foundation; June 6–11, 1994; Philadelphia, PA.

42. Wu BL, Sanders I, Biller FH. The human communicating nerve: an extension of the external superior laryngeal nerve which innervates the vocal cord. *Arch Otolaryngol.* 1994;120:1321–1328.

43. Vesalius A. *De corporis humani fabrica.* 1545.

44. Zaretsky L, Sanders I. The three bellies of the canine cricothyroid muscle. *Ann Otol Laryngol.* 1992;156(suppl):2.

45. Vilkman EA, Pitkanen R, Suominen H. Observations on the structure and the biomechanics of the cricothyroid articulation. *Acta Otol (Stockh).* 1987;103:117–126.

46. Stone RE, Nuttal AL. Relative movements of the thyroid and cricoid cartilages assessed by neural stimulation in dogs. *Acta Otolaryngol (Stockh).* 1974;78:135–140.

47. Ferrein A. De la formation de la voix de l'homme. *Mem Acad R Sci (Paris).* 1741;51:409–430.

48. Suzuki M, Kirschner JA, Murakami Y. The cricothyroid as a respiratory muscle. Its characteristics in bilateral re-

current laryngeal nerve paralysis. *Ann Otol Rhinol Laryngol.* 1970:79.

49. Konrad HR, Rattenborg CC. Combined action of laryngeal muscles. *Acta Otolaryngol (Stockh).* 1969;67:646–649.

50. Farnsworth DW. High speed motion pictures of the human vocal cords. *Bell Lab Record.* 1940;18:203–208.

51. Hiroto I, Hirano M, et al. Electromyographic investigation of the intrinsic laryngeal muscles related to speech sounds. *Ann Otol Rhinol Laryngol.* 1967;76:861–872.

52. Matsushita H. The vibratory mode of the vocal folds in the excised larynx. *Folia Phoniatr (Basel).* 1975;27:7–18.

53. Berke GS, Moore DM, Hantke DR, et al. Laryngeal modeling: theoretical, in vitro, in vivo. *Laryngoscope.* 1987;97:871–881.

54. Hirano M, Yoshida Y, Tanaka S. Vibratory behaviour of human vocal cords viewed from below. In: Gauffin J, Hammarberg B, eds. *Vocal Fold Physiology.* San Diego, CA: Singular; 1991:chap 1.

55. Yumoto E, Kadota Y, Kurokawah H. Infraglottic aspect of canine vocal fold vibration: affect of increase of mean air flow rate and lengthening of vocal fold. *J Voice.* 1993; 7(4):311–318.

56. Baer T. Measurement of vibration patterns of excised larynges. *J Acoust Soc Am.* 1983;54:318.

57. Pressman JJ. Physiology of the vocal cords in phonation and respiration. *Arch Otolaryngol.* 1942;35:355–398.

58. Van Den Berg J. On the role of the laryngeal ventricle in voice production. *Folia Phoniatr (Basel).* 1955;7:57–69.

59. Van Den Berg J. Myoelastic-aerodynamic theory of voice production. *Speech Hear Res.* 1958;1(3):227–243.

60. Miller RL. Nature of the vocal cord wave. *J Acoust Soc Am.* 1959;31(6):667–677.

61. Helmholtz H. *On the Sensations of Tone as a Physiologic Basis for the Theory of Music.* New York, NY: Dover; 1954.

62. Jiang JJ, Titze IR. Measurement of vocal fold intraglottal pressure and impact stress. *J Voice.* 1994;8:132–144.

63. Sanders I, Han Y, Wang J, Biller HF. Muscle spindles are concentrated in the superior vocalis subcompartment of the human thyroarytenoid muscle. *J Voice.* 1998;12:7–16.

64. Wang J, Han Y, Sanders I. The superior vocalis of the human thyroarytenoid muscle contains a specialized and possibly unique muscle fiber architecture. *Bull Am Acad Otolaryngol Head Neck Surg.* 1998;17:49.

65. Morgan DL, Proske U. Vertebrate slow muscle: I structure, pattern of innervation and mechanical properties. *Physiol Reviews.* 1984;64:103–168.

66. Hess A. Vertebrate slow muscle fibers. *Physiol Reviews.* 1970;50:40–62.

67. Simpson S. The distribution of tonic and twitch muscle fibers in the avian wing. *Am Zoologist.* 1979;19:925 (Abstract).

68. Fernand VSV, Hess A. The occurrence, structure and innervation of slow and twitch muscle fibers in the tensor tympani and stapedius of the cat. *J Physiol.* 1969;200:547–554.

6

Benign Vocal Fold Pathology Through the Eyes of the Laryngologist

John S. Rubin, MD, FACS, FRCS
Eiji Yanagisawa, MD, FACS

This chapter is dedicated to the memory of Steven Gray,
a great pioneer into the causes of benign vocal fold pathology.

There are numerous causes of benign vocal fold pathology. Because the laryngeal tract can only respond in certain ways, the symptoms produced are limited, and the resultant degree of clinical dysphonia depends more on the degree of air-wasting, amount of contact of the vocal folds, and alteration of vocal fold stiffness/mass effect, than on the specific disorder.

While the entire body must be looked upon as the vocal organ, this chapter will limit itself to benign processes directly affecting the vocal folds. It is being written by the laryngologist for the laryngologist. Thus, the primary focus will be on processes brought about by vocal misuse and abuse (eg, polyps, nodules, granulomas, cysts, Reinke's edema.)

Some of the confusion regarding etiology and pathogenesis of vocal abuse related processes is the result of failure of the pathologist to make crisp distinctions. Often, H&E stains of nodules and polyps look alike.[1] Some of the blame must also be laid on the

laryngologist for not giving adequate anatomic orientation of the lesion or clinical expectation. The pathologist and the laryngologist need to consider themselves a team. Much as with cancer specimens, the laryngologist should develop the habit of reviewing and orienting each specimen with the pathologist.

A representative series of benign pathology excised from the vocal folds is taken from Bouchayer (Table 6–1).[2]

RELEVANT ANATOMY OF THE VOCAL FOLD

The key to a reasoned approach to management of these lesions is a detailed understanding of the relevant anatomy of the vocal fold and, in particular, of the laryngeal "cover," as most of the pathology is found

Table 6–1. Example of Pathologic Specimens Removed at Surgery for Benign Vocal Fold Lesions. From Bouchayer M and Cornut G. Microsurgery for benign lesions of the vocal folds. *Ear Nose Throat J.* 1988;67:446-466.

Specimen	Percentage of Total
nodule	24%
cyst	17%
(14% epidermoid, 3% retention)	
sulcus	12%
polyp	11%
other	7%
pseudocyst	6%
Reinke's	6%
polypoid nodule	5%
chronic laryngitis	4%
postoperative scarring	3%
microweb	3%
granuloma	1%
papillomatosis	<1%
Total	**1283 lesions**

there. In previous chapters, Sasaki and Sato have already extensively described anatomic aspects relating to the vocal fold edge. Nonetheless, for orientation to the remainder of this chapter, certain anatomic aspects will be emphasized. Much of the following is attributable to Hirano and/or Gray.

The notion of cover and body fit well with studies of vocal fold vibration showing not only medial-lateral motion but also vertical motion.[3,4] The mucosal wave is caused by a mucosal upheaval, which starts low on the vocal fold and travels superiorly. The concept is that medial and superficial tissue glide over a more rigid body.[5]

The cover consists of the epithelium and superficial layer of the lamina propria (SLLP). The middle (MLLP) and deep (DLLP) layers of the lamina propria make up the vocal ligament. Whereas the SLLP is reasonably well-defined, the vocal ligament is not; at its depths, some collagenous fibers insert into the underlying vocalis muscle (Figure 6–1).[6,7] The MLLP and the DLLP constitute the transition and the muscle makes up the body.

Considerable work has detailed the lamina propria in humans to be composed of cells, mostly fibroblasts, and matrix substances excreted by these cells, including interstitial proteins (glycosaminoglycans and proteoglycans) and fibrous proteins (especially collagen and elastin).[8,9] Capillaries, veins, and macrophages are also found there.[8]

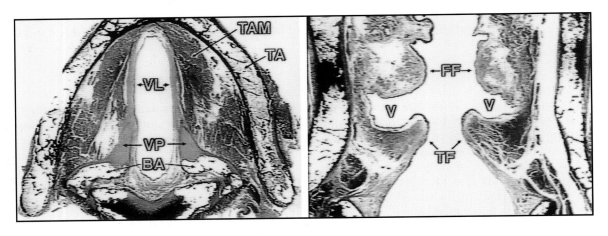

Figure 6-1. The whole organ sections of the mid larynx.
Left: Transverse section (stained for elastic tissues)
    VL   = vocal ligament
    VP   = vocal process of the arytenoid cartilage (the vocal process never ossifies)
    BA   = body of the arytenoid cartilage (the body usually ossifies)
    TAM = thyroarytenoid muscle
    TA   = thyroid ala
Right: Coronal section (hematoxylin and eosin)
    FF   = false fold
    V   = ventricle
    TF   = true fold
(Courtesy of John A. Kirchner, MD, Yale University, New Haven, CT)

Gray points out that the vast majority of the "cover" is extracellular and of the body, cellular. He considers the fibrous proteins to be scaffolding and the interstitial proteins to be "filling" by virtue of their location in the spaces between. In his view, the former are designed to handle stress and the latter to control tissue viscosity and water content.[10]

The larynx changes throughout life. There is, for example, a steady increase in elastin content of the lamina propria as we age, with a decrease in its distensibility caused by cross-branching.[11] There is also a thinning of the SLLP in the elderly.[11] Yet, as pointed out by Woo,[12] the vast majority of elderly patients with voice disorders have disease processes associated with aging rather than physiologic aging alone. Only 4% have bowing and breathiness consistent with presbylarynges.

In the normal adult male vocal fold, the mucosa is approximately 1.1 mm in thickness, and the length of the membranous segment is approximately 15 mm.[13] The vocal fold is classically described as being two-thirds membranous and one-third cartilaginous, although Hirano reports that the membranous to cartilaginous ratio is 3 to 2.[13] At the anterior and posterior ends of the membranous vocal fold, the intermediate layer condenses to form the anterior and posterior macula flava, connecting the vocal fold to the anterior commissure tendon and to the vocal process of the arytenoid, respectively. Hirano postulates that they serve as cushions against the trauma of vocal fold vibration.[6]

Epithelium

On coronal section of the membranous vocal fold, the most superficial layer encountered is stratified squamous epithelium. This layer is thin but stiff. Whereas most of the laryngopharynx consists of respiratory pseudostratified ciliated columnar epithelium, only the anterior surface of the epiglottis, superior margin of the aryepiglottic folds, and margins of the vocal folds are covered with stratified squamous epithelium.[14] This in itself affects distribution of neoplasms; for example, squamous papilloma have a predilection for stratified squamous epithelium (Figure 6–2).

The epithelium is 5 to 25 cell thickness deep and multilayered. Cells are mitotically active in the basal layer, and attached to the basement membrane by hemidesmosomes. Their nuclei are euchromatic denoting intense metabolic activity.[15] As they mature and migrate out, they are known as "pickle" cells. The most superficial layer consists of 1 to 3 flattened cells with small condensed nuclei; they are generally lost by surface abrasion.

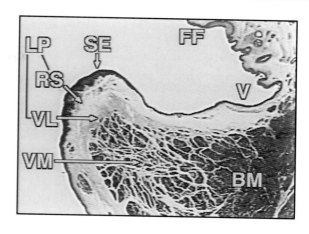

Figure 6-2. Enlarged view of coronal section of vocal fold.

SE	=	squamous epithelium
LP	=	lamina propria
RS	=	Reinke's space (superficial layer of lamina propria)
VL	=	vocal ligament (formed by intermediate and deep layers of lamina propria)
VM	=	vocalis muscle
BM	=	body of thyroarytenoid muscle
V	=	ventricle
FF	=	false fold

(Courtesy of John A. Kirchner, MD, Yale University, New Haven, CT)

The epithelium is mucus-coated derived not only from glands in the ventricles but also from special mucin-producing cells embedded in the epithelium.[16] Langerhan's cells, which are immunologically active, are found in the epithelium.[17]

Basement Membrane Zone

Gray has studied the basement membrane zone (BMZ), which mechanically links the epidermis and the SLLP.[18] He identified a chain-link fence arrangement of anchoring fibers which provide increased structural integrity and which he postulates allow for tissue compression and bending. Of interest, the population density of anchoring fibers is greatest in the mid-membranous region, an area subject to most stress.[18]

SLLP (Reinke's Space)

Just deep to the BMZ is the SLLP (Reinke's space). This layer contains loose tissue with sparse collagenous or mature elastin fibers, and few to no capillaries, seromucinous glands, or lymphatics. It does contain elastin precursors (elaunin and oxytalan) and a ground substance network of mucopolysaccharides, decorin and hyaluronic acid[8,11,18] allowing for a pliable consistency.[19]

Macrophages and myofibroblasts have also been found in about one-third of specimens studied by Catten et al. In that review, women had significantly more macrophages than men, suggesting an inflammatory response of the SLLP to trauma, the macrophages being involved in immunologic "mop-up" activities.[20] Similarly, fibroblasts are activated following trauma.[21]

Fibronectin is found in normal nondamaged vocal folds, maximally in the SLLP. It may be one determinant of tissue deformability in the SLLP.[1] Of interest, it is known to be deposited as a result of tissue injury.

The SLLP is sharply delimited by dense fibrous tissue in the anterior commissure, along the vocal process of the arytenoid and beneath the free margin of the vocal fold. The upper limit is not as well defined and may vary considerably in size, usually reaching to the inferior aspect of the ventricle and occasionally to the inferior surface of the ventricular fold. Use of the ventricular folds has been postulated to force fluid within Reinke's space toward the free edge of the vocal fold.[22]

Middle Layer of the Lamina Propria (MLLP)

The MLLP consists predominantly of longitudinally oriented, mature elastin fibers. Other proteins also responsible for its mechanical properties include hyaluronic acid and fibromodulin.[11] Hyaluronic acid is found in greater quantities in the MLLP than elsewhere in the lamina propria. Hyaluronic acid molecules are hydrophilic because of their inherent negative electrical charge. They are relatively inflexible molecules, and may act both as a space filler and as a "shock absorber," particularly in men in whom they are found to be more abundant than women.[8]

Deep Layer of the Lamina Propria (DLLP)

The DLLP consists primarily of collagenous fibers that are arrayed in a longitudinal pattern, parallel to both the vocal fold edge and the vocalis muscle. Fibroblasts are more abundant in this layer than other areas of the lamina propria.[20]

INJURY (GENERAL)

The cause of vocal fold injury and the pathologic response to that injury have been debated for years. Concepts of injury have included the following:

1. Microtrauma from excessive force during phonation causing vascular changes with interruption of the microcirculation. The temporary ischemia may be followed by disruption of capillaries and increased permeability, possibly with microhematomae, followed by rapid organization and then a fibrous mass. Once edema accumulates, it is difficult to dissipate as the lymphatic drainage of the vocal folds is so poor.[23]
2. Voice misuse. Examples might include prolonged use of intensity changes, rather than frequency changes for emphasis, use of a monotone, affectation of a low fundamental frequency. All of these could cause edema of the lamina propria.[24]
3. Direct compression on the vocal fold surface by the hammering effect of forceful vibrations during phonation, causing mucosal changes with a tendency toward parakeratosis, acanthosis, and development of rete ridges, especially in long-standing polyps and nodules. Hyaline changes seen therein may represent further degeneration in certain types of polyps and nodules.

    Epidermoid cysts may represent a form of implantation cyst because of the microtrauma, sending islets of squamous epithelium into the lamina propria.[25]
4. Effects of systemic/external factors. These are multifactorial and might include smoking, gastroesophageal reflux, environmental irritants, musculoskeletal issues, endocrine disorders, and allergy.

Inhalatory or nutritional allergy has been postulated to make the laryngeal mucosa more susceptible to all the above-mentioned factors.[26] Dixon has stated that nutritional allergy and chemical sensitivity are particularly common causes of laryngeal signs, including mild swelling and irritation of the vocal folds and increased mucus production.[27]

Any number of systemic illnesses, ranging from viral laryngitis to AIDS, can cause a state of increased capillary fragility and/or decreased platelet function. Similarly, systemic use of such medications as corticosteroids, aspirin or nonsteroidal anti-inflammatory drugs (NSAIDS), or hormonal changes surrounding menstruation could also contribute. See chapter 40 "Special Considerations for the Professional Voice User," or chapter 34, "Medications and the Voice" for further insights.

It should be recalled that the locus of vocal fold trauma, the junction of the anterior one-third and posterior two-thirds of the vocal fold, actually represents the midpoint of the membranous vocal fold, that is, the site of highest trauma on phonation.

Histopathologic Injury

Recently Gray et al have presented theories of injury patterns from electron microscopic and immunohisto-chemical investigations of benign vocal fold patholo-gy. Their research can be summarized as follows:

1. One type of injury pattern found included BMZ and SLLP disruption. The BMZ was characterized by marked thickening with disorientation and dis-array of the anchoring fibers. The SLLP was char-acterized by abnormally increased deposition of fi-bronectin (an early response to injury). This injury pattern is rarely seen in other body tissues, and is suggestive of repetitive injury.[1,18] This pattern was commonly seen in vocal fold nodules and in some vocal fold polyps.
2. Another type of injury pattern demonstrated the BMZ to be reasonably intact, but with a relative ab-sence of structural glycoproteins and fibrous pro-teins in the SLLP. This led to a propensity to in-creased deformability, or a "jelly-like" state, and was seen in some polyps and Reinke's ede-ma/polypoid corditis.[1]

NONSPECIFIC LARYNGITIS

Acute Nonspecific Laryngitis

Acute nonspecific laryngitis is an extremely common ailment, only rarely coming to the attention of the laryn-gologist. It can result from many causes: voice abuse, a viral exanthem or bacterial infection, laryngeal irrita-tion from smoke or chemicals, and others.

Clinical Presentation and Vocal Dynamics

The patient complains of a painful throat, often with the feeling of pain upon initiation of swallow. Progres-sive hoarseness is noted, occasionally even complete aphonia. The voice tends to improve somewhat after swallowing, gently clearing the throat or initiating speaking, and then worsens after prolonged speaking.

Usually, laryngoscopy demonstrates vocal fold edema to some degree. Erythema, especially along the vibratory aspects of the folds, and dilated mucosal blood vessels may be noted.

Treatment

Management is judicious voice rest, increased fluid in-take, and humidification. Generally acute nonspecific laryngitis is self-limited and will resolve in a few days unless it is bacterial in etiology, in which case antibi-otics may be indicated.

Chronic Nonspecific Laryngitis

Whereas the causes of this process are somewhat sim-ilar to acute laryngitis, the process is long-standing, with diffuse mucosal edema and occasionally with ep-ithelial hyperplasia. Smoking is often an underlying etiology. Mucosal changes may be irreversible.[28]

Clinical Presentation and Vocal Dynamics

The patient presents with chronic hoarseness and pain; laryngoscopy reveals thickened and dull vocal folds, usually with mild generalized edema. The mu-cosa may be redundant in association with areas of leukoplakia and hyperkeratosis. It may appear quite similar to early Reinke's edema.

Treatment

Management includes voice rest, humidification, and elimination of any irritant. Biopsy may be necessary to rule out a laryngeal malignancy. Kleinsasser recom-mends that surgery, when deemed necessary, be per-formed on one side first and then the other, with at least a 3-week interval between procedures to allow for adequate healing.[29]

LARYNGITIS ASSOCIATED WITH GASTROESOPHAGEAL REFLUX DISEASE (GERD): MORE RECENTLY TERMED LARYNGOPHARYNGEAL REFLUX

This subject is extensively described in the chapter by Koufman.

GERD was initially associated with laryngeal pathology by Chevalier Jackson.[30] The popularity of this concept among otolaryngologists waxed and waned until GERD was nearly forgotten. In 1968, Cherry and Margulies revived interest in it.[31] In the 1980s, it became more apparent to laryngologists that GERD plays an important role in patients with voice disorders. In fact, laryngopharyngeal manifestations of GERD represent laryngopharyngeal reflux, also called extra-esophageal reflux.

Clinical Presentation and Vocal Dynamics

Symptoms can be plebeian. The patient may complain of hoarseness, local irritation, cough or catarrh, throat clearing, pain upon initiation of swallow, and/or a lump in the throat.[32] In performers there may be no symptoms as the patient may be inured to the process. Heartburn and bilious taste in the mouth are classically described but uncommon to obtain in the history. Male predominance has been reported.

Physical findings most commonly observed are inflammation and edema of arytenoids and postcricoid mucosa.

Treatment

Management includes a change in eating and drinking habits, head of bed elevation, and a trial of H2 blockers or proton pump inhibitors. With the advent of laparoscopic surgery there may be more of a role in the future for surgical restoration of the sphincter. See the section on granuloma, Dr. Koufman's chapter on GERD, and Dr. Sataloff's chapter on medical management of benign voice disorders for further insights.

COMMON DISCRETE LARYNGEAL LESIONS SEEN BY THE VOICE SPECIALIST

Vocal Fold Polyp

Whereas vocal fold nodules have the greater overall prevalence, vocal fold polyps appear to be the more common benign surgical lesion removed.

In Kleinsasser's review of 900 cases of vocal fold polyps, he found that 76% of patients were males. The mean age was 40 years in males and 38 years in females. Ten percent of polyps were bilateral and 5% were both multiple and unilateral. Eighty to 90% of patients smoked cigarettes. Other contributing factors included inhaled allergens and irritants. All polyps occurred at the anterior one-third of the vocal fold.[33] In general, polyps develop on the free edge of the musculomembranous portion of the vocal fold, as this is the location of maximal aerodynamic and muscular forces (Figure 6–3).

Pathogenesis and Histology

Phonotrauma with mechanical stress causing localized subepithelial edema, the development and subsequent abrupt reduction of high subglottic pressure, and increased hyperemia of the vocal fold with vasodilation have all been linked to polyp formation.[33-35] Increased permeability of vessel walls then allows extravasation of edematous fluid, fibrin, and erythrocytes. Subsequently, labyrinthine thin-walled vascular

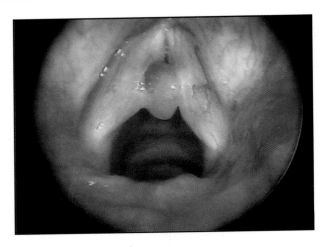

Figure 6-3. Pedunculated polyp arising from the midportion of the left true vocal fold (telescopic view).

spaces form. These are not vasoformative neoplasms, but reactive endothelial cells similar to a thrombus.[35,36]

Ultrastructural studies have demonstrated the BMZ to be more or less unaltered. Large clusters of angiomatous appearing vessels frequently disrupted the laminar pattern; fibronectin deposition clustered around these clusters. There was a relative decrease of collagen type IV in the surface epithelium and one author felt that perhaps this predisposed to polyp formation.[37] Another researcher found an 11-fold increase of Langerhans' cells in polyps compared to normal controls, suggesting a marked immune response, perhaps to the underlying injury.[38]

Polyps represent one extreme of a chronic edematous swelling of the vocal fold.[39] The gross appearance varies: it may be reddish or white, large or small, sessile or pedunculated. Most are small and sessile, however. Polyps are associated with other vocal fold lesions in 15% of cases.[40] As polyps become more advanced, there appear grapelike convolutions of blood vessels which become progressively pedunculated.[33]

On H&E, histology varies. There are 2 distinct subtypes and 1 combined group by light microscopy (Figure 6–4):

1. Gelatinous polyps: These have very loose edematous stroma, and sparse collagen fibers, between which lie small blood vessels, a few fibrocytes, histiocytes, and mast cells.
2. Telangiectatic polyps: These have homogeneous eosinophilic deposits and fibrin collections in the stroma. Characteristic are labyrinthine sinuslike channels lying between the homogeneous deposits or within the fibrin.[36]

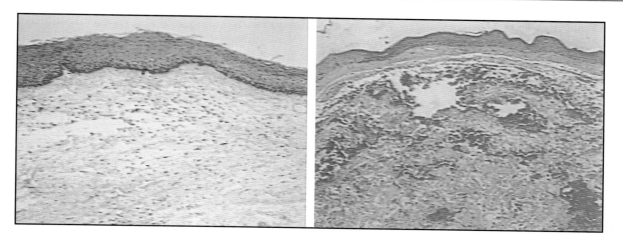

Figure 6-4 Histologic section showing two types of laryngeal polyps: (1) gelatinous polyp (*left*) and (2) telangiectatic polyp (*right*). (Courtesy of Romeo A. Vidone, MD, Hospital of St. Raphael, New Haven, CT)

3. Mixed type polyps: These have features of gelatinous and telangiectatic polyps. Polyps of mixed or transitional type are the most common type of polyp seen and contain a nucleus of tortuous vessels embedded in a gelatin substance and covered by squamous epithelium.[36]

Clinical Presentation and Vocal Dynamics

Vocal analysis of patients with vocal fold polyps have demonstrated: (1) the size of the polyp is negatively correlated to fundamental frequency; (2) the size of the polyp is positively correlated to the roughness of voice, the asymmetry and irregularity of vocal fold vibration, and the pitch and amplitude perturbation quotient; and (3) the glottic gap is negatively correlated to maximum phonation time and sound pressure level, but positively correlated to mean airflow rate.[41]

Clinically, initial symptoms are hoarseness and breathiness with reduced dynamic range and decreased vocal intensity. The lesion interferes with glottic closure causing decreased flexibility and elasticity of the free edge. It also interferes with vibratory movement of the contralateral fold.

The stiffness varies depending on the histologic type of polyp; stiffness increases when the main feature is hyaline degeneration and thrombosis, but decreases when the main feature is edema.[6] Increased mass of cover causes disturbance of periodicity and synchrony of vibration.[24]

A unilateral polyp may cause diplophonia because of the differing vibratory frequencies of the two folds.[42] Large polyps may cause dyspnea, intermittent dysphagia, and even airway embarrassment. They may rest on the subglottis and may cause a ball-valve effect during labored breathing.[43] Laryngoscopy is usually rapidly diagnostic; the typical polyp appears smooth, soft, and translucent with a broad base.

Treatment

Surgery is frequently required; voice therapy is less likely to be curative than for laryngeal nodules. Nonetheless, initial management with a course of voice therapy is warranted, in association with cessation of cigarette smoking and general removal of environmental irritants. Under these circumstances it is possible that resolution of underlying edema will occur and surgery may be avoided.

Surgical management depends on the size of the polyp. The base of the polyp, which often infiltrates the lamina propria, should generally be removed, preserving as much SLLP as possible and avoiding injury to the vocal ligament. Such an excision may leave a cavity. Often this is not a problem and will fill in without a notch.[40]

Chronic generalized polyps are treated like Reinke's edema with a lateral incision. Staged removal may be required in this setting. More discrete polyps are removed by grasping medially and excising (or lasering). In cases in which fibrous or hyaline infiltration has occurred, voice results will not be ideal. Postoperative voice therapy will be necessary.[39]

Vocal Fold Nodule

Vocal nodules are generally believed to be the most common discrete vocal fold lesion in both children and adults. The etiology is vocal abuse: in children screaming may produce nodules; in adults vocal misuse results from excessive muscle tension which may be related to anxiety, need for a loud voice, and so forth,[44,45] or just from excessive vocalizing. They are rarely seen in introverted bashful individuals. Other postulated etiologies include the use of an unnaturally low fundamental frequency. Men may adopt such fundamental frequency to give themselves an air of authority; women to make the voice more appealing or authoritative; and children may emulate their elders.[24]

When discussing vocal fold nodules, it must be remembered that many older series of vocal fold "nodules" were diagnosed without the benefit of the stroboscope. In fact "nodules" may well be much less common findings than previously believed.

Vocal nodules occur around the free edge of the vocal fold at the anteroposterior midpoint of the membranous fold. They typically are whitish, small, sessile, generally bilateral, and often symmetric (Figure 6–5).

All Kleinsasser's patients were female, between ages 20 and 40. Nearly all were schoolteachers, young mothers, amateur singers, or pop singers. None had studied singing.[46] He states that he has never seen a true singer's nodule in a man. In our experience nodules may occur in well-trained singers if they oversing or sing when they are ill, or if they misuse/abuse their voices while speaking. Nodules may occur in males as well as females. Nevertheless, we agree with Kleinsasser's basic premises.

Pathogenesis and Histology

Vocal nodules begin as edema and vasodilatation; depending on the chronicity of injury, the edema may differentiate into a hyalinized fibrous nodule.[24,39]

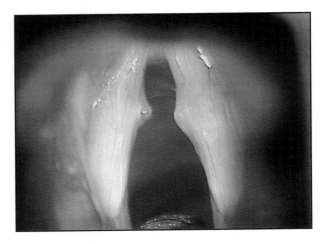

Figure 6-5. Laryngeal nodules (direct microlaryngoscopic view).

Kambic hypothesizes that if the condition persists as generalized edema and does not result in a nodule, it may degenerate into a polyp.[35] The nodule is confined to the superficial layer of the lamina propria.

Grossly, smaller nodules appear glassy-transparent and soft; larger nodules are more solid, conical, and usually asymmetric as they enlarge. This evolution represents stages in a process. Singers nodules have been likened to epithelial callus from phonotrauma.[46]

Histologically, nodules demonstrate:

1. The stratified squamous epithelium is hyperkeratotic and sometimes slightly acanthotic. There may also be parakeratosis. An increase in depth of rete ridges with a markedly thickened basement membrane is evident.
2. The subepithelial layer and core are infiltrated with dense irregularly arranged collagen fibers and abundant fibroblasts. It is only minimally vascularized and there are scarcely any inflammatory cells.
3. Edema is present in the connective tissue core; it may be subtle or be a dramatic finding.
4. No fibers in Reinke's space connect to or fix the epithelium to the muscular body of the vocal fold.[7,19,25,46]

Ultrastructural studies have demonstrated the BMZ to be up to three times normal in thickness. The fibronectin pattern was disordered with loss of laminar pattern and more dense than normal. It was seen throughout the lamina propria (rather than mostly in the SLLP as is seen in normals).[37]

Clinical Presentation and Vocal Dynamics

Nodules frequently interfere with complete closure of the glottis during phonation. Mass and stiffness of the cover are increased slightly, but the body is unaffected. The lesion may interfere slightly with the vibratory function of the contralateral fold. On stroboscopic evaluation, pronounced vibration of the anterior segment of the folds extending back to the nodules is seen. A small posterior glottic deficiency of closure is often noted. The clinical findings are hoarseness and breathiness. In singers, loss of frequency range is noted, especially loss of the higher frequencies.[6,24,46]

Treatment

The management of vocal fold nodules is nonsurgical, at least initially. The etiology of the vocal abuse should be carefully investigated and addressed. Voice therapy is the mainstay of therapy; at least 90% of vocal fold nodules will respond to appropriate treatment.

If surgery is eventually required, it should be recalled that this process is strictly superficial. The goal of surgery is a straight edge across the vibratory surface of the vocal fold with minimal disruption of the SLLP.

Reinke's Edema

Reinke's edema is also known as polypoid degeneration, chronic polypoid corditis, chronic edematous hypertrophy, and chronic hypertrophic laryngitis. There has been considerable interest in its pathogenesis and histology in recent years. Reinke's edema is an inflammatory process being the end result of chronic irritation by vocal abuse; it has been postulated that it may begin as polyps or nodules and then evolve with continued trauma.[42]

Pathogenesis and Histology

Etiologic agents have been investigated extensively. In general, smoking appears to be the major etiologic factor identified. In their series of patients with Reinke's edema, Fritzell found 98% of men and 94% of women studied to be smokers, and cessation of smoking improved the larynx, while neither surgery nor voice therapy helped if the patient continued smoking. They found no evidence for allergic disposition in their patients.[47] Other "caustic" exposures to the glottis considered have included gastroesophageal reflux and voice abuse.[48]

Abnormally high subglottic pressure has been noted in Reinke's edema (and certain other functional voice disorders). It has been postulated that this increased pressure together with the other caustic exposures may contribute to the superior distension of the SLLP and increased vascular permeability.[48]

Attempts to correlate thyroid dysfunction as a possible etiology for Reinke's edema have had varied success. Of three studies reviewed, two have not demonstrated any relationship[49,50] while one has.[51]

In general, Reinke's edema is an accumulation of fluid in the superior aspect of the SLLP along the entire length of the membranous fold. It remains localized because of dense anterior and posterior fibrous tissue connections and the poor lymphatic supply. It is almost always bilateral, but may be asymmetric (Figure 6–6).

Histologically, Vecerina-Volic et al have characterized two types of findings: "pale" (transparent) and "livid" (marked subepithelial vascularization.[52] In both types the lamina propria is very loose and edematous, filled with lakes of mucoid fluid interweaved with sheets or masses of immature young elastic fibers.[6,25,29,53]

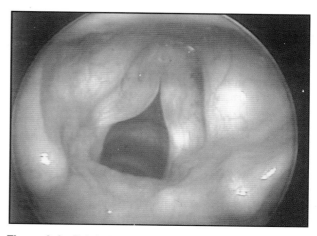

Figure 6-6. Reinke's edema of both vocal folds (telescopic view).

Authors vary regarding the relative thickness of the basement membrane. Some find it to be thickened[46,52] and the number of anchoring fibers increased.[54] Others differ.[1,37]

In the "pale" type (perhaps just early cases) a limited, fusiform, glazed swelling is noted. The epithelium is thin and the collection of clear watery fluid visible.

In the "livid" (advanced) type, the edematous masses increase, the color changes to yellow-gray, and the fluid thickens to gluelike consistency (Figure 6–6).[46]

Tillmann's studies[55,56] contradict earlier-held beliefs of distended lymphatics in the advanced type. His findings suggest that Reinke's edema has "hollow places" mostly lined by a layer of mesothelial fibroblast-like cell which develop like neobursae from mechanical strain.

Ultrastructurally and cytologically, studies have demonstrated few structural proteins and little fibronectin in the extracellular matrix.[1] The "pale" type demonstrates stromal cells with numerous intracytoplasmic granules, indicating high metabolic activity. The "livid" type has multiple dilated and irregularly spread vessels.[52] The endothelium has been characterized as having many fenestrae and vesicles, and to exude plasma. Vascular endothelial growth factor is also present.[52] All these features predispose to edema formation in Reinke's space.

Clinical Presentation and Vocal Dynamics

There is increased mass of cover but decreased stiffness. The body is not affected but the lesion interferes with the contralateral fold.[9] The glottis does usually close completely during phonation. On laryngoscopy, diffuse irregular vocal folds are noted with a ballooned appearance.

Clinically, the most common sign is lowering of pitch. The vocal quality is hoarse, harsh, gravelly, and breathy. The voice can also be diplophonic. Phonatory characteristics include: (1) an abnormally low mean speaking fundamental frequency; (2) severely reduced dynamic range affecting upper and lower extremes, (3) the highest sustainable tone at least one octave below normals.[57]

Treatment

Speech therapy is necessary to treat the underlying voice disorder. In early stages, and in association with cessation of cigarette smoking, aggressive nonsurgical therapy may be adequate. Most advanced cases will require surgery, however. A decision to operate is based on symptomatology and not the appearance of the folds.

When operating, the free margin must be respected and mucosa should be resected conservatively, if at all. The incision should be, if possible, placed superiorly and laterally, well away from the vibratory surface. The myxoid fluid can generally be bluntly eliminated while respecting the vocal ligament. The mucosa is redraped and excess mucosa trimmed. The patient must not smoke postoperatively.[39,40,58] Two recent studies, one with "cold" instruments and one with the laser have demonstrated a marked improvement in fundamental frequency, to near normal following surgery in most patients. In Zeitels' cases the average fundamental frequency in women rose from 123 to 154 Hz. There were failures, however, particularly in individuals who did not stop smoking.[48,59]

Vocal Fold Cyst

Intracordal cysts of the vocal fold are either mucus retention or epidermoid cysts. Hypotheses explaining pathogenesis include: (1) occlusion of one or a few mucus gland ducts of the inferior part of the vocal fold. The pressure of the secretions would then promote squamous metaplasia; (2) ingrowth of squamous elements from the free edge of the membranous vocal fold caused by microtrauma from vocal abuse; or (3) congenital anomaly.

Cysts occur equally in both sexes. They are located in the SLLP. Occasionally they will open into the laryngeal lumen or partly insert on the vocal ligament (Figure 6–7).[6,7]

Clinical Presentation and Vocal Dynamics

Milutinovic studied a series of patients with cysts and found functional hyperkinetic vocal abuse patterns, with increased muscular activity during phonation.[60]

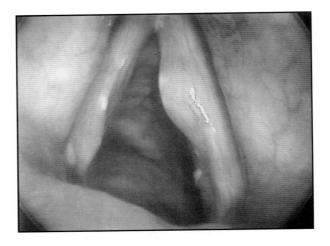

Figure 6-7. Laryngeal cyst involving the midportion of the right true vocal fold (telescopic view).

Colton has identified increased mass as well as stiffness of cover.[7]

Clinically the patient presents with hoarseness. On stroboscopy, unilateral submucosal swelling is noted with rigidity of the involved vocal fold and an asynchronous wave. Frequently edema of the contralateral fold is observed.[39]

Treatment

Cysts do not respond to nonsurgical management. The object of surgery is resection of the lesion with minimal injury to underlying tissue. Hirano suggests a technique whereby the incision is placed immediately posterior to the cyst at the mediolateral midpoint of the cyst. He emphasizes the difficulty of elevation of covering epithelium mucosa.[61]

Epidermoid Cysts

Epidermoid cysts are whitish structures, which tend to bulge out on the superior and medial aspect of the middle of the musculomembranous vocal fold. They are limited by a cyst wall in the superficial lamina propria and may be attached to connective tissue elements.

Grossly they contain pearly white epithelial debris. Histologically the cavity is bordered by a thin layer of keratinizing stratified squamous epithelium. The debris contains desquamated keratin and cholesterol crystals. The mass expands in a centripetal fashion. Dilated capillaries are sometimes noted converging toward the lesion on the superior aspect of the vocal fold.[40] There is usually no evidence of inflammation.[25]

Clinically it is not always easy to diagnose cysts by examination. In Bouchayer's series only 10% were obviously cysts. Another 55% were suspected to be cysts because of subtle fullness and dilated converging capillaries and stroboscopy showing absent or reduced vibratory pattern; however, 35% were only diagnosed at surgery.[62]

Mucus Retention Cysts

These present quite similarly to the epidermoid cyst; they are yellow cystic masses with mucoid contents caused by obstruction of a gland. They are also usually located in the middle of the musculomembranous vocal fold. As the free edge of the fold is typically devoid of glands, they tend to occur on the inferior aspect. The fold is distorted by the cyst and exhibits loss of vibration. The contralateral fold often develops a nodule.

Histologically in young cysts, the epithelium tends to be columnar and similar to terminal ducts of the small subglottic seromucous glands.[46]

Surgery involves meticulous dissection of the cyst wall from the underlying tissues. The membrane is delicate and often ruptures during removal. All cyst remnants must be removed and the mucous membrane repositioned, ideally without any resection of overlying epithelium.

Postoperatively there is usually no depression visible and the vocal fold returns to normal. Vocal quality is generally much improved but there may be residual huskiness with loss of resonance in the low frequencies.[2]

Other Types of Cysts and Pseudocysts

Other types of cysts and pseudocysts involving the larynx include pseudocysts, posthemorrhagic cysts, ventricular and saccular cysts, and epiglottic cysts. Relatively little has been written about pseudocysts or posthemorrhagic cysts, yet both are not infrequently seen in the busy voice clinic. In Bouchayer's surgical series, he noted a 6% incidence of pseudocysts (as compared with a 3% incidence of epidermoid cysts).[2] In the authors' experience, neither pseudocysts nor posthemorrhagic cysts represent true cysts, in that they do not have a true capsule. Rather they represent a localized area of polypoid degeneration. We have occasionally identified a small scar just below pseudocysts and have posited a relationship thereto (Tom Harris, FRCS, personal communication, 2000). We have been able to identify some pseudocysts as well as some mucus retention cysts of the true vocal fold with the use of ultrasound.[63]

Ventricular cysts, saccular cysts, and epiglottic cysts are all true cysts of the larynx. As these do not directly involve the true vocal folds they will not be discussed further here. That said, as ventricular cysts and saccular cysts enlarge, they can have an effect both on the voice and on the glottal airway.

Sulcus Vergeture and Sulcus Vocalis

Sulcus vergeture and sulcus vocalis are uncommon clinical conditions. Greisen reports 15 patients with sulcus out of a series of 1,400 referred with voice disorders.[64] Nakayama, however, identified shallow sulci in 4 of 20 larynges removed from random autopsy samples.[65] Thus subclinical sulcus may be more common than expected.

Bouchayer and Cornut distinguish sulcus vergeture from vocalis in the following manner: They consider sulcus vergeture to be a linear depression along the medial margin of the vocal fold which does not extend to the vocal ligament. They consider sulcus vocalis to be a focal invagination of the epithelium, attaching deeply to or through the vocal ligament.[40] Ford distinguishes sulcus into three types, 1 through 3, in which type 1 is a physiologic sulcus with preserved vibratory activity and anatomic layers of the lamina propria. He calls vergeture type 2 and sulcus vocalis type 3.[66] Lindestad and Hertegard do not distinguish them separately (Figure 6–8).[67]

Pathogenesis

Bouchayer has proposed a congenital basis of sulcus vocalis, resulting from faulty development of the 4th and 6th branchial arches. He has also suggested the possible occurrence of rupture of an epidermoid cyst.[62] In support of this concept, Bouchayer has not-

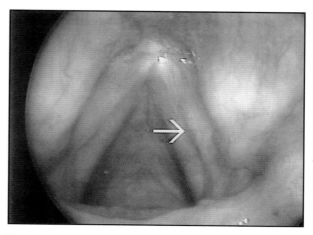

Figure 6-8. Sulcus vergeture. This is an atrophic depression along the free margin of the vocal fold (*arrow*) (telescopic view) and may be considered a variant of sulcus vocalis.

ed a small opening into the lumen in some cases.[2] Most patients with sulcus vocalis can trace their dysphonia to childhood.

The possibility of acquired sulcus has been raised by Nakayama et al,[65] who have identified sulcus deformities on the true folds, adjacent to cancer on 48% of their laryngeal specimens.

Histology

Sulcus vocalis is located in the region of the superficial layer of the lamina propria. From a histologic standpoint the sulcus creates a blind sac; the epithelial walls are thickened stratified squamous epithelium. Hyperkeratosis is a feature, particularly in the deeper aspect of the pit. Collagenous fibers are increased and capillaries decreased throughout.[2,7] The sulcus extends through the level of the superficial lamina propria (which is absent in the area of the sulcus) to adhere to the vocal ligament, the extent depending probably on the inflammatory reaction.

In Ford's series[66] of 20 cases of vergeture or sulcus, all were associated with bilateral abnormalities. In 10 of the cases of sulcus either an epidermoid cyst was identified (n = 9) or an open epidermoid pit was found (n = 1).

Clinical Presentation and Vocal Dynamics

Mechanically, the mass of cover is reduced while the stiffness is increased. The body is not affected.[7] At stroboscopy, a spindle-shaped closure defect may be seen, together with a medial furrow during inhalation, markedly impaired vibration, and frequently supraventricular hyperfunction.[40,64,65] (By contrast, on mirror laryngoscopy the larynx may actually look relatively normal.) Because of the compensatory hyperfunction, the condition is easy to overlook or confuse with the overlying vocal-abuse related pathology.

Clinically, the patient complains of a severely hoarse voice and vocal fatigue. The voice tends to be breathy and aesthenic, especially in males. It is typically effortful. Phonation time is invariably short.[64]

Treatment

Treatment is difficult. Voice therapy has limited success but is essential as an adjunct. Surgical intervention has included injection of teflon[68]; excision of the sulcus with microscissors,[2] or CO_2 laser[69]; incision with undermining, with or without steroid injection[2]; bioimplant[70-72]; medialization thyroplasty[73]; slicing, to break up linear tension.[66,74] Recently there has been considerable interest in fat implantation.[72] Rubin has begun using a deepithelialization technique with promising early results (J. Rubin, personal observation, 2005). The ideal surgical goal is replacement of the sulcus with normal tissue; currently no such procedure exists.[6] Consequently surgical procedures must be conservative.

Vocal Fold Scarring

Scarring can occur at any site along the vocal fold. The etiology may be trauma, intubation, inflammation, burn, or surgery. It can also occur in any layer.

Pathogenesis

Bouchayer notes 4 typical scar patterns as a result of excessive surgery. These are notches, webs, fibrous scars, and vocal fold rigidity, the latter especially after laser.[2,40]

Clinical Presentation and Vocal Dynamics

Postoperative vocal fold scarring poses a great therapeutic challenge. In essence, one must differentiate between dysphonia caused by the scarring versus that caused by the underlying pathology. Scar tissue, which is dense collagen, is much stiffer than normal tissue. This stiffness will be increased in the layer involved. Mass will vary depending on the amount and extent of injury.[7] Stroboscopy or high-speed photography is extremely important to assess vocal fold vibration. Scarring is likely to cause areas of adynamism and stiffness, interfere with or even obliterate the layered structure and the mucosal wave, and thereby alter phonation. It may also cause dysphonia by mechanical restriction, either of vocal fold vibration or of closure. This is particularly so in cases of dense web or fibrosis.[75]

Objective aerodynamic and acoustic assessment are valuable to diagnosis and documentation, therapy, and to evaluation of efficacy. (See chapter 16 by Korovin and Rubin, "Introduction to the Laboratory Diagnosis of Vocal Disorders" for further details.)

Treatment

The patient must understand the limitations of treatment. Similarly, before undertaking surgery, the voice team needs to understand the pathology, the vocal needs of the patient, and his or her motivation.

The speech-langauge pathologist must be involved before and after any surgical manipulation. Much as with sulcus vocalis, the patient will have developed compensatory voicing behaviors, which are usually hyperfunctional and counterproductive. The speech-language pathologist will need to work with the patient in an attempt to rid him or her of these behavioral patterns prior to consideration of any surgical intervention.

In general, surgical correction must be approached warily because the ideal procedure, that of replacement of the scarred area with normal tissue, does not yet exist. Procedures to restore the mucosal wave have included the following: steroid injection into the scar or vibratory margin; elevation of a microflap with or without steroid injection; injection of autologous fat into the underlying muscle; injection of collagen into the vocal ligament; and autologous fat implantation. Webs have been treated with excision, z-plasty, and stenting (Harvey Tucker, M.D, personal observation, 2000).[75-78]

Refer to the chapter by Woo for more insights into this problem.

Granuloma of the Larynx

A useful initial approach to vocal granuloma is a review of a study by Lehmann, who identified 61 cases out of 1,300 patients with voice disorders. Twenty-nine were post-traumatic (most caused by intubation), 28 were contact granuloma, and 4 were of unknown etiology. The mean age was 44. Forty-two out of 61 were unilateral, and 51 occurred on the vocal process of the arytenoid. Of the patients with contact granuloma 27 were male.[79] A third major etiology for granuloma is laryngopharyngeal reflux.[6]

Symptoms are mainly moderate or intermittent dysphonia, vocal fatigue, and decreased dynamic range. Less common symptoms include throat clearing, laryngeal pain, and a dry cough.

Contact Granuloma

These occur mainly in men of a certain vocal pattern and personality. Characteristics frequently noted include: (1) vocal abuse, especially seen in men trying to assume an unnaturally low fundamental frequency. This and laryngopharyngeal reflux are the most commonly accepted causative factors; (2) "en coups de glotte" attack, the achievement of high vocal intensity in a very brief period resulting in the clashing of arytenoids; and (3) a psychologic profile consisting of an aggressive personality, introversion, depression, emotional tension, and cancerophobia.[46]

Pathogenesis and Histology. Contact granuloma occur on the arytenoid process. They are unilateral and have a "2-lipped" form, fitting the vocal process of the contralateral side, which in turn develops slight epithelial hyperplasia.[46]

Histologically there is diversity. Lehmann noted 11 with simple pachydermia, 7 with surface ulceration, 10 with ulcerated granulation tissue.[79] Snow noted the base to be shaggy or granular with the healing process leading perhaps to a nonspecific granuloma.[24] Mossallam found dense connective tissue core with abundant collagen and fibroblasts, excessive vascularity but no edema or inflammation.[25]

Clinical Presentation and Vocal Dynamics. Clinically, the initial complaint is varying degrees of hoarseness and a low-pitched pressed quality to the voice, as well as frequent need to cough and clear the throat.[42] Stroboscopically the anterior folds do not close fully but the cartilaginous portions hammer together.

Treatment. Therapy is voice rest, voice therapy, and reflux treatment as discussed below. Surgery is only required if there is concern of malignancy, but it may be recommended in cases where the granuloma has not improved following several months of conventional therapy. There may also, particularly in recalcitrant cases, be a role for direct injection of steroid into the granuloma or of a dilute solution of botulinum toxin into the ipsilateral thyroarytenoid or lateral cricoarytenoid muscles.[80]

Granuloma from Laryngopharyngeal Reflux

Some controversy exists as to the role of laryngopharyngeal reflux in "contact granuloma." Ohman found 74% of patients with vocal fold granuloma to have esophageal dysmotility versus 30% in the general population.[81] Lehmann, on the other hand, only identified reflux in 1/32 patients with contact granulomas.[79] Feder postulates that both hyperfunctional and hyperacidic granuloma have vocal abuse as the primary etiologic factor.[82] This controversy notwithstanding, laryngopharyngeal reflux most likely represents a separate etiology for granuloma. We believe that antireflux therapy is an appropriate management plan in this group of patients. (See chapter 28 for further insights into this subject.)

Intubation Granuloma

The incidence of intubation granuloma is low, varying from 1:100 to 1:20,000 procedures. There is no direct correlation between duration of intubation and occurrence; it has been postulated that an overly large tube, excessive motion of tube or patient, and secondary infection in a debilitated patient are all etiologic factors,[28] and many laryngologists believe that reflux is usually a factor. Unlike contact granuloma, the incidence of intubation granuloma incidence is similar in women and men (women represented 4% of patients with contact granuloma but 44% of patients with intubation granuloma in Lehmann's series were women) (Figure 6–9).[79]

Histology. Histologic studies have demonstrated: (1) the epithelial covering is often eroded with a thick fibrin layer; (2) the connective tissue stroma is filled with abundant fibroblast and collagen fibers; (3) the stroma is much more vascular (hemangioma-like) than the stroma of contact granuloma.[25,46] The lesion is initially broad-based and then develops a mushroom-like configuration. Symptoms are similar to those of other laryngeal granulomata.

Treatment. Some authors[28,64] suggest surgical removal followed by voice therapy; others, including us, suggest medical and/or voice therapy primarily. It should be recalled that these granulomata not infrequently resolve on their own, without referral to any medical personnel.

Nonspecific and Other Granulomatous Conditions

There are a variety of other conditions characterized by granuloma which can affect the larynx.

Postsurgical Granuloma

These have to a large extent been described in the post-trauma section. It should be noted, however, that granulomatous changes can occur on the larynx in locations other than the arytenoid processes when ex-

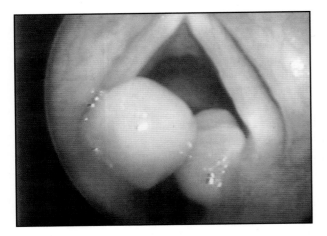

Figure 6-9. Bilateral postintubation granuloma (telescopic view).

cessive tissue, especially including muscle, has been removed, or for other reasons (such as reflux) that have not always been identified. This was the case in 6 patients with granulomata in Lehmann's series.[79]

Post-Teflon-Injection Granuloma

As more experience has accrued with long-term results from endolaryngeal Teflon injection, so has more experience with Teflon granuloma. Teflon paste injection causes early, brief-onset inflammatory reaction. On a longer-term basis, a foreign body granuloma forms around the teflon. Usually this is self-limited and the short- and long-term results of injection are satisfactory. If the injection is too superficial or too extensive, a foreign body granuloma can cause severe dysphonia with increase in both mass and stiffness (Figure 6–10). Granulomas may occur even when technique has been perfect. Sometimes they develop many years after initially successful Teflon injection, which is one of the reasons why this substance has been largely abandoned since the latter 1980s.

Surgical removal is extremely difficult, and the postsurgical voice result is unpredictable.[83] Endoscopic or external techniques may be used.

Inflammatory Arthritis

The cricoarytenoid joint is a synovial joint; hence, it can become involved by a variety of inflammatory processes, including rheumatoid arthritis, gouty arthritis, mumps, tuberculosis, syphilis, gonorrhea, Tietze's syndrome, lupus erythematosus, and so forth.[28] The most common of these etiologies is rheumatoid arthritis, which will be described.

Clinical

Symptoms include hoarseness (most commonly), a feeling of a lump in the throat, odynophagia, dysphonia, and pharyngeal fullness. The patient may complain of difficulty swallowing pills. Physical examination reveals acute inflammation and edema of the mucosa overlying the arytenoid cartilage. There is usually some motion, but frequently the mobility is severely diminished. The arytenoid process is tender to palpation. CT demonstrates subluxation of the cricoarytenoid joint.

Treatment

Therapy is aimed at the underlying condition. If the airway is compromised, an arytenoidopexy or arytenoidectomy might be indicated, or even tracheotomy.

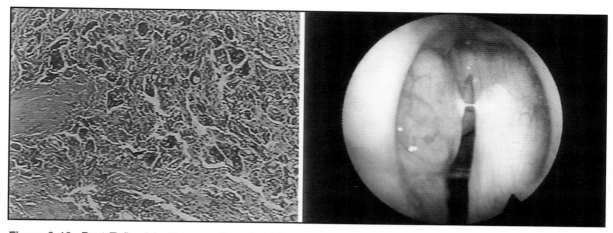

Figure 6-10. Post-Teflon injection granuloma involving the left true vocal fold. (*Right*) telescopic view; (*Left*) histologic section of Teflon granuloma showing multiple foreign bodies. (Courtesy of Richard N. Eisen MD, Yale University, New Haven, CT and Greenwich Hospital, Greenwich CT)

Sarcoidosis

Laryngeal involvement is uncommon but can occur. A large series identified it in 1.3% of cases.[84] The lesion is usually supraglottic, sparing the vocal fold. It can also occur in the subglottic larynx. In Neel's series, the appearance of the larynx was strikingly similar in all patients with supraglottic involvement. The supraglottic larynx was chronically edematous and pale pink. The rim of the epiglottis had a turban-like thickening. When the true vocal folds were involved, it was a reflection of the more extensive subglottic disease. Vocal fold mobility was intact in this series.[85]

Diagnosis is made by biopsy, demonstrating epithelioid tubercles and noncaseating granuloma with giant cells and macrophages. The angiotensin-converting enzyme level frequently is elevated and there may be hyperglobulinemia and hypercalcemia.[86]

Sarcoidosis can also cause vocal fold palsy by mediastinal compression of the left recurrent laryngeal nerve[87,88] or by cranial neuropathy.[28]

Symptoms are frequently mild but progressive airway obstruction can occur, either by diffuse edema or exophytic masses, especially if there is subglottic involvement.[89]

Autoimmune Processes

Systemic lupus erythematosus (SLE) is associated with mucous membrane lesions in 16% of patients and occasionally may involve the larynx. SLE may cause a multitude of processes, including: arthritis of the cricoarytenoid joint, vocal fold hyperplasia, mucosal nodularity, ulceration, inflammation, edema, as well as necrotizing vasculitis with airway obstruction. These latter lesions may mimic acute epiglottitis. Teitel et al have recently reviewed 4 personal cases and 97 cases reported in the literature. They note 28% with laryngeal edema and 11% with vocal fold palsy. The majority of symptoms in patients, including hoarseness, dyspnea, and even vocal fold palsy, resolved following therapy with corticosteroids.[90]

Another uncommon autoimmune disease entity that can affect the larynx is relapsing polychondritis. This disorder involves cartilaginous structures, the most common being the ear (which is affected in 75% of patients), followed by the nose. What is frequently not appreciated is that at some time during the course of the disease process the larynx and trachea can be affected in up to 50% of patients.[91] Involvement is manifested by progressive upper airway obstruction. Symptoms are pain and hoarseness and the findings are erythema and edema.

Laryngotracheal involvement is the most serious consequence of relapsing polychondritis. Airway obstruction may be caused by either destruction of the cartilaginous support or encroachment on the lumen by granulation tissue. This is not an easy diagnosis to make and generally is not made until more than two sites containing cartilage are affected. Two patients in McCaffrey's series of 29 had airway obstruction as their initial presention caused by subglottic involvement and requiring tracheotomy.[28,91]

Idiopathic Granulomata

Idiopathic granulomata and their involvement of the larynx (eg, Wegener's granulomatosis, polymorphic reticulosis, and idiopathic midline granuloma) are all covered well by Lebovics in his chapter.

SUMMARY

This chapter has limited itself to benign non-neoplastic processes affecting the vocal folds. It has mainly investigated processes which are commonly seen by the laryngologist specializing in care of voice disorders. In this fashion, an attempt has been made to outline laryngeal pathology from the viewpoint of the laryngologist.

It is clear that the majority of such processes seen by the laryngologist relate to the basement membrane zone and to the superficial layer of the lamina propria, and tend to either be self-induced or caused by local irritants.

The vocal dynamics vary depending on the mass and stiffness of the underlying process, as well as the degree of air-wasting caused by the process. Treatment tends to be conservative; management of the underlying self-abusive pattern or irritant is as important as surgical therapy, or even more important.

Goals of surgery in this group of patients are minimal disturbance of underlying tissues and replacement of tissue with tissue which is as near to normal as possible; as has been shown, in some processes the ideal treatment is still not available.

REFERENCES

1. Gray SD, Hammond E, Hanson DF. Benign pathologic responses of the larynx. *Ann Otol Rhinol Laryngol.* 1995; 104:13–18.
2. Bouchayer M, Cornut G: Microsurgery for benign lesions of the vocal folds. *Ear Nose Throat J.* 1988;67:446–466.
3. Hirano M. Phonosurgery: basic and clinical investigations. *Otol Fukuoka.* 1975;21:239–242.
4. Sato S. Phonosurgery: basic study on the mechanism of phonation and endolaryngeal microsurgery. *Otol Fukuoka.* 1977;23:171–184.
5. Hirano M, Yoshida T, Tanaka S. Vibratory behavior of human vocal folds viewed from below. In: Gauffin J, Hammarberb B, eds. *Vocal Fold Physiology.* San Diego, CA: Singular Publishing; 1991:1–6.
6. Hirano M. Phonosurgical anatomy of the larynx. In: Ford CN, Bless DM, eds. *Phonosurgery: Assessment and Surgical Management of Voice Disorders.* New York, NY: Raven Press; 1991:25–41.
7. Colton RH, Casper JK. *Understanding Voice Problems. A Physiological Perspective for Diagnosis and Treatment.* Baltimore, MD: Williams & Wilkins; 1990:51–69.
8. Hammond TH, Zhou R, Hammond EH, Pawlak A, Gray SD. The intermediate layer: a morphologic study of the elastin and hyaluronic acid constituents of normal vocal folds. *J Voice.* 1997;11:59–66.
9. Hirano M. Structure of the vocal fold in normal and disease states: Anatomical and physical studies. In: Ludlow C, ed. *Proceedings of the Conference on the Assessment of Vocal Pathology.* ASHA Report # 11; 1981.
10. Gray SD, Titze IR, Alipour F, Hammond TH. Biomechanical and histologic observations of vocal fold fibrous proteins. *Ann Rhinol Laryngol.* 2000;109:77–85.
11. Hammond TH, Gray SD, Butler J, Zhou R, Hammond E. Age and gender-related elastin distribution changes in human vocal folds. *Otolaryngol Head Neck Surg.* 1998;119: 314–322.
12. Woo P, Casper J, Colton R, Brewer D. Dysphonia in the aging: physiology versus disease. *Laryngoscope.* 1992; 102:139–144.
13. Kurita S, Nagata K, Hirano M. Comparative histology of mammalian vocal folds. In: Kirchner JA, ed. *Vocal Fold Histopathology: A Symposium.* San Diego, CA: College-Hill Press; 1986:1–10.
14. Meller SM. Functional anatomy of the larynx. In: Fried MP, ed. *Otolaryngol Clin North Am.* 1984;17:3–12.
15. Stiblar-Martincic D. Histology of laryngeal mucosa. *Acta Otolaryngol (Stockh).* 1997;527(suppl):138–141.
16. Gipson IK, Spurr-Michaud SJ, Tisdale AS. Stratified squamous epithelia produce mucin-like glycoproteins. *Tissue Cell.* 1995;27:397–405.
17. Thompson AC, Griffin NR. Langerhan cells in normal and pathological vocal cord mucosa. *Acta Otolaryngol (Stockh).* 1995;115:830–832.
18. Gray SD, Pignatari SSN, Harding P. Morphologic ultrastructure of anchoring fibers in normal vocal fold basement zone. *J Voice.* 1994;8:48–52.
19. Hirano M, Kurita S. Histological structure of the vocal fold and its normal and pathological variations. In: Kirchner JA, ed. *Vocal Fold Histopathology: A Symposium.* San Diego, CA: College-Hill Press; 1986:17–24.
20. Catten M, Gray SD, Hammond TH, Zhou R, Hammond E. Analysis of cellular location and concentration in vocal fold lamina propria. *Otolaryngol Head Neck Surg.* 1998;118:663–667.
21. Hirano M, Sato K, Nakashima T. Fibroblasts in human vocal fold mucosa. *Acta Otolaryngol.* 1999;119:271–276.
22. Kambic V, Gale N, Radsel Z. Anatomical markers of Reinke's space and the etiopathogenesis of Reinke edema. *Laryngo-Rhino-Otologie.* 1989;68(4):231–235.
23. Hiroto J. The etiology of polyp and polypoid degeneration of the vocal fold. *IALP Congress Proceedings. Special paedagogisk Forlag.* Copenhagen; 1977.
24. Snow JB. Surgical therapy for vocal dysfunction. *Otolaryngol Clin North Am.* 1984;17:91–100.
25. Mossallam I, Kotby MN, Ghaly AF, et al. Histopathological aspects of benign vocal fold lesions associated with dysphonia. In: Kirchner JA, ed. *Vocal Fold Histopathology: A Symposium.* San Diego, CA: College-Hill Press; 1986:65–80.
26. Hocevar-Boltezar I, Radsel Z, Zargi M. The role of allergy in the etiopathogenesis of laryngeal mucosal lesions. *Acta Otolaryngol (Stockh).* 1997;527(suppl):134–137.
27. Dixon HS. Allergy and laryngeal disease. *Otolaryngol Clin North Am.* 1992;25:239–250.
28. Fried MP, Shapiro J. Acute and chronic laryngeal infections. In: Paparella MM, Shumrick DA, Gluckman JL, et al, eds. *Otolaryngology.* 3rd ed. Philadelphia, PA: WB Saunders; 1991:2245–2256.

29. Kleinsasser O. *Microlaryngoscopy and Endolaryn-geal Microsurgery.* Philadelphia, PA: WB Saunders; 1968.

30. Jackson C: Contact ulcer of the larynx. *Ann Otol Rhinol Laryngol.* 1928;37:227–230.

31. Cherry J, Margulies SI. Contact ulcer of the larynx. *Laryngoscope.* 1968;73:1937–1940.

32. Sataloff RT, Castell DO, Katz PO, Sataloff DM. *Reflux Laryngitis and Related Disorders.* San Diego, CA: Plural Publishing Inc; 2005.

33. Kleinsasser O. Pathogenesis of vocal cord polyps. *Ann Otol Rhinol Laryngol.* 1982;91:378–381.

34. Roch JB, Cornut G, Bouchayer M. Modes of appearance of vocal cord polyps. *Rev Laryngol Otol Rhinol (Bord).* 1989;110:389–390.

35. Kambic V, Radsel Z, Zargi M, et al. Vocal cord polyps: incidence, histology and pathogenesis. *J Laryngol Otol.* 1981;95:609–618.

36. Frenzel H. Fine structural and immunohistological studies on polyps of human vocal folds. In: Kirchner JA, ed. *Vocal Fold Histopathology: A Symposium.* San Diego, CA: College-Hill Press; 1986:39–50.

37. Courey MS, Shohet JA, Scott MA, Ossoff RH. Immunohistochemical characterization of benign laryngeal lesions. *Ann Otol Rhinol Laryngol.* 1996;105:525–531.

38. Melgarejo-Moreno P, Helin-Meseguer D. Estudio mediante anticuerpos policlonales S-100 de las células de Langerhans en los polipos de cuerda vocal. *Acta Otorrinolaringol Esp.* 1999;50:203–204.

39. Werkhaven J, Ossoff RH. Surgery for benign lesions of the glottis. In: Koufman JA, Isaacson G, eds. *Otolaryngol Clin North Am.* 1991;24:1179–1199.

40. Bouchayer M, Cornut G. Instrumental microscopy of benign lesions of the vocal folds. In: Ford CN, Bless DM, eds. *Phonosurgery: Assessment and Surgical Management of Voice Disorders.* New York, NY: Raven Press; 1991:143–165.

41. Sanada T, Tanaka S, Hibi S, et al. Relationship between the degree of lesion and that of vocal dysfunction in vocal cord polyp. *Nippon Jibiinkoka Gakkai Kaiho.* 1990;93:388–392.

42. Stringer SP, Schaefer SD. Disorders of laryngeal function. In: Paparella MM, Shumrick DA, Gluckman JL, et al, eds. *Otolaryngology.* 3rd ed. Philadelphia, PA: WB Saunders; 1991:2257–2272.

43. Yanagisawa E, Hausfeld JN, Pensak ML. Sudden airway obstruction due to pedunculated laryngeal polyps. *Ann Otol Rhinol Laryngol.* 1983;92:340–343.

44. McFarlane SC. Treatment of benign laryngeal disorders with traditional methods and techniques of voice therapy. *Ear Nose Throat J.* 1988;67:425–435.

45. Kauffmann I, Lina-Granade G, Truy E, et al. Chronic hoarseness in children. Evaluation based on personal series of 64 cases. *Pediatrics.* 1992;47:313–319.

46. Kleinsasser O. Microlaryngoscopic and histologic appearances of polyps, nodules, cysts, Reinke's edema, and granulomas of the vocal cords. In: Kirchner JA, ed. *Vocal Fold Histopathology: A Symposium.* San Diego, CA: College-Hill Press; 1986:51–55.

47. Fritzell B, Hertegard S. A retrospective study of treatment for vocal fold edema: A preliminary report. In: Kirchner JA, ed. *Vocal Fold Histopathology: A Symposium.* San Diego, CA: College-Hill Press; 1986:57–61.

48. Zeitels SM, Hillman RE, Bunting GW, Vaughn T. Reinke's edema: phonatory mechanisms and management strategies. *Ann Otol Rhinol Laryngol.* 1997;106:533–543.

49. White A, Sim DW, Maran AGD. Reinke's oedema and thyroid function. *J Laryngol Otol.* 1991;105:291–292.

50. Wedrychowicz B, Nijander D, Betkowski A, Jastrzebski J. Obrzek reinkego a niedoczynnosec tarczycy. *Otolaryngol Pol.* 1992;46:538–542.

51. Benfari G, Carluccio F, Murgiano S, Lentini A. Test di stimolazione della ghiandola tiroide nell'edema di Reinke. Studio in 28 pazienti. *An Clinica Otorrinolaringol Ibero Am.* 1992;19:485–491.

52. Vecerina-Volic S, Kirincic N, Markov D. Some morphological, histological, cytological and histochemical aspects of Reinke's oedema. *Acta Otolaryngol.* 1996;116:322–324.

53. Remenar E, Elo J, Frint T. The morphologic basis for development of Reinke's oedema. *Acta Otolaryngol (Stockh).* 1984;97:169–176.

54. Knobber D. Die basalmembran bei erkrankungen der stimmlippen: elektronenmikroskopische und immunmorphologische befunde. *Laryngorhino-otologie.* 1994;73:642–646.

55. Tillmann B, Rudert H. Licht und elektronenmikroskopische untersuchungen zum reinkeodem. *HNO.* 1982;30:280–284.

56. Tillmann B, Rudert H, Schunke M, Werner JA. Morphological studies on the pathogenesis of Reinke's edema. *Eur Arch Otorhinolaryngol.* 1995;252:469–474.

57. Bennett S, Bishop S, Lumpkin SMM. Phonatory characteristics associated with bilateral diffuse polypoid degeneration. *Laryngoscope.* 1987;97:446–450.

58. Bouchayer M, Cornut G. Microsurgical treatment of benign vocal fold lesions: indications, technique, results. *Folia Phoniatr.* 1992;44:155–184.

59. Murry T, Abitbol J, Hersan R. Quantitative assessment of voice quality following laser surgery for Reinke's edema. *J Voice.* 1999;13:257–264.

60. Milutinovic Z, Vasiljevic J. Contribution to the understanding of the etiology of vocal fold cysts: a functional and histologic study. *Laryngoscope.* 1992;102:568–571.

61. Hirano M, Yoshida T, Hirade Y, et al. Improved surgical technique for epidermoid cysts of the vocal fold. *Ann Otol Rhinol Laryngol.* 1989;98:791–795.

62. Bouchayer M, Cornut G, Witzig E, et al. Epidermoid cysts, sulci and mucosal bridges of the true vocal cord: a report of 157 cases. *Laryngoscope.* 1985;95:1087–1094.

63. Rubin, JS, Lee S, McGuiness J, et al. The potential role of ultrasound in differentiating solid and cystic swellings of the true vocal fold. *J Voice.* 2004;18;231–235.

64. Greisen O. Vocal cord sulcus. *J Laryngol Otol.* 1984;98:293–296.

65. Nakayama M, Ford CN, Brandenburg JH, Bless DM. Sulcus vocalis in laryngeal cancer: a histopathologic study. *Laryngoscope.* 1994;104:16–24.

66. Ford CN, Inagi K, Bless D, Khidr A, Gilchrist KW. Sulcus vocalis: a rational analytical approach to diagnosis and management. *Ann Otol Rhinol Laryngol.* 1996;105:189–200.

67. Lindestad PA, Hertegard S. Spindle-shaped glottal insufficiency with and without sulcus vocalis: a retrospective study. *Ann Otol Rhinol Laryngol.* 1994;103:547–553.

68. Lee ST, Niimi S: Vocal fold sulcus. *J Laryngol Otol.* 1990;104:876–878.

69. Remacle M, Declaye X, Hamoir M, et al. CO_2 laser treatment of the glottic sulcus and of epidermoid cyst. Technic and results. *Acta Otorhino-laryngol Belg.* 1989;43:343–350.

70. Cornut G, Bouchayer M. Phonosurgery for singers. *J Voice.* 1989;3:269–276.

71. Ford CN, Bless DM. Selected problems treated by vocal fold injections of collagen. *Am J Otolaryngol.* 1993;14:257–261.

72. Sataloff RT. *Professional Voice: The Science and Art of Clinical Care.* 2nd ed. San Diego, CA: Singular Publishing Group; 1997:627–628.

73. Sataloff RT. Vocal fold scar. In: Sataloff RT. *Professional Voice: The Science and Art of Clinical Care.* 2nd ed. San Diego, CA: Singular Publishing Group; 1997:555–559.

74. Ford CN, Bless DM, Prehn RB. Thyroplasty as primary and adjunctive treatment of glottic insufficiency. *J Voice.* 1992;6:277–285.

75. Pontes P, Behlau M. Treatment of sulcus vocalis: auditory perceptual and acoustic analysis of the slicing mucosa surgical technique. *J Voice.* 1993;7:365–376.

76. Mikaelian D, Lowry LD, Sataloff RT. Lipoinjection for unilateral vocal cord paralysis. *Laryngoscope.* 1991;101:465–468.

77. Ford CN, Bless DM. Selected problems treated by vocal fold injection of collagen. *Am J Otolaryngol.* 1993;14:257–261.

78. Sataloff RT, Spiegel JR, Hawkshaw M, Rosen DC, Heuer RJ. Autologous fat implantation for vocal fold scar: a preliminary report. *J Voice.* 1997;11:238–246.

79. Lehmann W, Widman JJ. Nonspecific granulomas of the larynx. In: Kirchner JA, ed. *Vocal Fold Histopathology: A Symposium.* San Diego, CA: College-Hill Press; 1986:97–107.

80. Sataloff RT, Castell DO, Katz PO, Sataloff DM. *Reflux Laryngitis and Related Disorders.* San Diego, CA: Singular Publishing Group; 1999:48–49.

81. Ohman L, Oloffson J, Tibbling L, et al. Esophageal dysfunction in patients with contact ulcer of the larynx. *Ann Otol Rhinol Laryngol.* 1983;92:228–230.

82. Feder RJ, Mitchell MJ. Hyperfunctional hyperacidic and intubation granulomas. *Arch Otolaryngol.* 1984;110:582–584.

83. Benjamin B, Robb P, Clifford A, et al. Giant Teflon granuloma of the larynx. *Head Neck.* 1991;13:453–456.

84. Carasso B. Sarcoidosis of the larynx causing airway obstruction. *Chest.* 1974;65:693–695.

85. Neel HB Jr, McDonald TJ. Laryngeal sarcoidosis report of 13 patients. *Ann Otol Rhinol Laryngol.* 1982;91:359–362.

86. Kirchner, JA. Nonepithelial benign tumors of the larynx. In: Kirchner JA, ed. *Vocal Fold Histopathology: A Symposium.* San Diego, CA: College-Hill Press; 1986:81–91.

87. Povedano Rodriguez V, Seco Pinero MI, Jaramillo Perez J. Sarcoidosis as a cause of paralysis of the recurrent laryngeal nerve. Presentation of a case. *An Otorrinolaringol Ibero Am.* 1992;19:443–448.

88. Abramowicz MJ, Ninane V, Depierreux M, et al. Tumour-like presentation of pulmonary sarcoidosis. *Eur Respir J.* 1992;5:1286–1287.

89. Weisman RA, Canalis RF, Powell WJ. Laryngeal sarcoidosis with airway obstruction. *Ann Otol Rhinol Laryngol.* 1980;89:58–61.

90. Teitel AD, MacKenzie CR, Stern R, et al. Laryngeal involvement in systemic lupus erythematosus. *Semin Arthritis Rheum.* 1992;22:203–214.

91. McCaffrey TV, McDonald TJ, McCaffrey LA. Head and neck manifestations of relapsing polychondritis: review of 29 cases. *Otolaryngology.* 1978;86:473–478.

7

Laryngeal Function During Phonation

Ronald C. Scherer, PhD

The larynx performs many functions to aid communication and allow life. As an open flow valve, it permits breathing, blowing, and sucking, as well as yawning, voiceless consonant production, and musical instrument playing. As a transient closed valve, it produces coughing and throat clearing. As a prolonged closed valve, it participates in swallowing and effortful behaviors such as lifting and defecation. As a voiceless repetitive articulator, it valves airflow to produce staccato whistling. As a voiced repetitive articulator, it produces laughter, the singing ornament trillo, and repetitive glottalization of vowels such as the admonition with rising pitch and intensity "a-a-a-ah!" As an incompletely closed voiceless valve, it produces whisper. As a partially or completely closed voicing valve, the larynx produces vowels and prolonged voiced consonants, and as a speech coarticulator, it participates in the production of consonant-vowel strings. For example, the word "seat" begins with an open glottis for the /s/, the glottis acting as an open flow valve allowing airflow under lung pressure to travel through the glottis and through the anterior oral constriction. This is followed by vocal fold approximation for the /i/ vowel, the larynx acting as a partially or completely closed voicing valve. Finally, the glottis opens as an open flow valve to permit the impoundment of air pressure behind the anterior oral /t/-occlusion with the subsequent release of air, creating the characteristic aspiration.

The purpose of this chapter is to describe the larynx as a partially or completely closed voicing valve, that is, as the organ that produces phonation. Neuromuscular, biomechanic, and aeroacoustic characteristics determine phonation duration, pitch, loudness, quality, register, and vocal fold motion, through control of or changes in vocal fold length, mass and tension, vocal fold contour, arytenoid and vocal fold adduction, subglottal pressure, and vocal tract size and shape. This chapter emphasizes the reasonable hypothesis that effective interventions to help people with voice concerns (whether these involve prevention, rehabilitation, surgery, pharmacology, or training) can be improved by an understanding of basic vocal function.[1,2]

OVERVIEW OF BASIC CHARACTERISTICS OF PHONATION

The basic perceptual characteristics of phonation are the presence and change of duration, pitch, register, loudness, and quality. Each of these has one or two primary biomechanical control variables. These will be discussed briefly in this section, followed by discussions of selected topics in greater detail.

Duration of phonation refers to the length of time the vocal folds oscillate during the creation of sound. In the normal larynx, adduction is one of two main control variables for duration; the vocal folds must be sufficiently close to permit oscillation. Subglottal air pressure is also necessary to provide sufficient force to move the vocal folds at the beginning of each vibratory cycle. After phonation commences, to then cease phonation, the arytenoid cartilages can be moved apart (abducted), or moved further together (more highly adducted), both ceasing phonation if the degree of abduction or adduction is great enough. Additional ways to cause phonation to cease are to lower subglottal air pressure, or impound air pressure in the vocal tract above the glottis, until the pressure drop across the glottis is too low to sustain vocal fold vibration.

The perception of pitch, corresponding to the physical measure of fundamental frequency, and vocal register (the very low pitches of vocal fry, the conversational pitches of chest or modal register, and the very high pitches of falsetto), are highly dependent on vocal fold length[3,4] and the associated tension of the vocal fold mucosal cover. The string model for frequency,[5-8]

$$\text{(Equation 1)}, \quad F_0 = \left(\frac{1}{2L}\right)\left(\frac{T}{\rho}\right)^{0.5}$$

where T is the tension of the vocal fold mucosal cover, ρ is the density of the tissue, and L is the length of the vibrating vocal folds, is an explanatory model suggesting that tension of the vocal fold cover governs the fundamental frequency (tension T increases faster than vocal fold length L when the vocal folds are lengthened, and ρ is essentially constant regardless of phonatory condition).[8,9]

The loudness of sounds is related to their acoustic intensity, and phonation during speech is primarily dependent upon subglottal pressure. An increase in subglottal pressure changes the characteristics of the airflow that exits the glottis (the glottal volume velocity) during vocal fold vibration, creating an increase in acoustic intensity (see below).

At the glottal level, vocal quality variation, governed primarily by the closeness of the vocal folds, that is, by adduction (separate from tissue or neurologic abnormalities), is related primarily to the perception of normal, breathy, and pressed qualities. Breathiness occurs when the vocal folds are slightly abducted such that they do not close completely during each cycle, allowing some of the glottal volume

flow to be unmodulated and turbulent.[10] A breathy voice also can be created by full vocal fold closure (anterior to the vocal processes) but with the posterior glottis open, allowing turbulent air to flow between the arytenoid cartilages. If there is hyperadduction of the vocal folds, but with a significant opening of the posterior glottis, a pressed-breathy (or pressed-leakage) quality can result.[11,12] Pressed or constricted voice quality without breathiness results from full glottal adduction, and little air flows through the glottis.[13]

Intervention strategies to improve voice production require an appreciation of the basic mechanics of phonation. The remainder of this chapter offers a more thorough discussion of basic control characteristics of voice production.

DURATION OF PHONATION

Figure 7–1 illustrates the adductory range of phonation and the corresponding distances between the vocal processes of the arytenoid cartilages, the ventricular folds, and the superomedial eminences of the arytenoid cartilage apexes. Phonation takes place over only a small range of adduction (the *phonatory adductory range*) permitted by movement of the arytenoid cartilages (approximately 14% of the adductory range as shown in the single-subject example of Figure 7–1). From an adductory standpoint, therefore, duration of phonation depends on the potential for the vocal folds to be placed within the phonatory adductory range, and the length of time the vocal folds are actually placed within that range. To discontinue phonation, the arytenoid cartilages can be configured to produce sufficient overcompression of the vocal folds or, alternatively, sufficient abduction.

Phonation requires a certain minimal amount of subglottal air pressure to set the vocal folds into vibration (the *phonatory threshold pressure*[14]) and then to maintain phonation. If the vocal folds are placed in the phonatory adductory range, the subglottal pressure must coordinate with the tissue characteristics of the vocal folds (stiffness, mass, and damping) to cause them to move to begin the first cycle.[14] Lucero[15] suggests, using a theoretical approach, that the pressure threshold should reduce as the vocal folds are brought closer to each other, and as the glottal angle between the vocal folds comes closer to zero or slightly divergent, consistent with Titze[14] and Chan, Titze, and Titze.[16] The threshold pressure typically varies with fundamental frequency, ranging from about 3 cm H_2O (0.3 kPa) for lower pitches to about 6 cm H_2O (0.6 kPa) for higher pitches[17] because of greater tension of the vocal fold cover with vocal fold lengthening. The amount of subglottal pressure at phonation

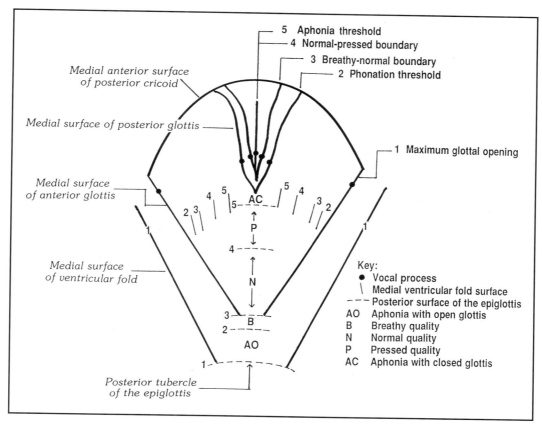

Figure 7–1. Adductory range of the larynx. This figure is a composite from photographs of glottal adductory positions obtained from a single adult male subject using rigid videolaryngoscopy. Positions of the medial surface of the anterior (membranous) glottis, posterior glottis, ventricular folds, and the posterior tubercle of the epiglottis are shown. Stages of glottal positioning include maximum glottal opening (position 1) to full adduction when phonation is not possible (position 5). The other positions (2, 3, and 4) are the position for adductory phonatory threshold and boundary locations between breathy, normal, and pressed voice qualities in this subject, perceptually judged and checked against electroglottograph (EGG) recordings. The adductory phonation range is only about 14% of the entire adductory range (see text).

offset is less than the onset pressure, not to exceed about half the onset pressure.[18-22] Because the phonatory threshold pressure is an important measure for glottal efficiency and clinical diagnostics, it is important that it be measured with care.[23]

There also may be an upper limit of subglottal pressure beyond which phonation is prevented or becomes unstable.[14] This upper limit may correspond to the upper limits of the *phonetogram,* a graph of the intensity range versus the fundamental frequency range of phonation for a particular person[24-28] (the recommendation of the term *voice range profile* for the phonetrogram was accepted by the Voice Committee of the International Association of Logopedics and Phoniatrics[29]). Subglottal pressures have been measured as high as 30 to 50 cm H_2O in loud phonation[30] (singing loudly at high pitches may produce even greater subglottal pressures[13]), but typically are below 10 cm H_2O for conversational speech.[30,31]

Intervention in voice surgery, therapy, and training often attempts to regain normal thresholds or to lower existing thresholds, the latter possibly creating less effortful phonation (relative to the employed forces of the respiratory system). Establishment of lower phonation thresholds may correspond to more physiologically efficient phonation and less voice fatigue.

The discussion directly above refers to the dependence that phonation has on subglottal pressure. More appropriately, phonation is dependent upon the *translaryngeal pressure,* defined as the subglottal air pressure minus the supraglottal air pressure for phonation on exhalation. Note that the translaryngeal pressure is the difference between the subglottal and supraglottal pressures acting on the inferior and superior surfaces of the vocal folds, respectively, as well as the pressure difference that drives the air through the glottis. If the translaryngeal air pressure were zero, the pressure would be equal on all surfaces of the vocal folds, air would not pass, and phonation would not occur. This can be approached, for example, with overly prolonged voiced consonants such as /b/, /d/, and /g/ during the complete occlusion of the vocal tract. Prolonging the voicing of these consonants creates buildup of supralaryngeal air pressure until that pressure nearly equals the subglottal pressure, causing cessation of phonation as the translaryngeal pressure drops below the minimum sustaining pressure difference.

Thus, the creation and duration of phonation depend upon how close the vocal folds are to each other and the amount of translaryngeal air pressure (disregarding tissue abnormality). To cease phonation, the vocal folds can be overadducted or overabducted, or the translaryngeal pressure can be lowered by decreasing the subglottal pressure or by increasing supraglottal pressure through supraglottal occlusion. All four methods most likely are used in normal speech production, and the ability of a patient to demonstrate all four methods is relevant diagnostically. These mechanisms for phonation cessation potentially can be compromised by arytenoidal, respiratory, or articulatory dysfunction, or by abnormal adductory configuration caused by vocal fold tissue change.

FUNDAMENTAL FREQUENCY OF PHONATION

Perceived pitch corresponds (nonlinearly) to the physical measure of fundamental frequency F_0,[32] which in turn corresponds to the number of cycles per second of the glottal motion during phonation. For normal phonation, the motion of the vocal folds is similar from cycle to cycle, giving rise to nearly equal periods of time between glottal closures.

Each phonatory cycle releases time-varying glottal flow (also called the glottal volume velocity) that generates sound. For normal phonation, acoustic excitation is created throughout the varying flow cycle, with a primary location giving the greatest excitation. Figure 7–2 shows two glottal volume velocity cycles of human phonation (top trace). The cycle period is T, which is 10 ms (and thus $F_0 = 1/T = 100$ Hz). The glottal volume velocity (usually given in liters per second, L/s, or cubic centimeters per second, cm^3/s) begins to exit the glottis gradually, rises to a peak, and then "shuts off" relatively abruptly. Air exits the glottis from time A to time B during the lateral then medial motion of the membranous vocal folds. The glottis is closed, or nearly so, from B to C. The amount of airflow during the interval B to C (seen as the offset from the horizontal baseline in Figure 7–2) corresponds to air "leakage" when the arytenoid cartilages are separated to some degree.

The lower trace of Figure 7–2 is the time derivative of the volume velocity signal of the upper trace. At any

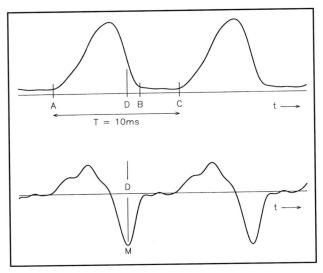

Figure 7–2. Glottal volume velocity waveforms and their derivatives. The top trace is a glottal volume velocity signal, and the bottom trace is the derivative of the top trace, showing the instantaneous slopes of the top trace. Cycle period is T (from time A to time C). "Open" glottis time is from A to B, and "closed" glottis time is from B to C. The moment of the maximum flow shutoff rate, or the maximum negative derivative of the glottal volume velocity signal, occurs at time D and corresponds to point M.

moment in time, the value on the lower trace equals the slope of the volume velocity signal at that moment. The fastest change of the volume velocity in the figure is at time D, and corresponds to the point M on the derivative waveform. The point M corresponds to the moment of time at which the greatest acoustic excitation is created.[33,34]

Perceptual judgments of an unclear voice (rather than confusion of pitch per se) occur when the more prominent moments of acoustic excitation during each cycle are not consistent from one cycle to the next (for a review of cyclic instabilities, see References 32, 35, 36). The time between primary acoustic excitations from one cycle to the next varies a small amount during normal phonation, helping to create a natural voice quality. However, the variation of periods can increase if there are tissue abnormalities such as swelling, nodules, polyps, unilateral stiffness, and so forth, causing kinematic (vocal fold motion) and glottal flow inconsistencies from cycle to cycle. Consecutively varying periods of primary acoustic excitations also can be created by turbulent airflow through the glottis (as in breathy voice), creating added noise to the acoustic signal. Aperiodicities can be measured by jitter, one definition being the average cycle-to-cycle difference in period or equivalent frequency, with large values of jitter corresponding to a sense of vocal roughness.[32] Figure 7–3 illustrates quasiperiodic cycles of the acoustic output of a prolonged vowel with a calculation of the segment's jitter value.

Jitter may be caused by or related to neuromuscular innervation abnormalities[37-40] as well as the structural and turbulence causes given above. Because tension of the vocal folds is highly dependent on the passive lengthening of the vocal fold cover, as suggested by Equation 1, relatively fast abnormal innervation changes to the cricothyroid muscles to lengthen the vocal folds and to the thyroarytenoid muscles to shorten the vocal folds may cause length and, therefore, ten-

sion changes, creating cycle-to-cycle fundamental frequency changes.

Pitch and vocal quality are also affected by changes that occur over longer time lengths than a phonatory cycle. Diplophonia (the existence of two pitches simultaneously[41]) and subharmonics (integer subdivisions of the fundamental frequency) come from multicycle length modulations of the volume velocity signal. These give rise to primary acoustic excitations at varying time intervals as well as about twice (or more) the primary phonatory period.[42-49] Figure 7–4

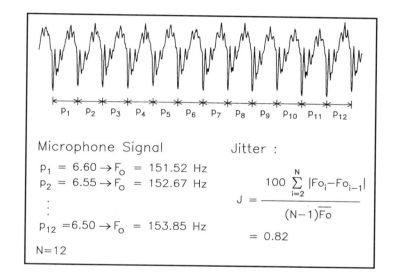

Figure 7–3. Aperiodicity of a microphone signal for a prolonged vowel. The periods of the microphone signal are indicated using the instants of the minimum values, and the calculation of the corresponding jitter is given. This is an example of a measure of voicing perturbation.

Microphone Signal

$p_1 = 6.60 \rightarrow F_o = 151.52$ Hz
$p_2 = 6.55 \rightarrow F_o = 152.67$ Hz
⋮
$p_{12} = 6.50 \rightarrow F_o = 153.85$ Hz

$N = 12$

Jitter :

$$J = \frac{100 \sum_{i=2}^{N} |Fo_i - Fo_{i-1}|}{(N-1)\overline{Fo}}$$

$= 0.82$

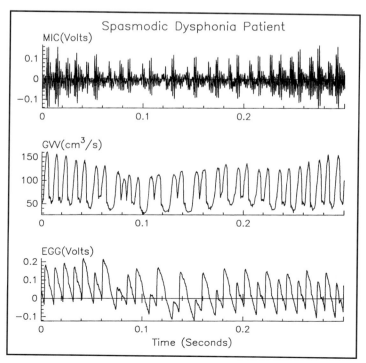

Figure 7–4. Voicing period alterations in a spasmodic dysphonia patient. Microphone, glottal volume velocity, and EGG signals are given, top to bottom. Notice the change from essentially single cycles to cycle clustering of two (and one case of three) cycles. The clustering of two cycles can be seen in all three signals: apparent motion variation of vocal fold contact, double flow pulsing, and double acoustic excitation seen in the microphone signal. (Data courtesy of Dr. Kimberly Fisher)

shows an example of the presence of cycle clustering in the glottal volume velocity signal of a spasmodic dysphonia patient. The cause of this dysfunction appears to be related to hyperadduction or asymmetry of laryngeal muscle function.

In vocal fry and "creaky" voice, pitch may be extremely low and the voice may have varied roughness qualities, depending on the complexity of the low frequency periodicities combined with higher frequency periodicities.[50-54] Figure 7–5 illustrates three different examples of vocal fry[53] (in Reference 53, 11 different types of vocal fry and creaky voice are illustrated). For each case, the microphone signal and the electroglottograph signal are displayed. These samples were created intentionally by a single normal adult male subject. The electroglottographic (EGG) signal may correspond to the contact area between the vocal folds when they touch each other during each cycle.[32,55] Figure 7–5A illustrates vocal fry of low and specific pitch. Each cycle shows a single primary acoustic excitation. This excitation corresponds to the fast upward movement of the EGG signal which corresponds to glottal closure and, therefore, to the glottal volume velocity "shutoff." Figure 7–5B illustrates the typical bimodal electroglottograph signal for vocal fry, with corresponding double acoustic excitations during each (low pitch) cycle. Figure 7–5C illustrates an extreme case of multiple cyclic motions of the vocal folds during each relatively long cycle, with corresponding acoustic excitations.

Pitch can be altered by fluid engorgement (edema). The usual explanation for pitch drop in edema cases is that greater mass creates lower natural frequencies. For example, computer modeling of phonation using biomechanical characteristics of tissue mass, stiffness, and damping relate fundamental frequency to the inverse of the vocal fold mass.[56] Figure 7–6 shows the results of increasing vocal fold mass (only) in a two-mass model of vocal fold function adapted from Ishizaka and Flanagan[57] by Smith.[58] Figure 7–6 shows a decrease in frequency by approximately 5.6 semitones for a doubling of the mass of the vocal folds. For example, for a subglottal pressure of 8 cm H_2O, the change in fundamental frequency for a doubling of the mass is approximately 134 Hz to 97 Hz in the figure.

Subglottal pressure plays a significant role in the control of pitch. Figure 7–6 suggests that an increase in subglottal pressure for a constant vocal fold mass will increase the fundamental frequency. The F_0 changes from 120 Hz to 156 Hz for a mass "M" and subglottal pressure from 4 to 16 cm H_2O for the conditions of Figure 7–6. The literature suggests that a change of 1 cm H_2O subglottal pressure results in a fundamental frequency change of 36 Hz.[59-62] The air pressure pushing against the undersurface of the vocal folds moves the vocal fold laterally and somewhat upwardly.[19,63-66] The extent of the lateral excursion is dependent upon the amount of the subglottal pressure and the length of the vocal folds.[6,67,68] Thus, for a constant anterior-posterior length of the glottis, a greater subglottal pressure will literally push the vocal folds to a greater lateral extent, creating a greater maximum *stretch* than for a lower subglottal pressure. Greater maximum stretch creates higher effective tension and thus a higher fundamental frequency.[6] Intonational (pitch) changes during conversational speech appear to be caused by a significant combination of the passive vocal fold

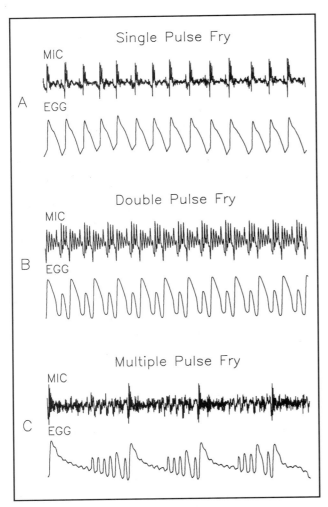

Figure 7–5. Three vocal fry examples. **A.** Single glottal pulses at 30 Hz; **B.** Double glottal pulses at 62 Hz for the period combining the two pulses; and **C.** a multiple pulse case with a low frequency of 7.5 Hz and a higher frequency of 93 Hz. In each grouping, the upper trace is the microphone signal and the lower trace is the electroglottograph signal. The examples were produced by a single adult male subject. See Reference 53.

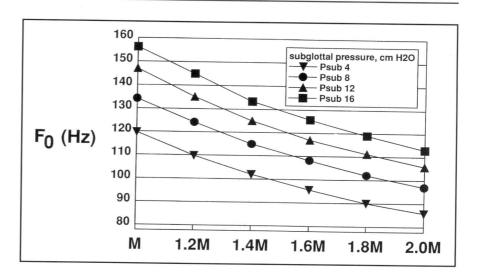

Figure 7–6. Vocal fold mass effect on fundamental frequency. As the amount of mass of the vocal fold in vibration increases, the fundamental frequency decreases. The abscissa ranges from a value of $M = 0.16$ g to twice that. The figure also indicates that fundamental frequency is dependent upon subglottal pressure. (Figure courtesy of Dr. Marshall Smith, who used an adaptation of the Ishizaka and Flanagan simulation.[57,58])

stretch by both the cricothyroid muscles and the subglottal pressure[69,70] (refer especially to the general discussion at the end of Reference 70).

Tension of the vocal fold cover may be changed (and therefore fundamental frequency changed) by external adjustments affecting the length of the vocal folds. Anterior pull of the hyoid bone by suprahyoid muscles may help tilt the thyroid cartilage forward to position its inferior border closer to the superior border of the anterior cricoid cartilage (similar to the function of the cricothyroid muscle), thus increasing vocal fold length and raising the fundamental frequency, as shown by Honda.[71] Alternatively, a suggestion is put forward by Sundberg et al[72] that the cricoid cartilage may be tilted down posteriorly, shortening the vocal fold length, by an inferior tracheal pull. This would come about by lowering the diaphragm with higher lung volume levels (or by coactivation of the diaphragm during phonation), inducing a pitch drop unless compensated for by increased cricothyroid muscle activity.

The above discussion emphasizes the contribution to pitch control through tension change of the vocal fold cover through passive stretch or by increasing subglottal pressure. The fundamental frequency is also dependent upon the activity of the vocalis (thyroarytenoid) muscle.[73,74] The vocalis muscle acts antagonistically to the cricothyroid muscle relative to length change of the cover.[73,75,76] Thus, if only the cover is vibrating, as in soft, high-pitch phonation, increase in vocalis contraction should shorten and reduce the tension of the mucosal cover, and thereby lower the fundamental frequency. However, if the vocalis muscle participates in the motion of the vocal fold to a significant degree, as in loud, low-pitch phonation,

increase in vocalis muscle contraction will increase the effective tension of the entire tissue in motion as a primary effect, and thereby raise the fundamental frequency. The effect on F_0 change related to vocalis muscle involvement conceptually depends on the relative amount of vocalis muscle participating in the vibratory mass, the tension within the vocalis muscle portion of the mass in motion, and the relative activity level of the vocalis muscle, as Titze, Jiang, and Drucker[73] analytically describe. In general then, pitch is controlled by many combinations of cricothyroid muscle contraction (to passively stretch the tissue in motion), vocalis muscle contraction (to passively shorten the cover and actively increase the tension of the vibratory vocalis portion), and subglottal pressure increase (to increase the amount of vocal fold mass placed into vibratory motion and passively stretch the tissue in motion). As a general rule, fundamental frequency would be expected to rise if there is greater tension (passive plus active) of the tissue in motion or less mass of the tissue in motion. Intervention strategies dealing with pitch alteration need to take into consideration these physiologic and aerodynamic bases.

As a segue to the next section on loudness and vocal quality, it is noted that various combinations of cricothyroid and vocalis muscle contraction, with adduction, may change vocal quality, especially relative to the medial shaping of the vocal fold. Greater vocalis muscle contraction tends to round (or medialize) the medial contour of the vocal fold,[74,77,78] potentially decreasing the vibratory threshold pressure[14] and creating a relatively longer closed time of the vocal folds each cycle,[79] which may change the voice spectra to reflect a brighter, louder sound.

LOUDNESS AND QUALITY OF PHONATION

Loudness and quality of phonation are perceptual correlates to the physical measures of intensity and acoustic spectra, respectively.[13,32,80,81] Both perceptions depend upon the glottal volume velocity waveform characteristics and vocal tract resonance structure. We will emphasize the glottal volume velocity here.

Figure 7–7 illustrates a typical glottal volume velocity waveform in modal register with corresponding schematized glottal motion. The general shape of the glottal volume velocity waveform shows that the flow typically begins more gradually than when it is shut off, and the flow maximum is produced after the time when the maximum of the glottal area occurs. This flow delay characteristic (or *skewing* to the right relative to the glottal area) is related to the inertance of the airway, glottal wall motion, and glottal shape. The inertive effect[82,83] refers to the fact that the air within the vocal tract has mass. When the glottis just opens, the air (being driven by the translaryngeal air pressure) moves through the glottis to meet the column of air of the vocal tract. The air coming through the glottis must literally move other air already within the vocal tract, and this requirement slows the motion of the air as it first comes out of the glottis.[2,84] Corresponding to this event is the increase in air pressure just above the glottis as air moves through the glottis into the air above, thus typically reducing the translaryngeal pressure drop.[2,85-89] If the vocal tract were modeled as a uniform tube, greater glottal airflow skewing would be created from greater inertance by elongating the vocal tract (through larynx lowering or lip protrusion) or by narrowing the cross-sectional vocal tract area.[89,90] Fant[86] showed analytically that skewing increases not only with an increase of the vocal tract inertance (which changes with certain vowels and is higher with a constriction at the false fold level), but also with an increase in the maximum glottal excursion during the phonatory cycle, a faster glottal closing time, a lower subglottal pressure, and a smaller glottal kinetic flow factor k (the latter is derived in detail in References 91 and 92), concepts fruitful for clinical and training considerations. After the moment of maximum flow, the airflow will reduce to zero or to its minimum value as the two vocal folds come together at the end of glottal closing.

Skewing of the glottal volume velocity is related to the motion of the vocal folds according to a numerical model by Alipour and Scherer.[93] The lower margin of the vibrating vocal fold may have a different amplitude of motion than the upper margin, and the two margins may vary in their relative phase during the cy-

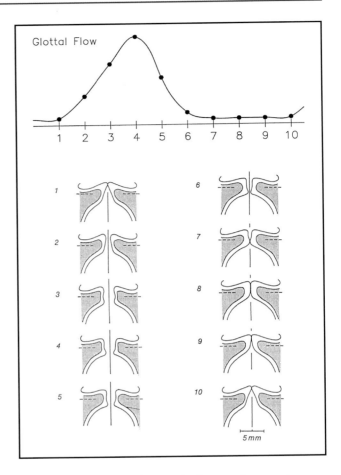

Figure 7–7. Glottal volume velocity waveform and corresponding glottal motion. The specific phases of the glottal cycle shown in the motion schematic are indicated on the glottal volume velocity waveform. (Adapted with permission from Hirano, M. *Clinical Examination of Voice*. Copyright 1981, Springer-Verlag.[30])

cle. Skewing of the glottal volume flow appears to increase as the amplitude of the lower margin increases relative to the upper margin, and decreases as the phase lead of the lower margin increases relative to the upper margin. This suggests that there may be an optimal compromise between amplitude and phase differences between the lower and upper glottal margins to maximize the skewing of the glottal volume velocity.

As Figure 7–7 shows, the glottis takes on a number of shapes during the vibratory cycle. A duct that expands in shape (a diffuser shape as suggested in steps 4, 5, and 6 of Figure 7–7) can have less resistance to flow than one of the same but constant (uniform) diameter.[91,92,94,95] The minimum flow resistance may occur when the glottis creates a diffuser shape of small angle (estimated to be between 5° and 10°[96-97]), which would most likely occur just past the time of the maximum glottal area. Therefore, when the glottis takes on the shape of a small-angled diffuser, the flow resistance may be less than at maximum glottal opening, and greater flow may then exit the glottis, to help skew the flow to the right relative to glottal area.

In general, then, if greater skewing of the glottal volume velocity is desired (as would be the case for any clinical or training condition needing greater energy in higher harmonic frequencies, see below), physiologic maneuvers should be considered to bring about the following: increase in the inertance of the vocal tract, increase in the lateral excursion of the vocal folds, decrease in the phase lead of the lower margin relative to the upper margin, and increase in the speed of glottal closure. These maneuvers would depend upon adjustments of the vocal tract shaping and length, level of glottal adduction (see below), level of subglottal pressure, and alteration in differential thyroarytenoid muscle contraction. These coordinations for optimal shaping and sizing of the glottal volume velocity waveform are central themes of needed research.

The qualities of the voice depend upon the glottal volume velocity waveform. Figure 7–8 shows an example of breathy (hypoadducted), normal, and pressed (hyperadducted) phonations in a normal adult male. The figure demonstrates typical variations of the glottal flow, the spectrum of the glottal flow, and the electroglottograph (EGG) waveforms for these qualities (the signals are not exactly time aligned). A Glottal Enterprises wide-band pneumotach system was used to acquire the inverse filtered (glottal) flow, and a Synchrovoice Laryngograph was used to obtain the EGG signal. Breathy voice is characterized by a more sinusoidal flow waveform than for normal phonation, with a significant flow bias. The flow bias is seen as a shift of the waveform away from the zero-flow baseline, indicating that there is always some flow exiting the glottis because of nonclosure throughout the cycle (the bias is also called the *DC flow*). In pressed phonation, the peaks of the flow are significantly smaller than for normal phonation, and the amount of time within the cycle during which the air exits the glottis is relatively short. Spectrally, the breathy quality example has energy primarily in the first two partials, whereas greater energy is distributed to higher harmonic frequencies in the normal and pressed quality examples. Up to 1000 Hz, the spectral slope is relatively steep at -17.3 dB/octave for breathy voice, less steep

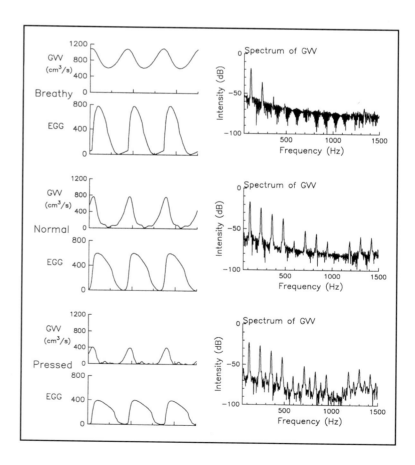

Figure 7–8. Breathy, normal, and pressed voice qualities. Glottal volume velocity and EGG waveforms are shown, as well as the spectrum of the glottal volume velocity waveforms. The subject was a normal adult male.

at -14.4 dB/octave for normal, and flattest at -10.8 dB/octave for the pressed condition for the examples in Figure 7–8. Notice the relative reduction in the level of the fundamental frequency compared to the first overtone from breathy to normal to pressed. The EGG waveforms suggest that there was a relatively large change of contact area between the surfaces of the two vocal folds during the breathy voicing, as seen by the relatively large amplitude (note that the greater the extent of the EGG waveform, the more vocal fold contact area change there is presumed to be[55]). However, the time during which the glottis was open, shown by the baseline length of the waveform, was relatively long in the breathy phonation compared to the other two qualities. The height of the pressed quality EGG waveform is shortest, suggesting relatively less dynamic contact of the vocal fold surfaces. This was explained by viewing the subject's larynx with stroboscopy; in pressed voice, the compression allowed only a restricted anterior glottal region to vibrate, thus resulting in the relatively short amplitudes because less of the total medial vocal fold surface participated in the vibration.

The overall intensity or sound pressure level (SPL) of the output sound may increase with increase in the maximum rate of change of the glottal volume velocity "shutoff" (the value M shown in Figure 7–2).[12,98-100] The maximum rate of change of the glottal flow is also the maximum negative slope, or *the maximum flow declination rate*. Greater maximum slope has the spectral effect of raising the energy of the partials primarily within the region of the first formant,[101] usually the most important spectral portion for overall SPL. This is like "turning [up] the volume control"[12(p.562)] (see also Reference 102). A doubling of the maximum negative slope corresponds empirically to an approximate increase of 5 to 9 dB in overall SPL.[12] Increased skewing of the glottal flow (discussed above) through increased vocal tract inertance and greater vocal fold motion should raise the overall SPL. For example, in their numerical study, Alipour and Scherer[93] found that increasing the amplitude of the lower glottal margin alone by 50% produced an increase in closing slope of more than 50%. These suggestions of acoustic (inertance) and kinematic (vocal fold motion) aides to enhance the desired characteristics of the glottal volume velocity need to be explored with human subject studies to eventually improve treatment and training of people with voice concerns.

It is of importance to note some other spectral effects of differences in the glottal volume velocity waveform. The amount of time the waveform shows air exiting the glottis (time A to time B in Figure 7–2) divided by the period of the cycle (time A to time C in Figure

7–2) is called the *open quotient*. The open quotient typically decreases when changing adduction from a more breathy to a more normal quality voice, and with increase in loudness.[14] When the open quotient decreases, there may be a minor reduction (a few dB) of the intensity of the fundamental frequency and possibly a minor boost (a few dB) of the intensity of the first overtone (an octave above the fundamental frequency).[102,103] Also, the greater the amplitude of the volume velocity waveform (or the greater the area under the volume velocity waveform), the greater is the amplitude of the fundamental frequency.[12,101,104] A doubling of the amplitude of the waveform corresponds to an increase of approximately 3 to 7 dB in the spectral level of the fundamental frequency. When the flow has nearly completely shut off, that is, when the flow has nearly reached the baseline just before glottal closure, there is a "shutoff corner." The sharpness of this corner is related to the energy generated in the overtones of the voice, according to the modeling by Fant and his colleagues.[101-103] A change from a well-rounded corner to a very sharp corner can cause the intensity of the overtones to increase by up to 10 to 20 dB, undoubtedly affecting the quality of the sound[102,103] (changing glottal adduction from a breathy voice quality to a normal quality would sharpen this flow shutoff corner considerably). This concept needs exploration relative to how the vocal folds come together and to the perception of vocal quality, especially taken in the context of clinical intervention and vocal performance instruction.

The intensity and spectra of the glottal airflow are dependent on subglottal air pressure and fundamental frequency. As subglottal air pressure increases for a constant level of glottal adduction, the maximum (peak) airflow through the glottis increases. This follows from the greater maximum glottal width that is created when subglottal air pressure increases (see discussion above) and the greater driving pressure across the larger opening (see, eg, Reference 105). As the maximum value of the volume velocity waveform increases, the intensity level of the fundamental frequency increases, as discussed above.[12] Also, if the peak flow increases, the maximum flow derivative should typically increase as the flow must reduce to zero (or near zero) from a greater value if the time during which the flow decreases remains the same.[100] An increase in the maximum flow derivative will increase the overall SPL and augment the spectrum, as indicated above. In addition, the increase in subglottal pressure may cause the vocal folds to come back together faster (or perhaps alter their dynamic phasing) after their larger maximum excursion, creating a sharper flow shutoff corner near the baseline, raising the overall spectrum of the overtones. Therefore, greater subglottal pressure may contribute to increasing the flow peak, increasing the maximum flow derivative, and sharpening the baseline flow shutoff corner. These effects change the flow spectrum shape by increasing the intensity level of the fundamental frequency and increasing the intensity of the overtones, thus raising the overall intensity of the voice. Titze and Sundberg[99] show explicitly how a doubling of subglottal pressure (more precisely, a doubling of the difference between subglottal pressure and threshold pressure) raises source acoustic power by 6 dB. Fant[86] broke down the intensity increase relative to the contributions of increased air velocity, increased maximum glottal area during the cycle, reduced time the glottis is open, faster glottal closing, and an increased flow derivative, totaling approximately 6 dB in intensity gain for a doubling of subglottal pressure. The early literature showed that voice intensity is strongly associated with subglottal pressure,[106-110] and this discussion has attempted to offer what has been suggested as an explanation as to how the subglottal pressure increase affects the sound source volume velocity waveform and the resultant increase of intensity.

Intensity is affected strongly by the fundamental frequency of voice production. Titze and Sundberg[99] show that the glottal power output will increase by 6 dB for an octave rise in fundamental frequency (all else the same), caused by the increase in the maximum flow derivative as the fundamental frequency rises (the same waveform shape with a shorter cycle period has a larger maximum flow derivative). At this point, one might ask why females, who speak at about 9 to 10 semitones above the fundamental frequency of men,[32] typically do not sound louder than men, and indeed do not differ substantially from men in intensity.[111] The just-mentioned effect of the higher frequency for women (about a ratio of 1.7 to 1) is potentially offset by a larger amplitude of glottal volume velocity for males (a ratio of about 2 to 1) so that the SPL for females is only 1 to 2 dB lower than for males.[99,111] In possible support, it is noted that Sapienza and Stathopoulos[112] found that the maximum flow derivative was essentially the same between men and women when they produced the same SPL values. Furthermore, Sulter and Wit[113] found that at normal and loud levels, the maximum flow derivative for untrained men was approximately double that for untrained women at comparable SPL levels. These conflicting data suggest that this area of study is unresolved.

Because vocal sound is created by the glottal volume velocity, intervention strategies should attempt to improve the glottal airflow waveform, as mentioned above. There may be combinations of voicing variables that produce optimally efficient voice production from acoustic and physiologic orientations. Titze[114] has reported maximal intensity production in excised dog larynges for vocal processes that are placed very near each other, with less intensity (ranging to a few dB) for greater and less adduction. Sundberg[13] (also see Reference 104) has proposed the term *flow mode*, a type of phonation in which the glottal volume velocity amplitude is relatively large with high efficiency of laryngeal function. This is further emphasized, perhaps diagnostically, by examining the value of the flow amplitude divided by the subglottal pressure (the *glottal permittance*[100]). This ratio allows a clear separation between a pressed (constricted) voice versus normal and "flow" phonations (for a limited number of subjects[100]) because of the greater flow amplitudes for the same subglottal pressure in the normal and "flow" types. It is of considerable importance (theoretically and clinically) that professional (classically trained) male singers may produce voiced sounds at higher intensity levels than male nonsingers for the same subglottal pressures, caused primarily by greater glottal flow amplitudes (from adjusted flow impedance).[14,99] In addition, performance training strategies have emphasized vocal tract adjustments to match lower voicing partials with the first formant[115] or to create an enhanced higher formant region[116,117] by clustering formants numbers 3, 4, and 5, strategies that boost the output energy of certain partials of the voice, creating a "bright" or "carrying" voice with desirable performance qualities. These tactics are not dissimilar to strategies employed in voice pathology (eg, References 118 and 119).

VOCAL FOLD MOTION DURING PHONATION

Although it is important to realize that the creation of the sound of voicing is within the airflow exiting the glottis, and not in the motion of the vocal folds per se, the motion of the vocal folds helps to determine the characteristics of the airflow.

Basic kinematic (motion) aspects of normal vocal folds include the effects of increased subglottal pressure, vocal fold elongation, and glottal adduction. Increased subglottal pressure produces increased lateral pressures on the medial surfaces and vertical pressures on the undersurface of the vocal folds, creating greater maximum excursion during the vibratory cycle (as discussed above). Elongation of the vocal folds by increased contraction of the cricothyroid muscles and/or decreased contraction of the thyroarytenoid muscles modifies the cross-sectional shape of the vocal fold (with no change of total vocal fold mass) to form a reduced vocal fold thickness (measured in the vertical direction),[120-123] giving rise to potentially less vocal fold tissue contact during vocal fold closure. For the same subglottal pressure and glottal adduction, vocal fold lengthening would affect the glottal volume velocity waveform by increasing the open quotient and decreasing the maximum flow derivative. Increased adduction will affect the motion of the vocal folds by creating more contact between the vocal folds and a longer glottal closed time within each cycle.[48,124-128] Any abnormality of tissue morphology (swelling, stiffness, or growth along the vocal fold), unilaterally or bilaterally, may alter the vibratory motion to create different glottal volume velocity waveforms from cycle to cycle, or from cycle group to cycle group (refer to the earlier discussion on perturbation). Severe laryngitis associated with extreme edema creates the well-known response of aphonia (inability to phonate or absence of phonation), which may be explained by the mass being too great to permit vibration, and the rounded glottal shaping causing less effective intraglottal pressures during phonation.[129] Refer to Hirano and Bless[130] for photographs of vibratory patterns for a number of vocal pathologies including nodules, polyps, cysts, and others.

These kinds of structural changes to the vocal folds lead to the question: How is the vibration of the vocal folds maintained? That is, what allows them to remain in oscillation? A response to this question will now be explored.

The mechanical phonatory motion of the vocal folds depends upon the folds being driven by air pressures within the glottis,[91,96,131-136] such air pressure forces working with the biomechanical characteristics of the vocal folds (mass, stiffness, damping) to overcome the damping losses within the tissue.[22,57,66,137-142] The *intraglottal pressures* are extremely important, then, in the maintenance of vocal fold oscillation.[2,8,142] If the intraglottal pressures are positive, they act to push the vocal folds away from each other. If the intraglottal pressures are negative, they pull the vocal folds toward each other. The polarity (positive or negative) of the intraglottal pressure depends upon both the dynamic air pressures directly above and below the glottis and the shape of the glottal airway, as will now be discussed (see References 2 and 90).

The acoustic air pressure just above the glottis may be important for maintaining vocal fold oscillation. As the glottis nears closure during a normal vibratory cycle, the airflow through the glottis decreases relatively quickly. The air that has already passed through the glottis continues to travel up the vocal tract, creating greater distance between itself (the air) and the glottis. This air momentum produces a negative rarefaction pressure directly above the glottis as the particles of air separate more and more from each other. Negative pressure at the glottal exit location would create pressures that are negative within the glottis (at least within the glottal duct near the exit) if the glottis has not closed at the lower glottal edge. The intraglottal negative pressure, located at least near the glottal exit, thus should facilitate the final closing of the glottis by pulling the two folds together (aided by the closing momentum of the tissue itself). The amount of the negative intraglottal pressure would depend upon the value of the maximum negative supraglottal pressure.

As the glottis opens during a vibratory cycle, the airflow through the glottis meets the mass of air directly above it, creating compression of the air and positive air pressure. The positive air pressure directly above the glottis creates positive air pressure within the glottis, at least near the glottal exit. The intraglottal positive pressure caused by the positive supraglottal pressure would therefore facilitate glottal opening by pushing on the vocal folds to help separate them. Thus, during opening, supraglottal positive pressure aids glottal opening, and during closing, supraglottal negative pressure aids glottal closing.

The glottis takes on two primary shapes during (exhalatory) phonation, *convergent* and *divergent* (see Figure 7–9).[18,143-145] During glottal opening, the convergent glottal shape is produced with a wider opening at glottal entrance and a narrower opening at glottal exit (Figure 7–7). Because of the convergent shape, a pressure drop (from a higher value to a lower value, Figure 7–9) is created from the positive tracheal pressure to the pressure existing at the glottal exit location,[96] which may be close to positive (as discussed above) or near atmospheric. Thus, the glottal convergent shape (itself) creates a positive pressure within the glottis, and this positive pressure pushes on the vocal folds, facilitating glottal opening. This pressure decrease within the converging glottis follows directly from the Bernoulli equation (for steady flow).

During glottal closing, the divergent glottal shape may be most prominent; the configuration has a narrower opening at glottal entrance than at glottal exit (Figure 7–9). Divergent glottal duct shapes are similar to mechanical diffusers in that the expanding area allows pressures within the duct to increase between the upstream inlet and the downstream outlet.[94,96,97] The pressure at glottal entry is, therefore, lower than at exit, and is negative within the glottis if the glottal exit pressure is atmospheric (zero) or negative (per the discussion above on glottal closing). This negative pressure is caused by the divergent shape of the glottis, with the minimal duct diameter formed at entry, creating the lowest pressure there (at entry) essentially in

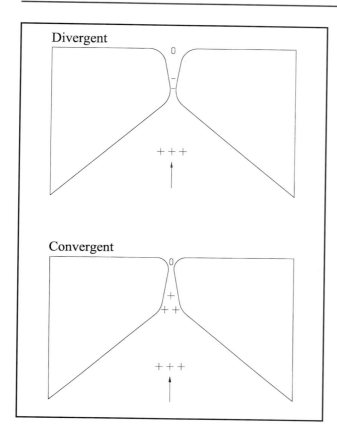

Divergent

Convergent

Figure 7–9. Pressures within the glottis relative to glottal shape. In the *convergent* glottis (*lower sketch*), the air pressures are positive in the entrance of the glottis and decrease to zero (or to the pressure just above the glottis). In the *divergent* glottis (*upper sketch*), the air pressures are negative in the entrance of the glottis and increase to zero (or to the pressure just above the glottis).

accordance with the Bernoulli equation. The negative intraglottal pressure would pull on the vocal fold surfaces, facilitating glottal closure.

The "Bernoulli effect" refers to the existence of negative pressure in a narrowed location of a duct through which air (fluid) is flowing. This is the result of the trade-off (described by the Bernoulli equation) between air pressure and air particle velocity for different size sections of the duct (lower pressure and higher velocity exist in a narrower section). The Bernoulli effect has been used historically to help "explain" phonation (Tonndorf was an important early proponent of this concept for the maintenance of vocal fold oscillation, see Reference 146). That is, as the air particles speed up as they enter the glottis from the trachea, the air pressure supposedly would become negative throughout the glottis because it would constitute a smaller opening than the trachea, and then the

negative pressure would suck the folds toward each other regardless of the glottal shape. This explanation is incomplete. During glottal opening, when the glottis has a convergent shape and the minimal glottal diameter is at the glottal exit, the Bernoulli energy equation does help to explain the pressure *reduction* from the glottal entrance to the glottal exit, but the intraglottal pressure is positive, not negative, despite the glottis being smaller than the trachea, because the pressure lowers from the positive tracheal value to the positive or near zero value at glottal exit. During glottal closing when the glottis forms a divergent (diffuser) shape, the pressure reduction from the trachea to glottal entry may follow the Bernoulli equation for the most part, but the application of the Bernoulli equation within the glottis would essentially apply only in the special case of no flow separation from the glottal walls. *Flow separation,* in which the air flows away from the glottal wall rather than staying close to the wall, occurs when there is a sufficient pressure rise in the diverging glottal duct. This creates a condition where the Bernoulli equation no longer applies beyond the flow separation point.[96,132,133,147] The pressure will increase from a negative value at the entrance to the glottis to a rather constant value (equal to the air pressure just downstream of the glottis) a short distance past the air separation location for these divergent glottis conditions.[147] These concepts are based on steady (constant) flow modeling with static glottal shapes of many angles.[97]

The pressure on the medial vocal folds during vibration is more complex than indicated above. During phonation the glottis viewed superiorly is rather elliptical in shape, with greatest amplitude of motion near the middle of the membranous glottis. Pressures appear to vary the most during the cycle within the glottis at the location of the maximum motion, with cyclic pressure variations decreasing anteriorly and posteriorly to this location.[136] These dynamic glottal pressure changes are called *bidirectional pressure gradients.*[136]

Another interesting complexity of glottal pressures is that, even when the glottis forms a symmetric convergent or divergent duct, the pressures on the two vocal folds may not be identical because of flow separation only on one side of the glottis and not the other side, or because the flow bends to one side downstream of the glottis.[97,147] However, there may not be time to develop these glottal wall pressure differences during phonation because the geometry changes so quickly.[148-150] When the glottal duct is slanted to one side, as can be seen in some normal and abnormal phonations in which the two vocal folds vibrate out of phase with each other,[151-153] the pressures on the two sides of the glottis may be substantially different.[147]

These pressure differences may promote the out-of-phase motion of the two vocal folds.

The actual interdependence among dynamic (time-varying) glottal shaping, translaryngeal pressures, and intraglottal pressures, and the application of equations of mechanics, require precise empirical measurement of glottal shaping, flows, and pressures during phonation, research yet to be adequately performed. In addition, the relationship among these aspects, the particle velocities that make up the glottal flow, and the resulting acoustic signal[33,154-164] extend this matter to the necessary and interfacing aeroacoustic level of phonation.

SUMMARY

This chapter has reviewed basic aspects of laryngeal function during phonation. The concepts underlying the understanding of duration, frequency, intensity, spectra, and vocal fold motion during phonation are the bases with which to make effective intervention decisions for laryngeal and voice change. These underlying concepts are applicable to both clinical and training practices.

Acknowledgments   The author is grateful to and would like to thank Chwen Guo and Daoud Shinwari for their help with the figures, Kimberly Fisher for the use of her spasmodic dysphonia data, Marshall Smith for his figure dealing with vocal mass and fundamental frequency change, Tamara Field for help in preparing Figure 7–1, and David Kuehn for an anatomical discussion. This project was prepared with support from NIDCD grants P60 DC00976 RTC and R01 DC03577, and is dedicated to the memory and mentorship of Dr. Wilbur James Gould.

REFERENCES

1. Scherer RC. Aerodynamic assessment in voice production. In: Cooper JA, ed. *Assessment of Speech and Voice Production: Research and Clinical Applications.* NIDCD Monograph Vol 1-1991. Bethesda, MD: National Institute on Deafness and Other Communication Disorders, NIH; 1991:112–123.
2. Scherer RC. Physiology of phonation: A review of basic mechanics. In: Ford CN, Bless DM, eds. *Phonosurgery: Assessment and Surgical Management of Voice Disorders.* New York, NY: Raven Press; 1991:77–93.
3. Hollien H, Moore GP. Measurement of the vocal folds during changes in pitch. *J Speech Hear Res.* 1960;3:157–165.
4. Nishizawa N, Sawashima M, Yonemoto K. In: Fujimura O, ed. *Vocal Physiology: Voice Production, Mechanisms, and Function.* New York, NY: Raven Press; 1988:75–82.
5. Backus J. *The Acoustical Foundations of Music.* 2nd ed. New York, NY: WW Norton & Co; 1977.
6. Titze IR, Durham PL. Passive mechanisms influencing fundamental frequency control. In: Baer T, Sasaki C, Harris KS, eds. *Laryngeal Function in Phonation and Respiration.* San Diego, CA: College-Hill Press; 1987:304–319.
7. Colton RH. Physiological mechanisms of vocal frequency control: the role of tension. *J Voice.* 1988;2(3):208–220.
8. Titze IR. *Principles of Voice Production.* Englewood Cliffs, NJ: Prentice Hall; 1994.
9. Perlman AL, Titze IR. Development of an in vitro technique for measuring elastic properties of vocal fold tissue. *J Speech Hear Res.* 1988;31/2:288–289.
10. Colton RH, Casper JK. *Understanding Voice Problems.* Baltimore, MD: Williams & Wilkins; 1990.
11. Hammarberg B, Fritzell B, Gauffin J, Sundberg J. Acoustic glottogram, subglottic pressure, and voice quality during insufficient vocal fold closure phonation. *Proceedings of the International Conference on Voice, Kurume, Japan.* 1986:28–35.
12. Gauffin J, Sundberg J. Spectral correlates of glottal voice source waveform characteristics. *J Speech Hear Res.* 1989;32:556–565.
13. Sundberg J. *The Science of the Singing Voice.* Dekalb, IL: Northern Illinois University Press; 1987.
14. Titze IR. Phonation threshold pressure: a missing link in glottal aerodynamics. *J Acoust Soc Am.* 1992;91(5):2926–2935.
15. Lucero JC. Optimal glottal configuration for ease of phonation. *J Voice.* 1998;12:151–158.
16. Chan RW, Titze IR, Titze MR. Further studies of phonation threshold pressure in a physical model of the vocal fold mucosa. *J Acoust Soc Am.* 1997;101:3722–3727.
17. Verdolini-Marston K, Titze I, Druker D. Changes in phonation threshold pressure with induced conditions of hydration. *J Voice.* 1990;4(2):142–151.
18. Baer T. *Investigation of Phonation Using Excised Larynges* [dissertation]. Cambridge, MA: Massachusetts Institute of Technology; 1975.
19. Baer T. Observation of vocal fold vibration: Measurement of excised larynges. In: Stevens KN, Hirano M, eds. *Vocal Fold Physiology.* Tokyo, Japan: University of Tokyo Press; 1981:119–133.
20. Draper MH, Ladefoged P, Whitteridge D. Expiratory pressures and air flow during speech. *British Med J.* 1960;18:1837–1843.
21. Berry DA, Herzel H, Titze IR, Story BH. Bifurcation in excised larynx experiments. *J Voice.* 1996;10:129–138.
22. Lucero JC. A theoretical study of the hysteresis phenomenon at vocal fold oscillation onset-offset. *J Acoust Soc Am.* 1999;105:423–431.
23. Fisher KV, Swank PR. Estimating phonation threshold pressure. *J Speech Hear Res.* 1997;40:1122–1129.
24. Coleman RF, Mabis JH, Hinson JK. Fundamental frequency-sound pressure level profiles of adult male and female voices. *J Speech Hear Res.* 1977;20:197–204.
25. Klingholz F, Martin F. Die quantitative Auswertung der Stimmfeldmessung. *Sprache-Stimme-Gehör.* 1983;7:106–110.
26. Titze IR. Acoustic interpretation of the voice range profile (phonetogram). *J Speech Hear Res.* 1992;35:21–34.

27. Coleman RF. Sources of variation in phonetograms. *J Voice.* 1993;7(1):1–14.

28. Gramming P. *The Phonetogram: An Experimental and Clinical Study.* Malmo, Sweden: Department of Otolaryngology, University of Lund; 1988.

29. Bless DM, Baken RJ, Hacki T, et al. International Association of Logopedics and Phoniatrics (IALP) Voice Committee discussion of assessment topics. *J Voice.* 1992;6(2):194–210.

30. Hirano M. *Clinical Examination of Voice.* New York, NY: Springer-Verlag; 1981.

31. Hirose H, Niimi S. The relationship between glottal opening and the transglottal pressure differences during consonant production. In: Baer T, Sasaki C, Harris KS, eds. *Laryngeal Function in Phonation and Respiration.* San Diego, CA: College-Hill Press; 1987:381–390.

32. Baken RJ. Clinical *Measurement of Speech and Voice.* Boston, MA: College-Hill Press, Little, Brown & Co; 1987.

33. Kakita Y. Simultaneous observation of the vibratory pattern, sound pressure, and airflow signals using a physical model of the vocal folds. In: Fujimura O, ed. *Vocal Physiology: Voice Production, Mechanisms, and Function.* New York, NY: Raven Press Ltd.; 1988:207–218.

34. Fant G. Some problems in voice source analysis. *Speech Commun.* 1993;13:7–22.

35. Kiritani S, Hirose H, Imagawa H. High-speed digital image analysis of vocal cord vibration in diplophonia. *Speech Commun.* 1993;13:23–32.

36. Pinto NB, Titze IR. Unification of perturbation measures in speech signals. *J Acoust Soc Am.* 1990;87(3):1278–1289.

37. Larson C, Kempster G, Kistler M. Changes in voice fundamental frequency following discharge of single motor units in cricothyroid and thyroarytenoid muscles. *J Speech Hear Res.* 1987;30:552–558.

38. Kempster GB, Larson CR, Kistler MK. Effects of electrical stimulation of cricothyroid and thyroarytenoid muscles on voice fundamental frequency. *J Voice.* 1988;2(3):221–229.

39. Titze IR. A model for neurologic sources of aperiodicity in vocal fold vibration. *J Speech Hear Res.* 1991;34(3):460–472.

40. Baer T. Vocal jitter: A neuromuscular explanation. In: Lawrence V, Weinberg B, eds. *Transcripts of the Eighth Symposium on Care of the Professional Voice.* New York, NY: The Voice Foundation; 1979:19–22.

41. Cavalli L, Hirson A. Diplophonia reappraised. *J Voice.* 1999;13:542–556.

42. Isshiki N, Ishizaka K. Computer simulation of pathological vocal cord vibration. *J Acoust Soc Am.* 1976;60:1193–1198.

43. Moon FC. *Chaotic Vibrations.* New York, NY: John Wiley & Sons; 1987.

44. Gerratt BR, Precoda K, Hanson D, Berke GS. Source characteristics of diplophonia. *J Acoust Soc Am.* 1988;83:S66.

45. Wong D, Ito MR, Cox NB, Titze IR. Observation of perturbations in a lumped-element model of the vocal folds with application to some pathological cases. *J Acoust Soc Am.* 1991;89:383–394.

46. Berke GS, Gerratt BR. Laryngeal biomechanics: an overview of mucosal wave mechanics. *J Voice.* 1993;7(2):123–128.

47. Titze IR, Baken RJ, Herzel H. Evidence of chaos in vocal fold vibration. In: Titze IR, ed. *Vocal Fold Physiology: Frontiers in Basic Science.* San Diego, CA: Singular Publishing Group; 1993:143–188.

48. Scherer R, Gould WJ, Titze I, Meyers A, Sataloff R. Preliminary evaluation of selected acoustic and glottographic measures for clinical phonatory function analysis. *J Voice.* 1988;2:230–244.

49. Omori K, Kojima H, Kakani R, Slavit DH, Blaugrund SM. Acoustic characteristics of rough voice: subharmonics. *J Voice.* 1997;1:40–47.

50. Hollien H, Moore P, Wendahl RW, Michel JF. On the nature of vocal fry. *J Speech Hear Res.* 1966;9:245–247.

51. Keidar A. *Vocal Register Change: An Investigation of Perceptual and Acoustic Isomorphism* [dissertation]. Iowa City: The University of Iowa; 1986.

52. Titze IR. A framework for the study of vocal registers. *J Voice.* 1988:2(3):183–194.

53. Scherer RC. Physiology of creaky voice and vocal fry. *J Acoust Soc Am.* 1989;86(S1):S25(A).

54. Blomgren M, Chen Y, Ng ML, Gilbert HR. Acoustic, aerodynamic, physiologic, and perceptual properties of modal and vocal fry registers. *J Acoust Soc Am.* 1998;103:2649–2658.

55. Scherer RC, Druker DG, Titze IR. Electroglottography and direct measurement of vocal fold contact area. In: Fujimura O, ed. *Vocal Physiology: Voice Production, Mechanisms, and Function.* New York, NY: Raven Press, Ltd; 1988:279–291.

56. Ishizaka K, Matsudaira M. Analysis of the vibration of the vocal cords. *J Acoust Soc Jap.* 1968;24:311–312.

57. Ishizaka K, Flanagan JL. Synthesis of voiced sounds from a two-mass model of the vocal cords. *Bell Sys Tech J.* 1972;51(6):1233–1268.

58. Smith ME, Berke GS, Gerratt BR, Kreiman J. Laryngeal paralysis: theoretical considerations and effects on laryngeal vibration. *J Speech Hear Res.* 1992;35:545–554.

59. Rothenberg M, Mahshie J. Induced transglottal pressure variations during voicing. *Speech Commun.* 1986;14(3)-4:365–371.

60. Baer T. Reflex activation of laryngeal muscles by sudden induced subglottal pressure changes. *J Acoust Soc Am.* 1979;65:1271–1275.

61. Cheng YM, Guerin B. Control parameters in male and female glottal sources. In: Baer T, Sasaki C, Harris KS, eds. *Laryngeal Function in Phonation and Respiration.* San Diego, CA: College-Hill Press; 1987:219–238.

62. Baken RJ, Orlikoff RF. Phonatory response to step-function changes in supraglottal pressure. In: Baer T, Sasaki C, Harris KS, eds. *Laryngeal Function in Phonation and Respiration.* San Diego, CA: College-Hill Press; 1987:273–290.

63. Saito S, Fukuda H, Isogai Y, Ono H. X-ray stroboscopy. In: Stevens KN, Hirano M, eds. *Vocal Fold Physiology.* Tokyo, Japan: University of Tokyo Press; 1981:95–106.

64. Saito S, Fukuda H, Kitahara S, et al. Pellet tracking in the vocal fold while phonating—experimental study using canine larynges with muscle activity. In: Titze IR, Scherer RC, eds. *Vocal Fold Physiology: Biomechanics, Acoustics and Phonatory Control.* Denver, CO: The Denver Center for the Performing Arts; 1985:169–182.

65. Fukuda H, Saito S, Kitahara S, et al. Vocal fold vibration in excised larynges viewed with an x-ray stroboscope and an ultra-high-speed camera. In: Bless DM, Abbs JH, eds. *Vocal Fold Physiology, Contemporary Research and Clinical Issues.* San Diego, CA: College-Hill Press; 1983: 238–252.

66. Alipour-Haghighi F, Titze IR. Simulation of particle trajectories of vocal fold tissue during phonation. In: Titze IR, Scherer RC, eds. *Vocal Fold Physiology: Biomechanics, Acoustics and Phonatory Control.* Denver, CO: The Denver Center for the Performing Arts; 1985:183–190.

67. Muta H, Fukuda H. Pressure-flow relationship in the experimental phonation of excised canine larynges. In: Fujimura O, ed. *Vocal Physiology: Voice Production, Mechanisms, and Function.* New York, NY: Raven Press, Ltd; 1988:239–247.

68. Titze IR, Luschei ES, Hirano M. Role of the thyroarytenoid muscle in regulation of fundamental frequency. *J Voice.* 1989;3(3):213–224.

69. Gelfer CE, Harris KS, Collier R, Baer T. Is declination actively controlled? In: Titze IR, Scherer RC, eds. *Vocal Fold Physiology: Biomechanics, Acoustics and Phonatory Control.* Denver, CO: The Denver Center for the Performing Arts; 1985:113–126.

70. Gelfer CE, Harris KS, Baer T. Controlled variables in sentence intonation. In: Baer T, Sasaki C, Harris KS, eds. *Laryngeal Function in Phonation and Respiration.* San Diego, CA: College-Hill Press; 1987:422–435.

71. Honda K. Relationship between pitch control and vowel articulation. In: Bless DM, Abbs JH, eds. *Vocal Fold Physiology, Contemporary Research and Clinical Issues.* San Diego, CA: College-Hill Press; 1983:286–297.

72. Sundberg J, Leanderson R, von Euler C. Activity relationship between diaphragm and cricothyroid muscles. *J Voice.* 1989;3(3):225–232.

73. Titze IR, Jiang J, Drucker DG. Preliminaries to the body-cover theory of pitch control. *J Voice.* 1988;1(4):314–319.

74. Choi HS, Berke GS, Ye M, Kreiman J. Function of the thyroarytenoid muscle in a canine laryngeal model. *Ann Otol Rhinol Laryngol.* 1993;102:769–776.

75. Arnold GE. Physiology and pathology of the cricothyroid muscle. *Laryngoscope.* 1961;71:687–753.

76. Fujimura O. Body-cover theory of the vocal fold and its phonetic implications. In: Stevens KN, Hirano M, eds. *Vocal Fold Physiology.* Tokyo, Japan: University of Tokyo Press; 1981:271–288.

77. Hirano M. Phonosurgery: Basic and clinical investigations. *Otologia (Fukuoka).* 1975;21:239–442.

78. Hirano M. The laryngeal muscles in singing. In: Hirano M, Kirchner JA, Bless DM, eds. *Neurolaryngology, Recent Advances.* Boston, MA: A College-Hill Publication, Little, Brown & Co; 1987:209–230.

79. Titze IR. A four-parameter model of the glottis and vocal fold contact area. *Speech Commun.* 1989;8:191–201.

80. Plomp R. *Aspects of Tone Sensation.* New York, NY: Academic Press; 1976.

81. Strong WJ, Plitnik GR. *Music Speech Audio.* Provo, UT: Soundprint; 1992.

82. Rothenberg M. Acoustic interaction between the glottal source and the vocal tract. In: Stevens KN, Hirano M, eds. *Vocal Fold Physiology.* Tokyo, Japan: University of Tokyo Press; 1981:305–328.

83. Rothenberg M. An interactive model for the voice source. In: Bless DM, Abbs JH, eds. *Vocal Fold Physiology, Contemporary Research and Clinical Issues.* San Diego, CA: College-Hill Press; 1983:155–165.

84. Titze IR. The physics of small-amplitude oscillation of the vocal folds. *J Acoust Soc Am.* 1988;83:1536–1552.

85. Kitzing P, Lofqvist A. Subglottal and oral pressures during phonation—preliminary investigation using a miniature transducer system. *Medical and Biological Eng.* 1975;13(5):644–648.

86. Fant G. Preliminaries to analysis of the human voice source. *STL-QPRS.* 1983;(4)1982:1–27.

87. Miller DG, Schutte HK. Characteristic patterns of sub- and supra-glottal pressure variations within the glottal cycle. In: Lawrence VL, ed. *Transcripts of the XIIIth Symposium: Care of the Professional Voice.* New York, NY: The Voice Foundation; 1984:70–75.

88. Cranen B, Boves L. A set-up for testing the validity of the two mass model of the vocal folds. In: Titze IR, Scherer RC, eds. *Vocal Fold Physiology: Biomechanics, Acoustics and Phonatory Control.* Denver, CO: The Denver Center for the Performing Arts; 1985:500–513.

89. Olson HF. *Solutions of Engineering Problems by Dynamical Analogies.* 2nd ed. New York, NY: D Van Nostrand Co; 1966.

90. Titze IR. Mean intraglottal pressure in vocal fold oscillation. *J Phonetics.* 1986;14:359–364.

91. Scherer RC, Guo CG. Laryngeal modeling: translaryngeal pressure for a model with many glottal shapes. *ICSLP Proceedings, 1990 International Conference on Spoken Language Processing.* Vol 1. The Acoustical Society of Japan, Japan; 1990:3.1.1–3.1.4.

92. Scherer RC, Guo CG. Generalized translaryngeal pressure coefficient for a wide range of laryngeal configurations. In: Gauffin J, Hammarberg B, eds. *Vocal Fold Physiology: Acoustic, Perceptual, and Physiological Aspects of Voice Mechanisms.* San Diego, CA: Singular Publishing Group; 1991:83–90.

93. Alipour F, Scherer RC. Pulsatile flow within an oscillating glottal model. *J Iran Mech Eng.* 1998:3;73–81.

94. Kline SJ. On the nature of stall. *ASME J Basic Eng.* 1959;81:305–320.

95. Miller DS. *Internal Flow, a Guide to Losses in Pipe and Duct Systems.* Cranfield, UK: British Hydromechanics Research Association; 1971.

96. Guo CG, Scherer RC. Finite element simulation of glottal flow and pressure. *J Acoust Soc Am.* 1993;94(2)(pt 1): 688–700.

97. Scherer RC, Shinwari D. Glottal pressure profiles for a diameter of 0.04 cm. *J Acoust Soc Am.* 2000;107(5)(pt 2): 2905.

98. Scherer R, Sundberg J, Titze I. Laryngeal adduction related to characteristics of the flow glottogram. *J Acoust Soc Am.* 1989;85(S1):S129(A).

99. Titze IR, Sundberg J. Vocal intensity in speakers and singers. *J Acoust Soc Am.* 1992;91:2936–2946.

100. Sundberg J, Titze I, Scherer R. Phonatory control in male singing: a study of the effects of subglottal pressure, fundamental frequency, and mode of phonation on the voice source. *J Voice.* 1993;7(1):15–29.

101. Fant G, Liljencrants J, Lin Q. A four-parameter model of glottal flow. *STL-QPSR.* 1985;(4)1985:1–13.

102. Gobl C, Karlsson I. Male and female voice source dynamics. In: Gauffin J, Hammarberg B, eds. *Vocal Fold Physiology: Acoustic, Perceptual, and Physiological Aspects of Voice Mechanisms.* San Diego, CA: Singular Publishing Group; 1991:121–128.

103. Fant G, and Lin Q. Comments on glottal flow modeling and analysis. In: Gauffin J, Hammarberg B, eds. *Vocal Fold Physiology: Acoustic, Perceptual, and Physiological Aspects of Voice Mechanisms.* San Diego, CA: Singular Publishing Group; 1991:47–56.

104. Sundberg J, Gauffin J. Waveform and spectrum of the glottal voice source. In: Lindblom B, Ohman S, eds. *Frontiers of Speech Communication Research.* New York, NY: Academic Press; 1979:301–322.

105. Scherer RC, Titze IR, Curtis JF. Pressure-flow relationships in two models of the larynx having rectangular glottal shapes. *J Acoust Soc Am.* 1983;73:668–676.

106. Ladefoged P, McKinney NP. Loudness, sound pressure, and subglottal pressure in speech. *J Acoust Soc Am.* 1963;35:454–460.

107. Isshiki N. Regulatory mechanism of voice intensity variations. *J Speech Hear Res.* 1964;7:17–29.

108. Isshiki N. Remarks on mechanism for vocal intensity variation. *J Speech Hear Res.* 1969;12:665–672.

109. Rubin HJ, LeCover M, Vennard W. Vocal intensity, subglottic pressure, and airflow relationships in singers. *Folia Phoniatr.* 1967;19:393–413.

110. Bouhuys A, Mead J, Proctor D, Stevens K. Pressure-flow events during singing. *Ann NY Acad Sci.* 1968;155: 165–176.

111. Holmberg EB, Hillman RE, Perkell J. Glottal airflow and transglottal air pressure measurements for male and female speakers in soft, normal, and loud voice. *J Acoust Soc Am.* 1988;84:511–529.

112. Sapienza CM, Stathopoulos ET. Comparison of maximum flow declination rate: children versus adults. *J Voice.* 1994;8:240–247.

113. Sulter AM, Wit H. Glottal volume velocity waveform characteristics in subjects with and without vocal training, related to gender, sound intensity, fundamental frequency, and age. *J Acoust Soc Am.* 1996;100:3360–3373.

114. Titze IR. Regulation of vocal power and efficiency by subglottal pressure and glottal width. In: Fujimura O, ed. *Vocal Physiology: Voice Production, Mechanisms, and Function.* New York, NY: Raven Press, Ltd; 1988: 227–238.

115. Raphael BN, Scherer RC. Voice modifications of stage actors: Acoustic analyses. *J Voice.* 1987;1:83–87.

116. Bartholomew WT. A physical definition of "good voice quality" in the male voice. *J Acoust Soc Am.* 1934;6: 25–33.

117. Sundberg J. Articulatory interpretation of the "singing formant." *J Acoust Soc Am.* 1974;55:838–844.

118. Perkins WH. *Voice Disorders.* New York, NY: Thieme-Stratton Inc; 1983.

119. Verdolini K, Druker DG, Palmer PM, Samawi H. Laryngeal adduction in resonant voice. *J Voice.* 1998;12: 315–327.

120. Hollien HF, Curtis JF. A laminagraphic study of vocal pitch. *J Speech Hear Res.* 1960;3:361–371.

121. Hollien HF. Vocal fold thickness and fundamental frequency of phonation. *J Speech Hear Res.* 1962;5(3):237–243.

122. Hollien HF, Colton RH. Four laminagraphic studies of vocal fold thickness. *Folia Phoniatr.* 1969;21:179–198.

123. Hollien HF, Coleman RF. Laryngeal correlates of frequency change: A STROL study. *J Speech Hear Res.* 1970;13(2):271–278.

124. Scherer RC, Vail VJ, Rockwell B. Examination of the laryngeal adduction measure EGGW. In: Bell-Berti F, Raphael LJ, eds: *Producing Speech: Contemporary Issues: A Festshrift for Katherine Safford Harris.* Woodbury, NY: American Institute of Physics; 1995:269–290.

125. Hess Mm, Verdolini K, Bierhals W, Mansmann U, Gross M. Endolaryngeal contact pressure. *J Voice.* 1998; 12:50–67.

126. Verdolini K, Chan R, Titze IR, Hess M, Bierhals W. Correspondence of electroglottographic closed quotient to vocal fold impact stress in excised canine larynges. *J Voice.* 1998;12:415–423.

127. Verdolini K, Hess MH, Titze IR, Bierhals W, Gross M. Investigation of vocal fold impact stress in human subjects. *J Voice.* 1999;13:184–202.

128. Yamana T, Kitajima K. Laryngeal closure pressure during phonation in humans. *J Voice.* 2000;14:1–7.

129. Scherer RC, DeWitt K, Kucinschi BR. Effect of vocal radii on pressure distributions in the convergent glottis. *J Acoust Soc Am.* 2001;110:2267–2269.

130. Hirano M, Bless DM. *Videostroboscopic Examination of the Larynx.* San Diego, CA: Singular Publishing Group; 1993.

131. Berg Jw van den, Zantema JT, Doornenbal P Jr. On the air resistance and the Bernoulli effect of the human larynx. *J Acoust Soc Am.* 1957;29:626–631.

132. Scherer RC. Pressure-flow relationships in a laryngeal airway model having a diverging glottal duct. *J Acoust Soc Am.* 1983;73(S1):S46(A).

133. Scherer RC, Titze IR. Pressure-flow relationships in a model of the laryngeal airway with a diverging glottis. In: Bless DM, Abbs JH, eds. *Vocal Fold Physiology, Contemporary Research and Clinical Issues.* San Diego, CA: College-Hill Press; 1983:179–193.

134. Gauffin J, Binh N, Ananthapadmanabha TV, Fant G. Glottal geometry and volume velocity waveform. In: Bless DM, Abbs JH, eds. *Vocal Fold Physiology: Contemporary Research and Clinical Issues.* San Diego, CA: College-Hill Press; 1983:194–201.

135. Ishizaka K. Air resistance and intraglottal pressure in a model of the larynx. In: Titze IR, Scherer RC. eds. *Vocal Fold Physiology: Biomechanics, Acoustics and Phonatory Control.* Denver, CO: The Denver Center for the Performing Arts; 1985:414–424.

136. Alipour R, Scherer RC. Dynamic glottal pressures in an excised hemilarynx model. *J Voice.* 2000;14(4):443–454.

137. Ishizaka K, Matsudaira M. *Fluid mechanical considerations of vocal cord vibration.* SCRL Monograph No. 8, April 1972.

138. Titze IR. The human vocal cords: A mathematical model. Part I. *Phonetica.* 1973;28:129–170.

139. Titze IR. The human vocal cords: A mathematical model. Part II. *Phonetica.* 1974;29:1–21.

140. Titze IR. On the mechanics of vocal fold vibration. *J Acoust Soc Am.* 1976;60(6):136–1380.

141. Titze IR. Biomechanics and distributed-mass models of vocal fold vibration. In: Stevens KN, Hirano M, eds. *Vocal Fold Physiology.* Tokyo, Japan: University of Tokyo Press; 1981:245–270.

142. Alipour F, Titze IR. A finite element simulation of vocal fold vibration. In: *Proc. Fourteenth Annual Northeast Bioeng.* Conf. Durham; IEEE publications #88-CH2666-6; 1988:86–189.

143. Schonharl E. *Die Stroboskopie in der praktischen Laryngologie.* Stuttgart, Germany: Thieme; 1960.

144. Stevens KN, Klatt DH. Current models of sound sources for speech. In: Wyke B, ed. *Ventilatory and Phonatory Control Systems, an International Symposium.* New York, NY: Oxford University Press; 1974:279–292.

145. Hirano M. Structure and vibratory behavior of the vocal folds. In: Sawashima M, Cooper FS, eds. *Dynamic Aspects of Speech Production.* Tokyo, Japan: University of Tokyo Press; 1977:13–27.

146. Cooper DS. Voice: a historical perspective (Woldemar Tonndorf and the Bernoulli effect in voice production). *J Voice.* 1989;3(1):1–6.

147. Scherer RC, Shinwari D, DeWitt K, Zhang C, Kucinschi B, Afjeh A. Intraglottal pressure profiles for a symmetric and oblique glottis with a divergence angle of 10 degrees. *J Acoust Soc Am.* 2001;109:1616–1630.

148. Pelorson X, Hirschberg A, van Hassel RR, Wijnands APJ. Theoretical and experimental study of quasi-steady-flow separation within the glottis during phonation. Application to a modified two-mass model. *J Acoust Soc Am.* 1994;96:3416–3431.

149. Pelorson X, Hirschberg A, Wijnands APJ, Bailliet H. Description of the flow through in vitro models of the glottis during phonation. *Acta Acustica.* 1995;3:191–202.

150. Hofmans GCJ. *Vortex Sound in Confined Flows* [dissertation]. Eindhoven: CIP-Data Library Technische Universiteit Eindhoven; 1998.

151. von Leden H, Moore P, Timcke R. Laryngeal vibrations: measurements of the glottic wave. Part III: the pathologic larynx. *Arch Otolaryngol.* 1960;71:16–35.

152. Koike Y, Imaizumi S. Objective evaluation of laryngostroboscopic findings. In: Fujimura O, ed. *Vocal Physiology: Voice Production, Mechanisms and Functions.* New York, NY: Raven Press, Ltd; 1988:433–442.

153. Svec JG, Schutte HK. Videokymography: high-speed line scanning of vocal fold vibration. *J Voice.* 1996;10:201–205.

154. Kaiser J. Some observations on vocal tract operation from a fluid flow point of view. In: Titze IR, Scherer RC, eds. *Vocal Fold Physiology: Biomechanics, Acoustics and Phonatory Control.* Denver, CO: The Denver Center for the Performing Arts; 1985:358–386.

155. Teager H, Teager S. Active fluid dynamic voice production models, or there is a unicorn in the garden. In: Titze IR, Scherer RC, eds. *Vocal Fold Physiology: Biomechanics, Acoustics and Phonatory Control.* Denver, CO: The Denver Center for the Performing Arts; 1985:387–401.

156. McGowan RS. An aeroacoustic approach to phonation. *J Acoust Soc Am.* 1988;88:696–704.

157. McGowan RS. Phonation from a continuum mechanics point of view. In: Gauffin J, Hammarberg B, eds. *Vocal Fold Physiology: Acoustic, Perceptual, and Physiological Aspects of Voice Mechanisms.* San Diego, CA: Singular Publishing Group; 1991:65–72.

158. Berke GS, Moore DM, Monkewitz PA, Hanson DG, Gerratt BR. A preliminary study of particle velocity during phonation in an in vivo canine model. *J Voice.* 1989;3(4):306–313.

159. Shadle CH, Barney AM, Thomas DW. An investigation into the acoustic and aerodynamics of the larynx. In: Gauffin J, Hammarberg B, eds. *Vocal Fold Physiology: Acoustic, Perceptual, and Physiological Aspects of Voice Mechanisms.* San Diego: Singular Publishing Group; 1991:73–80.

160. Alipour F, Fan C. Pulsatile flow in a three-dimensional model of larynx. In: Biewener AA, Goel VK, eds. *Proceedings of 1993 ASB Meeting.* 1993:221–222.

161. Davies POAL, McGowan RS, Shadle CH. Practical flow duct acoustics applied to the vocal tract. In: Titze IR, ed. *Vocal Fold Physiology: Frontiers in Basic Science.* San Diego, CA: Singular Publishing Group; 1993:93–134.

162. Scherer R. Practical flow duct acoustics applied to the vocal tract: Response. In: Titze IR, ed. *Vocal Fold Physiology: Frontiers in Basic Science.* San Diego, CA: Singular Publication Group; 1993:134–142.

163. Alipour F, Scherer RC. Pulsatile airflow during phonation: an excised larynx model. *J Acoust Soc Am.* 1995; 97:1241–1248.

164. Zhao W. *A Numerical Investigation of Sound Radiated from Subsonic Jet with Application to Human Phonation,* [dissertation]. West Lafayette, IN: Purdue University; 2000.

8

Laryngeal Neurophysiology

Michael S. Benninger, MD
Glendon M. Gardner, MD
Craig Schwimmer, MD
Venu Divi, MD

The larynx provides the basic functions of airway protection, respiration, and voice. These are accomplished via a delicate balance of sensation, reflexes, and voluntary movement, all mediated through an intricate neurologic system. The ability to evaluate and treat a patient with neurologic dysfunction of the larynx requires an understanding of the complicated neuroanatomy of the larynx. Neurologic vocal fold immobility can result from insults that affect the motor input from the nucleus ambiguus to the final neuromuscular junction. Sensory disruption can affect the mechanical, tactile, thermal, pH, and other receptors necessary for the maintenance of reflexive pathways, resulting in alterations of normal laryngeal function.

This chapter describes the neuroanatomy and neurophysiology of the larynx and identifies key laryngeal reflexes.

NEUROANATOMY OF THE LARYNX

The vagus nerve (cranial nerve X), named for its wandering course, is the longest cranial nerve. It contains somatic sensory (skin near the ear and posterior external auditory canal), visceral afferent (from heart, pancreas, stomach, esophagus, and upper respiratory tract), somatic motor, autonomic afferent, and taste fibers.[1] The afferent fibers (visceral, taste, and somatic sensory) have cells that originate in the nodose and jugular ganglions, which are the sensory ganglia of the nerve. They enter the medulla and divide into descending and ascending branches.

Somatic motor fibers arise in the nucleus ambiguus to innervate the striated muscles of the larynx and a portion of the pharynx.[2] Intracranial or supranodose ganglion sectioning of the vagal nerve fibers results in degeneration of "large" and "intermediate" myelinated fibers of the recurrent laryngeal nerve, which consist of laryngeal motor axons originating in the nucleus ambiguus.[3] The nucleus ambiguus receives collaterals that control voluntary muscle movement of the larynx from the opposite pyramidal tract (Figure 8–1). Reflex pathways from terminal sensory nuclei are part of the reticular formation.

Taste fibers from the epiglottis and larynx pass in the vagus to join the tractus solitarius to terminate in

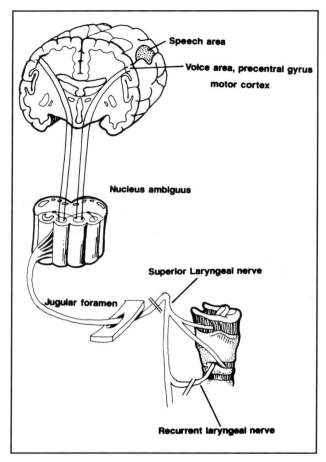

Figure 8-1. Central neural schema of vagus nerve.

the nucleus of the tractus solitarius, which contacts with the motor centers of the medulla oblongata, pons, and spinal cord for mastication and deglutition.

The superficial origin of the vagus is from eight to ten rootlets attached to the medulla oblongata (Figure 8–1). These lie in the groove between the olive and inferior peduncle with the roots of the glossopharyngeal nerve coursing superiorly and the spinal accessory nerve inferiorly. The rootlets unite to pass beneath the flocculus of the cerebellum. The vagus leaves the cranial vault through the jugular foramen along with the glossopharyngeal nerve, the spinal accessory nerve, and the internal jugular vein. The internal carotid artery and hypoglossal nerve exit in adjacent canals. It lies in the same dural sheath as the spinal accessory nerve but is separated from the glossopharyngeal nerve by a septum.[1]

The jugular ganglion or superior ganglion of the vagus nerve lies in the jugular foramen (Figure 8–2). These sensory ganglion cells enter the medulla just dorsal to the motor units. Some of the peripheral processes are distributed to the pharynx. The nodose

ganglion or inferior ganglion lies just distal to the jugular foramen (Figure 8–2). The central processes of these cells pass through the jugular ganglion to enter the medulla along with the jugular cell rootlets. The peripheral processes of these ganglion cells make up the internal branch of the superior laryngeal nerves, other vagal branches to the larynx, trachea, esophagus, bronchi, and thoracic and abdominal viscera.

The cranial portion of the spinal accessory nerve joins the vagus near the nodose ganglion to supply motor branches of the vagus to the larynx and pharynx. The vagus nerve trunk passes within the carotid sheath deep to, and between, the internal jugular vein and carotid artery as they descend in the neck. The left vagus nerve enters the thorax deep to the innominate vein between the subclavian and carotid arteries and passes between the aorta and the left pulmonary artery to give off the recurrent laryngeal nerve (RLN) branch as the vagus crosses the left side of the arch of the aorta (Figure 8–2). The RLN loops under the arch of the aorta just distal to the ligamentum arteriosum to pass on the side of the trachea to ascend deep to the carotid artery in the tracheoesophageal groove. It runs medial to the deep surface of the thyroid gland under the lower border of the inferior constrictor muscle to enter the larynx through the cricothyroid membrane behind the articulation of the inferior cornua of the thyroid cartilage with the cricoid cartilage. It supplies motor input to all the muscles of the larynx other than the cricothyroid muscle. The terminal branch of the RLN communicates with the fibers of the SLN and is called the ansa galeni.[4]

The right vagus nerve enters the thorax to cross superficial to the subclavian artery between the artery and the innominate vein. Here it loops under the subclavian and ascends behind it to lie in the tracheoesophageal groove. A rare nondescending right RLN occurs in less than 1% of humans. The intimate relation of the RLNs to the aorta, subclavian, thyroid, and cricothyroid joints allows for injury from surgery or neoplasms in these areas.

The diameter of the myelinated fibers has been found to be greater in the left RLN than the right.[5,6] This has led to the theory that the bundle size difference allows for almost simultaneous activation of the laryngeal muscles on the two sides, despite the left RLN being longer.[3] Nerve topographic studies have shown that nerve fiber content is divided between laryngeal and nonlaryngeal groups of nerve fibers in the RLN with laryngeal motor axons usually found in the largest fascicles of the nerve.[3] Laryngeal motor axons have been found in the anterior position in the vagus superior to the hyoid bone and in the medial position inferior to the hyoid.[6]

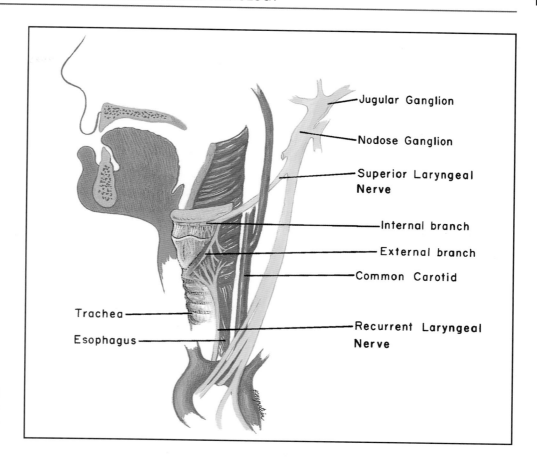

Figure 8-2. Extracranial course of vagus, with superior and recurrent laryngeal nerves detailed.

The superior laryngeal nerve (SLN) arises from the vagus just caudal to the nodose ganglion and descends posteriorly to the internal carotid artery where it splits into internal and external branches near the greater cornua of the thyroid cartilage after communicating with a branch or the cervical sympathetics (Figure 8–2).

The internal branch, the larger of the two superior nerve branches, passes through the thyrohyoid membrane along with the superior laryngeal artery. This branch supplies parasympathetic secretory motor fibers to the glands of the larynx down to the level of the true vocal fold, the aryepiglottic folds, epiglottis, and base of tongue. It supplies sensory fibers to these areas and terminates in a small branch that communicates with a branch of the RLN.[7] The internal branch of the SLN has also been found to send bilateral innervation to the interarytenoid muscles.[7,8] The communication between the SLN and RLN are also by nerve branches other than Galen's anastomosis.[9] The external branch of the SLN runs along the larynx to pass deep to the sternothyroid muscle to supply motor fibers to the cricothyroid muscle and a portion of the inferior constrictor. It supplies fibers to the pharyngeal plexus and has communication with the superior sympathetic cardiac nerve.[1]

Sensation from the supraglottic areas is transmitted via the SLN and sensation from the glottic and subglottic areas are transmitted via the RLN to the nodose ganglion and the tractus solitarius. Sensory and proprioreceptive nerve endings are denser on the laryngeal surface of the epiglottis than on the true vocal folds and are greater at the posterior portion of the true vocal fold than the anterior commissure.[4,7]

LARYNGEAL CHEMOREFLEXES

The human larynx serves four basic functions: airway protection, respiration, phonation, and facilitating increases in intrathoracic pressure for lifting, coughing, defecating, and so forth.[10-13] Protective reflex closure of the human larynx has been described as its most basic and primitive function.[10] Simple, reflexive closure of the glottis during deglutition is referred to as the glottic closure reflex. In addition to local effects, chemical stimulation of the larynx elicits reflexive changes in the respiratory and cardiovascular systems. These effects include apnea, bradycardia, hypertension, bronchoconstriction, coughing, and changes in peripheral vascular resistance.[10-14] Such systemic responses to laryngeal stimulation are referred to as laryngeal chemoreflexes (LCR). Laryngospasm refers to reflexive muscular contraction that persists despite removal of the eliciting stimulus.

Anatomy and Physiology

A wide variety of receptor nerve endings, including subepithelial plexuses, intraepithelial nerve endings (myelinated and unmyelinated), epiglottal taste bud-like structures, and others have been described in the hypopharynx and larynx.[12-18] Laryngeal receptors sensitive to decreases in temperature have been reported in dogs. These receptors have been localized to the mucosa of the vocal folds in proximity to the vocal processes of the arytenoid cartilages. Their firing is rapidly blocked by topical application of lidocaine, suggesting a superficial location. Such receptors are specifically responsive to cold and are not responsive to mechanical changes such as transmural pressure, airflow, or local probing and are silent near body temperature.[16] The cooling effect of increased airflow, however, makes them indirectly sensitive to respiration. Laryngeal reflex effects can be reproduced by stimulation of the superior laryngeal nerves (SLN), and abolished by sectioning the SLN, suggesting that afferent stimuli are carried by the SLN.[10-12,14,16]

A wide variety of chemical substances have been studied across numerous species regarding elicitation of laryngeal chemoreflexes. The reflex effects caused by laryngeal instillation of water, milk, acidic substances, ammonia, cigarette smoke, graphite dust, capsaicin, glucose solutions, and others have been described, often with species-specific results.[12-16] For example, laryngeal cooling has been shown to result in increased lower airway resistance and bronchoconstriction in dogs,[16,19] as does mechanical stimulation of the larynx in cats.[20] Laryngeal instillation of water is known to cause bradycardia and to decrease the respiratory rate in dogs, piglets, lambs, and human infants.[21-25] It has been suggested that a common characteristic of apnea-inducing substances is a chloride concentration lower than that normally found in extracellular fluid, although this theory has recently been questioned.[23,25]

LARYNGEAL MECHANORECEPTORS

Laryngeal mechanoreceptors detect various physical changes within the larynx. The information from the mechanoreceptors acts as the afferent limb for many reflex arcs responsible for maintaining patency of the larynx. The afferent information is transmitted via the internal branch of the superior laryngeal nerve. Mechanoreceptors are characterized by the stimuli to which they respond.

Pressure receptors respond to either positive or negative airway pressure, with a vast majority (85%) responding to negative pressure. These receptors are active during respiration and have a high gain, meaning a small pressure change from baseline results in a high receptor output. These receptors have features of both slow- and fast-adapting receptors, meaning they have both a steady firing rate (slow) and demonstrate an on/off response to stimuli (fast).

Drive receptors respond to rhythmic contraction of upper airway respiratory muscles. Paralysis of laryngeal muscles decreases firing from these receptors. They are located within the laryngeal muscle fibers. The afferent signals from these receptors are inhibited with the administration of topical anesthesia, suggesting a superficial location. During airway collapse, the receptors respond to passive stretch of the muscle and initiate a reflexive contraction of the posterior cricoarytenoid muscle and extralaryngeal dilators.[26]

Mechanoreceptors have also been found to modulate muscle contraction during vocalization. These are divided into frequency-following fibers and frequency-nonfollowing fibers. The discharge from frequency-following receptors varies to match the vibratory rate in a 1:1 or 1:2 relationship. These receptors are thought to play a role in aiding the central nervous system in maintaining a pitch. The frequency-nonfollowing receptors respond to phonation but do not vary with changes in frequency and are speculated to deliver information on laryngeal position.[27] Cold receptors, those that respond to a decrease in temperature, have been identified along the rim of the vocal fold and along the vocal process of the arytenoid. Cooling of the larynx inhibits other respiration modulated mechanoreceptors.

Developmental Aspects of Laryngeal Chemoreflexes

Laryngeal chemoreflexes appear to be age-dependent. For instance, when adult canine larynges were perfused with agents that induce apnea in puppies, little or no effect on breathing was noted, but reflex coughing and swallowing did occur.[22] A study of piglets showed that stimulating SLN in animals younger than 1 month yielded only a slight decrease in respiratory rate and depth.[28] It has been noted that, "In no species has a fatal or sustained apneic response been elicited in an adult animal or even an immature animal after a certain developmental period."[11]

It has been suggested that the maturation of central, antagonistic respiratory drive mechanisms prevents laryngeal chemostimulation from inducing apnea.[29] An anatomic basis for this supposition has been proposed. The superior laryngeal nerve, which carries the afferent arc of the laryngeal chemoreflex, terminates in the area of the solitary tract and dorsal nuclei. The motor fibers of vagus nerve responsible for the efferent reflex arc originate in the nucleus ambiguus and nucleus retroambigualus. These nuclei lie near the nuclei of the reticular system and could conceivably interact.[29,30]

Laryngeal Chemoreflexes and Sudden Infant Death Syndrome (SIDS)

SIDS is defined as the sudden death of any child or infant that is unexpected by history and in which a thorough postmortem examination fails to demonstrate an adequate cause for death. SIDS is the most common cause of death between 2 weeks and 1 year of age and has a peak incidence between the second and fourth months of life.[31]

Several lines of evidence suggest a link between LCR and SIDS. First, the LCR is an age-dependent reflex. Stimuli capable of producing fatal apneas in immature animals have been shown to elicit only reflexive swallowing in mature animals.[30,32,33] Second, a relationship has been shown between gastroesophageal reflux (GER) and infantile apneas. Infants who present with life-threatening apneas have a higher rate of significant GER events, longer periods of esophageal acidification, and increased risk for SIDS.[34] Additionally, apneic spells immediately following documented GER have been reported. It was recently demonstrated that stimulation of distal esophageal sensory nerves in young puppies causes laryngospasm. This suggests that vagal pathways other than LCR might contribute to the relationship between GER and SIDS.[35]

Central Neuroanatomy

A comprehensive discussion of the central neuroanatomy and physiology of phonation is beyond the scope of this chapter. However, the reader should be aware that substantial advances have been made in our understanding of the importance of the cortex, subcortex, periaqueductal gray matter, and other areas in the phonatory process. The reader is encouraged to consult other sources. Much of this research is based on animal studies.[36,37]

SUMMARY

Many factors are involved in the physiology, reflexes, and pathology of neurolaryngeal disorders. Recent studies have advanced our understanding of the basic laryngeal neuroanatomic pathways, vocal fold proprioception, and laryngeal reflexes; and these concepts will likely play major roles in future investigation, assessment, and treatment of laryngeal neural dysfunction.

REFERENCES

1. Goss, CM, ed. *Gray's Anatomy of the Human Body.* 28th ed. Philadelphia, Pa: Lea & Febiger; 1959:1012–1020.
2. Yoshida Y, Miyazaki T, Hirano M, et al. Arrangement of motoneurons innervating intrinsic laryngeal muscles of cats as demonstrated by horseradish peroxidase. *Acta Otolaryngol.* 1982;94:329–334.
3. Malmgren L, Gacek R. Peripheral motor innervation of the larynx. In: Blitzer A, Brin M, Sasaki C, et al, eds. *Neurologic Disorders of the Larynx.* New York, NY: Thieme Medical; 1992:36–43.
4. Tucker H. *The Larynx.* 2nd ed. New York, NY: Thieme Medical; 1993:17.
5. Harrison D. Fibre size frequency in the recurrent laryngeal nerves of man and giraffe. *Acta Otolaryngol.* 1981;91:383–389.
6. Shin T, Rabuzzi D. Conduction studies of the canine recurrent laryngeal nerves. *Laryngoscope.* 1971;81:586–596.
7. Sasaki C, Isaacson G. Functional anatomy of the larynx. *Otolaryngol Clin North Am.* 1988;21:595–612.
8. Sanders I, Mu L. Anatomy of the human internal superior laryngeal nerve. *Anat Rec.* 1998;252:646–656.
9. Sanders I, Wu B, Mu L, et al. The innervation of the human larynx. *Arch Otolaryngol Head Neck Surg.* 1993;119:934–939.
10. Sasaki C, Suzuki M. Laryngeal reflexes in cat, dog, and man. *Arch Otolaryngol.* 1976;102:400–402.
11. Cooper D, Lawson W. Laryngeal sensory receptors. In: Blitzer A, Brin M, Sasaki C, et al, eds. *Neurologic Disorders of the Larynx.* New York, NY: Thieme Medical; 1992:16.
12. Boushey H, Richardson P, Widdicombe J, Wise Jl. The response of laryngeal afferent fibers to mechanical and chemical stimuli. *J Physiol.* 1974;240:153–175.
13. Mathew O, Sant'Ambrogio G, Fisher J, Sant'Ambrogio F. Laryngeal pressure receptors. *Respir Physiol.* 1984;57:113–122.
14. Suzuki M, Kirchner J. Afferent nerve fibers in the external branch of the superior laryngeal nerve in the cat. *Ann Otol Rhinol Laryngol.* 1968;77:1059–1070.
15. Palecek F, Matthew O, Sant'Ambrogio F, et al: Cardiorespiratory responses to inhaled laryngeal irritants. *Inhalation Toxicol.* 1990;2:93–104.
16. Sant'Ambrogio G, Mathew O, Sant'Ambrogio F. Characteristics of laryngeal cold receptors. *Respir Physiol.* 1988;71:287–297.

17. Abo-el-Enein M. Laryngeal myotatic reflexes. *Nature.* 1966;209:682–685.

18. Sant'Ambrogio F, Tsubone H, Mathew O, Sant'Ambrogio G. Afferent activity in the external branch of the superior laryngeal and recurrent laryngeal nerves. *Ann Otol Rhinol Laryngol.* 1991;100:944–950.

19. Jammes Y, Barthelemy P, Delpierre S. Respiratory effects of cold air breathing in anesthetized cats. *Respir Physiol.* 1983;54:41–54.

20. Tomori Z, Widdicomb J. Muscular, bronchomotor and cardiovascular reflexes elicited by mechanical stimulation of the respiratory tract. *J Physiol.* 1969;200:25–49.

21. Goding G, Richardson M, Trachy R. Laryngeal chemoreflex: anatomic and physiologic study by use of the superior laryngeal nerve in the piglet. *Otolaryngol Head Neck Surg.* 1987;97:28–38.

22. Woodson G, Brauel G. Arterial chemoreceptor influences on the laryngeal chemoreflex. *Otolaryngol Head Neck Surg.* 1992;107:775–782.

23. Davies A, Koenig J, Thatch B. Upper airway chemoreflex responses to saline and water in preterm infants. *J Appl Physiol.* 1988;64:1412–1420.

24. Davies A, Koenig J, Thatch B. Characteristics of upper airway chemoreflex prolonged apnea in human infants. *Am Rev Resp Dis.* 1989;139:668–673.

25. Boggs D, Bartlett D Jr. Chemical specificity of a laryngeal apneic reflex in puppies. *J Appl Physiol.* 1982;53:455–462.

26. Sant'Ambrogio G, Tsubone H, Sant'Ambrogio F. Sensory information from the upper airway: role in the control of breathing. *Respir Physiol.* 1995;102:1–16.

27. Gozaine TC, Clark KF. Function of the laryngeal mechanoreceptors during vocalization. *Laryngoscope.* 2005;115:81–88.

28. Lee J, Stoll B, Downing S. Properties of the laryngeal chemoreflex in neonatal piglets. *Am J Physiol.* 1977;233:R30–R36.

29. Van Vliet B, Uenishi M. Antagonistic interaction of laryngeal and central chemoreceptor respiratory reflexes.*J Appl Physiol.* 1992;72:643–649.

30. Rimell F, Goding G Jr, Johnson K. Cholinergic agents in the laryngeal chemoreflex model of sudden infant death syndrome. *Laryngoscope.* 1993;103:623–630.

31. Beers MH, Berkow R, eds. *Merck Manual of Diagnosis and Therapy.* 17th ed. Whitehouse Station, NJ: Merck & Co Inc; 1999. Available online at http://www.merck.com/pubs/mmanual/

32. Sasaki C. Development of laryngeal function: etiologic significance in the sudden infant death syndrome. *Laryngoscope.* 1979;89:1964–1981.

33. Downing S, Lee J. Laryngeal chemosensitivity: a possible mechanism for sudden infant death. *Pediatrics.* 1975;55:640–649.

34. Kelly D, Shannon D. Sudden infant death syndrome and near sudden infant death syndrome: a review of the literature 1964–1982. *Pediatr Clin North Am.* 1982;19:1241–1261.

35. Bauman N, Sandler A, Schmidt C, et al. Reflex laryngospasm induced by stimulation of distal esophageal afferents. *Laryngoscope.* 1994;104:209–214.

36. Yoshida Y, Mitsumasu T, Miyazaki T, Hirano M, Kaneseki T. Distribution of motoneurons in the brain stem of monkeys, innervating the larynx. *Brain Res Bull.* 1984;13:413–419.

37. Fukuyama T, Umezaki T, Shin T. Origin of laryngeal sensory evoked potentials (LSEPs) in the cat. *Brain Res Bull.* 1993;31:381–392.

9

The Neurology of Stuttering

Rebecca Spain, MD
Steven Mandel, MD
Robert Thayer Sataloff, MD, DMA

What do singer Carly Simon, Chicago Bulls basketball player Bob Love, NBA all-star and sports broadcaster Bill Walton, actress Marilyn Monroe, author John Updike, and politician Sir Winston Churchill have in common? All were stutterers, and all were able to achieve successful public careers.[1] It is well known that even people with severe stuttering often can sing fluently. Although stuttering is really a speech disorder rather than a voice disorder, voice care professionals often are involved in the care of people who stutter and may be called on to participate in their diagnostic and therapeutic care team. Consequently, it is useful for laryngologists, speech pathologists, singing teachers, and other voice professionals to remain familiar with current concepts in and research on this complex disorder.

Stuttering is a common problem, affecting approximately 4 to 10% of children and 1% of adults.[2] It can have a profound impact on those affected by it, both emotionally and socially, and on those who live and work with them. Although it was once thought that stuttering was caused by stress and anxiety, current thinking takes a more scientific approach. Researchers study developmental stutterers for anatomic differ-

ences, genetic factors, and associated disorders. Individuals who acquire stuttering later in life provide clues into the anatomic locations controlling speech and suggest roles for neurotransmitters in the cause and treatment of stuttering. Taken together, current research in stuttering points to the existence of multiple neural networks that work together to control initiation, production, and modulation of normal speech. These networks can help explain why a stutterer such as Carly Simon can nonetheless achieve a successful singing career; and by better understanding normal mechanisms of speech, we can better target our therapies for stuttering.

STUTTERING DEFINED

Stuttering is a disturbance in the normal fluency and time patterning of speech that is inappropriate for the person's age.[3] The vast majority of stuttering behaviors are "developmental," meaning that the problem begins in childhood usually between the ages of 2 and 5 years during a period of highly intensive speech and language development.[4] In the normal speech and language learning process, babbling begins at 6 to 10 months, spoken words at 1 year, two-word phrases at 14 to 24 months, and three-word phrases by age 3 years. Clear syntax, the grammatical arrangement of words in sentences, emerges by age 4 years.[5] It is normal for preschoolers to have certain levels of dysfluencies as they learn both to translate ideas into words and to gain the fine motor control of muscles necessary for speech production. It is estimated that about 10% of preschool-aged children go through a period of dysfluency severe enough to warrant evaluation by a speech-language pathologist.[6] Types of dysfluencies include sound and syllable repetition ("ca-ca-ca-cat"), prolongations ("sssss-salad," "fffffff-fish"), and complete blockages of airflow. Additional dysfluencies include interjections ("we went to the . . . uh . . . store") and revisions or incomplete phrases ("I lost my . . . where did daddy go?"). It is normal for adults and children to have a certain level of dysfluency, but anything greater than 10%, that is 10 words spoken dysfluently per 100 words, is considered concerning.

DEVELOPMENTAL STUTERING

Although it is has been estimated that 50% to 80% of developmental stuttering (DS) will resolve by puberty with or without treatment, investigation can be warranted because some stuttering is associated with other neurologic and/or psychiatric disorders. DS can be associated with Tourette's disease, a disorder of motor and vocal tics.[3] Indeed, some of the secondary behaviors of stuttering—including grimacing, eye-blinking, and social anxiety—are reminiscent of tics. Congenital and developmental disorders such as Down syndrome and autism may also be associated with stuttering. Anxiety and depression can coexist with or even result from stuttering. In addition, stuttering should be distinguished from other types of language disturbances that may warrant different investigations or treatments. Cluttering, which involves excessive breaks in the normal flow of speech that seem to result from disorganized speech planning, talking too fast or in spurts, or simply being unsure of what one wants to say, is one such disturbance.[1] Cluttering can be associated with the genetic disorder fragile X syndrome. Spastic dysphonia occurs in middle-aged adults who sound like they are being strangled. Spastic dysphonia coexists with breathing abnormalities and has no known cause.[3]

Speech-language pathologists are often the first specialists to evaluate children referred by parents, teachers, and doctors for speech problems.[7] They can help distinguish between isolated stuttering and global stuttering, which is associated with other speech,

language, developmental, neurologic, and psychiatric problems and may require additional diagnosis and treatments.

ACQUIRED STUTTERING

Acquired stuttering is far less common than DS and can be divided into neurogenic and psychogenic causes. Acquired stuttering tends to begin in older, previously fluent individuals and should prompt a thorough neurologic investigation. Neurogenic stuttering is caused by specific underlying brain pathology. A sudden onset of stuttering suggests events such as stroke or trauma, whereas a gradual onset is more likely due to a tumor or to degenerative diseases such as Parkinson's disease or Alzheimer's disease. Less commonly reported neurogenic causes of stuttering include seizures, medications, toxins such as copper, or systemic disease such as renal failure. In most cases, neurogenic stuttering is distinguished from DS by the lack of associated movement disorders (eg, grimacing, eye-blinking) or anxiety that can accompany developmental stuttering. Additional deficits based on the location of the injury, such as weakness, personality changes, or cognitive decline, may be noted. Neurogenic stuttering is distinguished also by being less amenable to improvement by standard techniques of repetition, choral reading, and singing.[3]

Psychogenic stuttering is a rare. Although normal dysfluencies of speech increase during stressful events, psychogenic stuttering occurs suddenly after an emotional trauma, is persistent rather than fluctuating, and is not accompanied by other neurological dysfunction. Psychogenic stutterers tend to have only one type of dysfluency (usually repetition of the initial syllable), never have the usual fluctuations of dysfluency, and can appear indifferent to the problem.[3] Although there are rare case reports of stuttering occurring as a manifestation of a seizure, stuttering is actually far more predictive of a nonepileptic seizure, another psychogenic neurologic condition. Roughly one quarter to one third of patients admitted to epilepsy monitoring units that simultaneously record electroencephalograms (EEGs) and video have nonepileptic seizures.[8] One study found that, among 230 cases reviewed from a video-EEG monitoring unit, 117 cases with psychogenic nonepileptic seizures and 113 with true epileptic seizures, all the patients who stuttered as part of their seizure were found to have psychogenic nonepileptic seizures. These patients were also noted to have other features inconsistent with true seizures and were dealing with severe emotional traumas. Psychogenic stuttering, like psychogenic seizures, is best treated with counseling and psychological support.

NORMAL BRAIN ANATOMY OF SPEECH AND LANGUAGE

Much is already known about the anatomic locations in the brain responsible for spoken language (Figure 9–1). Many of these discoveries came from the work of 19th century neurologists who studied first the clinical deficits of their patients after a stroke and later the postmortem brains for the location of the stroke lesion. Both Broca's area and Wernicke's area (named for the neurologists Paul Broca and Carl Wernicke) were found in this manner. Lesions of these areas in one hemisphere of the brain (the left hemisphere in over 90% of people) caused characteristic language disturbances called *aphasias* and led to the discovery that language is predominantly located in the dominant hemisphere. In the 1930s, surgeon Wilder Penfield mapped the primary motor cortex of the brain (part of the sensorimotor area of Figure 9–1) by electrically stimulating the cerebral cortex and observing the motor responses of the alert subject (this is possible because of the lack of sensory nerve endings on the exposed cortex). These experiments led to the foundation of our knowledge of speech production, the sequence of which is as follows: Auditory information is processed first in the primary auditory cortex of the superior temporal lobe and then sent to the primary auditory association area that includes Wernicke's area. This auditory information is then sent by a discrete bundle of fibers called the arcuate fasciculus (not shown in

Figure 9–1) to Broca's area in the prefrontal association area of the frontal lobe. Broca's area, which is responsible for the motor planning of speech, then sends signals to the primary motor cortex of the sensorimotor area. The motor cortex sends signals via the corticospinal tracts, another discrete nerve fiber bundle that travels deep into the brain and through the brainstem. In the brainstem, some of the corticospinal nerves branch off and synapse, or make connections, with specific nerves that extend to the muscles of the tongue, pharynx, vocal folds, and lips in order to produce speech. The remaining corticospinal tract fibers either branch from the tract at the level of the brainstem to synapse on other facial muscles or continue into the spinal cord where they synapse on nerves destined for the muscles of the neck, arms, trunk, and legs. In summary, speech involves a series of steps and connections throughout the brain including reception of auditory information, comprehension, planning of the content of the response, planning of the motor action of the response, signals to the appropriate muscles, and finally production of speech.[9]

APHASIAS

Diseases that affect any of the regions of the brain described above will result in disorders of language termed *aphasias*. A lesion in Broca's area is characterized by difficulty with speech production and repetition but with relatively preserved comprehension of written and spoken language. These people will know what they want to say but cannot "get the words out" with varying degrees of severity, even to the point of

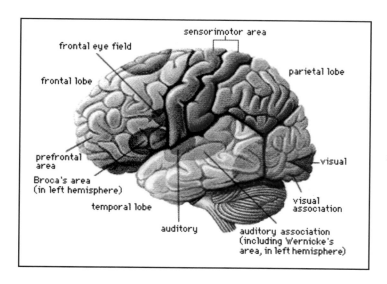

Figure 9–1. Gross anatomy of the brain: frontal lobe (*purple, blue*), parietal lobe (*dark and light red*), occipital lobe (*orange*), temporal lobe (*yellow*), and cerebellum (*striped orange*) shown. Also marked are the areas receiving primary sensory information: auditory, visual, somatosensory (touch, etc). Areas receiving smell and taste information are hidden from view. Wernicke's area, which is involved in auditory processing, is shown in the posterior, superior temporal lobe, and Broca's area, which is involved in motor production of speech, is shown in the posterior, inferior frontal lobe. (Reproduced with permission from: http://www.emc.maricopa.edu/faculty/farabee/BIOBK/brain.gif)

total muteness. Although their speech may have a stuttering quality, a Broca's aphasia (sometimes called an *expressive* aphasia) can be distinguished from developmental stuttering by associated problems such as right-sided weakness due to nearby destruction of other motor planning areas in the frontal lobe or possibly eye deviation from involvement of the nearby frontal eye field.

A Wernicke's (or *receptive*) aphasia, again a disorder of language, will present with difficulties in comprehension of language as well as impaired repetition. However, the meaningless speech that is produced will be fluent and without pauses or halting qualities. People with Wernicke's aphasia are usually unaware of their language deficit. Variations of these aphasias are found with lesions in the arcuate fasciculus or other nearby anatomic locations. In contrast to developmental stuttering, aphasias may have associated impairments of writing and reading language. However the greatest distinction between aphasias and developmental stuttering lies in the fact that aphasias are acquired lesions, usually due to a stroke, tumor, or traumatic injury to the left side of the brain. Therefore, there is a decline from previously attained levels of speech and language. Although children with developmental stuttering may have minor fluctuations in abilities due to anxiety or while attaining more complex skills, they do not experience significant or permanent declines in function. Strokes and tumors are certainly possible in children (although fortunately rare), but the lack of weakness, alterations in consciousness, or decline in cognitive function should all point away from these causes of language disturbance in children.[3]

CAUSES OF ACQUIRED STUTTERING

Strokes

Although rare, there are case reports of lesions in the brain that cause stuttering but are not located in the classic Broca's and Wernicke's areas. Grant et al described four patients who developed stuttering in association with an acute ischemic (ie, nonhemorrhagic, or nonbleeding) stroke, only two of which involved the typical left-sided language areas. The third involved a left-handed man with severe but transient stuttering after a right parietal infarct. Another was a right-handed man who began stuttering after a left occipital infarction. Two of the people who acquired stuttering had been childhood stutterers but had "grown out" of their stuttering years before the strokes.[10] Although it could be argued that the left-handed man might have had his language area in the right side of his brain (approximately 10% of left-

handed are right-hemisphere dominant, the rest are left dominant as are all right-handed people), a parietal location is not typically associated with stuttering. These cases raise the possibility of a right parietal contribution to fluent speech and introduce the idea that there may be something different about the brains of childhood stutterers that makes them susceptible to stuttering again after a stroke.

Reports of other strokes that produced stuttering from lesions in unexpected areas are described by Ciabarra et al.[11] One patient had a pontine infarct (a brainstem location), a second had a left basal ganglia stroke (located deep within the brain), and a third had a left-sided stroke near the language cortex but deeper than normally found (Figure 9–2). Previously, all language processing was thought to occur in the cortex of the

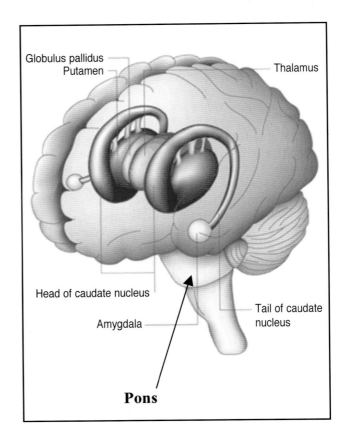

Figure 9–2. Deep structures of the brain. The basal ganglia are comprised of right- and left-sided groups of deep nuclei including the globus pallidus, putamen, caudate nucleus, and thalamus. The pons is part of the brainstem, the phylogenetically oldest part of the brain. Lesions in these areas have been implicated in the cause of acquired stuttering in three case reports. (Reproduced with permission from: http://general.rau.ac.za/psych/Resources/Honours/Neuropsych/Downloads/downloadstr/Lect2-opt/basalganglia.jpg)

brain, the outer 3 mm of the brain's surface, but these cases implicate areas located deep within the brain instead of in the cortex. The cortex varies from 1.3 mm to 4.5 mm in thickness and follows the convolutions of the surface of the brain. Most of the connections, or synapses, between neurons occur in the cortex, which is estimated to contain 14 billion nerve cells.[12] The subcortical regions affected in the strokes described are known to be involved in regulation of other motor activities, but previously were not known to affect speech. The authors proposed that the pontine stroke may have affected connections between the brainstem and prefrontal motor planning areas. The basal ganglia are involved in timing and amplitude of movement of head and body, thus lesions might similarly affect control of the mouth, tongue, and so on. Finally, the subcortical stroke provides evidence of a connection between deep structures, such as the basal ganglia, and known cortical pathways. Interestingly, there is one case report of a 66-year-old man with severe, lifelong stuttering whose stuttering suddenly ceased after simultaneous strokes to both thalami (Figure 9–2) due to a heart arrhythmia, again implicating pathways involving the basal ganglia in stuttering.[13] Patients who have suffered a thalamic stroke with impairment in language, like this man, tend to have other associated problems related to the territory of the artery involved in the stroke.[14]

Strokes, usually thought to cause single lesions, may also be the result of diffuse cerebral vascular disease leading to multiple areas of stroke. Heuer et al present two such cases that both led to stuttering due to multiple and bilateral hemispheric lesions.[15] The first case was a 40-year-old woman with multiple complaints over several weeks including difficulty walking, shifting leg pain, balance problems, and severe stuttering. After multiple imaging techniques, she was diagnosed with Moya Moya, a disease that causes narrowing of the cerebral arteries leading to multiple cortical and subcortical areas of low blood flow. Following vascular surgery, some of the symptoms improved' unfortunately, others did not, indicating strokes in the distribution of the blood vessels affected by the moya moya disease. In a second case, a 53-year-old man who had initially developed stuttering after a stroke in the left basal ganglia, suddenly worsened after 1 year. Further neuroimaging revealed an abnormally small cerebral vessel and multiple small strokes throughout both cerebral hemispheres in the cortex and subcortical structures.

Degenerative Diseases

Diseases of the basal ganglia provide other insights into stuttering. Parkinson's disease is a progressive, degenerative disorder affecting parts of the basal ganglia

and causing the classic signs of rigidity, slowness of movement (bradykinesia), postural imbalance, and tremor. Repetitive speech phenomena are well known in patients with Parkinson's disease and were studied in detail by Benke et al.[16] They observed two types of speech disorders: hyperfluent, poorly articulated iterations with an increasing rate and a decreasing volume and nonfluent, well-articulated iterations with constant rate and volume. Both types of speech disorders were relatively common among their sample of Parkinson's patients (28%), and were more prevalent among those with advanced disease. Furthermore, the speech problems were persistent and did not fluctuate with the levels of levodopa taken for symptom control as previously theorized to be the cause of the speech problems.[17] Benke et al proposed that the close association between repetitive speech and advancing Parkinson's disease may result from the same mechanism of neuron degeneration.

Several theories regarding the contribution of the basal ganglia to fluent speech are proposed by these authors. One is that the normal stimulation of speech by the basal ganglia breaks down in a general fashion causing apparent blocks and hesitations. Another is that the same problem of "freezing," a sudden and short-lasting break in the midst of preprogrammed, overlearned motor tasks such as walking, also occurs in speech leading to problems in initiating, executing, and switching tasks when talking. A third hypothesis is that the stuttering occurs because of impairment at a prearticulatory level, causing difficulty assembling the correct words and organizing them serially to form a sentence. Finally, any combination of the above hypotheses may be at play leading to the breakdown of fluent speech in patients with Parkinson's disease. Interestingly, 10 patients who received stimulation from surgically implanted devices in their basal ganglia (specifically in the subthalamic nucleus) had significant improvement of their speech disorders in addition to the intended improvement in motor function.[18] Deep brain stimulation also has been reported to improve vocal tremor, a condition that can also cause apparent interruptions in speech.[19]

Other degenerative disease processes, including progressive supranuclear palsy and Alzheimer's disease, can result in stuttering or similar language disturbances. Renal failure and dialysis are metabolic insults that can sometimes cause stuttering. Toxic processes like Wilson's disease, which, if untreated, causes an accumulation of copper in the basal ganglia, also cause stuttering.[3]

The Role of Neurotransmitters

Other inferences regarding the production of fluent speech can be drawn from Parkinson's disease. Not only is there degeneration of neurons in the basal ganglia, but there is also a specific loss of the neurotransmitter dopamine. Replacement of dopamine in the form of the drug levodopa is believed by some to help relieve of the speech problems in patients with Parkinson's disease.[15] No known neurotransmitter disorder is associated with developmental stuttering, but drugs such as haloperidol that block certain dopamine receptors in the brain can sometimes improve fluency. Haloperidol is also used in Tourette's disease, attention deficit-hyperactive disorder, and oppositional defiant and conduct disorders, which all have, among other things, abnormalities in three dopaminergic genes. Positron emission tomography (PET) scans of stutterers have shown an increased uptake in labeled dopamine (6-FDOPA) in cortical and subcortical areas of the brain indicating an abnormality of dopamine balance and providing further evidence of subcortical involvement in stuttering.[3]

A variety of other possible neurotransmitters is suggested by case reports involving antiepileptic medications. Reversible language regression was noted in three children after treatment with the antiepileptic medication topiramate, a medication that affects the neurotransmitter gamma aminobutyric acid (GABA), which affects sodium and calcium channels and blocks glutamate receptors. In another case, the antiepileptic medication gabapentin that affects inhibitory GABA receptors induced stuttering in a patient being treated for seizures.[20] The stuttering resolved when gabapentin therapy was stopped. By contrast, two other antiepileptic drugs, divalproex sodium and levetiracetam, were fortuitously discovered to be useful in the management of stuttering when they were used in the treatment of seizures.[21,22] The precise neurotransmitters and/or receptor channels affected by these medications are as yet unknown. However, despite the numerous case reports, the evidence for involvement of dopamine in stuttering is by far the strongest and has helped direct medical therapies using newer drugs (eg, risperidone, olanzapine) that affect dopamine balance without some of the undesirable side effects of haloperidol.[1,23]

CAUSES OF DEVELOPMENTAL STUTTERING

Despite all the information about stuttering gained from strokes and other acquired lesions, the vast majority of people who stutter, an estimated 4 to 10% of preschoolers and 1% of the adult population, are developmental stutterers without any history of strokes or brain diseases. In contrast to acquired stutterers, roughly three quarters of people with DS are male; 50% to 80% recover spontaneously with or without treatment; and most have a better response to many of the currently used speech and medical therapies.[3] In attempts to tease out the differences between developmental stuttering, acquired stuttering, and fluent speakers, research has delved into anatomic differences using magnetic resonance imaging (MRI) techniques and positron emission tomography (PET) studies. Genetic studies attempt to find patterns of inheritance within families and locate gene defects common to DS and its associated disorders. Examinations of traditionally used treatment modalities for developmental stuttering have led to hypotheses regarding how they might work physiologically.

Anatomic Differences

Much of the current work investigating anatomic differences in the brains of developmental stutterers employs up-to-date imaging techniques rather than postmortem examinations. One such technique, PET, is able to detect functional differences in addition to volumetric differences in brain regions. Changes in regional metabolism due to increased brain activity are demonstrated by using labeled metabolites such as glucose or oxygen. Localized brain activity is generated by having the subject perform specific tasks while being scanned. These tasks can be either motor tasks, such as moving a finger, or cognitive tasks, such as *thinking* about moving a finger or solving a math equation. Other methods include sending sensory stimuli (visual, auditory, sensory, etc) or having the subject speak, read, or sing. Fox et al used PET to identify the regions of the brain activated during paragraph reading, stuttering, and induced fluency.[24] They discovered that. in normal subjects, paragraph reading resulted in activation of the motor cortex representing the mouth, motor planning areas, auditory regions, visual systems, and the cerebellum. These activations were predominantly left-lateralized, consistent with the fact that language resides mainly in the left hemisphere for nearly all people. In contrast, stuttered reading produced extensive hyperactivity of the motor system with a *right* lateralization. Some left-sided areas thought to be involved in self-monitoring were absent during stuttering. Several other left-sided areas, predominantly in the frontal-temporal regions, also failed to activate or had diminished activation compared to controls.

Choral reading, reading aloud in unison with others, is a phenomenon well-known to temporarily suspend stuttering. Choral reading was thus used to induce fluency among the stuttering subjects and in fact was able to completely eliminate the stuttering of all 10 subjects who stuttered. Choral reading also reduced the abnormalities seen on PET scans during the stuttering. However, choral reading did not fully reverse the right-sided lateralization in the motor and motor-planning areas. The authors concluded that stuttering involves diffuse overactivity of the cerebral and cerebellar motor systems, a right dominance of the cerebral motor system, a lack of "self-monitoring" activations in the left hemisphere, and reduction in left cortical frontal-temporal "verbal-fluency" circuits.

Sandak et al discussed the data from PET studies and added further evidence that stutterers show a reverse pattern of brain activation when reading single words aloud.[25] Rather than first activating the visual area, then Broca's linguistic processing area, and finally the premotor and motor cortices for motor programming of speech, stutterers during normal speech initiate motor programming first before the articulatory code is prepared. However, while performing tasks that minimize their stuttering such as choral reading or singing, different circuitries are activated in their brains, ones that rely less on planned linguistic programming and more on automatic processes. Thus Sendak proposes that stuttering is a state-dependent continuum based on the type of task involved; dysfluency-invoking tasks (eg, conversational speech) involve controlled language processing whereas fluency-invoking tasks (eg, singing, choral reading) involve automatic processing. This proposal raises interesting clinical questions: Do fluency-invoking therapies like singing help stutterers to become more fluent in conversational speech by repairing an abnormal linguistic programming circuit or do they subvert the task to a better-functioning automatic circuit? Neuroimaging stutterers before and after various types of speech therapies may help us select the most effective therapy based on the resultant patterns of neural activations. Furthermore, patterns of activation may help identify children who will spontaneously stop stuttering from those who need more intensive therapies.

In a 2001 issue of *Neurology*, Foundas et al published a frequently quoted study titled, "Anomalous anatomy of speech-language areas in adults with persistent developmental stuttering."[26] Based on the knowledge that regions of the brain can grow in size or atrophy based on patterns of use or disuse, they hypothesized that differences would exist in the size of the speech-language regions between individuals who stutter

and normal controls reflecting the altered patterns of use. Quantitative techniques were used to evaluate regions of interest (ROI) on MRI scans to detect an atypical size of the ROI within its hemisphere, for atypical, reduced, or reversed asymmetry between hemispheres, for extreme asymmetry, and finally for aberrant gyral patterns. The ROI were centered on classical speech-language areas including Broca's area, Wernicke's area, and the region connecting the two areas. The major finding was that the planum temporale (PT), which is comprised of the auditory association cortex and includes Wernicke's area (Figure 9–1), differed significantly both in size and asymmetry between the two groups. Both the left and right PT size was larger in adults with persistent developmental stuttering, and the normal left dominant asymmetry was reduced, making the size of the right PT relatively similar in size to the left. Thus, they concluded that the anomalous anatomy puts some people at risk for stuttering.

In a 2004 follow-up study, Foundas et al attempted to relate the differences in brain anatomy among stutterers to the phenomena of delayed auditory feedback.[27] Delayed auditory feedback (DAF) is a technique that can both improve stuttering in some stutterers and can induce stuttering in some nonstutterers. DAF devices, worn over the ear or as a headphone, delay sound from reaching the ears by a matter of milliseconds. The mechanism of action has not been fully elucidated, but is proposed to work by altering the auditory input in a way that diminishes an underlying auditory perceptual defect. Many devices based on DAF are marketed with variable success.* Foundas proposed that the anomalous anatomy found in stutterers, that is, the lack of normal asymmetry in the auditory PT region of the left and right hemispheres, might induce atypical activation-deactivation patterns that change the timing patterns needed for the coordination of the neural networks involved in speech. Alternatively, DAF might cause auditory perceptual defects that disrupt auditory self-monitoring.

To explore the relationship between anomalous anatomy and fluency under altered feedback conditions, 14 adults with developmental stuttering and normal controls matched for age, sex, educational level, and hand preference were asked to read aloud under normal and delayed auditory feedback conditions. Brain MRI scans were then acquired for evaluation of the PT sizes and symmetry. Both groups

---

*In a survey published online by The Stuttering Foundation, 800 questionnaires were sent to people who requested information about delayed auditory feedback devices. Of the 149 responders, 82.5% did not purchase a device for a variety of reason. Over half of those who did purchase the device were not using it 8 months later.

were found to have a similar mix of leftward and rightward PT asymmetry as expected based on handedness. However, the developmental stutterers who had the atypical rightward PT asymmetry had significantly more dysfluency at baseline and were more likely to have induced fluency under DAF conditions that the developmental stutterers with the more typical leftward PT. Furthermore, stuttering was induced under DAF conditions in normal controls only if they also had the atypical rightward PT asymmetry. Based on these findings, the researchers concluded that fluency among stutterers and dysfluency among normals were more likely to be affected under DAF conditions if an atypical rightward PT was present.

This presumption that abnormal anatomy yields abnormal function has been criticized as a kind of chicken-versus-egg argument. Cortical regions representing body parts are known to diminish due to disuse (eg, the area representing the arm while immobilized in a cast). Similarly, other areas enlarge when actively used such as the finger representations in a piano player. Size reflects the number of connections, or synapses, with other neurons that will increase (or decrease) the more (or less) that function is used. Thus PT asymmetry may be the result and not the cause of underlying neural abnormalities. Additionally, Perkins argues that the PT regions are involved in voluntary speech perception and speech planning and not in the high-speed and involuntary mechanisms needed for synchronization of speech in process.[28] Therefore, any size abnormalities in regional areas are secondary results of abnormalities in subcortical underlying circuits that affect speed and timing. In response, Rosenfield maintains that the Foundas' article points out only risk factors for stuttering, and that grouping subsets of stutterers based on anomalous underlying structure points the way to novel genetic, imaging, clinical, and therapeutic approaches.[29]

Genetics

The role of genetics in stuttering has been alluded to several times in this chapter and, as genetic information and techniques grow, may have an increasingly important place in diagnosis and therapy. Genetics are clearly at play in the fact that developmental stuttering is three to four times more common in boys than girls, with a similar ratio among the adult persistent developmental stuttering group. Stuttering is more frequent among monozygotic (from a single fertilized egg) individuals than among dizygotic twins (from two fertilized eggs) and does run in families. There is an association between developmental stuttering and other disorders that have a genetic basis such as Down syndrome, autism, and Tourette's disorder. The ab-

normalities in several dopamine genes seen in developmental stuttering, Tourette's, and other related disorders occurs too often to believe that these disorders are due to spontaneous gene mutations rather than inherited disorders. Work at the National Institutes of Health is looking at sites on chromosomes 18, 13, and 7 as potential candidates for stuttering genes.[1]

Multiple Neural Networks Involved in Fluent Speech

Despite the debates regarding the application of research about acquired stuttering to developmental stuttering, or the relevance of anatomic differences in brain regions, a gradually emerging theory combining anatomy, genetics, and brain chemistry is gaining general acceptance and is forming the basis of future research. The hypothesis maintains that fluent speech depends on several nested neural networks that control the initiation and production of speech and are involved in the on-line, moment-by-moment processing of speech. Several authors have proposed the existence of two specific neural circuits that must coordinate to produce fluent speech (Figure 9–3).[1,24,30] One is the outer "linguistic" circuit involved with phonologic, lexical, syntactic, and semantic language functions, and elemental auditory processing including selecting and monitoring speech sounds. In other words, the outer "linguistic" circuit chooses the correct sounds, words, and word order to produce speech in addition to self-monitoring the speech produced for comparison to what was intended. The second circuit, the inner "phonatory" circuit is involved with the motor programs of the vocal apparatus. The terms "outer" and "inner" generally correspond to the cortex and the subcortex of the brain, but the progression of signals does not always occur in adjacent locations and may occur in parallel as well as sequential events. The linguistic circuit begins with auditory processing by the primary auditory cortex in the temporal lobe (specifically in the planum temporale and Wernicke's area). Higher order processing occurs in the auditory association area located in the superior marginal gyrus and angular gyrus of the parietal lobe. Motor planning for speech output occurs in the premotor planning area, or Broca's area, of the frontal lobe. Signals then travel to the precentral sulcus of the frontal lobe that contains the primary motor cortex. The phonatory circuit is a reciprocal loop between the primary motor cortex and the basal ganglia located deep in the brain. There are connections between the outer and inner loops mentioned previously that involve other subcortical areas of the brain, which are not shown in Figure 9–3. The final output is speech production, which, in turn, gets

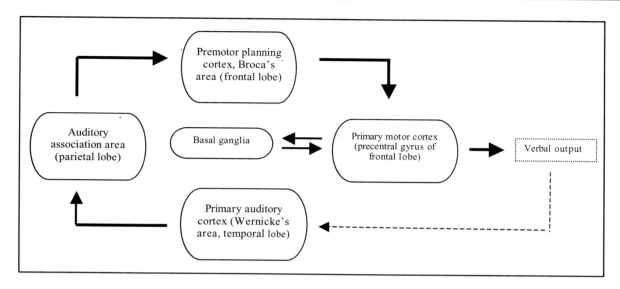

Figure 9–3. Proposed neural networks involved in production of fluent speech. The outer "linguistic" circuit starts with auditory processing by the primary auditory cortex in the temporal lobe. Further processing occurs in the auditory association area of the parietal lobe. Information then goes to the motor planning area of the frontal lobe and then to the primary motor cortex of the frontal lobe. The inner "phonatory" circuit, involved in regulating motor control of speech, is reciprocal between the motor cortex and the basal ganglia. The final verbal output is directed by the motor cortex. The resultant speech is again picked up as auditory information in a process of continual self-monitoring.

processed in the primary auditory cortex. Any disturbance of timing or momentary instability of activation in these systems can lead to stuttering.

SUMMARY

The neural networks controlling fluency traverse nearly the entire brain. It is not surprising, then, that stuttering is found in a wide variety of disease states. Furthermore, it is easy to imagine a multitude of events affecting these networks during development causing the common, and usually transient, developmental stuttering. Most certainly, stuttering is the final, common symptom of a heterogeneous group of defects. Current research—using PET scans, looking for genetic markers, identifying neurotransmitters and receptors—is searching for these defects. By identifying specific defects, stutterers could be subdivided into groups better able to respond to therapies targeted to their particular problem. For example, developmental stuttering that will resolve spontaneously could be identified and treated with speech therapy, support, and encouragement. Those who will go on to have persistent adult stuttering would be identified early and evaluated for specific genetic defects that may be more amenable to medical or even genetic therapies. Acquired stuttering, albeit rare, would also benefit from

knowledge of the normal mechanisms of fluent speech by targeting speech therapies and medication based on the location of the lesion or the mechanisms of the diseases involved. It is useful for voice professionals to be familiar with this complex disorder and to remain active in the diagnosis and treatment team involved in the management of patients with stuttering.

REFERENCES

1. The Stuttering Foundation; 3100 Walnut Grove Road, Ste 603, P.O. Box 11749, Memphis, TN 38111-0749; 1-800-992-9392; www.stutteringhelp.org
2. Foundas AL, Bollich AM, Feldman J, et al. Aberrant auditory processing and atypical planum temporale in developmental stuttering. *Neurology.* 2004;63(9):1640–1646.
3. Costa D, Kroll, R. Stuttering: an update for physicians. *CMAJ.* 2000;162(13):1849–1855.
4. National Stuttering Association. 119 W. 40th Street, 14th floor, New York, NY 10018; 1-800-937-8888; www.nastutter.org
5. Busari JO, Weggelaar NM. How to investigate and manage the child who is slow to speak. *Br Med J.* 2004; 328(7434):272–276.
6. Weir E, Bianchet S. Developmental dysfluency: early intervention is key. *CMAJ.* 2004;170(12):1790–1791.
7. Brown J, Hasselkus A, Tenenholtz E. Speech-language pathologists add value to home care. *Home Healthcare Nurse.* 2002;20(6): 393–398.

8. Vossler DG, Haltiner AM, Schepp SK, Friel PA, Caylor LM, Morgan JD, Doherty, MJ. Ictal stuttering: a sign suggestive of psychogenic nonepileptic seizures. *Neurology.* 2004;63(3):516–519.

9. Bradley WG, Daroff RB, Fenichel GM, Jankovic J. *Neurology in Clinical Practice.* 4th ed. New York, NY: Butterworth/Heinmann, Elsevier; 2004.

10. Grant AC, Biousse V, Cook AA, Newman NJ. Stroke-associated stuttering. *Arch Neurol.* 1999;56(5):624–627.

11. Ciabarra AM, Elkind MS, Roberts JK, Marshall RS. Subcortical infarction resulting in acquired stuttering. *J Neurol Neurosurg Psychiatry.* 2000;69(4):546–549.

12. Gilman S, Newman SW. *Manter and Gatz's Essentials of Clinical Neuroanatomy and Neurophysiology.* 10th ed. Philadelphia, PA: F.A. Davis Co; 2003:4.

13. Muro A, Hirayama K, Tanno Y, et al. Cessation of stuttering after bilateral thalamic infarction. *Neurology.* 1999; 53(4):890–891.

14. Schmahmann JD. Vascular syndromes of the thalamus. *Stroke.* 2003;34(9):2264–2278.

15. Heuer RJ, Sataloff RT, Mandel S, Travers N. Neurogenic stuttering: further corroboration of site of lesion. *Ear Nose Throat J.* 1996;75(3):161–168.

16. Benke T, Hohenstein C, Poewe W, Butterworth B. Repetitive speech phenomena in Parkinson's disease. *J Neurol Neurosurg Psychiatry.* 2000;69(3):319–325.

17. Anderson JM, Hughes JD, Rothi LJ, et al. Developmental stuttering and Parkinson's disease: the effects of levodopa treatment. *J Neurol Neurosurg Psychiatry.* 1999;66(6): 776–778.

18. Pinto S, Thobois S, Costes N, et al. Subthalamic nucleus stimulation and dysarthria in Parkinson's disease: a PET study. *Brain.* 2004;127(3):602–615.

19. Sataloff RT, Heuer RJ, Munz M, Yoon MS, Spiegel JR. Vocal tremor reduction with deep brain stimulation: a preliminary report. *J Voice.* 2002;16(1):132–135.

20. Nissani M, Sanchez EA. Stuttering caused by gabapentin. *Ann Intern Med.* 1997;126(5):410.

21. Mulder L, Spierings EH. Stuttering relieved by divalproex sodium. *Neurology.* 2003;61(5):714.

22. Paola Canevini M, Chifari R, Piazzini A. Improvement of a patient with stuttering on levetiracetam. *Neurology.* 2002;59(8):1288.

23. Maguire GA, Riley GD, Franklin DL, Gottschalk LA. Risperidone for the treatment of stuttering. *J Clin Psychopharmacol.* 2000;20(4):479–482.

24. Fox PT, Ingham RJ, Ingham JC, et al. A PET study of the neural systems of stuttering. *Nature.* 1996;382(6587):158–162.

25. Sandak R, Fiez JA. Stuttering: a view from neuroimaging. *Lancet.* 2000;356(9228):445–446.

26. Foundas AL, Bollich AM, Corey DM. Hurley M, Heilman KM Anomalous anatomy of speech-language areas in adults with persistent developmental stuttering. *Neurology.* 2001;57(2):207–215.

27. Foundas AL, Bollich AM, Feldman J, et al. Aberrant auditory processing and atypical planum temporale in developmental stuttering. *Neurology.* 2004;63(9):1640–1646.

28. Perkins WH. Anomalous anatomy of speech-language areas in adults with persistent developmental stuttering. *Neurology.* 2002;58(2):332–333.

29. Rosenfield DB. Anomalous anatomy of speech-language areas in adults with persistent developmental stuttering. *Neurology.* 2002;58(2):333.

30. Nudelman HB, Herbich RD, Hess KR, et al. A model of phonatory response time of stutters and fluent speakers to frequency-modulated tones. *J Acoust Soc Am.* 1992;92: 1882–1888.

10

Dynamical Disorders of Voice: A Chaotic Perspective on Vocal Irregularities

R. J. Baken, PhD

The modern era of voice research might fairly be said to have begun about 50 years ago, with the elaboration of a crucial understanding: phonation results from and is governed by the biomechanical characteristics of vocal fold tissue interacting with glottal aerodynamic properties. That insight was the heart of the myoelastic-aerodynamic theory of phonation,[1-3] a construct that physiologic observation of vocal fold behavior has amply validated. Numerous mathematical models of vocal fold function that were founded upon it[4-5] have generally had extraordinarily impressive predictive and explanatory power. As a result, the process of normal phonation is quite well understood.

Unfortunately, despite very serious efforts by many of our best researchers over a significant period of time, there are still large gaps in our comprehension of laryngeal phonatory behavior. Nowhere are these lacunae wider than in our understanding of many of the anomalies encountered in abnormal vocal function, and (when one actually looks for them)

even in the normal voice.[6] The increase of frequency and amplitude perturbation that is so characteristic of dysphonia, for example, remains only poorly explained, despite several hypotheses of varying attractiveness.[7-13] The "pitch breaks" of the adolescent also lack a coherent explanatory model, as has the "biphonation" of the infant's cry.[14-15]

Even less well explained is the kind of situation illustrated in Figure 10–1A, which shows the fundamental frequency (F_0) of successive periods during a sustained vowel by an 81-year-old female with a diagnosis of spasmodic dysphonia. Her F_0 undergoes a relatively slow cyclic variation at a rate of about 4 cycles per second, most likely caused by tremor of the laryngeal muscles. There is also, however, a much faster frequency variation that is sometimes observable at the peaks of the slower oscillations. This is harder to explain. However, most striking are the outbreaks of "diplophonia"—more properly, subharmonic oscillation—that occur in the "valleys" of the F_0 pattern and

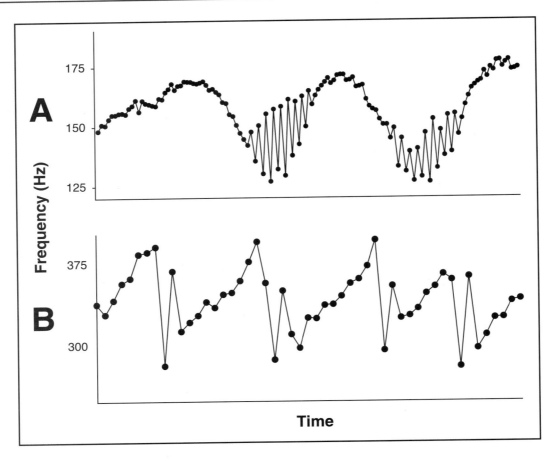

Figure 10–1. Fundamental frequency of successive periods during sustained vowels. **A.** An aged spasmodic dysphonic woman, showing subharmonic oscillation during the low parts of a tremor cycle; **B.** very complex patterns of F_0 change in the voice of a dysphonic patient.

that persist halfway up the next peak. We have had no easy explanation for this kind of behavior. Even less have we been able to offer coherent and parsimonious explanations for the more complex patterns of F_0 change, like that of Figure 10–1B, that are not uncommon in dysphonic voices. While we have developed a fairly clear picture of the mechanisms of the phonationally regular, we have not done nearly as well in elucidating the vocally complex or erratic.

The fact is, of course, that we have not done much worse in dealing with oscillatory misbehavior than most of the broader sciences of which we are a part. All have been impeded by a paucity of scientific tools for describing disorder, modeling instability, and characterizing capriciousness.

The outlook improved dramatically about 20 years ago with the recognition of the pivotal importance, broad applicability, and enormous explanatory power of a radically different way of considering natural phenomena. The new discipline is formally known as the *theory of nonlinear dynamics,* but it is more popularly called *chaos theory.* It offers a different way of look-

ing at life functions[16-18] that has begun to have a significant impact in the biomedical world. Cochlear function,[19] abnormal motor behavior,[20] cardiac electrical instability,[21-25] Cheyne-Stokes respiration,[26] cerebral electrophysiology,[27] and even menopausal hot flashes[28] have been explored with the new tools—both qualitative and quantitative—that it provides. The application of chaos theory to voice production is now well underway.[29-45] It holds the promise of important breakthroughs in understanding those erratic phenomena of voice, normal and disordered, that have thus far proved so intractable.

The purpose of this chapter is to consider a few of the most basic concepts of chaos theory, and to show how they might profitably be applied to problems of vocal dysfunction. The theory itself is intensely mathematical, and the mathematics can be quite difficult and counterintuitive. It is, therefore, useful to take a very informal concept-oriented approach even though doing so greatly circumscribes the extent to which important areas can be developed. The purpose is not to provide a tutorial introduction to applied chaos theory so much as to suggest something of the flavor of this relatively new branch of the sciences and to suggest why it holds such promise. To do this, some conjectures will be proposed that might explain the sudden appearance of phonatory anomalies that are so characteristic of disordered voices. Insofar as possible, we will proceed in a completely nonmathematical (and consequently nonrigorous) way, because it seems likely that doing so will meet the needs of most readers who would like to understand the general tenor of what is involved, but who are unlikely to want to tackle nonlinear dynamical analyses themselves (at least not yet). Numerophiles and those who wish really to explore the area should consult a good general text.*

CHAOS DEFINED

The very term "chaos" has become trendy, a fashionable buzzword that is too often dropped into discussions as a synonym for "erratic," "unpredictable," or "very complex." But the word *chaos* has, in fact, a very specific definition. If it is to be a useful concept, it is important to specify exactly what "chaos" really means.

Basically, behavior can be said to be chaotic **if and only if:**

- *It is the product of a deterministic system.* "Deterministic" means that the observed behavior is governed by a rule. We may not understand what that rule is but we must know that it does, in fact, exist and that it is controlling the system. The fact that there is a governing nonlinear rule is the sine qua non of a chaotic system.
- *The system is nonlinear.* In the simplest sense, a linear system is one whose function can be plotted as a straight line on a graph. Figure 10–2A is an example. All other things being equal, it shows that airflow through the vocal tract is directly and linearly proportional to the pressure in the lungs. A nonlinear function, on the other hand, is represented by a curved line (which can be quite complex). Figure 10–2B is illustrative. It shows the relationship that has been observed[60] between subglottal pressure and the intensity of the vocal signal.
- Despite the determinism (rule-based operation) of the generating system, the *output is nonetheless unpredictable*. This requirement needs to be understood carefully. It does, of course, imply that the be-

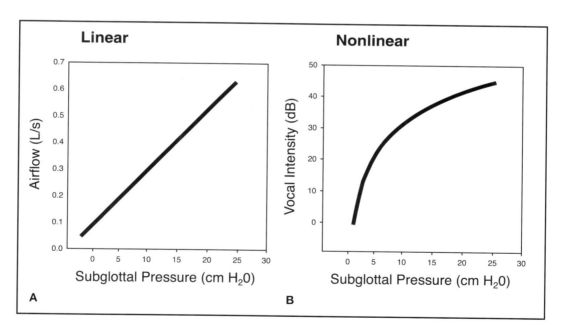

Figure 10–2. Linear and nonlinear functions.

*The classic source of understanding for numerophobes is Gleick (1987),[46] a volume that appeared for many weeks on the best-seller lists. A very brief nontechnical presentation is Crutchfield, Farmer, et al (1986)[47] For those who can tolerate a minimal mathematical exposition, Abraham and Shaw[48-51] offer an excellent—and lighthearted—starting point that calls for no background at all. More mathematically rigorous introductions are provided by Rasband,[52] Baker and Golub,[53] Moon,[54] and Thompson and Stewart.[55] Eubank and Farmer (1990)[56] is a classic, and is surprisingly approachable. A good overview of chaos in several scientific disciplines is available in Cvitanovic (1984),[57] while Glass and Mackey[58] explore nonlinear dynamics of various biological systems, and West[59] concisely reviews nonlinear dynamics considered in pathophysiology.

havior might be random-looking. But it also allows, for example, for the system to produce a number of different patterns of response (within each of which a succession of output states might be completely predictable). If one is not able to specify, to any arbitrarily specified level of precision, which *pattern* will be produced at any given time, the system may validly be described as chaotic (provided, of course, that the other requirements are met).

- The system must have a relatively small number of parameters. That is, it must be controlled by only a few factors. Put another way, a chaotic system, however much it behaves in complex ways, must nonetheless be a fairly simple system. For reasons that will shortly become clear, it is described as a "low dimensional" system.

- *Finally, the behavior of the system must be "exquisitely sensitive to initial conditions."* What this means is that extremely small differences in some controlling parameter can have dramatically large effects on the qualitative aspects of the system's behavior. Note, in Figure 10–3, how changing the coefficient a in the function $x_{n+1} = ax_n(1-x_n)$ by a mere 0.005, from $a = 3.855$ to $a = 3.860$, alters the qualitative nature of the output dramatically.**

In fact, radical shifts in the output of a chaotic system can be produced by changes that are *infinitesimally* small. "Infinitesimal" is used here in its literal, mathematical sense. Therefore, we can never have enough decimal places in our specification of the con-

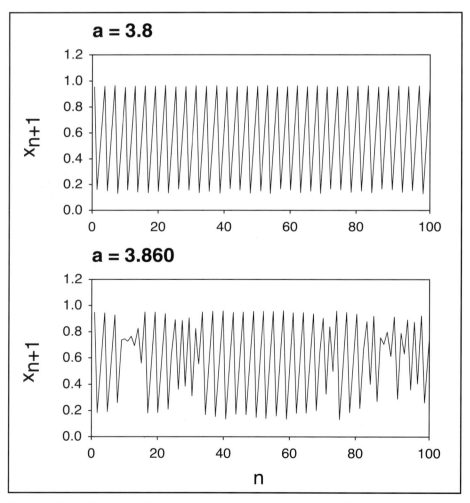

Figure 10–3. Output of the "logistic equation" can be dramatically altered by tiny changes of its coefficient "a."

**Known as the "logistic equation" this is a favorite example of a chaotic generator. Despite its extreme simplicity, its output can be astoundingly complex. Any of the texts cited in the previous footnote will provide more information about this "simple" system.

trolling variable to be able to predict the resultant behavior of the system with absolute certainty. Furthermore, an infinitesimally small difference is, from a practical point of view, a difference of zero. This implies that a chaotic system can change its behavior for no measurable reason at all.

DYNAMICS OF A SYSTEM

It is vital to understand that one cannot tell if a system is behaving in a chaotic manner just by looking at its output. Consider the two data sets plotted in Figure 10–4. One was produced by a chaotic system (that is, by a system that has the defining characteristics just discussed). The other, as best one can tell, is simply random. Which is the chaotic one? There are often ways to find out, but looking is not one of them. Not everything that looks random is chaotic.

Trajectories in State Space

How can one describe the dynamics (the behavior) of a system? One of the best ways is to plot its behavior in *state space* (often called *phase space*). It is easier to understand what this means from an example than from a definition, and the example will prove useful in developing some further concepts.

Consider a pendulum—like one that hangs from a clock, illustrated in Figure 10–5. Give it, for the sake of our example, the rather special property that it is not subject to friction, so that once started, it swings forever. It turns out that the dynamics of this extraordinarily simple (linear) system can be fully described in terms of the position and velocity of the pendulum. We can show their relationship graphically, as in Figure 10–6.

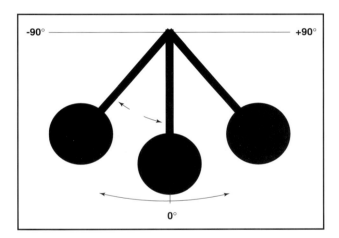

Figure 10–5. Simple pendulum, swinging through an angle q.

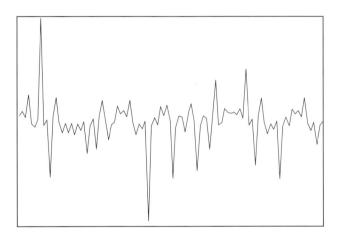

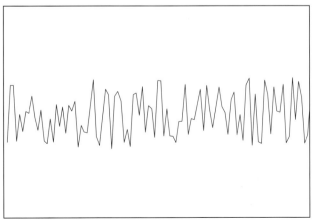

Figure 10–4. Only one of these patterns was produced by a chaotic system. Which one?

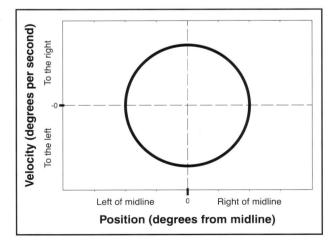

Figure 10–6. Relationship of the position and velocity of the pendulum of Figure 10–5. The plane of the graph is the "state space" of the pendulum system.

The position of the pendulum (in degrees, q) to the left or right of midline is plotted on the horizontal axis, while its speed (in degrees per second, toward the left or right) is plotted on the vertical axis. The (two-dimensional) space that these axes create is one example of a *state space* (also called a *phase space*). The ellipse that results is a *trajectory* that passes through all the points in this space that are possible for a simple pendulum. It, therefore, demarcates all the combinations of position and speed that this uncomplicated dynamic system can have. As it happens, the pendulum is so simple that a two-variable state space is enough to define its dynamics *completely*. That is, there is nothing else that we need to know (or would have to derive) about this system to understand all its operation.

If the pendulum were free to swing not only from side to side, but also front-to-back (so that its motion described not an arc, but a circle) then we would need another axis to describe its motion in this direction, as in Figure 10–7. Adding an axis creates a three-dimensional space, which is the minimum necessary to describe this system. Hence, it could be called a three-dimensional dynamical system. "Dimension" is the way in which we specify the number of axes, each representing an independent variable, that is necessary to describe the dynamics of a system.

Attractors

Real pendulums, of course, are subject to friction. With each oscillation a little energy is lost and the width of the swing decreases, until finally the pendulum hangs at rest. To counter this, pendulum clocks have a mechanism that gives the pendulum a little "kick" when it passes a certain position in its swing cycle, adding back the energy that it lost during the previous oscillation. Because of the kick the trajectory of the pendulum system in state space has a little "glitch" in it, as in Figure 10–8.

Now, the amount of energy added by each kick is constant, and is just enough to keep the pendulum's arc at a given width. Suppose, therefore, that the pendulum is started by pulling it very far from the midline—to a position much further out than it would normally swing. Remembering that the once-per-cycle kick only provides enough energy for a swing of moderate width, it is clear that the amount of energy lost to friction on the initial huge swing will not be fully made up by the kick. Therefore, the next swing will be a little less energetic, and a little less wide. In fact, more energy is lost during each wider-than-normal swing than is restored by the kick, and so the swings will constantly become less wide until the arc is just the right size—the size at which the energy lost is exactly made up by the energy that the kick adds. Because, at this arc width, the energy loss and addition are exactly balanced, the pendulum will continue to oscillate in an arc of that width forever (or as long as the clock is kept

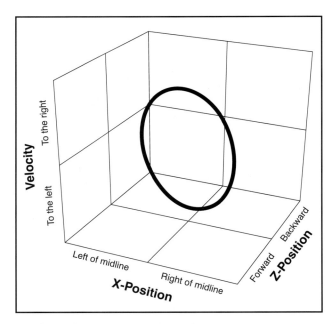

Figure 10–7. A third axis is required to describe the movement of a pendulum that can swing not only side-to-side, but also front-to-back. The state space of such a pendulum is three-dimensional.

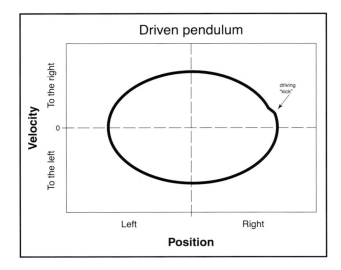

Figure 10–8. A real pendulum needs a small "kick" during each swing to make up for frictional losses. The kick produces a glitch in the trajectory in phase space, but delivers the energy that keeps the system going.

wound up). The situation is illustrated in Figure 10–9A.

A similar situation prevails, in reverse, if we start the pendulum swinging from a position that is not as far out as it usually goes. Each swing, being smaller than usual, loses less energy than the standard-sized once-per-cycle kick delivers, so with each swing there is a net gain of energy, and each oscillation is a bit larger than the one before (Figure 10–9B). Finally, the swing is large enough that the energy lost equals the energy gained, and thereafter the pendulum follows the same trajectory in phase space "forever."

The final trajectory, then, has an important property. Starting the pendulum from almost anywhere in the state space—with however much displacement from the midline, and with however strong a push one might give it—it will always end up swinging with the same frequency and arc width. All paths seem to be compelled to head for the same final trajectory, which is therefore called an *attractor*.

Model Behavior

The human vocal system is extraordinarily complex and is largely inaccessible to direct observation. Fur-

thermore, there is a very limited number of ways in which one can manipulate it for experimental purposes. One means of getting around these problems is to use a mathematical model of the vocal folds (and sometimes of other elements of the vocal tract as well). A respectable number of models have been developed, each expressing its creator's conceptualization of the nature of the forces driving phonatory oscillation. One of the least complex and best known is the Ishizaka-Flanagan (1972)[61] model. It simplifies each vocal fold to an upper and a lower mass. They are more or less tightly coupled to each other but each is free to move toward or away from the glottis. The user chooses such important biomechanical and aerodynamic parameters as the size and stiffness of each mass, the length of the glottis, the subglottal pressure, and so on. Despite its very significant simplification of a complex system, it does provide a useful portrayal—validated by comparison to real phonation—of vocal fold oscillation under a wide range of physiologic conditions. Furthermore, its simplicity is ideal for present purposes, because it makes it possible to explore the potential for chaotic behavior in a "phonatory apparatus" that has only a few controlling variables, and hence in a system that should be easily understandable.

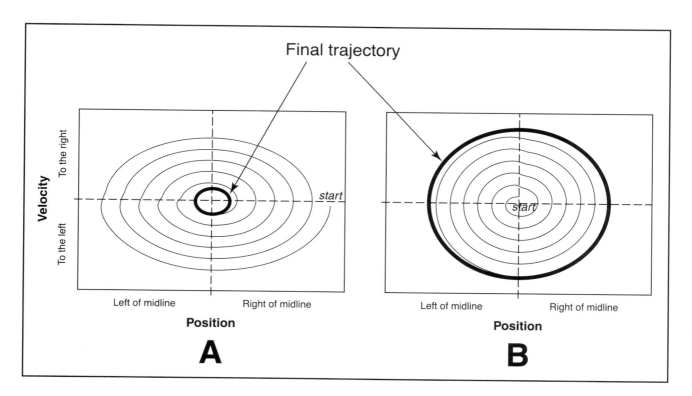

Figure 10–9. The constant-sized kick provides just enough energy to keep the pendulum swinging with an arc of only a certain size—no bigger and no smaller. No matter how the pendulum is started, it will end up swinging with an arc of that certain size. The system is *attracted* to a special trajectory in state space.

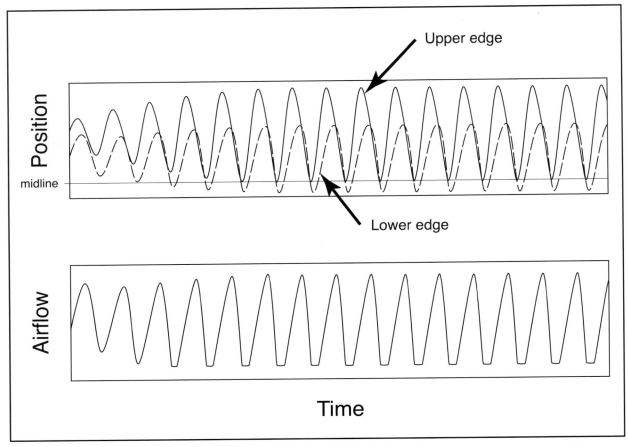

Figure 10–10. Typical oscillation just after onset of the vocal folds in the two-mass model. *Top:* Position of the vocal fold's upper and lower edges. *Bottom:* Transglottal airflow.

Model Phonation

If we set parameters for the two-mass model to some reasonable values—say moderate stiffness and subglottal pressure—and let it run, it oscillates quite well. Typical vibration is shown in Figure 10–10. The shaded area in the plot is the region where this vocal fold moves past the midline, and hence overlaps the opposite fold. Obviously, in real life this cannot happen. Instead, the vocal folds collide and deform each other. However, in the purely mathematical world of the model all things are possible, and the position trace has been allowed to extend into this realm of impossibility to provide some sense of how much deformation there would be.

Note that, as in the living larynx, there is a phase difference between the upper and lower lips of the vocal fold. Also, again as in nature, it takes a few oscillatory cycles for full vibratory amplitude to be achieved. The record of airflow through the modeled glottis shows a regular train of pulses, although their shape is not a precise representation of that of real voice.

One way to show the dynamics of the model's vocal fold in a state space is to plot the position of the upper mass of the vocal fold against the position of the lower mass, as in Figure 10–10. The trajectory of the system in this state space bears an obvious resemblance to the outward-spiraling trajectory of a simple pendulum shown in Figure 10–9B. That is, driven by the energy boost from the subglottal pressure, the trajectory spirals out from the starting condition until ultimately it reaches and is held by an attractor. The attractor itself is quite different, however. Instead of being a single line in state space, it appears to be "unstable" in that it is a *cluster* of lines. An enlargement of a small region of the attractor, shown on the right of Figure 10–11, reveals that the lines of the attractor show signs of being "bundled." In fact, although not shown here, each "bundle" of lines could be shown to be itself composed of bundles, and those bundles of still other bundles, and so on, ad infinitum. With a little mathematical trickery—the details of which are beyond our present discus-

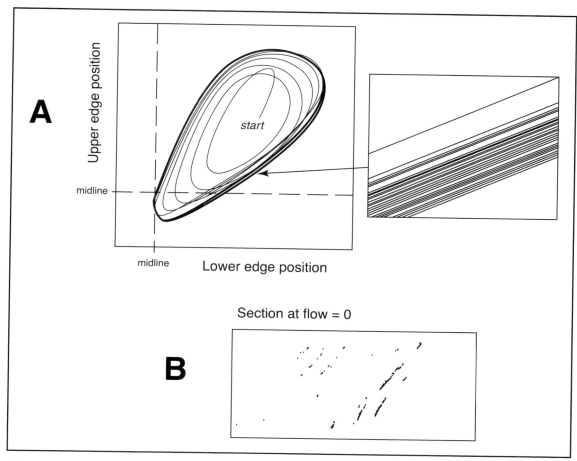

Figure 10–11. Oscillation of the vocal fold of the two-mass model shown in an "Upper-edge/lower-edge" state space. **A.** After start-up the system seems to be drawn to an attractor. However, magnifying that attractor shows that it is really a bundle of separate lines. Increasing the magnification would reveal ever-smaller bundles of lines. **B.** Plotting a "cross-section" of the attractor shows that the bundles of lines that compose it are arranged in layers. This is, therefore, a "strange attractor" that has fractal properties.

sion[†]—it is possible to "cut" across these bundles, something like chopping across a fistful of spaghetti, and then to look at the cut surface. If we do this, as in Figure 10–11B, we find that not only are the lines "bundled," but the bundles are arranged in layers. As it happens, if we were to repeatedly enlarge each layer, we would see that each layer is itself composed of layers—layers within layers, ad infinitum. In short, the appearance of the attractor at every magnification would have very much the appearance of any other magnification. This property of any small part being a miniature version of the whole—technically referred to as "self-similarity at all scales"—makes the attractor a "fractal" structure.[‡] An attractor that is fractal is said—in the technical jargon of nonlinear dynamics—to be *strange*. Strange attractors are characteristic of chaotic systems.

The Ishizaka-Flanagan two-mass model, and other simple models of the vocal folds have, in fact, been shown to be chaotic systems,[30,37,64,65] and thus can serve us well in our present exploration of the role of chaos in vocal dysfunction.

---

†Except, perhaps, to note that the result is termed as Poincaré section, and to suggest that the techniques for doing this and for interpreting the results are found in numerous introductory texts in the field of nonlinear dynamical systems theory.

‡Because fractal shapes are often surprisingly and intriguingly beautiful they have captured the imagination of many in recent years. Accordingly, there are many excellent books for neophytes who would like to learn more about them. The best known is by Mandelbrot (1977),[62] who founded the field of fractal geometry. A somewhat more useful text—complete with computer algorithms for generating fractal images—is Peitgen and Saupe, 1988.[63]

A Moment's Consideration of an Important Bias

Although oscillation of the model's vocal folds is governed by an attractor, that attractor, by being fractal, allows each cycle—in fact, it *requires* each cycle—to be slightly different from every other one. That is worth thinking about for a moment, because the oscillation we are dealing with here is generated by an equation. An equation does not change while the model is running. An equation does not involve perturbing factors—variations in subglottal pressure, small alterations of muscle tension, minuscule shifts of mucus, or shifts of vocal tract posture. Despite this, the output shows observable perturbation.

Our bias is to believe that any effect—such as the radical shifts of F_0 of Figure 10–1—must have a proximate cause which is, in principle, identifiable. That bias accounts for several theories and speculations concerning the origins of, for example, frequency and amplitude perturbation. However, perturbation in the output of a mathematical model is a common observation (for example Wong, Ito, et al, 1991)[64] and can only be an inherent result of the equations that form it. It cannot, in a model, be the product of immediate outside causes. The question naturally arises: How much of the perturbation of the normal (real) vocal signal is caused by small pressure variations, little muscle twitches, and the like. How much is simply inherent in the vocal fold dynamics—as shown by a strange attractor? Similarly, the theory of nonlinear dynamics makes it clear that the behavior of a system can alter in the absence of any external influence. Effects do not necessarily have immediate causes.

Basin of Attraction: The Attractor's Realm

It is worthwhile to look at the dynamics of the pendulum once again. Recall that it gets a little push whenever it passes a given point in its swing, and this little boost is just sufficient to replace the energy lost to friction. Figure 10–12 recapitulates some things that were said about this system earlier. That is, if the pendulum is started from a position either more than or less than its usual displacement, oscillations either diminish or enlarge until their amplitude represents an equilibrium between the energy gain and loss. The final trajectory that represents this equilibrium state is an attractor, because the dynamics of the system seem—in some metaphorical sense—to be drawn to it.

The plane of the state space of Figure 10–12 contains all the possible combinations of position and velocity that, in principle, a pendulum could have. A reasonable

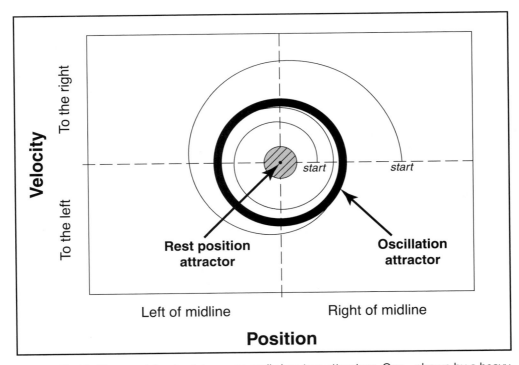

Figure 10–12. The pendulum's state space really has two attractors. One—shown by a heavy line—is an oscillation, but the other—represented by a dot in the middle of the plane—is hanging motionless. Most starting points on the plane lead to the oscillation attractor, but some lead to the motionless condition. There are two "basins of attraction" in the state space.

26. Kryger MH, Millar T. Cheyne-Stokes respiration: stability of interacting systems in heart failure. *Chaos.* 1991;1: 265–269.

27. Rapp PE, Bashore TR, Martinerie JM, Albano AM, Zimmerman ID, Mees AI. *Brain Topogr.* 1989;2:99–118.

28. Kroenenberg F. Menopausal hot flashes: randomness or rhythmicity? *Chaos.* 1991;1:271–278.

29. Pickover CA, Khorsani A. Fractal characterization of speech waveform graphs. *Comput Graphics.* 1986;10:51–61.

30. Awrejcewicz J. Bifurcation portrait of the human vocal cord oscillations. *J Sound Vibration.* 1990;136:151–156.

31. Baken RJ. Irregularity of vocal period and amplitude: a first approach to the fractal analysis of voice. *J Voice.* 1990;4:185–197.

32. Mende W, Herzel H, Wermke K. Bifurcations and chaos in newborn cries. *Physics Lett A.* 1990;145:418–424.

33. Herzel H, Steinecke I, Mende W, Wermke K. Chaos and bifurcations in voiced speech. In: Mosekilde E. ed. *Complexity, Chaos, and Biological Evolution.* New York, NY: Plenum Press; 1991.

34. Titze IR, Baken RJ, Herzel H. Evidence of chaos in vocal fold vibration. In: Titze IR, ed. *Vocal Fold Physiology: Frontiers in Basic Science.* San Diego, CA: Singular Publishing; 1993:143–188.

35. Baken RJ. The aged voice: a new hypothesis. *Voice* (Journal of the British Voice Association). 1994;3:57–73.

36. Kakita Y, Okamoto H. Visualizing the characteristics of vocal fluctuation from the viewpoint of chaos: An attempt toward qualitative quantification. In: Fujimura O, Hirano M, eds. *Vocal Fold Physiology: Voice Quality Control.* San Diego, CA: Singular Publishing; 1994:235–348.

37. Steinecke I, Herzel H. Bifurcations in an asymmetric vocal-fold model. *J Acoust Soc Am.* 1995;97:1874–1884.

38. Herzel H, Berry D, Titze IR, Steinecke I. Nonlinear dynamics of the voice: signal analysis and biomechanical modeling. *Chaos.* 1995;5:30–34.

39. Berry DA, Herzel H, Titze IR, Story BH. Bifurcations in excised larynx experiments. *J Voice.* 1996:10;129–138.

40. Fletcher, NH. Nonlinearity, complexity, and control in vocal systems: In: Davis PJ, Fletcher NH, eds. *Vocal Fold Physiology: Controlling Complexity and Chaos.* San Diego, CA: Singular Publishing; 1996:3–16.

41. Herzel H. Possible mechanisms of vocal instabilities. In: Davis PJ, Fletcher NH, eds. *Vocal Fold Physiology: Controlling Complexity and Chaos.* San Diego, CA: Singular Publishing; 1996:63–75.

42. Kumar A, Mullick SK. Nonlinear dynamical analysis of speech. *J Acoust Soc Am.* 1996;100:615–629.

43. Behrman A, Baken RJ. Correlation dimension of electroglottographic data from healthy and pathologic subjects. *J Acoust Soc Am.* 1997;102:2371–2379.

44. Ouaknine M, Giovanni A, Guelfucci B, Teston B, Triglia JM. Nonlinear behavior of vocal fold vibration in an experimental model of asymmetric larynx: role of coupling between the two folds. *Rev Laryngol Otol Rhinol.* 1998; 119:249–252.

45. Behrman A. Global and local dimensions of vocal dynamics. *J Acoust Soc Am.* 1999;106:432–443.

46. Gleick J. *Chaos: Marking a New Science.* New York, NY: Viking Penguin; 1987.

47. Crutchfield JP, Farmer JD, Packard NH, Shaw RS. Chaos. *Sci Am.* December 1986;46–57.

48. Abraham RH, Shaw CD. *Dynamics—The Geometry of Behavior. Part One: Periodic Behavior.* The Visual Mathematics Library: VisMath Vol 1. Santa Cruz, CA: Aerial Press; 1982.

49. Abraham RH, Shaw, CD. *Dynamics—The Geometry of Behavior. Part Two: Chaotic Behavior.* The Visual Mathematics Library: VisMath Vol 2. Santa Cruz, CA: Aerial Press; 1983.

50. Abraham RH, Shaw CD. *Dynamics—The Geometry of Behavior. Part Three: Global Behavior.* The Visual Mathematics Library: VisMath Vol 3. Santa Cruz, CA: Aerial Press; 1985.

51. Abraham RH, Shaw CD. Dynamics—*The Geometry of Behavior. Part Four: Bifurcation Behavior.* The Visual Mathematics Library: VisMath Vol 4. Santa Cruz, CA: Aerial Press; 1982.

52. Rasband SN. *Chaotic Dynamics of Nonlinear Systems.* New York, NY: Wiley; 1990.

53. Baker GL, Golub JP. *Chaotic Dynamics: An Introduction.* New York, NY: Cambridge University Press; 1990.

54. Moon FC. *Chaotic Vibrations: An Introduction for Applied Scientists and Engineers.* New York, NY: Wiley; 1987.

55. Thompson JMT, Stewart HB. *Nonlinear Dynamics and Chaos: Geometrical Methods for Engineers and Scientists.* New York, NY: Wiley; 1986.

56. Eubank S, Farmer D. *An Introduction to Chaos and Randomness.* Boston, MA: Addison-Wesley; 1990.

57. Cvitanovic P, ed. *Universality in Chaos.* 2nd ed. New York, NY: Adam Hilger (IOP Publishing, Ltd.); 1984.

58. Glass L, Mackey MC. *From Clocks to Chaos.* Princeton, NJ: Princeton University Press; 1988.

59. West BJ. *Fractal Physiology and Chaos in Medicine.* Singapore: World Scientific; 1990.

60. Isshiki N. Regulatory mechanism of voice intensity variation. *J Speech Hear Res.* 1964;7:17–29.

61. Ishizaka K, Flanagan JL. Synthesis of voiced sounds from a two-mass model of the vocal cords. *Bell Sys Tech J.* 1972;51:1233–1268.

62. Mandelbrot BB. *The Fractal Geometry of Nature.* New York, NY: Freeman; 1977.

63. Peitgen H-O, Saupe D, eds. *The Science of Fractal Images.* New York, NY: Springer-Verlag; 1988.

64. Wong D, Ito M, Cox NB, Titze IR. Observation of perturbations in a lumped-element model of the vocal folds with application to some pathological cases. *J Acoust Soc Am.* 1991;89:383–394.

65. Lucero JC. Dynamics of the two-mass model of the vocal folds: equilibria, bifurcations, and oscillation region. *J Acoust Soc Am.* 1993;94:3104–3111.

66. Mackey MC, Glass L. Oscillations and chaos in physiological control systems. *Science.* 1977;197:287–289.

67. Goldberger AL, West BJ. Chaos in physiology: Health or disease. In: Holton A, Olsen LF, eds. *Chaos in Biological Systems.* New York, NY: Plenum Press; 1987:1–5.

68. Mackey MC, Milton JC. Dynamical diseases. *Ann NY Acad Sci.* 1987;504;16–32.

11

Research in Laryngology

Gayle E. Woodson, MD

The birth of laryngology as a specialty was enabled by the introduction of a new technology: mirror laryngoscopy. This indirect means of viewing the larynx was developed by a singing teacher, but was quickly adopted by physicians. Suddenly, the phonatory mechanism could be studied. It was possible to detect a physical basis for hoarseness in many patients and to observe changes in response to treatment.

Throughout its history, the development of laryngology as a specialty has largely been spurred by advances in laryngeal examination. In the late 20th century, the development of rod lens telescopes and fiberoptics greatly enhanced the ability to observe laryngeal function and pathology. But visualization alone was not sufficient. Sustained, meaningful progress has been the result of "bridging" research: the collaborative efforts of clinicians who seek better ways to care for their patients and basic scientists who seek to understand structure and function. Some of the fruits of such research include sound principles of vocal hygiene, improved methods of voice therapy, and the emergence of phonosurgical techniques. More recently, advances in molecular biology have provided new directions for laryngeal research. Many important questions that could improve the care of patients with laryngeal disorders remain. If properly harnessed, the current exponential increase in medical knowledge and technology could provide answers that would transform drastically the field in the coming years.

CRUCIAL RESEARCH ISSUES IN LARYNGOLOGY

The primary need is for information that can be directly applied to the management of serious clinical problems, such as disabling voice disorders, laryngeal airway impairment, and dysphagia. However, there are also many significant gaps in our fundamental knowledge of the physiology of phonation, respiration, and deglutition; and these deficiencies limit clinical progress. The gross anatomy of the larynx has been described well for centuries, but the complexity of laryngeal motion and the importance of the microscopic architecture of the vocal fold have been appreciated only in recent years. Developments in experimental techniques and molecular biology may provide important tools for elucidating structure-function relationships, but are likely to raise new questions that will change the direction and focus of research interest. Thus, it is impossible to predict what future investigations will accomplish. This chapter reviews some important developments in laryngeal research and considers the implications of each for future research directions.

Hirano described the unique layered structure of connective tissue in the vocal fold cover, and pointed out the crucial role of this tissue in normal phonation.[1] Consequently, entirely new research questions arose. What factors are responsible for the development and maintenance of this layered structure? What biologic processes and factors are involved in laryngeal scarring? How can the normal structure be restored for a scarred vocal fold? Surgery is by far the most frequent cause of scarring that limits vocal fold mobility. What surgical techniques or medical therapy can be used to prevent scarring?

Improving phonation in a scarred vocal fold requires restoration of the mobility of the epithelium, so that it vibrates without constraint by underlying tissue. Techniques using injections or grafts to separate the epithelium from underlying tissue have had disappointing results. It has become clear that the superficial layer of vocal fold lamina propria is dynamic tissue that requires constant maintenance. It cannot be replaced by simple introduction of some static material. Thus, current research into vocal scarring addresses the biologic processes that maintain and repair the lamina propria. The maculae flavae are dense masses of stellate cells at the anterior and posterior ends of the membranous vocal folds. The maculae flavae appear to be "factories" for generating the proteins necessary to maintain the lamina propria.[2] A number of growth factors have been shown to stimulate the production of hyaluronan by fibroblasts.[3] Animal experiments suggest that application of growth factors could improve vocal healing.[4] An alternate strategy for restoration of the lamina propria could be accomplished by implantation of cultured tissue.[5] Another potential solution could be found in stem cell research.

More is being learned about the development of the lamina propria. Recent data indicates that the layered structure of the human vocal fold lamina propria does not exist at birth, but is initially a monolayer of cells. The layered structure observed in adults does not begin to develop until the age of 13. Additional information about the development of vocal fold structure will enhance the treatment of voice disorders in children and could give us further insight into how to restore damaged lamina propria.[6]

Laryngeal motion is more complex than previously recognized. The vocal folds do not merely open and close, lengthen and shorten. The cricoarytenoid joints, and hence the vocal folds, are capable of moving in three dimensions. Moreover, the intrinsic laryngeal muscles appear to be divided into functional compartments with different functions. For example, the human posterior cricoarytenoid muscle has two bellies, with different vectors of force on the arytenoid cartilage and separate nerve branches.[7,8] The thyroarytenoid muscle can be divided into regions with different myosin composition.[9] The functional significance of compartmentalization and complex motion has not been established. Activation patterns may be significantly different for speech, deglutition, and respiratory tasks. Control of pitch and vocal quality undoubtedly requires precise adjustments in glottic configuration. Further research in vivo and in excised human larynges could address these issues.

Complexity in motor control could account for some of the difficulties in regaining normal motion after regeneration or repair of the recurrent laryngeal nerve. Lack of normal vocal fold motion, despite reinnervation, has been attributed to synkinesis, the simultaneous contraction of opposing muscles. Research in animals has confirmed the inappropriate reinnervation of laryngeal muscles after nerve injury.[10-12] However, immobility caused by synkinesis would require that opposing forces exactly cancel each other out. This implies precisely orthogonal vectors with exactly equal strength—not the most likely outcome of a random process. Therefore, other factors, such as mechanical reduction of joint mobility, or irreversible muscle changes, should be investigated.

Spasmodic dysphonia is currently treated by peripheral intervention, such as chemodenervation of muscles or surgical disruption of nerves or muscles. However, it is generally regarded to be a focal dystonia, and hence a central neurologic disorder. There is very little understanding of the central neuropathology in this disorder, but some recent findings give hope that we will learn more. In one patient with adductor spasmodic dysphonia, PET scanning showed abnormal activation of auditory association areas during reading aloud. This activity significantly decreased after successful response to thyroplasty.[13] Also, research indicates that, in normal subjects, repeated air stimulation of the laryngeal mucosa induces central suppression of laryngeal adductor muscle activity. It is possible that in spasmodic dysphonia, this suppression of reflexes is abnormal.[14]

The first successful laryngeal transplant, performed in January of 1998, has generated more questions about reinnervation, because of some unexpected findings. Not only did the larynx survive, but its function was better than anticipated.[15] The patient, who received a transplant to replace a severely traumatized larynx, still requires a tracheotomy because of deficient inspiratory abduction. However, he is able to eat normally and has a surprisingly functional voice. Despite the fact that only one recurrent laryngeal nerve was reanastomosed both vocal folds have become reinnervated and have good muscle tone. Initially, the patient was unable to swallow because of severe aspiration; however, months after the transplant, he regained laryngeal sensation and was able to swallow. If phonation involves complex motor control, why has this patient recovered this much vocal function? Why are both vocal folds essentially equally reinnervated when the nerve was reanastomosed on only one side? This case does demonstrate that laryngeal transplantation is technically possible. Whether it is economically feasible remains to be seen.

The neural control of voice in speech is not well understood but is clearly complex. The spectrum of vocal dysfunction in patients with neurologic disorders is broad, implying the existence of various pathways susceptible to impairment. Patients with spasmodic dysphonia (SD) (presumably a midbrain disorder) have significant variation in symptom severity with task, implying differing levels of midbrain control or perhaps different feedback mechanisms.[16] In fact, it is possible that impaired sensory feedback could be involved in the pathophysiology of SD. Research to elucidate the neural pathways involved in speech control ultimately could lead to effective interventions for patients with neurogenic dysphonia.

It is well recognized that phonation is only one component of voice production. Resonance of the vocal tract, including the pharynx, skull, and chest, is an important determinant of vocal quality. In fact, resonant characteristics may be key factors in determining vocal register and imbuing singers with an exceptional voice. Classical voice training focuses attention on resonant structures. However, the physical basis for source and tract interactions, and the potential for volitional modification of resonance, are not well understood. Information about these relationships could eventually empower interventions to improve vocal function, not only for performance, but also for everyday use.

Vocal function may be impaired by a variety of systemic illnesses. Therapeutic drugs can also affect the voice, although there is very little available objective information on their effects. The precise mechanism of impairment or site of lesion is not always apparent. For example, rheumatoid arthritis occasionally involves the cricoarytenoid joint. More often, hoarseness in patients with rheumatoid arthritis is caused by irritation by gastroesophageal reflux, promoted by steroid or anti-inflammatory medication. Medications that inhibit angiotensin-converting enzyme have been reported to cause an irritative cough, which can damage the larynx. The mechanism of this effect is not known. Studies of drug effects on the larynx may have

relevance to mechanisms in patients with idiopathic chronic cough.

The larynx is an organ that differs profoundly with gender, apparently in response to changes in hormone status. The male larynx grows dramatically during puberty with the onset of increases in testosterone. With menopause, submucosal edema accumulates in the female larynx.[17] Thus, it is not surprising that endocrine disorders can profoundly affect the larynx. Myxedema of hypothyroidism is manifested in the larynx. Masculinizing tumors, male hormone therapy, pregnancy, or menopause can deepen the voice. The vocal changes appear to be irreversible, but the mechanism is unknown. It could involve increases in connective tissue or muscle bulk. Research in frogs has indicated a sex-linked difference in laryngeal muscle myosin.[18] Research on hormonal effects could provide very useful information about laryngeal function.

Gastroesophageal reflux is extremely common and can have far-reaching effects on the voice. It is one of the most common causes of chronic laryngitis. It is not clear why some patients with significant reflux develop laryngeal pathology and others do not. Abusive vocal habits have been implicated, but it is likely there are other cofactors. Research into the epidemiology and pathogenesis of reflux laryngitis could provide useful information not only for treatment of laryngitis, but also for potentially preventing more severe sequelae that have been attributed to reflux, such as cancer or laryngotracheal stenosis. Multidsciplinary research indicates that it is not only acid that damages the larynx, but that pepsin plays a key role. The presence of pepsin in patients with laryngeal reflux disease also correlates with depletion of carbonic anhydrase, implicating deficiencies in mucosal defense.[19] A gene for susceptibility to pediatric reflux also has been identified, opening a whole new avenue for research.[20]

Laryngotracheal stenosis itself is a problem that merits careful study. Most often it is the result of endotracheal intubation and/or tracheotomy; however, the majority of intubated patients are not affected. Previously, excessive cuff pressure and prolonged intubation were identified as cofactors. Modification of the cuff to reduce pressure and changes in intubation practices have diminished, but not eliminated, stenosis. Patients who are affected may have some underlying impairment of wound healing, as surgery to correct the stenosis is plagued by high failure rates. Recent research has suggested that the use of topical mitomycin can reduce the rate of restenosis following corrective surgery.[21] This is encouraging evidence that therapeutic intervention could be effective in prevention and treatment of stenosis. Research is needed to identify the responsible mechanisms, to guide the development of effective therapy and prevention, and to permit prospective identification of patients at high risk for developing stenosis.

EFFICACY OF VOICE THERAPY

A major problem in caring for patients with voice disorders is the lack of data regarding the efficacy of treatment and, in particular, the efficacy of voice therapy. Wide clinical experience and numerous small studies support the efficacy of various voice therapy regimens for specific voice disorders. Extrapolations can also be made from the results of vocal pedagogy. It is well known that breath control is crucial in singing. Classical voice training focused on breath support long before the myoelastic theory of phonation was developed. Nevertheless, the importance of breath support in conversational speech is grossly undervalued. In conversational speech, most humans use the larynx very inefficiently, converting less than 1% of the aerodynamic power of the lungs into sound. Although such an inefficient vocal mechanism may be adequate for minimal use situations, it is likely to fail in conditions of prolonged vocalization, noisy environment, and/or psychologic duress. Inadequate breath support is widely recognized as one of the most common causes of functional dysphonia. However, further research is required to elucidate the mechanisms involved, so that effective intervention can be developed.

Vocal training can greatly enhance vocal efficiency. It has been noted that the larynges of trained singers age less rapidly. Trained singers can also compensate for many variations in physiologic or environmental conditions and can often produce a normal-sounding voice in the presence of laryngeal pathology, such as edema or nodules. The study of vocal mechanism in gifted or exceptional singers or speakers can demonstrate the range of human capacity and identify specific strategies to improve vocal efficiency in patients with inadequate phonation.

Although experience and logic support the value of voice therapy, definitive clinical trials are rare. Ironically, a major factor limiting progress in studying the efficiency of voice disorders is the very lack of outcomes data. Definitive data cannot be generated without funding; funding requires pilot data; and pilot data cannot be generated without some source of funding, either start-up funding, or third-party reimbursement for treatment. The catch-22 situation is that third parties frequently do not pay for voice therapy or significantly restrict indications for therapy. It is difficult to reverse this policy in the absence of hard data.

Another limitation to studying the efficiency of treatment is the lack of consensus regarding objective measures for documenting improvement. Despite decades of research, there is still no gold standard of vocal function measures analogous to the audiogram for hearing. Acoustic measures are relatively easy to obtain, but are not clinically reliable in severe voice disorders. Perceptual analyses are more valid across the spectrum of vocal function, yet such measures are inherently subjective and only semiquantitative. Furthermore, reliable perceptual analysis requires listener training and, ideally, blinded evaluation. Perceptual data are not practical for routine clinical use or large studies. Aerodynamic measures provide physiologic data that correlate with the effort of speaking: however, this data collection is more difficult and less widely used. A promising development is the use of a questionnaire, the Vocal Handicap Index. Research is urgently needed to establish standards and to acquire a database of normal and pathologic function. We also do not really know the limits to vocal performance in normal individuals. Normative acoustic and aerodynamic data are lacking for children across development. Carefully planned and well-supported studies are needed to collect this information.

In laryngology, there is no lack of questions significant to research. Where the next 20 years of research will take us is unknown. The only certainty is that thoughtful bridging research will continue to improve the care of patients with voice disorders.

REFERENCES

1. Hirano M. Phonosurgical anatomy of the larynx. In: Ford CN, Bless DM, eds. *Phonosurgery.* New York, NY: Raven Press; 1991.
2. Sato K, Hirano.M, Nakashima T. 3D structure of the macula flava in the human vocal fold. *Acta Otolaryngol.* 2003;123:269–273.
3. Hirano S, Bless DM, Heisey D, Ford CN. Effect of growth factors on hyaluronan production by canine vocal fold fibroblasts. *Ann Otol Rhinol Laryngol.* 2003;112: 617–625.
4. Hirano S, Bless DM, Nagai H, et al. Growth factor therapy for vocal fold scarring in a canine model. *Ann Otol Rhinol Laryngol.* 2004;113:777–785.
5. Chhetri DK, Head C, Revazova E, et al. Lamina propria replacement therapy with cultured autologous fibroblasts for vocal fold scars. *Otolaryngol Head Neck Surg.* 2004;131:864–870.
6. Hartnick CJ, Rehbar R, Prasad V. Development and maturation of the pediatric human vocal fold lamina propria. *Laryngoscope.* 2005;115:4–15.
7. Bryant NJ, Woodson GE, Kaufman K, et al. Human posterior cricoarytenoid muscle compartments: anatomy

12

Patient History

Robert Thayer Sataloff, MD,/DMA
Mary J. Hawkshaw, BSN, RN, CORLN
Joseph Anticaglia, MD

A comprehensive history and physical examination usually reveals the cause of voice dysfunction. Effective history taking and physical examination depend on a practical understanding of the anatomy and physiology of voice production.[1-3] Because dysfunction in virtually any body system may affect phonation, medical inquiry must be comprehensive. The current standard of care for all voice patients evolved from advances inspired by medical problems of voice professionals such as singers and actors. Even minor problems may be particularly symptomatic in singers and actors, because of the extreme demands they place on their voices. However, a great many other patients are voice professionals. They include teachers, sales people, attorneys, clergy, physicians, politicians, telephone receptionists, and anyone else whose ability to earn a living is impaired in the presence of voice dysfunction. Because good voice quality is so important in our society, the majority of our patients are voice professionals; and all patients should be treated as such.

The scope of inquiry and examination for most voice patients is similar to that required for singers and actors, except that performing voice professionals have unique needs, which require additional history and examination. Questions must be added regarding performance commitments, professional status and voice goals, the amount and nature of voice training, the performance environment, rehearsal practices, abusive habits during speech and singing, and many other matters. Such supplementary information is essential to proper treatment selection and patient counseling of singers and actors. However, analogous factors must also be taken into account for stockbrokers, factory shop foremen, elementary school teachers, homemakers with several noisy children, and many others. Physicians familiar with the management of these challenging patients are well equipped to evaluate all patients with voice complaints.

PATIENT HISTORY

Obtaining extensive historical background information is necessary for thorough evaluation of the voice patient, and the otolaryngologist who sees voice professionals (especially singers) only occasionally cannot reasonably be expected to remember all the pertinent questions. Although some laryngologists consider a lengthy inquisition helpful in establishing rapport, many of us who see a substantial number of voice patients each day within a busy practice need a thorough but less time-consuming alternative. A history questionnaire can be extremely helpful in documenting all of the necessary information, helping the patient sort out and articulate his or her problems, and saving the clinician time recording information. The author has developed a questionnaire[4] that has proven helpful (see Appendix 12-1). The patient is asked to complete the relevant portions of the form at home prior to his or her office visit or in the waiting room before seeing the doctor. A similar form has been developed for voice patients who are not singers.

No history questionnaire is a substitute for direct, penetrating questioning by the physician. However, the direction of most useful inquiry can be determined from a glance at the questionnaire, obviating the need for extensive writing, which permits the physician greater eye contact with the patient and facilitates rapid establishment of the close rapport and confidence that are so important in treating voice patients. The physician is also able to supplement initial impressions and historical information from the questionnaire with seemingly leisurely conversation during the physical examination. The use of the history questionnaire has added substantially to the efficiency, consistent thoroughness, and ease of managing these delightful, but often complex, patients. A similar set of questions is also used by the speech-language pathologist with new patients and by many enlightened singing teachers when assessing new students.

How Old Are You?

Serious vocal endeavor may start in childhood and continue throughout a lifetime. As the vocal mechanism undergoes normal maturation, the voice changes. The optimal time to begin serious vocal training is controversial. For many years, most singing teachers advocated delay of vocal training and serious singing until near puberty in the female and after puberty and voice stabilization in the male. However, in a child with earnest vocal aspirations and potential, starting specialized training early in childhood is reasonable. Initial instruction should teach the child to vocalize without straining and to avoid all forms of voice abuse. It should not permit premature indulgence in operatic bravado. Most experts agree that taxing voice use and singing during puberty should be minimized or avoided altogether, particularly by the male. Voice maturation (attainment of stable adult vocal quality) may occur at any age from the early teenage years to the fourth decade of life. The danger-

ous tendency for young singers to attempt to sound older than their vocal years frequently causes vocal dysfunction.

All components of voice production are subject to normal aging. Abdominal and general muscular tone frequently decrease, lungs lose elasticity, the thorax loses its distensibility, the mucosa of the vocal tract atrophies, mucous secretions change character and quantity, nerve endings are reduced in number, and psychoneurologic functions change. Moreover, the larynx itself loses muscle tone and bulk and may show depletion of submucosal ground substance in the vocal folds. The laryngeal cartilages ossify, and the joints may become arthritic and stiff. Hormonal influence is altered. Vocal range, intensity, and quality all may be modified. Vocal fold atrophy may be the most striking alteration. The clinical effects of aging seem more pronounced in female singers, although vocal fold histologic changes may be more prominent in males. Excellent male singers occasionally extend their careers into their 70s or beyond.[5,6] However, some degree of breathiness, decreased range, and other evidence of aging should be expected in elderly voices. Nevertheless, many of the changes we typically associate with elderly singers (wobble, flat pitch) are due to lack of conditioning, rather than inevitable changes of biological aging. These esthetically undesirable concomitants of aging often can be reversed.

What Is Your Voice Problem?

Careful questioning as to the onset of vocal problems is needed to separate acute from chronic dysfunction. Often an upper respiratory tract infection will send a patient to the physician's office; but penetrating inquiry, especially in singers and actors, may reveal a chronic vocal problem that is the patient's real concern. Identifying acute and chronic problems before beginning therapy is important so that both patient and physician may have realistic expectations and make optimal therapeutic selections.

The specific nature of the vocal complaint can provide a great deal of information. Just as dizzy patients rarely walk into the physician's office complaining of "rotary vertigo," voice patients may be unable to articulate their symptoms without guidance. They may use the term hoarseness to describe a variety of conditions that the physician must separate. Hoarseness is a coarse or scratchy sound that is most often associated with abnormalities of the leading edge of the vocal folds such as laryngitis or mass lesions. Breathiness is a vocal quality characterized by excessive loss of air during vocalization. In some cases, it is due to improper technique. However, any condition that prevents full approximation of the vocal folds can be responsible. Possible causes include vocal fold paralysis, a mass lesion separating the leading edges of the vocal folds, arthritis of the cricoarytenoid joint, arytenoid dislocation, scarring of the vibratory margin, senile vocal fold atrophy (presbyphonia), psychogenic dysphonia, malingering, and other conditions.

Fatigue of the voice is inability to continue to speak or sing for extended periods without change in vocal quality and/or control. The voice may show fatigue by becoming hoarse, losing range, changing timbre, breaking into different registers, or exhibiting other uncontrolled aberrations. A well-trained singer should be able to sing for several hours without vocal fatigue.

Voice fatigue may occur through more than one mechanism. Most of the time, it is assumed to be due to muscle fatigue. This is often the case in patients who have voice fatigue associated with muscle tension dysphonia. The mechanism is most likely to be peripheral muscle fatigue and due to chemical changes (or depletion) in the muscle fibers. "Muscle fatigue" may also occur on a central (neurologic) basis. This mechanism is common in certain neuropathic disorders, such as some patients with multiple sclerosis; may occur with myasthenia gravis (actually neuromuscular junction pathology); or may be associated with paresis from various causes. However, the voice may also fatigue due to changes in the vibratory margin of the vocal fold. This phenomenon may be described as "lamina propria" fatigue. It, too, may be related to chemical or fluid changes in the lamina propria or cellular damage associated with conditions such as phonotrauma and dehydration. Excessive voice use, suboptimal tissue environment (eg, dehydration, effects of pollution, etc), lack of sufficient time of recovery between phonatory stresses, and genetic or structural tissue weaknesses that predispose to injury or delayed recovery from trauma all may be associated with lamina propria fatigue.

Although it has not been proven, this author (RTS) suspects that fatigue may also be related to the linearity of vocal fold vibrations. The principles behind this belief are discussed elsewhere. However, briefly, voices have linear and nonlinear (chaotic) characteristics. As the voice becomes more trained, vibrations become more symmetric; and the system becomes more linear. In many pathologic voices, the nonlinear components appear to become more prominent. If a voice is highly linear, slight changes in the vibratory margin may have little effect on the output of the system. However, if the system has substantial nonlinearity due to vocal fold pathology, poor tissue environment, or other causes, slight changes in the tissue (slight swelling, drying, surface cell damage) may cause substantial changes in the acoustic output of the system (the butterfly effect), causing vocal quality changes and fatigue much more quickly with much smaller changes in initial condition than in more linear vocal systems.

Fatigue is often caused by misuse of abdominal and neck musculature or oversinging, singing too loudly, or too long. However, we must remember that vocal fatigue also may be a sign not only of general tiredness or vocal abuse (sometimes secondary to structural lesions or glottal closure problems), but also of serious illnesses such as myasthenia gravis. So, the importance of this complaint should not be understated.

Volume disturbance may manifest as inability to sing loudly or inability to sing softly. Each voice has its own dynamic range. Within the course of training, singers learn to sing more loudly by singing more efficiently. They also learn to sing softly, a more difficult task, through years of laborious practice. Actors and other trained speakers go through similar training. Most volume problems are secondary to intrinsic limitations of the voice or technical errors in voice use, although hormonal changes, aging, and neurologic disease are other causes. Superior laryngeal nerve paralysis impairs the ability to speak or sing loudly. This is a frequently unrecognized consequence of herpes infection (cold sores) and Lyme disease and may be precipitated by any viral upper respiratory tract infection.

Most highly trained singers require only about 10 minutes to half an hour to "warm up the voice." Prolonged warm-up time, especially in the morning, is most often caused by reflux laryngitis. Tickling or choking during singing is most often a symptom of an abnormality of the vocal fold's leading edge. The symptom of tickling or choking should contraindicate singing until the vocal folds have been examined. Pain while singing can indicate vocal fold lesions, laryngeal joint arthritis, infection, or gastric acid reflux irritation of the arytenoid region. However, pain is much more commonly caused by voice abuse with excessive muscular activity in the neck rather than an acute abnormality on the leading edge of a vocal fold. In the absence of other symptoms, these patients do not generally require immediate cessation of singing pending medical examination. However, sudden onset of pain (usually sharp pain) while singing may be associated with a mucosal tear or a vocal fold hemorrhage and warrants voice conservation pending laryngeal examination.

Do You Have Any Pressing Voice Commitments?

If a singer or professional speaker (eg, actor, politician) seeks treatment at the end of a busy performance season and has no pressing engagements, management of the voice problem should be relatively conservative and designed to insure long-term protection of the larynx, the most delicate part of the vocal mechanism. However, the physician and patient rarely have this luxury. Most often, the voice professional needs treatment within a week of an important engagement and sometimes within less than a day. Younger singers fall ill shortly before performances, not because of hypochondria or coincidence, but rather because of the immense physical and emotional stress of the preperformance period. The singer is frequently working harder and singing longer hours than usual. Moreover, he or she may be under particular pressure to learn new material and to perform well for a new audience. The singer may also be sleeping less than usual because of additional time spent rehearsing or because of the discomforts of a strange city. Seasoned professionals make their living by performing regularly, sometimes several times a week. Consequently, any time they get sick is likely to precede a performance. Caring for voice complaints in these situations requires highly skilled judgment and bold management.

Tell Me About Your Vocal Career, Long-Term Goals, and the Importance of Your Voice Quality and Upcoming Commitments

To choose a treatment program, the physician must understand the importance of the patient's voice and his or her long-term career plans, the importance of the upcoming vocal commitment, and the consequences of canceling the engagement. Injudicious prescription of voice rest can be almost as damaging to a vocal career as injudicious performance. For example, although a singer's voice is usually his or her most important commodity, other factors distinguish the few successful artists from the multitude of less successful singers with equally good voices. These include musicianship, reliability, and "professionalism." Canceling a concert at the last minute may seriously damage a performer's reputation. Reliability is especially critical early in a singer's career. Moreover, an expert singer often can modify a performance to decrease the strain on his or her voice. No singer should be allowed to perform in a manner that will permit serious injury to the vocal folds; but in the frequent borderline cases, the condition of the larynx must be weighed against other factors affecting the singer as an artist.

How Much Voice Training Have You Had?

Establishing how long a singer or actor has been performing seriously is important, especially if his or her active performance career predates the beginning of vocal training. Active untrained singers and actors frequently develop undesirable techniques that are difficult to modify. Extensive voice use without training or premature training with inappropriate repertoire may underlie persistent vocal difficulties later in life. The number of years a performer has been training his or her voice may be a fair index of vocal proficiency. A person who has studied voice for 1 or 2 years is somewhat more likely to have gross technical difficulties than is someone who has been studying for 20 years. However, if training has been intermittent or discontinued, technical problems are common, especially among singers. In addition, methods of technical voice use vary among voice teachers. Hence, a student who has had many teachers in a relatively brief period of time commonly has numerous technical insecurities or deficiencies that may be responsible for vocal dysfunction. This is especially true if the singer has changed to a new teacher within the preceding year. The physician must be careful not to criticize the patient's current voice teacher in such circumstances. It often takes years of expert instruction to correct bad habits.

All people speak more often than they sing, yet most singers report little speech training. Even if a singer uses the voice flawlessly while practicing and performing, voice abuse at other times can cause damage that affects singing.

Under What Kinds of Conditions Do You Use Your Voice?

The Lombard effect is the tendency to increase vocal intensity in response to increased background noise. A well-trained singer learns to compensate for this tendency and to avoid singing at unsafe volumes. Singers of classical music usually have such training and frequently perform with only a piano, a situation in which the balance can be controlled well. However, singers performing in large halls, with orchestras, or in operas early in their careers tend to oversing and strain their voices. Similar problems occur during outdoor concerts because of the lack of auditory feedback. This phenomenon is seen even more among "pop" singers. Pop singers are in a uniquely difficult position; often, despite little vocal training, they enjoy great artistic and financial success and endure extremely stressful demands on their time and voices. They are required to sing in large halls or outdoor arenas not designed for musical performance, amid smoke and other environmental irritants, accompanied by extremely loud background music. One fre-

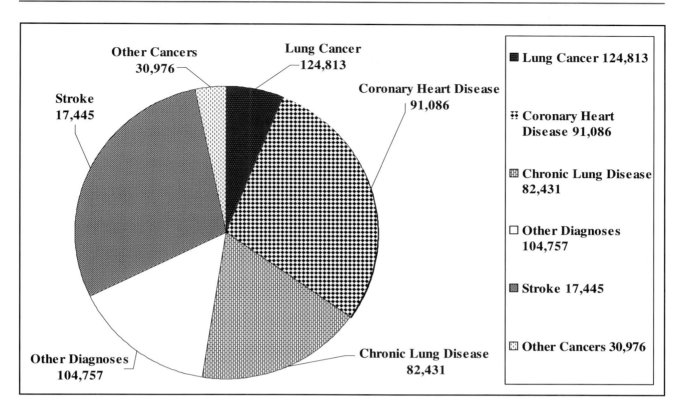

Figure 12–1. Average annual number of deaths attributable to cigarette smoking, 1995–1999.

Any condition that adversely affects lung function, such as chronic exposure to smoke or uncontrolled asthma, can contribute to dysphonia by impairing the strength, endurance and consistency of the airstream responsible for establishing vocal fold oscillation. Any lesion that compromises vocal fold vibration and glottic closure can cause hoarseness and breathiness. Inflammation of the cover layer of the vocal folds and/or the mucosal lining of the nose, sinuses, and oral or nasopharyngeal cavities can affect the quality and clarity of the voice.

Tobacco smoke can damage the lungs' parenchyma and the exchange of air through respiration. Cigarette manufacturers add hundreds of ingredients to their tobacco products to improve taste, to make smoking seem milder and easier to inhale and to prolong burning and shelf life.[14] More than 3000 chemical compounds have been identified in tobacco smoke, and more than 60 of these compounds are carcinogens.[15]

The tobacco plant, *Nicotiana tabacum*, is grown for its leaves, which can be smoked, chewed, or sniffed with various effects. The nicotine in tobacco is the addictive component and rivals crack cocaine in its ability to enslave its users. Most smokers want to stop; yet only a small percentage are successful in quitting cigarettes; and the majority who quit relapse into smoking once

again.[16] Tars and carbon monoxide are among the disease-causing components in tobacco products. The tar in cigarettes exposes the individual to a greater risk of bronchitis, emphysema, and lung cancer. These chemicals affect the entire vocal tract as well as the cardiovascular system (Table 12–1).

Cigarette smoke in the lungs can lead also to increased vascularity, edema, and excess mucus production, as well as epithelial tissue and cellular changes. The toxic agents in cigarette smoke have been associated with an increase in the number and severity of asthma attacks, chronic bronchitis, emphysema, and lung cancer, all of which can interfere with the lungs' ability to generate the stream of air needed for voice production.

Chronic bronchitis due to smoking has been associated with an increase in the number of goblet (mucous) cells, an increase in the size (hyperplasia) of the mucous-secreting glands, and a decrease in the number of ciliated cells, the cells used to clean the lungs. Chronic cough and sputum production are seen more commonly in smokers compared to nonsmokers. Also, the heat and chemicals of unfiltered cigarette and marijuana smoke are especially irritating to the lungs and larynx.

An important component of voice quality is the symmetrical, unencumbered vibration of the true vo-

Table 12–1. Chemical Additives Found in Tobacco and Commercial Products

Tobacco Chemical Additives	Also Found In
Acetic acid	vinegar; hair dye
Acetone	nail polish remover
Ammonia	floor cleaner, toilet cleaner
Arsenic	poison
Benzene	a leukemia-producing agent in rubber cement
Butane	cigarette lighter fluid
Cadmium	batteries, some oil paints
Carbon monoxide	car exhaust
DDT	insecticides
Ethanol	alcohol
Formaldehyde	embalming fluid, fabric, lab animals
Hexamine	barbecue lighter
Hydrazine	jet fuel, rocket fuel
Hydrogen cyanide	gas chamber poison
Methane	swamp gas
Methanol	rocket fuel
Naphthalene	explosives, mothballs, paints
Nickel	electroplating
Nicotine	insecticides
Nitrobenzene	gasoline additive
Nitrous oxide phenols	disinfectant
Phenol	disinfectants, plastics
Polonium-210	a radioactive substance
Stearic acid	candle wax
Styrene	insulation materials
Toluene	industrial solvent, embalmer's glue
Vinyl chloride	plastic manufacturing; garbage bags

cal folds. Anything that prevents the epithelium covering the vocal folds from vibrating or affects the loose connective tissue under the epithelium (in the superficial layer of the lamina propria known as Reinke's space) can cause dysphonia. Cigarette smoking can cause the epithelium of the true vocal folds to become red, swollen, develop whitish discolorations (leukoplakia), undergo chronic inflammatory changes, or develop squamous metaplasia or dysplasia (tissue changes from normal to a potentially malignant state).

In chronic smokers, the voice may become husky due to the accumulation of fluid in Reinke's space (Reinke's edema). These alterations in structure can interfere with voice production by changing the biomechanics of the vocal folds and their vibratory characteristics. In severe cases, cancer can deform and paralyze the vocal folds.

Vocal misuse often follows in an attempt to compensate for dysphonia and an altered self-perception of one's voice. The voice may feel weak, breathy, raspy or strained. There may be loss of range, vocal breaks, long warm-up time, and fatigue. The throat may feel raw, achy, or tight. As the voice becomes unreliable, bad habits increase as the individual struggles harder and harder to compensate vocally.

As selected sound waves move upward, from the larynx toward and through the pharynx, nasopharynx, mouth, and nose (the resonators), sounds gain a unique richness and timbre. Exposing the pharynx to cigarette smoke aggravates the linings of the oropharynx, mouth, nasopharynx, sinuses, and nasal cavities. The resulting erythema, swelling, and inflammation predispose one to nasal congestion and increased mucous production. With nasal congestion and impaired mucosal function, there may be predisposition to sinusitis and pharyngitis, in which the voice may become hyponasal, the sinuses achy, and the throat painful.

Although relatively rare in the United States, cancer of the nasopharynx has been associated with cigarette smoking,[17] and one of the presenting symptoms is unilateral hearing loss due to fluid in the middle ear caused by eustachian tube obstruction from the cancer. Smoking-induced cancers of the oral cavity, pharynx, larynx and lung are common throughout the world, including in the United States.

The palate, tongue, cheeks, lips, and teeth articulate the sound modified by the resonators into speech. Cigarette, cigar, or pipe smoking can cause a "black hairy tongue," precancerous oral lesions (leukoplakia), and/or cancer of the tongue and lips.[18] Any irritation that causes burning or inflammation of the oral mucosa can affect phonation; and all tobacco products are capable of causing these effects.

Smokeless "Spit" tobacco is highly addictive, and users who dip 8 to 10 times a day may get the same nicotine exposure as those who smoke 1½ to 2 packs of cigarettes per day.[19] Smokeless tobacco has been associated with gingivitis, cheek carcinoma, and cancer of the larynx and hypopharynx.

Exposure to environmental tobacco smoke (ETS), also called secondhand smoke, sidestream smoke, or passive smoke, accounts for an estimated 3000 lung cancer deaths, and approximately 35,000 deaths in the United States from heart disease in nonsmoking adults.[20]

Secondhand smoke is the "passive" inhalation of tobacco smoke from environmental sources such as smoke given off by pipes, cigars, cigarettes (sidestream), or the smoke exhaled from the lungs of smokers and inhaled by other people (mainstream). This passive smoke contains a mixture of thousands of chemicals some of which are known to cause cancer. The National Institutes of Health (NIH) lists ETS as a "known" carcinogen, and the more you are exposed to secondhand smoke, the greater your risk.[21]

Infants and young children are affected particularly by secondhand smoke with increased incidences of otitis media (ear infections), bronchitis, and pneumonia. If small children are exposed to secondhand smoke, the child's resulting illness can have a stressful effect on the parent who frequently catches the child's illness. Both the illness and the stress of caring for the sick child may interfere with voice performance. People who are exposed routinely to secondhand smoke are at risk for lung cancer, heart disease, respiratory infection, and an increased number of asthma attacks.[22]

There is an intricate relationship between the lungs, larynx, pharynx, nose, and mouth in the production of speech and song. Smoking can have deleterious effects on any part of the vocal tract, causing the respiratory system to lose power, damaging the vibratory margins of the vocal folds, and detracting from the richness and beauty of a voice.

The deleterious effects of tobacco smoke on mucosa are indisputable. Anyone concerned about the health of his or her voice should not smoke. Smoking causes erythema, mild edema, and generalized inflammation throughout the vocal tract. Both smoke itself and the heat of the cigarette appear to be important. Marijuana produces a particularly irritating, unfiltered smoke that is inhaled directly, causing considerable mucosal response. Voice patients who refuse to stop smoking marijuana should at least be advised to use a water pipe to cool and partially filter the smoke. Some vocalists are required to perform in smoke-filled environments and may suffer the same effects as the smokers themselves. In some theaters, it is possible to place fans upstage or direct the ventilation system so as to create a gentle draft toward the audience, clearing the smoke away from the stage. "Smoke eaters" installed in some theaters are also helpful.

Do Any Foods Seem to Affect Your Voice?

Various foods are said to affect the voice. Traditionally, singers avoid milk and ice cream before performances. In many people, these foods seem to increase the amount and viscosity of mucosal secretions. Allergy and casein have been implicated, but no satisfactory explanation has been established. In some cases, restriction of these foods from the diet before a voice performance may be helpful. Chocolate may have the same effect and should be viewed similarly. Chocolate also contains caffeine, which may aggravate reflux or cause tremor. Voice patients should be asked about eating nuts. This is important not only because some people experience effects similar to those produced by milk products and chocolate, but also because they are extremely irritating if aspirated. The irritation produced by aspiration of even a small organic foreign body may be severe and impossible to correct rapidly enough to permit performance. Highly spiced foods may also cause mucosal irritation. In addition, they seem to aggravate reflux laryngitis. Coffee and other beverages containing caffeine also aggravate gastric reflux and may promote dehydration and/or alter secretions and necessitate frequent throat clearing in some people. Fad diets, especially rapid weight reducing diets, are notorious for causing voice problems. Lemon juice and herbal teas are considered beneficial to the voice. Both may act as demulcents, thinning secretions, and may very well be helpful. Eating a full meal before a speaking or singing engagement may interfere with abdominal support or may aggravate upright reflux of gastric juice during abdominal muscle contraction.

Do You Have Morning Hoarseness, Bad Breath, Excessive Phlegm, a Lump in Your Throat, or Heartburn?

Reflux laryngitis is especially common among singers and trained speakers because of the high intra-abdominal pressure associated with proper support and because of lifestyle. Singers frequently perform at night. Many vocalists refrain from eating before performances, because a full stomach can compromise effective abdominal support. They typically compensate by eating heartily at postperformance gatherings late at night and then going to bed with a full stomach. Chronic irritation of arytenoid and vocal fold mucosa by reflux of gastric secretions may occasionally be associated with dyspepsia or pyrosis. However, the key features of this malady are bitter taste and halitosis on awakening in the morning, a dry or "coated" mouth, often a scratchy sore throat or a feeling of a "lump in the throat," hoarseness, and the need for prolonged vocal warm-up. The physician must be alert to these symptoms and ask about them routinely; otherwise, the diagnosis will often be overlooked; because people who have had this problem for many years or a lifetime do not even realize it is abnormal

Do You Have Trouble With Your Bowels or Belly?

Any condition that alters abdominal function, such as muscle spasm, constipation, or diarrhea, interferes with support and may result in a voice complaint. These symptoms may accompany infection, anxiety, various gastroenterologic diseases, and other maladies.

Are You Under Particular Stress or in Therapy?

The human voice is an exquisitely sensitive messenger of emotion. Highly trained voice professionals learn to control the effects of anxiety and other emotional stress on their voices under ordinary circumstances. However, in some instances, this training may break down or a performer may be inadequately prepared to control the voice under specific stressful conditions. Preperformance anxiety is the most common example; but insecurity, depression, and other emotional disturbances are also generally reflected in the voice. Anxiety reactions are mediated in part through the autonomic nervous system and result in a dry mouth, cold clammy skin, and thick secretions. These reactions are normal, and good vocal training coupled with assurance that no abnormality or disease is present generally overcomes them. However, long-term, poorly compensated emotional stress and exogenous stress (from agents, producers, teachers, parents, etc) may cause substantial vocal dysfunction and result in permanent limitations of the vocal apparatus. These conditions must be diagnosed and treated expertly. Hypochondriasis is uncommon among professional singers, despite popular opinion to the contrary.

Recent publications have highlighted the complexity and importance of psychological factors associated with voice disorders.[23] A comprehensive discussion of this subject is also presented in chapter 33. It is important for the physician to recognize that psychological problems may not only cause voice disorders, but they may also delay recovery from voice disorders that were entirely organic in etiology. Professional voice users, especially singers, have enormous psychological investment and personality identification associated with their voices. A condition that causes voice loss or permanent injury often evokes the same powerful psychological responses seen following death of a loved one. This process may be initiated even when physical recovery is complete if an incident (injury or surgery) has made the vocalist realize that voice loss is possible. Such a "brush with death" can have profound emotional consequences in some patients. It is essential for laryngologists to be aware of these powerful factors and manage them properly if optimal therapeutic results are to be achieved expeditiously.

Do You Have Problems Controlling Your Weight? Are You Excessively Tired? Are You Cold When Other People Are Warm?

Endocrine problems warrant special attention. The human voice is extremely sensitive to endocrinological changes. Many of these are reflected in alterations of fluid content of the lamina propria just beneath the laryngeal mucosa. This causes alterations in the bulk and shape of the vocal folds and results in voice change. Hypothyroidism[24-28] is a well-recognized cause of such voice disorders, although the mechanism is not fully understood. Hoarseness, vocal fatigue, muffling of the voice, loss of range, and a sensation of a lump in the throat may be present even with mild hypothyroidism. Even when thyroid function test results are within the low normal range, this diagnosis should be entertained, especially if thyroid-stimulating hormone levels are in the high normal range or are elevated. Thyrotoxicosis may result in similar voice disturbance.[25]

Do You Have Menstrual Irregularity, Cyclical Voice Changes Associated with Menses, Recent Menopause, or Other Hormonal Changes or Problems?

Voice changes associated with sex hormones are encountered commonly in clinical practice and have been investigated more thoroughly than have other hormonal changes.[29,30] Although a correlation appears to exist between sex hormone levels and depth of male voices (higher testosterone and lower estradiol levels in basses than in tenors),[29] the most important hormonal considerations in males occur during or are related to puberty.[31,32] Voice problems related to sex hormones are more common in female singers.[33-49]

Do You Have Jaw Joint or Other Dental Problems?

Dental disease, especially temporomandibular joint (TMJ) dysfunction, introduces muscle tension in the head and neck, which is transmitted to the larynx directly through the muscular attachments between the mandible and the hyoid bone and indirectly as generalized increased muscle tension. These problems often result in decreased range, vocal fatigue, and change in the quality or placement of a voice. Such tension often is accompanied by excess tongue muscle activity, especially pulling of the tongue posteriorly. This hyperfunctional behavior acts through hyoid attachments to disrupt the balance between the intrinsic and extrinsic laryngeal musculature. TMJ problems are also problematic for wind instrumentalists and some string players, including violinists. In some cases, the problems may actually be caused by instrumental technique. The history should always include information about musical activities, including instruments other than the voice.

Do You or Your Blood Relatives Have Hearing Loss?

Hearing loss is often overlooked as a source of vocal problems. Auditory feedback is fundamental to speaking and singing. Interference with this control mechanism may result in altered vocal production, particularly if the person is unaware of the hearing loss. Distortion, particularly pitch distortion (diplacusis) may also pose serious problems for the singer. This appears to be due not only to aesthetic difficulties in matching pitch, but also to vocal strain that accompanies pitch shifts.[50]

In addition to determining whether the patient has hearing loss, inquiry should also be made about hearing impairment occurring in family members, roommates, and other close associates. Speaking loudly to people who are hard-of-hearing can cause substantial, chronic vocal strain. This possibility should be investigated routinely when evaluating voice patients.

Have You Suffered Whiplash or Other Bodily Injury?

Various bodily injuries outside the confines of the vocal tract may have profound effects on the voice. Whiplash, for example, commonly causes changes in technique, with consequent voice fatigue, loss of range, difficulty singing softly, and other problems. These problems derive from the neck muscle spasm, abnormal neck posturing secondary to pain, and consequent hyperfunctional voice use. Lumbar, abdominal, head, chest, supraglottic, and extremity injuries may also affect vocal technique and be responsible for the dysphonia that prompted the voice patient to seek medical attention.

Did You Undergo Any Surgery Prior to the Onset of Your Voice Problems?

A history of laryngeal surgery in a voice patient is a matter of great concern. It is important to establish exactly why the surgery was done, by whom it was done, whether intubation was necessary, and whether voice therapy was instituted pre- or postoperatively if the lesion was associated with voice abuse (vocal nodules). If the vocal dysfunction that sent the patient to the physician's office dates from the immediate postoperative period, surgical trauma must be suspected.

Otolaryngologists frequently are asked about the effects of tonsillectomy on the voice. Singers especially may consult the physician after tonsillectomy and complain of vocal dysfunction. Certainly removal of tonsils can alter the voice.[51,52] Tonsillectomy changes the configuration of the supraglottic vocal tract. In addition, scarring alters pharyngeal muscle function, which is trained meticulously in the professional singer. Singers must be warned that they may have permanent voice changes after tonsillectomy; however, these changes can be minimized by dissecting in the proper plane to lessen scarring. The singer's voice generally requires 3 to 6 months to stabilize or return to normal after surgery, although it is generally safe to begin limited singing within 2 to 4 weeks following surgery. As with any procedure for which general anesthesia may be needed, the anesthesiologist should be advised preoperatively that the patient is a professional singer. Intubation and extubation should be performed with great care, and the use of nonirritating plastic rather than rubber or ribbed metal endotracheal tubes is preferred. Use of a laryngeal mask may be advisable for selected procedures for mechanical reasons; but this device is often not ideal for tonsillectomy; and it can cause laryngeal injury such as arytenoid dislocation.

Surgery of the neck, such as thyroidectomy, may result in permanent alterations in the vocal mechanism through scarring of the extrinsic laryngeal musculature. The cervical (strap) muscles are important in maintaining laryngeal position and stability of the laryngeal skeleton; and they should be retracted rather than divided whenever possible. A history of recurrent or superior laryngeal nerve injury may explain a hoarse, breathy, or weak voice. However, in rare cases, even a singer can compensate for recurrent laryngeal nerve paralysis and have a nearly normal voice.

Thoracic and abdominal surgery interfere with respiratory and abdominal support. After these procedures, singing and projected speaking should be prohibited until pain has subsided and healing has occurred sufficiently to allow normal support. Abdominal exercises should be instituted before resumption of vocalizing. Singing and speaking without proper support are often worse for the voice than not using the voice for performance at all.

Other surgical procedures may be important factors if they necessitate intubation or if they affect the musculoskeletal system so that the person has to change stance or balance. For example, balancing on one foot after leg surgery may decrease the effectiveness of the support mechanism.

What Medications and Other Substances Do You Use?

A history of alcohol abuse suggests the probability of poor vocal technique. Intoxication results in incoordination and decreased awareness, which undermine vocal discipline designed to optimize and protect the voice. The effect of small amounts of alcohol is controversial. Although many experts oppose its use because of its vasodilatory effect and consequent mucosal alteration, many people do not seem to be adversely affected by small amounts of alcohol such as a glass of wine with a meal. However, some people have mild sensitivities to certain wines or beers. Patients who develop nasal congestion and rhinorrhea after drinking beer, for example, should be made aware that they probably have a mild allergy to that particular beverage and should avoid it before voice commitments.

Patients frequently acquire antihistamines to help control "postnasal drip" or other symptoms. The drying effect of antihistamines may result in decreased vocal fold lubrication, increased throat clearing, and irritability leading to frequent coughing. Antihistamines may be helpful to some voice patients, but they must be used with caution.

When a voice patient seeking the attention of a physician is already taking antibiotics, it is important to find out the dose and the prescribing physician, if any, as well as whether the patient frequently treats himself or herself with inadequate courses of antibiotics often supplied by colleagues. Singers, actors, and other speakers sometimes have a "sore throat" shortly before important vocal presentations and start themselves on inappropriate antibiotic therapy, which they generally discontinue after their performance.

Diuretics are also popular among some performers. They are often prescribed by gynecologists at the vocalist's request to help deplete excess water in the premenstrual period. They are not effective in this scenario, because they cannot diurese the protein-bound water in the laryngeal ground substance. Unsupervised use of these drugs may cause dehydration and consequent mucosal dryness.

Hormone use, especially use of oral contraceptives, must be mentioned specifically during the physician's inquiry. Women frequently do not mention them routinely when asked whether they are taking any medication. Vitamins are also frequently not mentioned. Most vitamin therapy seems to have little effect on the voice. However, high-dose vitamin C (5 to 6 g/day), which some people use to prevent upper respiratory tract infections, seems to act as a mild diuretic and may lead to dehydration and xerophonia.[53]

Cocaine use is common, especially among pop musicians. This drug can be extremely irritating to the nasal mucosa, causes marked vasoconstriction, and may alter the sensorium, resulting in decreased voice control and a tendency toward vocal abuse.

Many pain medications (including aspirin and ibuprofen), psychotropic medications, and many others may be responsible for a voice complaint. So far, no adverse vocal effects have been reported with selective COX-2 inhibiting anti-inflammatory medications (which do not promote bleeding, as do other nonsteroid anti-inflammatory medicines and aspirin), such as selecoxib (Celebrex, Pfizer Inc, New York, NY) and valdecoxib (Bextra, Pharmacia Corp, New York, NY). The effects of other new medications such as sildenafil citrate (Viagra, Pfizer Inc, New York) and medications used to induce abortion remain unstudied and unknown; but it seems plausible that such medication may affect voice function, at least temporarily. Laryngologists must be familiar with the laryngologic effects of the many substances ingested medically and recreationally. These are reviewed elsewhere in this book and in other literature.

REFERENCES

1. Sataloff RT. Professional singers: the science and art of clinical care. *Am J Otolaryngol.* 1981;2:251–266.
2. Sataloff RT. The human voice. *Sci Am.* 1992;267:108–115.
3. Sundberg J. *The Science of the Singing Voice.* DeKalb, IL: Northern Illinois University Press; 1987:1–194.
4. Sataloff RT. Efficient history taking in professional singers. *Laryngoscope.* 1984;94:1111–1114.
5. Ackermann R, Pfau W. Gerontology studies on the susceptibility to voice disorders in professional speakers. *Folia Phoniatr (Basel).* 1974;26:95–99.
6. von Leden H. Speech and hearing problems in the geriatric patient. *J Am Geriatr Soc.* 1977;25:422–426.
7. Schiff M. Comment. Presented at the Seventh Symposium on Care of the Professional Voice; June 15–16, 1978; The Juilliard School, New York, NY.
8. Spiegel JR, Cohn JR, Sataloff RT, et al. Respiratory function in singers: medical assessment, diagnoses, treatments. *J Voice.* 1988;2:40–50.
9. Cohn JR, Sataloff RT, Spiegel JR, et al. Airway reactivity-induced asthma in singers (ARIAS). *J Voice.* 1991;5:332–337.
10. Feder RJ. The professional voice and airline flight. *Otolaryngol Head Neck Surg.* 1984;92:251–254.
11. Anticaglia A, Hawkshaw M, Sataloff RT. The effects of smoking on voice performance. *J Singing.* 2004;60:161–167.
12. Centers for Disease Control (CDC). Annual smoking-attributable mortality, years of potential life lost, and economic costs, United States—1995–1999. *Morbidity & Mortality Weekly Report (MMWR).* 2002;51(14):300–303.
13. World Health Organization. *World Health Report 1999.* Geneva, Switzerland: WHO; 1999.
14. United States Department of Health and Human Services, (USDHHS). *Tobacco Products Fact Sheet, 2000.* Washington, DC: Government Printing Office; 2000.
15. National Cancer Institute. Environmental tobacco smoke. Fact sheet 3.9; 1999. Available at: http//cis.nci.nih.gov/fact/3_9htm

16. Centers for Disease Control and Prevention. Cigarette smoking among adults—United States, 1993. *Morbidity & Mortality Weekly Report (MMWR).* 1994;3:925–929.
17. Chow WH, McLaughlin JK, Hrubec Z, et al. Tobacco use and nasopharyngeal carcinoma in a cohort of US veterans. *Int J Cancer.* 1993;55(4):538–540.
18. Casiglia J, Woo, SB. A comprehensive view of oral cancer. *Gen Dent.* 2001;49(1):72–82.
19. Centers for Disease Control. Determination of nicotine, pH and moisture content of six U.S. commercial moist snuff products. *Mortality & Morbidity Weekly Review (MMWR).* 1999;48 (19):398.
20. American Cancer Society. *Cancer Facts and Figures 2002.* Atlanta, GA: ACS; 2002.
21. US Dept Health and Human Services, Public Health Service, National Toxicology Program (NTP). *Report on Carcinogens.* 10th ed. 2002. Available at: http://ehp.niehs.nih.gov/roc/toc10.html.
22. Academy of Pediatrics, Committee on Environmental Health. Environmental tobacco smoke: a hazard to children. *Pediatrics.*1997;99(4): 639–642.
23. Rosen DC, Sataloff RT. *Psychology of Voice Disorders.* San Diego, CA: Singular Publishing Group; 1997:1–261.
24. Gupta OP, Bhatia PL, Agarwal MK, et al. Nasal pharyngeal and laryngeal manifestations of hypothyroidism. *Ear Nose Throat J.* 1977;56:10–21.
25. Malinsky M, Chevrie-Muller, Cerceau N. Etude clinique et electrophysiologique des alterations de la voix au cours des thyrotoxioses. *Ann Endocrinol* (Paris). 1977;38:171–172.
26. Michelsson K, Sirvio P. Cry analysis in congenital hypothyroidism. *Folia Phoniatr (Basel).* 1976;28:40–47.
27. Ritter FN. The effect of hypothyroidism on the larynx of the rat. *Ann Otol Rhinol Laryngol.* 1964;67:404–416.
28. Ritter FN. Endocrinology. In: Paparella M, Shumrick D, eds. *Otolaryngology.* Vol I. Philadelphia, PA: Saunders; 1973:727–734.
29. Meuser W, Nieschlag E. [Sex hormones and depth of voice in the male.] *Dtsch Med Wochenschr.*1977:102: 261–264.
30. Schiff M. The influence of estrogens on connective tissue. In: Asboe-Hansen G, ed. *Hormones and Connective Tissue.* Coopenhagen, Denmark: Munksgaard Press; 1967:282–341.
31. Brodnitz F. The age of the castrato voice. *J Speech Hear Disord.* 1975;40:291–295.
32. Brodnitz F. Hormones and the human voice. *Bull N Y Acad Med.* 1971;47:183–191.
33. Carroll C. Personal communication with Dr. Hans von Leden; 1992; Arizona State University at Tempe.
34. van Gelder L. Psychosomatic aspects of endocrine disorders of the voice. *J Commun Disord.* 1974;7:257–262.
35. Lacina O. Der Einfluss der Menstruation auf die Stimme der Sangerinnen. *Folia Phoniatr (Basel).* 1968;20:13–24.
36. Wendler J. [The influence of menstruation on the voice of the female singer.] *Folia Phoniatr (Basel).* 1972;24:259–277.
37. Brodnitz F. Medical care preventive therapy (panel). In: Lawrence VL, ed. *Transcripts of the Seventh Annual Sym-*

posium. Care of the Professional Voice. New York, NY: The Voice Foundation; 1978;3:86.

38. Dordain M. Etude Statistique de l'influence des contraceptifs hormonaux sur la voix. *Folia Phoniatr (Basel).* 1972;24:86–96.

39. Pahn J, Goretzlehner G. [Voice changes following the use of oral contraceptives.] *Zentralbl Gynakol.* 1978;100: 341–346.

40. Schiff M. "The pill" in otolaryngology. *Trans Am Acad Ophthalmol Otolaryngol.* 1968;72:76–84.

41. von Deuster CV. [Irreversible vocal changes in pregnancy.] *HNO.* 1977;25:430–432.

42. Flach M, Schwickardi H, Simen R. Welchen Einfluss haben Menstruation und Schwangerschaft auf die augsgebildete Gesangsstimme? *Folia Phoniatr (Basel).* 1968;21: 199–210.

43. Arndt HJ. Stimmstorungen nach Behandlung mit Androgenen und anabolen Hormonen. *Munch Med Wochenschr.* 1974;116:1715–1720.

44. Bourdial J. Les troubles de la voix provoques par la therapeutique hormonale androgene. *Ann Otolaryngol Chir Cervicofac.* 1970;87:725–734.

45 Damsté PH. Virilization of the voice due to the use of anabolic steroids. *Ned Tijdschr Geneeskd.* 1963;107:891–892.

46. Damsté PH. Voice changes in adult women caused by virilizing agents. *J Speech Hear Disord.* 1967;32:126–132.

47. Saez S, Sakai F. Recepteurs d'androgenes: mise en evidence dans la fraction cytosolique de muqueuse normale et d'epitheliomas pharyngolarynges humains. *C R Acad Sci Hebd Seances Acad Sci D.* 1975;280:935–938.

48. Vuorenkoski V, Lenko HL, Tjernlund P, et al. Fundamental voice frequency during normal and abnormal growth, and after androgen treatment. *Arch Dis Child.* 1978;53:201–209.

49. Imre V. Hormonell bedingte Stimmstorungen. *Folia Phoniatr (Basel).* 1968;20:394–404.

50. Sundberg J, Prame E, Iwarsson J. Replicability and accuracy of pitch patterns in professional singers. In: Davis PJ, Fletcher NH, eds. *Vocal Fold Physiology: Controlling Chaos and Complexity.* San Diego, CA: Singular Publishing Group Inc; 1996:291–306.

51. Gould WJ, Alberti PW, Brodnitz F, Hirano M. Medical care preventive therapy. [Panel.] In: Lawrence VL, ed. *Transcripts of the Seventh Annual Symposium. Care of the Professional Voice.* New York, NY: The Voice Foundation; 1978;3:74–76.

52. Wallner LJ, Hill BJ, Waldrop W, Monroe C. Voice changes following adenotonsillectomy. *Laryngoscope.* 1968;78:1410–1418.

53. Lawrence VL. Medical care for professional voice (panel). In: Lawrence VL, ed. *Transcripts from the Annual Symposium. Care of the Professional Voice.* New York, NY: The Voice Foundation; 1978;3:17–18.

APPENDIX 12-1. PATIENT HISTORY FORM FOR PROFESSIONAL VOICE USERS

Name _____ **Age** _____ **Sex** _____ **Race** _____

Height _____ **Weight** _____ **Date** _____

How long have you had your present voice problem?

Who noticed it?

Do you know what caused it?   Yes   No

If so, what?

Did it come on slowly or suddenly?   Slowly   Suddenly

Is it getting: Worse,   Better,   Same?

Which symptoms do you have? (Please check all that apply)

Hoarseness (coarse or scratchy sound)

Fatigue (voice tires or changes quality after speaking for a short period of time)

Volume disturbance: (trouble speaking) softly,   loudly

Loss of range: high,   low

Prolonged warm-up time (over 1/2 hr to warm up voice)

Breathiness

Tickling or choking sensation while speaking

Pain in throat while speaking

Other (Please specify):

Have you ever had training for your singing voice?

Yes   No

Have there been periods of months or years without lessons in that time?

Yes   No

How long have you studied with your present teacher?

Teacher's name:

Teacher's address:

Teacher's telephone number:

Please list previous teachers and years during which you studied with them:

In what capacity do you use your voice professionally?

Actor

Announcer (television/radio/sports arena)

Attorney

Clergy

Politician

Salesperson

Teacher

Telephone operator or receptionist

Other (Please specify):

Do you have an important performance soon?

Yes   No

Date(s):

Do you do regular voice exercises?

Yes   No

If yes, describe:

Do you play a musical instrument?

Yes   No

If yes, please check all that apply:

  Keyboard (Piano, Organ, Harpsichord, Other _____)

  Violin, Viola, Cello

  Bass

  Plucked Strings (Guitar, Harp, Other _____)

  Brass

  Wind with single reed

  Wind with double reed

  Flute, Piccolo

  Percussion

  Bagpipe

  Accordion

  Other (Please specify):

Do you warm up your voice before practice or performance?

  Yes   No

Do you cool down after using it?

  Yes   No

How much are you speaking at present (average hours per day)?

  Rehearsal   Performance   Other

Please check all that apply to you:

  Voice worse in the morning

  Voice worse later in the day, after it has been used

  Sing performances or rehearsals in the morning

  Speak extensively (teacher, clergy, attorney, telephone, work, etc.)

  Cheerleader

  Speak extensively backstage or at postperformance parties

Choral conductor

Frequently clear your throat

Frequent sore throat

Jaw joint problems

Bitter or acid taste; bad breath or hoarseness first thing in the morning

Frequent "heartburn" or hiatal hernia

Frequent yelling or loud talking

Frequent whispering

Chronic fatigue (insomnia)

Work around extreme dryness

Frequent exercise (weight lifting, aerobics, etc.)

Frequently thirsty, dehydrated

Hoarseness first thing in the morning

Chest cough

Eat late at night

Ever use antacids

Under particular stress at present (personal or professional)

Frequent bad breath

Live, work, or perform around smoke or fumes

Traveled recently:

    When:

    Where:

Your family doctor's name, address, and telephone number:

Your laryngologist's name, address, and telephone number:

Recent cold?

Yes   No

Current cold?

Yes   No

Have you been evaluated by an allergist?

Yes   No

If yes, what allergies do you have?

[none, dust, mold, trees, cats, dog, foods, other]

If yes, give name and address of allergist:

Are you allergic to any medications?   Yes   No

If yes, please list:

How many packs of cigarettes do you smoke per day?

Smoking history:

Never

Quit. When?

Smoked about_____packs per day for_____years.

Smoked_____packs per day. Have smoked for_____years.

Do you work in a smoky environment?

Yes   No

How much alcohol do you drink?

none,   rarely,   a few times per week,   daily

If daily, or few times per week, on the average, how much do you consume?

1, 2, 3, 4, 5, 6, 7, 8, 9, 10, more glasses per day,   week of beer,   wine,   liquor

Did you use to drink more heavily?

Yes   No

How many cups of coffee, tea, cola, or other caffeine-containing drinks do you drink per day?

List other recreational drugs you use:

[marijuana, cocaine, amphetamines, barbiturates, heroin, other_____]

Have you noticed any of the following? (Check all that apply)

Hypersensitivity to heat or cold

Excessive sweating

Change in weight: gained/lost_____lb. In_____weeks/_____months

Change in your voice

Change in skin or hair

Palpitation (fluttering) of the heart

Emotional lability (swings of mood)

Double vision

Numbness of the face or extremities

Tingling around the mouth or face

Blurred vision or blindness

Weakness or paralysis of the face

Clumsiness in arms or legs

Confusion or loss of consciousness

Difficulty with speech

Difficulty with swallowing

Seizure (epileptic fit)

Pain in the neck or shoulder

Shaking or tremors

Memory change

Personality change

For females:

Are you pregnant?   Yes   No

Are your menstrual periods regular? Yes   No

Have you undergone hysterectomy?   Yes   No

Were your ovaries removed?   Yes   No

At what age did you reach puberty?

Have you gone through menopause?   Yes   No

Have you ever consulted a psychologist or psychiatrist?

Yes   No

Are you currently under treatment?

Yes   No

Have you injured your head or neck (whiplash, etc.)?

Yes   No

Describe any serious accidents related to this visit:

Are you involved in legal action involving problems with your voice?

Yes   No

List names of spouse and children:

Brief summary of ENT problems, some of which may not be related to your present complaint.

Hearing loss

Ear pain

Ear noises

Facial pain

Lump in face or head

Lump in neck

Dizziness

Stiff neck

Facial paralysis

Nasal obstruction

Nasal deformity

Nosebleeds

Mouth sores

Trouble swallowing

Trouble breathing

Eye problem

Excess eye skin

Excess facial skin

Jaw joint problem

Other (Please specify):

Do you have or have you ever had:

Diabetes

Seizures

Hypoglycemia

Psychologic therapy or counseling

Thyroid problems

Frequent bad headaches

Syphilis

Ulcers

Gonorrhea

Kidney disease

Herpes

Urinary problems

Cold sores (fever blisters)

Arthritis or skeletal

High blood pressure problems

Severe low blood pressure

Cleft palate

Intravenous antibiotics or diuretics

Asthma, lung or breathing problems

Heart attack

Angina

Irregular heartbeat

Rheumatic fever

Other heart problems

Unexplained weight loss

Cancer of _____

Other tumor _____

Blood transfusions

Hepatitis

Tuberculosis

AIDS

Glaucoma

Meningitis

Multiple sclerosis

Other illnesses (Please specify):

Do any blood relatives have:

Diabetes

Hypoglycemia

Cancer

Heart disease

Other major medical problems such as those listed above.

Please specify:

Describe serious accidents unless directly related to your doctor's visit here.

    None

    Occurred with head injury, loss of consciousness, or whiplash

    Occurred without head injury, loss of consciousness, or whiplash

    Describe:

List all current medications and doses (include birth control pills and vitamins).

    None

    Aspirin

    Codeine

    Medication for allergies

    Novocaine

    Penicillin

    Sulfamides

    Tetracycline

    Erythromycin

    Keflex/Ceclor/Ceftin

    Iodine

    X-ray dyes

    Adhesive tape

    Other: (Please specify)

List operations:

    Tonsillectomy   (age_____)

    Adenoidectomy (age_____)

    Appendectomy (age_____)

    Heart surgery   (age_____)

    Other: (Please specify)

List toxic drugs or chemicals to which you have been exposed:

Streptomycin, Neomycin, Kanamycin

Lead

Mercury

Other: (Please list)

Have you had x-ray treatments to your head or neck (including treatments for acne or ear problems as a child), treatments for cancer, etc.?

Yes   No

Describe serious health problems of your spouse or children

13

Physical Examination

Robert Thayer Sataloff, MD, DMA

PHYSICAL EXAMINATION

A detailed history frequently reveals the cause of a voice problem even before a physical examination is performed. However, a comprehensive physical examination, often including objective assessment of voice function, also is essential.[1-3] In response to feedback from readers of the previous editions, this chapter has been expanded to include a brief overview of objective voice assessment and other subjects covered more comprehensively in subsequent chapters. This overview is provided here for the reader's convenience.

Physical examination must include a thorough ear, nose, and throat evaluation and assessment of general physical condition. A patient who is extremely obese or appears fatigued, agitated, emotionally stressed, or otherwise generally ill has an increased potential for voice dysfunction. This could be due to any number of factors: altered abdominal support, loss of fine motor control of laryngeal muscles, decreased bulk of the submucosal vocal fold ground substance, change in the character of mucosal secretions, or other similar mechanisms. Any physical condition that impairs the normal function of the abdominal musculature is suspect as a cause for dysphonia. Some conditions, such as pregnancy, are obvious; however, a sprained ankle or broken leg that requires a singer or actor to balance in an unaccustomed posture may distract him or her from maintaining good abdominal support and thereby result in voice dysfunction. A tremorous neurologic disorder, endocrine disturbances such as thyroid dysfunction or menopause, the aging process, and other systemic conditions also may alter the voice. The physician must remember that maladies of almost any body system may result in voice dysfunction, and the doctor must remain alert for conditions outside the head and neck. If the patient uses his or her voice professionally for singing, acting, or other vocally demanding professions, physical examination should also include assessment of the patient during typical professional vocal tasks. For example, a singer should be asked to sing. Evaluation techniques for assessing performance are described in greater detail elsewhere in this book.

Complete Ear, Nose, and Throat Examination

Examination of the ears must include assessment of hearing acuity. Even a relatively slight hearing loss may result in voice strain as a singer tries to balance his or her vocal intensity with that of associate performers. Similar effects are encountered among speakers, but they are less prominent in the early stages of hearing loss. This is especially true of hearing losses acquired after vocal training has been completed. The effect is most pronounced with sensorineural hearing loss. Diplacusis, distortion of pitch perception, makes vocal strain even worse. With conductive hearing loss, singers tend to sing more softly than appropriate rather than too loudly; and this is less harmful.

During an ear, nose, and throat examination, the conjunctivae and sclerae should be observed routinely for erythema that suggests allergy or irritation, for pallor that suggests anemia, and for other abnormalities such as jaundice. These observations may reveal the problem reflected in the vocal tract even before the larynx is visualized. Hearing loss in a spouse may be problematic as well if the voice professional strains vocally to communicate.

The nose should be assessed for patency of the nasal airway, character of the nasal mucosa, and nature of secretions, if any. A patient who is unable to breathe through the nose because of anatomic obstruction is forced to breathe unfiltered, unhumidified air through the mouth. Pale gray allergic mucosa or swollen infected mucosa in the nose suggests abnormal mucosa elsewhere in the respiratory tract.

Examination of the oral cavity should include careful attention to the tonsils and lymphoid tissue in the posterior pharyngeal wall, as well as to the mucosa. Diffuse lymphoid hypertrophy associated with a complaint of "scratchy" voice and irritative cough may indicate infection. The amount and viscosity of mucosal and salivary secretions also should be noted. Xerostomia is particularly important. The presence of scalloping of the lateral aspects of the tongue should be noted. This finding is caused commonly by tongue thrust and may be associated with inappropriate tongue tension and muscle tension dysphonia. Dental examination should be focused not only on oral hygiene but also on the presence of wear facets suggestive of bruxism. Bruxism is a clue to excessive tension and may be associated with dysfunction of the temporomandibular joints, which should also be assessed routinely. Thinning of the enamel of the central incisors in a normal or underweight patient may be a clue to bulimia. However, it may also result from excessive ingestion of lemons, which some singers eat to help thin their secretions.

The neck should be examined for masses, restriction of movement, excess muscle tension and/or spasm, and scars from prior neck surgery or trauma. Laryngeal vertical mobility is also important. For example, tilting of the larynx produced by partial fixation of cervical muscles cut during previous surgery may produce voice dysfunction, as may fixation of the trachea to overlying neck skin. Particular attention should be paid to the thyroid gland. Examination of posterior neck muscles and range of motion should not be neglected. The cranial nerves should also be examined. Diminished fifth nerve sensation, diminished gag re-

flex, palatal deviation, or other mild cranial nerve deficits may indicate cranial polyneuropathy. Postviral, infectious neuropathies may involve the superior laryngeal nerve(s) and cause weakness of the vocal fold muscle secondary to decreased neural function resulting in ineffective compensatory efforts in attempts to overcome diminished neural input, fatigability, and loss of range and projection of the voice. The recurrent laryngeal nerve is also affected in some cases. More serious neurologic disease may also be associated with such symptoms and signs.

Laryngeal Examination

Examination of the larynx begins when the singer or other voice patient enters the physician's office. The range, ease, volume, and quality of the speaking voice should be noted. If the examination is not being conducted in the patient's native language, the physician should be sure to listen to a sample of the patient's mother tongue, as well. Voice use is often different under the strain or habits of foreign language use. Rating scales used to describe the speaking voice more consistently may be helpful.[4,5] The classification proposed by the Japanese Society of Logopedics and Phoniatrics is one of the most widely used. It is known commonly as the GRBAS Voice Rating Scale and is discussed below in the section on psychoacoustic evaluation.[6]

Physicians are not usually experts in voice classification. However, physicians should at least be able to discriminate substantial differences in range and timbre, such as between bass and tenor or alto and soprano. Although the correlation between speaking and singing voices is not perfect, a speaker with a low, comfortable bass voice who reports that he is a tenor may be misclassified and singing inappropriate roles with consequent voice strain. This judgment should be deferred to an expert, but the observation should lead the physician to make the appropriate referral. Excessive volume or obvious strain during speaking clearly indicates that voice abuse is present and may be contributing to the patient's singing complaint. The speaking voice can be evaluated more consistently and accurately using standardized reading passages (Appendix 13-1); and such assessments are performed routinely by speech-language pathologists, phoniatricians, and sometimes by laryngologists.

Any patient with a voice complaint should be examined by indirect laryngoscopy at least (Figure 13–1A). It is not possible to judge voice range, quality, or other vocal attributes by inspection of the vocal folds. However, the presence or absence of nodules, mass lesions, contact ulcers, hemorrhage, erythema, paralysis, arytenoid erythema (reflux), and other anatomic abnormalities must be established. Erythe-

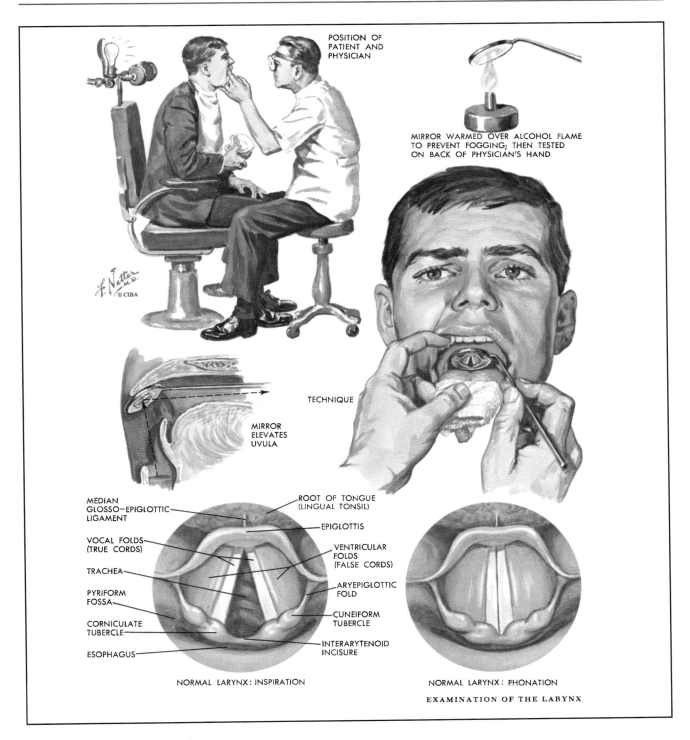

POSITION OF PATIENT AND PHYSICIAN

MIRROR WARMED OVER ALCOHOL FLAME TO PREVENT FOGGING; THEN TESTED ON BACK OF PHYSICIAN'S HAND

TECHNIQUE

MIRROR ELEVATES UVULA

MEDIAN GLOSSO–EPIGLOTTIC LIGAMENT

ROOT OF TONGUE (LINGUAL TONSIL)

EPIGLOTTIS

VOCAL FOLDS (TRUE CORDS)

VENTRICULAR FOLDS (FALSE CORDS)

TRACHEA

ARYEPIGLOTTIC FOLD

PYRIFORM FOSSA

CUNEIFORM TUBERCLE

CORNICULATE TUBERCLE

INTERARYTENOID INCISURE

ESOPHAGUS

NORMAL LARYNX: INSPIRATION

NORMAL LARYNX: PHONATION

EXAMINATION OF THE LARYNX

Figure 13–1. A. Traditional laryngeal examination. The laryngologist uses a warmed mirror to visualize the vocal fold indirectly. The tongue is grasped between the thumb and third finger. The thumb is placed as far posteriorly as possible in the middle third of the tongue (farther back than illustrated). The grip optimizes tongue depression and rotation. If the third finger is held firmly against the lower teeth and used to pivot rather than pull, discomfort along the frenulum can be avoided. The mirror is placed against the soft palate while the patient phonates on the vowel /i/. Placing the mirror during the phonation decreases the tendency to gag, and the vowel /i/ puts the larynx in the best position for visualization. (From the Larynx, *Clinical Symposia*, New Jersey: CIBA Pharmaceutical Company, 1964;16(3): Plate VI. Copyright 1964. Icon Learning Systems, LLC, a subsidiary of MediMedia USA Inc. Reprinted with permission from Icon Learning Systems, LLC, illustrated by Frank H. Netter, MD. All rights reserved.) *(continued)*

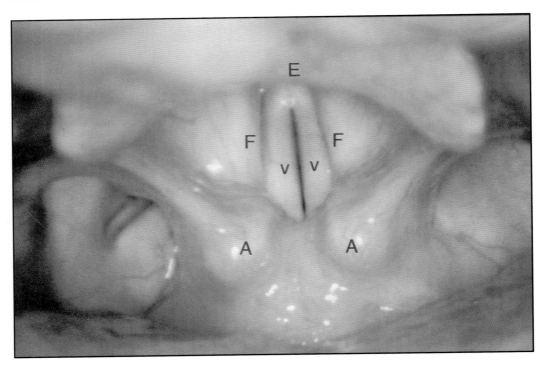

Figure 13–1. *(continued)* **B.** Photograph of normal larynx showing the true vocal folds (*V*), false vocal folds (*F*), arytenoids (*A*), and epiglottis (*E*).

ma and edema of the laryngeal surface of the epiglottis is seen often in association with muscle tension dysphonia and with frequent coughing or clearing of the throat. It is caused by direct trauma from the arytenoids during these maneuvers. The mirror or a laryngeal telescope often provides a better view of the posterior portion of the endolarynx than is obtained with flexible endoscopy. Stroboscopic examination adds substantially to diagnostic abilities (Figure 13–1B), as discussed below. Another occasionally helpful adjunct is the operating microscope. Magnification allows visualization of small mucosal disruptions and hemorrhages that may be significant but overlooked otherwise. This technique also allows photography of the larynx with a microscope camera. Magnification may also be achieved through magnifying laryngeal mirrors or by wearing loupes. Loupes usually provide a clearer image than do most of the magnifying mirrors available.

A laryngeal telescope may be combined with a stroboscope to provide excellent visualization of the vocal folds and related structures. The author usually uses a 70-degree laryngeal telescope, although 90-degree telescopes are required for some patients. The combination of a telescope and stroboscope provides optimal magnification and optical quality for assessment of vocal fold vibration. However, it is generally per-

formed with the tongue in a fixed position; and the nature of the examination does not permit assessment of the larynx during normal phonatory gestures.

Flexible fiberoptic laryngoscopy can be performed as an office procedure and allows inspection of the vocal folds in patients whose vocal folds are difficult to visualize indirectly. In addition, it permits observation of the vocal mechanism in a more natural posture than does indirect laryngoscopy, permitting sophisticated dynamic voice assessment. In the hands of an experienced endoscopist, this method may provide a great deal of information about both speaking and singing techniques. The combination of a fiberoptic laryngoscope with a laryngeal stroboscope may be especially useful. This system permits magnification, photography, and detailed inspection of vocal fold motion. Sophisticated systems that permit flexible or rigid fiberoptic strobovideolaryngoscopy are currently available commercially. They are invaluable assets for routine clinical use. The video system also provides a permanent record, permitting reassessment, comparison over time, and easy consultation. A refinement not currently available commercially is stereoscopic fiberoptic laryngoscopy, which is accomplished by placing a laryngoscope through each nostril, fastening the two together in the pharynx, and observing the larynx through the eyepieces.[7] This method allows visualization of laryngeal motion in three dimensions. However, it is used primarily in a research setting.

Rigid endoscopy under general anesthesia may be reserved for the rare patient whose vocal folds cannot be assessed adequately by other means or for patients who need surgical procedures to remove or biopsy laryngeal lesions. In many cases, this can be done with local anesthesia, avoiding the need for intubation and the traumatic coughing and vomiting that may occur even after general anesthesia administered by mask. Coughing after general anesthesia can be minimized by using topical anesthesia in the larynx and trachea. However, topical anesthetics act as severe mucosal irritants in a small number of patients. They may also predispose the patient to aspiration in the postoperative period. If a patient has had difficulty with a topical anesthetic administered in the office, it should not be used in the operating room. When used in general anesthesia cases, topical anesthetics should usually be applied at the end of the procedure. Thus, if inflammation occurs, it will not interfere with performance of microsurgery. Postoperative duration of anesthesia is also optimized. The author has had the least difficulty with 4% Xylocaine.

OBJECTIVE TESTS

Reliable, valid, objective analysis of the voice is extremely important and is an essential part of a comprehensive physical examination.[2] It is as valuable to the laryngologist as audiometry is to the otologist.[8,9] Familiarity with some of the measures and technologic advances currently available is helpful. This information is covered in greater detail elsewhere but is included here as a brief overview for the convenience of the reader.

Strobovideolaryngoscopy

Integrity of the vibratory margin of the vocal fold is essential for the complex motion required to produce good vocal quality. Under continuous light, the vocal folds vibrate approximately 250 times per second while phonating at middle C. Naturally, the human eye cannot discern the necessary details during such rapid motion. The vibratory margin may be assessed through high-speed photography, strobovideolaryngoscopy, high-speed video, videokymography, electroglottography (EGG), or photoglottography. Strobovideolaryngoscopy provides the necessary clinical information in a practical fashion. Stroboscopic light allows routine

slow-motion evaluation of the mucosal cover layer of the leading edge of the vocal fold. This state-of-the-art physical examination permits detection of vibratory asymmetries, structural abnormalities, small masses, submucosal scars, and other conditions that are invisible under ordinary light.[10-11] Documentation of the procedure by coupling stroboscopic light with the video camera allows later re-evaluation by the laryngologist or other health care providers.

Stroboscopy does not provide a true slow-motion image, as is obtained through high-speed photography (Figure 13–2). The stroboscope actually illuminates different points on consecutive vocal fold waves, each of which is retained on the retina for 0.2 seconds. The stroboscopically lighted portions of the successive waves are fused visually, thus the examiner is actually evaluating simulated cycles of phonation. The slow-motion effect is created by having the stroboscopic light desynchronized with the frequency of vocal fold vibration by approximately 2 hertz. When vocal fold vibration and the stroboscope are synchronized exactly, the vocal folds appear to stand still, rather than move in slow motion (Figure 13–3). In most instances, this approximation of slow motion provides all of the clinical information necessary.

We currently use a Kay Elemetrics (Lincoln Park, NJ) digital stroboscope. In virtually all cases, we examine patients with both an Olympus flexible ENFL-3 or Pentax chip-tip laryngoscope and a rigid magnifying telescope. We have both 70° and 90° telescopes available, but we find the 70° telescope more useful in most cases. Examination with the flexible nasolaryngoscope is possible in virtually all cases, and this technique provides good information about vocal habits, vocal fold motion during speech and singing, and vi-

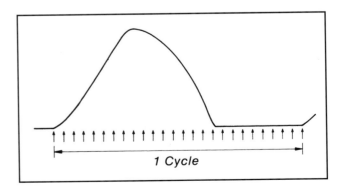

Figure 13–2. The principle of ultrahigh-speed photography. Numerous images are taken during each vibratory cycle. This technique is a true slow-motion representation of each vocal fold vibration.

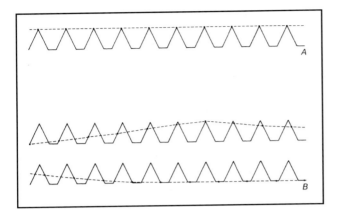

Figure 13–3. The principle of stroboscopy. The stroboscopic light illuminates portions of successive cycles. The eye fuses the illuminated points into an illusion of slow motion. **A.** If the stroboscope is synchronized with vocal fold vibration, a similar point is illuminated on each successive cycle and the vocal fold appears to stand still. **B.** If the stroboscope is slightly desynchronized, each cycle is illuminated at a slightly different point, and the slow-motion effect is created.

bratory margin characteristics under stroboscopic light in virtually every case. Examination with the telescope provides higher image quality and a larger image with a better light, and it occasionally reveals subtle abnormalities that are missed with the flexible laryngoscope.

Fundamental frequency can be influenced by various vocal fold parameters. For example, fundamental frequency is increased with increasing vocal fold tension or stiffness, increased subglottal pressure, or a shortened length of vibrating vocal fold. Fundamental frequency decreases as vocal fold mass increases.

Symmetry is assessed by observing both vocal folds simultaneously. In a trained voice, they are mirror images, opening with the same lateral excursions (symmetry of amplitude) and mirror-image waves (symmetry of phase). In untrained voices, phase asymmetry is common. Clearly, significant asymmetries may be caused by differences between the vocal folds in position, tension, elasticity, viscosity, shape, mass, or other mechanical properties.

Periodicity refers to the regularity of successive vibrations. Regular periodicity requires balanced control of expiratory force and the mechanical characteristics of the vocal folds. Irregular periodicity may be caused by an inability to maintain a steady expiratory stream of air, an inability to sustain steady laryngeal muscle contraction (as in neuromuscular disease), or marked differences in the mechanical properties of the vocal folds. Periodicity is assessed by locking the stro-

boscope in phase with vocal fold vibration. This should result in vocal folds that appear to stand still. If they move, vibration is aperiodic. Failure of glottic closure may be caused by vocal fold paresis or paralysis, an irregular vocal fold edge, a mass (or masses) separating the vocal fold edges, stiffness of a vibratory margin, cricoarytenoid joint dysfunction, falsetto singing, psychogenic dysphonia, and other causes. It is helpful to describe failures of glottic closure more specifically. They may be complete or incomplete, constant or intermittent, and may involve a posterior glottic chink, a specific small portion of the vocal folds, or as much as the entire vocal fold.

Amplitude of vibration and mucosal wave characteristics are assessed looking at the vocal folds one at a time. Small amplitude is associated with short vibrating segments of the vocal fold, increased stiffness, increased mass, and vocal fold motion. Amplitude is increased by increasing subglottal pressure, such as that occurring with loud phonation. Amplitude is not generally affected very much by soft masses such as cysts and nodules.

The mucosal wave is affected by many factors. It is diminished by dryness, scar, mucosal stiffness or edema, hyperplasia, masses, dehydration, and falsetto phonation. It also varies with pitch. The mucosal wave is also increased with loud phonation (increased subglottal pressure) and altered by hypofunctional or hyperfunctional voice technique. If there is an area of stiffness on the vocal fold, this will impede the traveling mucosal wave. This situation is encountered with small scars, some mass lesions, and sulcus vocalis.

Nonvibrating (adynamic) segments are often signs of serious vocal fold injury involving scar that obliterates the complex anatomy of the lamina propria and mucosa. Adynamic segments are seen only under stroboscopic light or in high-speed motion pictures. They are found typically on vocal folds that have undergone previous surgery, hemorrhage, or other trauma. Often the vocal folds look normal under continuous light, but the voice is hoarse and breathy. The reason is obvious when the adynamic segment is revealed under stroboscopic light. Adynamic segments may also occur temporarily, as seen sometimes in acute vocal fold hemorrhage with submucosal edema.

Other Techniques to Examine Vocal Fold Vibration

Other techniques to examine vocal fold vibration include ultrahigh-speed photography, EGG, photoelectroglottography and ultrasound glottography, and most recently videokymography[14] and high-speed video (digital or analog). Ultrahigh-speed photography provides images that are in true slow motion, rather than simulated. High-speed video offers similar advantages without most of the disadvantages of high-speed motion pictures. Videokymography offers high speed imaging of a single line along the vocal fold. EGG uses two electrodes placed on the skin of the neck above the thyroid laminae. It traces the opening and closing of the glottis and can be compared with strobo-scopic images.[15] EGG allows objective determination of the presence or absence of glottal vibrations and easy determination of the fundamental period of vibration and is reproducible. It reflects the glottal condition more accurately during its closed phase. Photo-electroglottography and ultrasound glottography are less useful clinically.[16]

Measures of Phonatory Ability

Objective measures of phonatory ability are easy to use, readily available to the laryngologist, helpful in treatment of professional vocalists with specific voice disorders, and quite useful in assessing the results of surgical therapies. Maximum phonation time is measured with a stopwatch. The patient is instructed to sustain the vowel /a/ for as long as possible after deep inspiration, vocalizing at a comfortable frequency and intensity. The frequency and intensity may be determined and controlled by an inexpensive frequency analyzer and sound level meter. The test is repeated three times, and the greatest value is recorded. Normal values have been determined.[16] Frequency range of phonation is recorded in semitones and documents the vocal range from the lowest note in the modal register (excluding vocal fry) to the highest falsetto note. This is the physiologic frequency range of phonation and disregards quality. The musical frequency range of phonation measures lowest to highest notes of musically acceptable quality. Tests for maximum phonation time, frequency ranges, and many of the other parameters discussed later (including spectrographic analysis) may be preserved on a tape recorder or digitized and stored for analysis at a convenient future time and used for pre- and post-treatment comparisons. Recordings should be made in a standardized, consistent fashion.

Frequency limits of vocal register also may be measured. The registers are (from low to high) vocal fry, chest, mid, head, and falsetto. However, classification of registers is controversial, and many other classifications are used. Although the classification listed above is common among musicians, at present, most voice scientists prefer to classify registers as pulse, modal, and loft. Overlap of frequency among registers occurs routinely.

Testing the speaking fundamental frequency often reveals excessively low pitch, an abnormality associated with chronic voice abuse and development of vocal nodules. This parameter may be followed objectively throughout a course of voice therapy. Intensity range of phonation (IRP) has proven a less useful measure than frequency range. It varies with fundamental frequency (which should be recorded) and is greatest in the middle frequency range. It is recorded in sound pressure level (SPL) re: 0.0002 microbar. For normal adults who are not professional vocalists, measuring at a single fundamental frequency, IRP averages 54.8 dB for males and 51 dB for females.[17] Alterations of intensity are common in voice disorders, although IRP is not the most sensitive test to detect them. Information from these tests may be combined in a fundamental frequency-intensity profile,[16] also called a phonetogram.

Glottal efficiency (ratio of the acoustic power at the level of the glottis to subglottal power) provides useful information but is not clinically practical because measuring acoustic power at the level of the glottis is difficult. Subglottic power is the product of subglottal pressure and airflow rate. These can be determined clinically. Various alternative measures of glottic efficiency have been proposed, including the ratio of radiated acoustic power to subglottal power,[18] airflow intensity profile,[19] and ratio of the root mean square value of the AC component to the mean volume velocity (DC component).[20] Although glottal efficiency is of great interest, none of these tests is used in routine clinical circumstances.

Aerodynamic Measures

Traditional pulmonary function testing provides the most readily accessible measure of respiratory function. The most common parameters measured include: (1) tidal volume, the volume of air that enters the lungs during inspiration and leaves during expiration in normal breathing; (2) functional residual capacity, the volume of air remaining in the lungs at the end of inspiration during normal breathing, which can be divided into expiratory reserve volume (maximal additional volume that can be exhaled) and residual volume (the volume of air remaining in the lungs at the end of maximal exhalation); (3) inspiratory capacity, the maximal volume of air that can be inhaled starting at the functional residual capacity; (4) total lung capacity, the volume of air in the lungs following maximal inspiration; (5) vital capacity, the maximal volume of air that can be exhaled from the lungs following maximal inspiration; (6) forced vital capacity, the rate of airflow with rapid, forceful expiration from total lung capacity to residual volume; (7) FEV_1, the forced expiratory volume in 1 second; (8) FEV3, the forced expiratory volume in 3 seconds; (9) maximal mid-expiratory flow, the mean rate of airflow over the middle half of the forced vital capacity (between 25% and 75% of the forced vital capacity).

For singers and professional speakers with an abnormality caused by voice abuse, abnormal pulmonary function tests may confirm deficiencies in aerobic conditioning or reveal previously unrecognized asthma.[21] Flow glottography with computer inverse filtering is also a practical and valuable diagnostic for assessing flow at the vocal fold level, evaluating the voice source, and imaging the results of the balance between adductory forces and subglottal pressure.[22] It also has therapeutic value as a biofeedback tool.

The spirometer, readily available for pulmonary function testing, can also be used for measuring airflow during phonation. However, the spirometer does not allow simultaneous display of acoustic signals, and its frequency response is poor. A pneumotachograph consists of a laminar air resistor, a differential pressure transducer, and an amplifying and recording system. It allows measurement of airflow and simultaneous recording of other signals when coupled with a polygraph. A hot-wire anemometer allows determination of airflow velocity by measuring the electrical drop across the hot wire. Modern hot-wire anemometers containing electrical feedback circuitry that maintains the temperature of the hot wire provide a flat response up to 1 kHz and are useful clinically.

The four parameters traditionally measured in the aerodynamic performance of a voice are: subglottal pressure (P_{sub}), supraglottal pressure (P_{sup}), glottal impedance, and the volume velocity of airflow at the glottis. These parameters and their rapid variations can be measured under laboratory circumstances. However, clinically their mean value is usually determined as follows:

$$P_{sub} - P_{sup} = MFR \times GR$$

where MFR is the mean (root mean square) flow rate and GR is the mean (root mean square) glottal resistance. When vocalizing the open vowel /ɑ/, the supraglottic pressure equals the atmospheric pressure, reducing the equation to:

$$P_{sub} = MFR \times GR$$

The mean flow rate is a useful clinical measure. While the patient vocalizes the vowel /ɑ/, the mean flow rate is calculated by dividing the total volume of air used during phonation by the duration of phonation. The subject phonates at a comfortable pitch and loudness either over a determined period of time or for a maximum sustained period of phonation.

Air volume is measured by the use of a mask fitted tightly over the face or by phonating into a mouthpiece while wearing a nose clamp. Measurements may be made using a spirometer, pneumotachograph, or hot-wire anemometer. The normal values for mean flow rate under habitual phonation, with changes in intensity or register, and under various pathologic circumstances were determined in the 1970s.[16] Normal values are available for both adults and children. Mean flow rate also can be measured and is a clinically useful parameter to follow during treatment for vocal nodules, recurrent laryngeal nerve paralysis, spasmodic dysphonia, and other conditions.

Glottal resistance cannot be measured directly, but it can be calculated from the mean flow rate and mean subglottal pressure. Normal glottal resistance is 20 to 100 dyne seconds/cm^5 at low and medium pitches and 150 dyne seconds/cm^5 at high pitches.[18] The normal values for subglottal pressure under various healthy and pathologic voice conditions have also been determined by numerous investigators.[16] The phonation quotient is the vital capacity divided by the maximum phonation time. It has been shown to correlate closely with maximum flow rate[23] and is a more convenient measure. Normative data determined by various authors have been published.[16] The phonation quotient provides an objective measure of the effects of treatment and is particularly useful in cases of recurrent laryngeal nerve paralysis and mass lesions of the vocal folds, including nodules.

Acoustic Analysis

Acoustic analysis of voice signals is both promising and disappointing. The skilled laryngologist, speech-language pathologist, musician, or other trained listener frequently infers a great deal of valid information from the sound of a voice. However, clinically useful technology for analyzing and quantifying subtle acoustic differences is still not ideal. In many ways, the tape recorder (analog or digital, traditional or minidisk) is still one of the laryngologist's most valuable tools for acoustic analysis. Recording a patient's voice under controlled, repeatable circumstances before, during, and at the conclusion of treatment allows both the physician and the patient to make a qualitative, subjective acoustic analysis. Objective analysis with instruments may also be made from recorded voice samples.

Acoustic analysis equipment can determine frequency, intensity, harmonic spectrum, cycle-to-cycle perturbations in frequency (jitter), cycle-to-cycle perturbations in amplitude (shimmer), harmonics-to-noise ratios, breathiness index, and many other parameters. The DSP Sona-Graph Sound Analyzer Model 5500 (Kay Elemetrics, Lincoln Park, NJ) is an integrated voice analysis system. It is equipped for sound spectrography capabilities. Spectrography provides a visual record of the voice. The acoustic signal is depicted using time (x axis), frequency (y axis), and intensity (z axis), shading of light versus dark. Using the band pass filters, generalizations about quality, pitch, and loudness can be made. These observations are used in formulating the voice therapy treatment plan. Formant structure and strength can be determined using the narrow-band filters, of which a variety of configurations are possible. In clinical settings in which singers and other professional voice users are evaluated and treated routinely, this feature is extremely valuable. A sophisticated voice analysis program (an optional program) may be combined with the Sona-Graph and is an especially valuable addition to the clinical laboratory. The voice analysis program (Computer Speech Lab, Kay Elemetrics, Lincoln Park, NJ) measures speaking fundamental frequency, frequency perturbation (jitter), amplitude perturbation (shimmer), harmonics-to-noise ratio, and provides many other useful values. An electroglottograph may be used in conjunction with the Sona-Graph to provide some of these voicing parameters. Examining the EGG waveform alone is possible with this setup, but its clinical usefulness has not yet been established. An important feature of the Sona-Graph is the long-term average (LTA) spectral capability, which permits analysis of longer voice samples (30-90 seconds). The LTA analyzes only voiced speech segments, and may be useful in screening for hoarse or breathy voices. In addition, computer interface capabilities (also an optional program) have solved many data storage and file maintenance problems.

In analyzing acoustic signals, the microphone should be placed at the level of the mouth or positioned in or over the trachea, although intratracheal recordings are used for research purposes only. The position should be standardized in each office or laboratory.[24] Various techniques are being developed to improve the usefulness of acoustic analysis. Because of the enormous amount of information carried in the acoustic signal, further refinements in objective acoustic analysis should prove particularly valuable to the clinician.

Laryngeal Electromyography

Electromyography (EMG) requires an electrode system, an amplifier, an oscilloscope, a loudspeaker, and a recording system.[25] Electrodes are placed transcutaneously into laryngeal muscles. EMG can be extremely valuable in confirming cases of vocal fold paresis, differentiating paralysis from arytenoid dislocation, distinguishing recurrent laryngeal nerve paralysis from combined recurrent and superior nerve paralysis, diagnosing other more subtle neurolaryngologic pathology, and documenting functional voice disorders and malingering. It is also recommended for needle localization when using botulinum toxin for treatment of spasmodic dysphonia and other conditions.

Psychoacoustic Evaluation

Because the human ear and brain are the most sensitive and complex analyzers of sound currently available, many researchers have tried to standardize and quantify psychoacoustic evaluation. Unfortunately, even definitions of basic terms such as hoarseness and breathiness are still controversial. Psychoacoustic evaluation protocols and interpretations are not standardized. Consequently, although subjective psychoacoustic analysis of voice is of great value to individual skilled clinicians, it remains generally unsatisfactory for comparing research among laboratories or for reporting clinical results.

The GRBAS scale[6] helps standardize perceptual analysis for clinical purposes. It rates the voice on a scale from 0 to 3, with regard to grade, roughness, asthenia, breathiness, and strain. Grade 0 is normal; 1 is slightly abnormal; 2 is moderately abnormal; and 3 is extremely abnormal. Grade refers to the degree of hoarseness or voice abnormality. Roughness refers to the acoustic/auditory impression of irregularity of vibration and corresponds with gear and shimmer. Asthenic evaluation assesses weakness or lack of power and corresponds to vocal intensity and energy in higher harmonics. Breathiness refers to the acoustic/auditory impression of air leakage and corresponds to turbulence. Strain refers to the acoustic/auditory impression of hyperfunction and may be related to fundamental frequency, noise in the high-frequency range, and energy in higher harmonics. For example, a patient's voice might be graded as G2, R2, B1, A1, S2.

OUTCOME ASSESSMENT

Measuring the impact of a voice disorder has always been challenging. However, recent advances have begun to address this problem. Validated instruments such as the Voice Handicap Index (VHI)[26] are currently in clinical use, and are likely to be utilized widely in future years. Chapter 21 reviews current trends and future directions in measuring voice treatment outcomes.

VOICE IMPAIRMENT AND DISABILITY

Quantifying voice impairment and assigning a disability rating (percentage of whole person) remain controversial. This subject is still not addressed comprehensively even in the most recent editions (2001, 5th ed) of the American Medical Association's *Guides to the Evaluation of Permanent Impairment* (The Guides).The Guides still do not take into account the person's profession when calculating disability. Alternative approaches have been proposed,[27] and advances in this complex arena are anticipated over the next few years. This subject is discussed in greater detail in chapter 22.

EVALUATION OF THE SINGING VOICE

The physician must be careful not to exceed the limits of his or her expertise especially in caring for singers. However, if voice abuse or technical error is suspected, or if a difficult judgment must be reached on whether to allow a sick singer to perform, a brief observation of the patient's singing may provide invaluable information. This is accomplished best by asking the singer to stand and sing scales either in the examining room or in the soundproof audiology booth. Similar maneuvers may be used for professional speakers, including actors (who can vocalize and recite lines), clergy and politicians (who can deliver sermons and speeches), and virtually all other voice patients. The singer's stance should be balanced, with the weight slightly forward. The knees should be bent slightly and the shoulders, torso, and neck should be relaxed. The singer should inhale through the nose whenever possible allowing filtration, warming, and humidification of inspired air. In general, the chest should be expanded, but most of the active breathing is abdominal. The chest should not rise substantially with each inspiration, and the supraclavicular musculature should not be involved obviously in inspiration. Shoulders and neck muscles should not be tensed even with deep inspiration. Abdominal musculature should be contracted shortly before the initiation of the tone. This may be evaluated visually or by palpation (Figure 13–4). Muscles of the neck and face should be relaxed. Economy is a basic principle of all art forms. Wasted energy and motion and muscle tension are incorrect and usually deleterious.

The singer should be instructed to sing a scale (a five-note scale is usually sufficient) on the vowel /a/, beginning on any comfortable note. Technical errors are usually most obvious as contraction of muscles in the neck and chin, retraction of the lower lip, retraction of the tongue, or tightening of the muscles of mastication. The singer's mouth should be open widely but comfortably. When singing /a/, the singer's tongue should rest in a neutral position with the tip of the tongue lying against the back of the singer's mandibular incisors. If the tongue pulls back or demonstrates obvious muscular activity as the singer performs the scales, improper voice use can be confirmed on the basis of positive evidence (Figure 13–5). The position of the larynx should not vary substantially with pitch changes. Rising of the larynx with ascending pitch is evidence of technical dysfunction. This examination

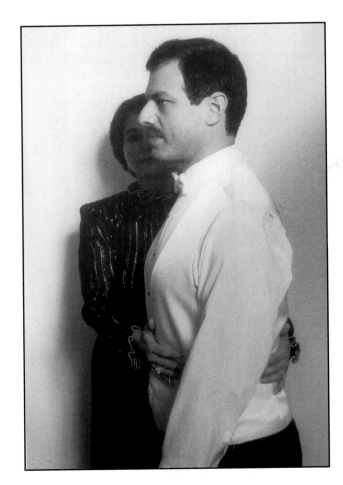

Figure 13–4. Bimanual palpation of the support mechanism. The singer should expand posteriorly and anteriorly with inspiration. Muscles should tighten prior to onset of the sung tone.

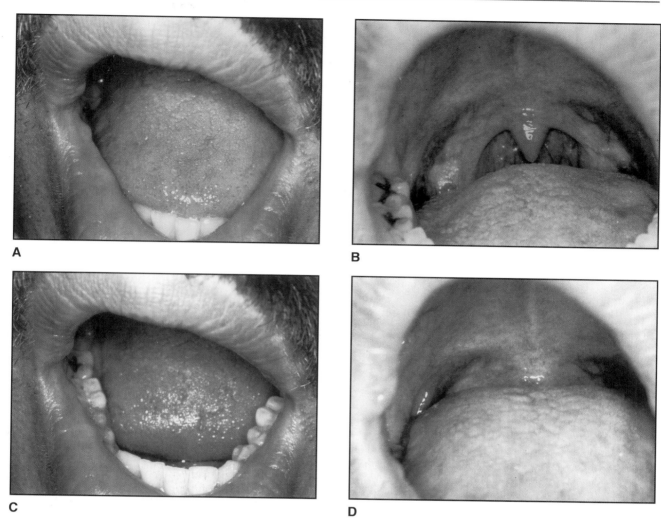

Figure 13–5. Proper relaxed position of the anterior (**A**) and posterior (**B**) portions of the tongue. Common improper use of the tongue pulled back from the teeth (**C**) and raised posteriorly (**D**).

also gives the physician an opportunity to observe any dramatic differences between the qualities and ranges of the patient's speaking voice and the singing voice. A physical examination summary form has proven helpful in organization and documentation.[3]

Remembering the admonition not to exceed his or her expertise, the physician who examines many singers often can glean valuable information from a brief attempt to modify an obvious technical error. For example, deciding whether to allow a singer with mild or moderate laryngitis to perform is often difficult. On the one hand, an expert singer has technical skills that allow him or her to compensate safely. On the other hand, if a singer does not sing with correct technique and does not have the discipline to modify volume, technique, and repertoire as necessary, the risk of vo-

cal injury may be increased substantially even by mild inflammation of the vocal folds. In borderline circumstances, observation of the singer's technique may greatly help the physician in making a judgment.

If the singer's technique appears flawless, the physician may feel somewhat more secure in allowing the singer to proceed with performance commitments. More commonly, even good singers demonstrate technical errors when experiencing voice difficulties. In a vain effort to compensate for dysfunction at the vocal fold level, singers often modify their technique in the neck and supraglottic vocal tract. In the good singer, this usually means going from good technique to bad technique. The most common error involves pulling back the tongue and tightening the cervical strap muscles. Although this increased muscular activity gives the singer the illusion of making the voice more secure, this technical maladjustment undermines vocal efficiency and increases vocal strain. The physician may ask the singer to hold the top note of a five-note scale; while the note is being held, the singer may simply be told, "Relax your tongue." At the same time the physician points to the singer's abdominal musculature. Most good singers immediately correct to good technique. If they do, and if upcoming performances are particularly important, the singer may be able to perform with a reminder that meticulous technique is essential. The singer should be advised to "sing by feel rather than by ear," to consult his or her voice teacher, and conserve the voice except when it is absolutely necessary to use it. If a singer is unable to correct from bad technique to good technique promptly, especially if he or she uses excessive muscle tension in the neck and ineffective abdominal support, it is generally safer not to perform with even a mild vocal fold abnormality. With increased experience and training, the laryngologist may make other observations that aid in providing appropriate treatment recommendations for singer patients. Once these skills have been mastered for the care of singers, applying them to other patients is relatively easy, so long as the laryngologist takes the time to understand the demands of the individual's professional, avocational, and recreational vocal activities.

If treatment is to be instituted, making at least a tape recording of the voice is advisable in most cases and essential before any surgical intervention. The author routinely uses strobovideolaryngoscopy for diagnosis and documentation in virtually all cases as well as many of the objective measures discussed. Pretreatment testing is extremely helpful clinically and medicolegally.

ADDITIONAL EXAMINATIONS

A general physical examination should be performed whenever the patient's systemic health is questionable. Debilitating conditions such as mononucleosis may be noticed first by the singer as vocal fatigue. A neurologic assessment may be particularly revealing. The physician must be careful not to overlook dysarthrias and dysphonias, which are characteristic of movement disorders and of serious neurologic disease. Dysarthria is a defect in rhythm, enunciation, and articulation that usually results from neuromuscular impairment or weakness such as may occur after a stroke. It may be seen with oral deformities or illness, as well. Dysphonia is an abnormality of vocalization usually caused by problems at the laryngeal level.

Physicians should be familiar with the six types of dysarthria, their symptoms, and their importance.[28,29]

Flaccid dysarthria occurs in lower motor neuron or primary muscle disorders such as myasthenia gravis and tumors or strokes involving the brainstem nuclei. Spastic dysarthria occurs in upper motor neuron disorders (pseudobulbar palsy) such as multiple strokes and cerebral palsy. Ataxic dysarthria is seen with cerebellar disease, alcohol intoxication, and multiple sclerosis. Hypokinetic dysarthria accompanies Parkinson's disease. Hyperkinetic dysarthria may be spasmodic, as in Gilles de la Tourette's disease, or dystonic, as in chorea and cerebral palsy. Mixed dysarthria occurs in amyotrophic lateral sclerosis (ALS) or Lou Gehrig's disease. The preceding classification actually combines dysphonic and dysarthric characteristics but is very useful clinically. The value of a comprehensive neurolaryngologic evaluation[30] cannot be overstated. More specific details of voice changes associated with neurologic dysfunction and their localizing value are available in chapter 30.[2,32]

It is extremely valuable for the laryngologist to assemble an arts-medicine team that includes not only a speech-language pathologist, singing voice specialist, acting voice specialist, and voice scientist, but also medical colleagues in other disciplines. Collaboration with an expert neurologist, pulmonologist, endocrinologist, psychologist, psychiatrist, internist, physiatrist, and others with special knowledge of, and interest in, voice disorders is invaluable in caring for patients with voice disorders. Such interdisciplinary teams have not only changed the standard of care in voice evaluation and treatment, but are also largely responsible for the rapid and productive growth of voice as a subspecialty.

REFERENCES

1. Sataloff RT. Professional singers: the science and art of clinical care. *Am J Otolaryngol.* 1981;2:251–266.
2. Rubin JS, Sataloff RT, Korovin GS. *Diagnosis and Treatment of Voice Disorders.* 2nd ed. Albany, NY: Delmar Thomson Learning; 2003:137–284.
3. Sataloff RT. The professional voice: part II, physical examination. *J Voice.* 1987;1:91–201.
4. Fuazawa T, Blaugrund SM, El-Assuooty A, Gould WJ. Acoustic analysis of hoarse voice: a preliminary report. *J Voice.* 1988;2(2):127–131.
5. Gelfer M. Perceptual attributes of voice: development and use of rating scales. *J Voice.* 1988;2(4):320–326.
6. Hirano M. *Clinical Examination of the Voice.* New York, NY: Springer-Verlag; 1981:83–84.
7. Fujimura O. Stereo-fiberoptic laryngeal observation. *J Acoust Soc Am.* 1979;65:70–72.
8. Sataloff RT, Spiegel JR, Carroll LM, Darby KS, Hawkshaw MJ, Rulnick RK. The clinical voice laboratory: practical design and clinical application. *J Voice.* 1990;4:264–279.
9. Sataloff RT, Heuer RH, Hoover C, Baroody MM. Laboratory assessment of voice. In: Gould WJ, Sataloff RT,

Spiegel JR. *Voice Surgery.* St. Louis, MO: Mosby; 1993: 203–216.

10. Sataloff RT, Spiegel JR, Carroll LM, Schiebel BR, Darby KS, Rulnick RK. (1988) Strobovideolaryngoscopy in professional voice users: results and clinical value. *J Voice.* 1986;1:359–364.

11. Sataloff RT, Spiegel JR, Hawkshaw MJ. Strobovideolaryngoscopy: results and clinical value. *Ann Otol Rhinol Laryngol.* 1991;100:725–727.

12. Bless D, Hirano M, Feder RJ. Video stroboscopic evaluation of the larynx. *Ear Nose Throat J.* 1987;66:289–296.

13. Hirano M. Phonosurgery: basic and clinical investigations. *Otologia (Fukuoka).* 1975;21:239–442.

14. Svec J, Shutte H. Videokymography: high-speed line scanning of vocal fold vibration. *J Voice.* 1996;10:201–205.

15. Leclure FLE, Brocaar ME, Verscheeure J. Electroglottography and its relation to glottal activity. *Folia Phoniatr (Basel).* 1975;27:215–224.

16. Hirano M. *Clinical Examination of the Voice.* New York, NY: Springer-Verlag; 1981:25–27, 85–98.

17. Coleman RJ, Mabis JH, Hinson JK. Fundamental frequency sound pressure level profiles of adult male and female voices. *J Speech Hear Res.* 1977;20:197–204.

18. Isshiki N. Regulatory mechanism of voice intensity variation. *J Speech Hear Res.* 1964;7:17–29.

19. Saito S. Phonosurgery: basic study on the mechanisms of phonation and endolaryngeal microsurgery. *Otologia (Fukuoka).* 1977;23:171–384.

20. Isshiki N. Functional surgery of the larynx. In: *Report of the 78th Annual Convention of the Oto-Rhino-Laryngological Society of Japan.* Fukuoka: Kyoto University; 1977.

21. Cohn JR, Sataloff RT, Spiegel JR, Fish JE, Kennedy K. Airway reactivity-induced asthma in singers (ARIAS). *J Voice.* 1991;5:332–337.

22. Sundberg J. *The Science of the Singing Voice.* Dekalb, IL: Northern Illinois University Press; 1987:11, 66, 77–89

23. Hirano M, Koike Y, von Leden H. Maximum phonation time and air usage during phonation. *Folia Phoniatr (Basel).* 1968;20:185–201.

24. Price DB, Sataloff RT. A simple technique for consistent microphone placement in voice recording. *J Voice.* 1988; 2:206–207.

25. Sataloff RT, Mandel S, Mañon-Espaillat R, et al. *Laryngeal Electromyography.* 2nd ed. San Diego, CA: Plural Publishing; 2006.

26. Benninger MS, Gardner GM, Jacobson BH, Grywalski C. New dimensions in measuring voice treatment outcomes. In: Sataloff RT. *Professional Voice: The Science and Art of Clinical Care.* 3rd ed. San Diego, CA: Plural Publishing, Inc; 2005:471–477.

27. Sataloff RT. Voice and speech impairment and disability. In: Sataloff RT. *Professional Voice: The Science and Art of Clinical Care.* 3rd ed. San Diego, CA: Plural Publishing, Inc; 2005:1427–1432.

28. Darley FL, Aronson AE, Brown JR. Differential diagnostic of patterns of dysarthria. *J Speech Hear Res.* 1969;12(2): 246–249.

29. Darley FL, Aronson AE, Brown JR. Clusters of deviant speech dimensions in the dysarthrias. *J Speech Hear Res.* 1969;12(3):462–496.

30. Rosenfield DB. Neurolaryngology. *Ear Nose Throat J.* 1987;66:323–326.

31. Raphael BN, Sataloff RT. Increasing vocal effectiveness. In: Sataloff RT. *Professional Voice: Science and Art of Clinical Care.* 3rd ed. San Diego, CA: Plural Publishing, Inc; 2005:993–1004.

APPENDIX 13-1. READING PASSAGES

A classic passage including all the speech sounds of English.

The Rainbow Passage

When the sunlight strikes raindrops in the air, they act like a prism and form a rainbow. The rainbow is a division of white light into many beautiful colors. These take the shape of a long round arch, with its path high above, and its two ends apparently beyond the horizon. There is, according to legend, a boiling pot of gold at one end. People look but no one ever finds it. When a man looks for something beyond his reach, his friends say he is looking for the pot of gold at the end of the rainbow.

An all voiced passage.

Marvin Williams

Marvin Williams is only nine. Marvin lives with his mother on Monroe Avenue in Vernon Valley. Marvin loves all movies, even eerie ones with evil villains in them. Whenever a new movie is in the area, Marvin is usually an early arrival. Nearly every evening Marvin is in row one, along the aisle.

A general purpose passage useful for evaluating hard glottal attack, phrasing, and nasal resonance.

Towne-Heuer Vocal Analysis Reading Passage

If I take a trip this August, I will probably go to Austria. Or I could go to Italy. All of the places of Europe are easy to get to by air, rail, ship or auto. Everybody I have talked to says he would like to go to Europe also.

Every year there are varieties of festivals or fairs at a lot of places. All sorts of activities, such as foods to eat, sights to see occur. Oh, I love to eat ices seated outdoors! The people of each area are reported to like us . . . the people of the U.S.A. It is said that that is true except for Paris.

Aid is easy to get because the officials are helpful. Aid is always available if troubles arise. It helps to have with you a list of offices or officials to call if you do require aid. If you are lost, you will always be helped to locate your route or hotel. The local police will assist you, if they are able to speak as you do. Otherwise a phrase book is useful.

I have had to have help of this sort each trip abroad. However, it was always easy to locate. Happily, I hope, less help will be required this trip. Last trip every hotel was occupied. I had to ask everywhere for flats. Two earlier trips were hard because of heat or lack of heat at hotels.

On second thought, I may want to travel in autumn instead of in August. Many countries can be expensive in the summer months and much less so in autumn. November and December can make fine months for entertainment in many European countries. There may be concerts and musical events more often than during the summer. Milan, Rome, and Hamburg, not to mention Berlin, Vienna, and Madrid are most often mentioned for music.

Most of my friends and I wouldn't miss the chance to try the exciting, interesting, and appetizing menus at most continental restaurants. In many European countries food is inexpensive and interestingly prepared. Servings may be small but meals are taken more often so that there is no need to go hungry.

Maritime countries make many meals of seafood, such as mussels, clams, shrimp, flounder, and salmon or herring. Planning and making your own meals cannot be done even in most small, inexpensive hotels. One must eat in the dining room or in restaurants. Much fun can be had meeting the local natives during mealtimes. Many of them can tell you where to find amusing and interesting shops and sights not mentioned in tour manuals.

14

Evaluation of Laryngeal Biomechanics by Fiberoptic Laryngoscopy

Jamie A. Koufman, MD

Biomechanical analysis of the performance of athletes has become relatively common. It is accomplished by linking a video system to a computer system so that movement can be evaluated critically in ultraslow motion, frame-by-frame. With this approach, patterns of movement can be identified that are, at one extreme, optimally efficient and, at the other extreme, maladaptive, or even abusive. Using similar methods, laryngeal biomechanics also can be studied.

Like injured athletes, people with voice disorders often demonstrate patterns of abnormal biomechanics (abnormal laryngeal muscle tension), which voice clinicians can identify during laryngeal examination by transnasal fiberoptic laryngoscopy (TFL).[1,2] However, these same patterns sometimes are observed in people who have no problems with their voices; for example, they may be seen transiently in singers working at the limits of the voice in terms of loudness and/or pitch.[3]

What are the abnormal muscle tension patterns? How much laryngeal muscle tension is physiologic, that is, what's normal? When do observed muscle tension pat-

terns indicate a functional (nonorganic) voice disorder? When do they indicate compensation for an organic condition?

TFL is the first and single most important laryngeal examination for patients with laryngeal and voice disorders because assessment of laryngeal biomechanics holds the key to understanding the underlying glottal condition. Most dysfunctional states are associated with hyperkinetic laryngeal biomechanics (eg, supraglottic contraction); however, used properly, TFL distinguishes compensatory from intrinsic laryngeal behaviors. In the author's practice, the TFL findings often determine the type of diagnostic work-up and the initial approach to management.

LARYNGEAL EXAMINATION METHODS

For over a hundred years, indirect *mirror laryngoscopy* (ML) was the standard method for performing a laryngeal examination; but although clinicians could visualize the larynx using that technique, they could not visually assess (examine) vocal function. Approximately two decades ago, *telescopic laryngoscopy* (TL), *transnasal fiberoptic laryngoscopy* (TFL), and *videostroboscopy* became available in the United States, and for the first time, laryngeal biomechanics could be evaluated effectively in a clinical setting. Since then, a great deal has been learned about laryngeal function and the biomechanics of patients with voice disorders. Although each voice clinician may have preferred examination methods, there are specific indications for, and advantages and disadvantages of, each technique (ML, TL, and TFL); these are summarized in Table 14–1.

The technique of TL is similar to ML, but instead of a mirror, a rigid optical instrument is used. To perform TL, the examiner grasps the subject's tongue, pulls it forward, and inserts the telescope into the oropharynx. This method (as well as ML) limits the phonatory repertoire of the patient to producing a sustained vowel (eg, /a/ or /i/); connected speech and singing cannot be evaluated. In other words, grasping the tongue and inserting the instrument during TL significantly alters laryngeal biomechanics. In addition, TL may cause gagging, so that the technique is sometimes limited by subject intolerance, unless effective prior laryngopharyngeal topical anesthesia is established.

On the other hand, TFL is well tolerated by virtually all patients, alters laryngeal biomechanics very little, if at all, and provides essential diagnostic information in the vast majority of cases. TFL (with or without stroboscopy) is recommended at the first examination for all patients with voice disorders and TL with stroboscopy at the second, the latter for patients with specific vocal fold lesions for which enhanced optics (magnification) is needed. However, TFL with videostroboscopy will suffice in many patients.

These recommendations are based on use of state-of-the-art TFL systems. Although the optics (resolution and magnification) of currently available TFL systems are still not quite as good as those of TL systems, the gap has narrowed in recent years. Theoretically, when TFL optics improve to the level of current TL optics, the latter examination will become obsolete, because the TFL is more physiologic and permits a comprehensive examination of laryngeal function.

Technique of Transnasal Fiberoptic Laryngoscopy (TFL)

TFL is usually performed by spraying a topical anesthetic into one, or both, of the nasal passages; most patients have a best side based on the presence of some nasal septal abnormality, such as a spur. A standard

Table 14–1. Advantages and Disadvantages of Laryngeal Examination Methods

I. Mirror laryngoscopy

  A. Advantages

    1. Quick overview

    2. Prognostic for telescopic laryngoscopy

  B. Disadvantages

    1. Poorly tolerated (gagging)

    2. Can only assess sustained vowel sounds, eg, /i/

    3. Alters laryngeal biomechanics

II. Telescopic laryngoscopy

  A. Advantages

    1. Excellent optics; best for photography

    2. Magnification; best for videostroboscopic evaluation of free-edge lesions

  B. Disadvantages

    1. Poorly tolerated (gagging)

    2. Alters laryngeal biomechanics

    3. Can only assess vowel sounds, eg, /i/

    4. Cannot assess the entire vocal tract

    5. Cannot assess connected speech or singing

III. Transnasal fiberoptic laryngoscopy

  A. Advantages

    1. Best way to assess laryngeal biomechanics

    2. Can assess the entire vocal tract

    3. Well tolerated by almost all patients

    4. Can assess the voice across the dynamic and pitch ranges of the voice during connected speech and singing

    5. Good for videostroboscopy

  B. Disadvantages

    1. Magnification and optics inferior to that of the telescopic instruments

anesthetic such as Xylocaine may be used, but as an alternative, 2% cocaine with 1% ephedrine may be used. Although many subjects can tolerate TFL without any anesthetic, topical anesthesia is recommended.

There are many types of fiberscopes available, and, in general, the larger the external diameter, the better the light and optics; unfortunately, a fiberscope with

15

Transnasal Esophagoscopy

Anthony Sparano, MD
Natasha Mirza, MD

Traditional esophagoscopy is typically performed transorally with a flexible or rigid endoscope and the patient under conscious sedation or general anesthesia. Recent technologic advances now allow esophagoscopy to be comfortably performed transnasally in an unsedated patient. The technique for doing so is known as transnasal esophagoscopy (TNE).

The frequent occurrence of dysphagia, laryngopharyngeal reflux (LPR), and other pathologic esophageal lesions in patients with otolaryngologic complaints makes TNE a practical and useful addition to the otolaryngologist's diagnostic and therapeutic repertoire. Without TNE, the capacity to evaluate the esophagus below the piriform sinus is compromised and often necessitates some combination of barium esophagram, gastroenterology consultation, or general anesthesia. Given otolaryngologists' familiarity with in-office flexible endoscopic evaluation of the hypopharynx and larynx and rigid and flexible endoscopic evaluations of the esophagus in the operating room setting, the recent availability of ultrathin flexible endoscopes has made way for more economical, practical, and safer esophageal examination in TNE.

When compared with conventional upper endoscopy, transnasal esophagoscopy has demonstrated a shortened overall procedure time, a significantly shortened recovery period, a 65% reduction in the cost of consumable supplies, and a 92% reduction in the cost of pharmaceuticals.[1] Conscious sedation accounts for a significant portion of the cost of traditional upper endoscopy. These costs include procedural and postprocedural monitoring, use of requisite associated medications, and management of any cardiopulmonary complications, which have been attributed mostly to adverse effects of conscious sedation.[2-5] In addition, the societal costs associated with a missed day of work and the need for independently arranged separate transportation subsequent to conscious sedation and extended postprocedure recovery are significant when considering the relative cost-effectiveness of in-office TNE in an unsedated patient.

ESOPHAGEAL ANATOMY

The esophagus is a tubular organ originating at the level of the cricoid cartilage and ending after passage through the hiatus in the right crus of the diaphragm (Figure 15–1). Proximally, the esophagus begins where the inferior pharyngeal constrictor merges with the cri-

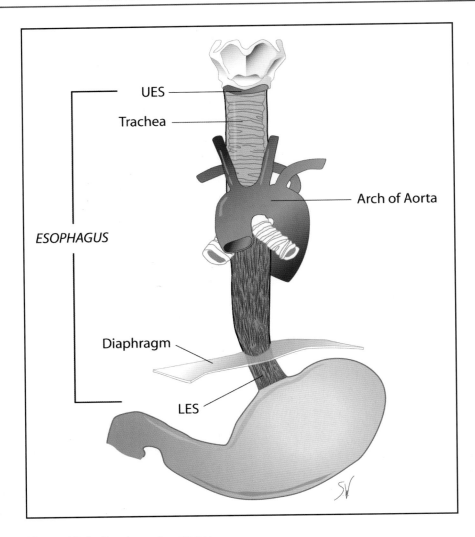

Figure 15–1. Esophageal anatomy.

copharyngeus muscle, making up the upper esophageal sphincter (UES). In the neck the esophagus lies posterior and leftward of the trachea. In the thorax it gradually reaches midline at about the level of the fifth thoracic vertebrae (T5). At about the T7 level it deviates leftward and passes through the diaphragm 2 to 3 cm left of center at T10 to enter the stomach.

The UES is contracted at rest, forming a high-pressure barrier to proximal air entry and distal esophageal reflux. It is a true sphincter that is attached to the cricoid cartilage. On electromyogram (EMG) study, the UES demonstrates tonic contractions temporarily inhibited by a swallow, with input control through fibers from the nucleus ambiguus to motor end plates in the cricopharyngeus muscle. Contractile forces are predominantly in the anterior-posterior direction and can measure up to 100 mm Hg. Lateral contractile forces are also present, but are weaker and usually

measure less than 40 mm Hg. The overall mean resting pressure of the UES is approximately 20 to 60 mm Hg.[6] The lower esophageal sphincter (LES) is formed at the level of the diaphragm, and functions as a physiologic sphincter only. Despite a lack of true circular sphincter muscle fibers, the LES demonstrates a high pressure zone with resting pressures averaging 10 to 20 mm Hg,[6] with minute-to-minute variations in tonic force by EMG analysis.

The body of the esophagus between the upper and lower sphincters generally ranges between 18 and 22 cm in length. The upper esophagus, just below the UES, measures approximately 18 cm from the nasal alar rim. The gastroesophageal junction (GE-junction) measures a distance of 26 to 50 cm in men and 22 to 41 cm in women from the nasal alar rim.[7] On endoscopic examination, the esophagus demonstrates three distinct areas of external compression: the first is from the left main stem bronchus as the esophagus passes posterior to it; the second is from the crossing of the aortic arch; and the third is from the crura of the diaphragm.

The esophagus is composed of four distinct layers: the innermost mucosal layer, the submucosa, the muscularis propria, and the outermost adventitia. The muscularis propria is responsible for the transport function inherent to the esophagus. Below the UES, the muscularis propria separates into inner circular and outer longitudinal muscular sublayers. The upper third of the muscularis is composed of skeletal muscle fibers, the distal third is composed of smooth muscle fibers, and there is a combination of the two in between. Efferent neural terminations are on motor end plates of the upper esophageal skeletal muscle and on a distinct neural plexus, known as Auerbach's plexus, between the circular and longitudinal smooth muscle fibers of the lower esophagus. A second neural network, Meissner's plexus, is an afferent sensory pathway located within the submucosal layer. The smooth muscle fibers of the esophagus are innervated by both parasympathetic and sympathetic nerves, with parasympathetic fibers from the vagus nerve controlling smooth muscle peristalsis.

The esophagus has a segmental arterial and venous blood supply, with the upper esophagus supplied by branches of the superior and inferior thyroid arteries. The mid-portion of the esophagus is supplied by the bronchial and right intercostal arteries and branches of the descending aorta. The lower esophagus is supplied by branches of the left gastric, left inferior phrenic, and splenic arteries. These vessels collectively anastamose to form a dense network of vasculature within the submucosal layer.

On endoscopic examination, the esophageal mucosa appears smooth and pink. The GE-junction is recognized by the presence of an irregularly shaped, whitish Z-line, known as the ora serrata, marking the transition from squamous to columnar epithelium. (Figure 15–2). A biopsy specimen of undisturbed esophageal mucosa would show a nonkeratinized, stratified squamous epithelial lining with long and flat cells with a small nuclear-to-cytoplasmic ratio on the surface and more densely packed cuboidal cells along the basal layer. Rete pegs, or dermal papillae, containing elements of the lamina propria, normally extend into the epithelium less than half the distance toward the esophageal lumen.

The main function of the esophageal phase of swallowing is transport. First, the longitudinal muscle fibers contract to shorten the esophagus and provide a structural base for circular muscle fiber contraction. The circular muscle fibers contract in a proximal-to-distal direction, generating the primary peristaltic wave to move a bolus at 3 to 5 cm/sec, so as to reach

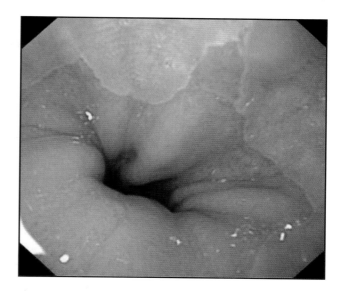

Figure 15–2. Gastroesophageal junction showing the Z-line, or ora serrata, marking the transition from squamous to columnar epithelium.

the stomach in 5 to 10 seconds.[8] Inadequately cleared or refluxed food matter distend the mid-esophagus to generate another peristaltic wave known as secondary peristalsis. Tertiary peristaltic waves usually occur in the distal esophagus, often in elderly individuals or in those with esophageal motility disorders. Tertiary peristalsis is nonpropulsive and has no physiologic function. It represents uncoordinated contractions of smooth muscle fibers and is responsible for the classic "corkscrew" appearance of esophageal spasm seen in barium swallow study.[8]

INSTRUMENTATION

Currently, the major companies producing ultrathin transnasal esophagoscopes have utilized traditional fiberoptic-based or, more recently, video-processor-based designs. The latter design utilizes a distal chip camera and provides brighter illumination, improved air insufflation, a larger screen image, and overall improved optical quality.[9] The general setup for TNE involves most of the elemental equipment used for conventional upper endoscopy, including a light source, an irrigation and pump unit, and a powered suction device. Although there are certainly slight differences between models, the currently more popular video-based transnasal esophagoscopes have an approximately 5-mm diameter, 60- to 65-cm length, 2-mm biopsy channel, air/water insufflation and suction controls, and a 210/120 degree up/down flexion capacity for close retroflexed assessment of the GE-junction when in the stomach (Figure 15–3). Along with the advanced technology inherent to the newer designs has arrived the requirement for more careful and protracted cleaning methods. Typical cleaning techniques involve a process of precleaning, leakage testing, manual cleaning, rinsing, disinfection, rerinsing, and then drying. In an attempt to minimize the reprocessing time between patients, sterile insertion tubes or sheaths have been introduced for the transnasal esophagoscope. Sterile insertion tubes or sheaths have the disadvantage of compromised visualization across the procedure.

EXAMINATION TECHNIQUE

The more patent nasal cavity is selected, decongested, and anesthetized first with aerosolized sprays typical-

ly used prior to office-based nasopharyngolaryngoscopy. These most commonly include aerosolized lidocaine, Pontocaine, oxymetazoline, and phenylephrine. Additional topical anesthesia is applied via cotton-tipped applicators impregnated with some variation of the same solution. Although cocaine has been previously used as an anesthetizing decongestant, lidocaine with oxymetazoline has been shown to be equally effective, is available as an unrestricted agent, and is significantly less costly.[10] Some advocate anesthesia of the oropharynx with a combination of 20% benzocaine spray and 1 to 2 benzonatate capsules (ie, Tessalon Perles); others believe this modality adds to an unnecessary abundance of secretions in the hypopharynx, causing frequent cough and occasional aspiration.[6] If benzonatate capsules are used, they should be allowed to dissolve on the back of the patient's tongue and then swallowed, 10 to 20 minutes prior to the procedure. An emphasis on adequate and

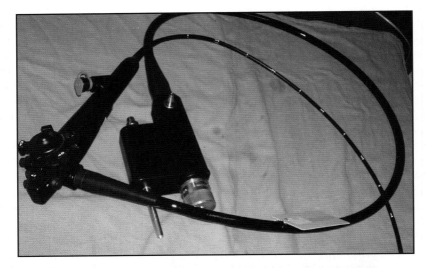

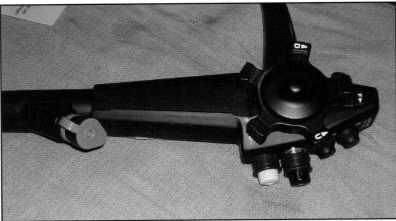

Figure 15–3. TNE equipment

careful nasal anesthesia cannot be overstated.

The distal portion of the esophagoscope is lubricated with 2 to 4% viscous lidocaine and passed along the floor of the nose, or between the inferior and middle turbinates, as is done for typical nasopharyngolaryngoscopy. Examination of the hypopharynx and larynx is performed as the scope is advanced to a level just above the larynx. The examiner should be careful not to depress the air insufflation or irrigation buttons while positioned just above the larynx. The patient is asked to flex his or her chin to the chest, and the scope is then advanced posterior to the laryngeal surface of the epiglottis toward the cricopharyngeus muscle. Once the scope is just above the cricopharyngeus, the patient is asked to either swallow or belch and, as the cricopharyngeus muscle relaxes, the scope is advanced into the proximal esophagus. After entry into the esophagus is confirmed, gentle air insufflation will expand the esophageal lumen, allowing easy advancement of the scope along the thoracic esophagus and through the GE-junction into the stomach. As the scope is advanced, attention is paid to note any mucosal abnormalities, masses, strictures, or diverticulae, and the squamocolumnar junction and lower esophageal sphincter are assessed. After examination of the stomach, a retroflexed view of the lower esophageal sphincter is performed prior to withdrawing the scope proximally into the esophagus. A slow withdrawal of the scope with careful examination of the esophagus is repeated. Biopsies of any endoscopic abnormalities can be easily performed through the biopsy channel with the appropriate flexible forceps.

Transnasal esophagoscopy by this general technique has been largely well-tolerated as an unsedated office-based procedure. In a large review of 611 consecutive patients who had TNE performed by an otolaryngology group, 17 procedures were aborted due to an inability to pass the esophagoscope through a tight nasal vault (3%), and 2 procedures were aborted due to self-limited vasovagal reactions. Of the 592 completed examinations, significant findings were noted in 50%.[11]

INDICATIONS FOR TRANSNASAL ESOPHAGOSCOPY

As the technology continues to develop and the otolaryngology community becomes more familiar with the technique of TNE and with the array of pathology associated with the esophagus in general, indications for TNE will continue to define themselves. Currently, the relative indications for TNE can be grouped into three categories: esophageal-based, extra-esophageal-based, and procedural-based (see Table 15–1).

A frequent esophageal-based indication involves use of TNE as a screening examination, for complicated gastroesophageal reflux disease (GERD). The demonstrated efficacy of appropriately dosed proton pump inhibitors has largely precluded the need for upper endoscopy in uncomplicated GERD. Patients who have demonstrated a poor response to varied attempts at medical therapy, with refractory symptoms (ie, more than 5 years) of dysphagia, heartburn, globus, odynophagia, or weight loss, and patients older than 40 years of age, should be seriously considered for TNE. It is now known that esophagoscopy performed without biopsy is weakly sensitive for the diagnosis of GERD, as only 50% of patients with significant symptoms have macroscopic evidence of esophagitis at the time of the screening examination.[7] Thus, it is recommended that single site biopsy of normal-appearing distal esophageal mucosa be performed in patients with symptoms of complicated GERD. Periodic four-quadrant biopsy surveillance is indicated for patients with either clinical evidence of or a previously established diagnosis of Barrett's esophagus. The American

TABLE 15–1. Indications for Transnasal Esophagoscopy

Esophageal	Extraesophageal	Procedural
Complicated GERD	Head and neck cancer screening	Foreign body removal
Refractory GERD	Refractory asthma	Dilation of strictures
Known Barrett's	Chronic cough	TEP placement
pH-documented LPR	Cervical dysphagia	Biopsy of esophageal lesions
Recurrent regurgitation		Assessment of flap reconstruction
Persistent dysphagia		
Upper GI bleeding		

College of Gastroenterologists guidelines for the frequency of biopsies is once every 3 years in cases that are negative for dysplasia. If high-grade dysplasia is found then a repeat biopsy is indicated and four-quadrant biopsies every 1 to 2 cm of the distal esophagus should be performed every three months.

Additional esophageal-based indications for TNE include a history of recurrent regurgitation, persistent dysphagia unexplained by a thorough laryngopharyngeal examination, and upper gastrointestinal bleeding with an unknown source.

When to perform TNE in patients with classic signs and symptoms of laryngopharyngeal reflux (LPR) remains controversial.[12] The possibilities of masking underlying esophageal pathology with antireflux medical therapy and of leaving esophageal metaplasia or dysplasia undiagnosed in patients with classic LPR, center on the diagnostic dilemma. One paradigm that has been suggested involves screening patients with significant symptoms and signs of LPR with ambulatory 24-hour dual-probe pH monitoring. A finding of abnormal acid exposure to the distal esophagus indicates a screening with TNE. Normal pH monitoring appears to correlate with a low risk of Barrett's metaplasia and does not warrant TNE.[7,13]

A relative extra-esophageal-based indication for TNE is as a screening examination of the esophagus in patients with a known primary head and neck malignancy. Other extra-esophageal-based indications for TNE include examination of patients with poorly controlled asthma, with a chronic cough of unknown etiology, and with refractory globus pharyngeus or cervical dysphagia. A review of TNE in patients with chronic cough has suggested that these patients demonstrate more significant esophageal inflammation, and thus may be at higher risk for Barrett's metaplasia even without classically described associated heartburn.[7] Patients with persistent globus pharyngeus or cervical dysphagia unresponsive to attempts at medical therapy may have other pathologic esophageal lesions accounting for their symptoms (eg, *Candida* esophagitis). TNE instrumentation and technique can also be used for office-based tracheoscopy to diagnose and possibly biopsy various tracheal abnormalities.

Procedural indications for TNE continue to present themselves. Current procedural indications include evaluation and potential treatment of possible esophageal foreign body, removal of pharyngeal foreign body, dilation of esophageal stricture,[14] replacement of a tracheoesophageal prosthesis (TEP) under direct vision,[11] secondary tracheoesophageal puncture,[15] biopsy of a known lesion in the upper aerodigestive tract,[16] and even office-based excisional/ablational laser-assisted laryngeal surgery.[16] TNE has also been used to evaluate the status of pharyngoesophageal flap reconstruction following resection of a malignancy.[17]

FINDINGS WITH TRANSNASAL ESOPHAGOSCOPY

The largest reviews of TNE performed by otolaryngologists report positive esophageal findings in 44 to 50% of patients, with esophagitis, Barrett's metaplasia, and hiatal hernia found most commonly.[9,18] Esophageal candidiasis, stricture, carcinoma, and esophageal polyps were also seen somewhat frequently. Less common findings included a patulous GE-junction, esophageal diverticulum, esophageal web, foreign body, and tracheoesophageal fistula.[11] Although a thorough description of the possible pathologic esophageal findings is beyond the scope of this chapter, a brief discussion of the more common findings is of interest.

Esophagitis involves inflammation of the esophageal mucosa from any of a number of causes. The most common cause by far is associated with gastroesophageal reflux disease. Esophagitis has been most commonly classified using the Savary-Miller grading system (Table 15–2). Infectious causes of esophagitis most commonly involve *Candida*, herpes, and cytomegalovirus.[7]

Barrett's metaplasia involves a change of the esophageal mucosa from normal squamous epithelium to spe-

TABLE 15–2. Savary-Miller Endoscopic Grading System for Esophagitis

Grade	Description
I	Single erosive lesion involving only one mucosal fold
II	Noncircular multiple erosive lesions involving more than one mucosal fold
III	Circular erosive lesion
IV	Chronic lesions with ulceration and/or stricture
V	Grades I–IV associated with Barrett's metaplasia

cialized columnar epithelium. The diagnosis is usually made easily across endoscopic examination by the presence of salmon-pink mucosal patches extending, usually in the proximal direction, from the lower esophageal sphincter. These regions should be biopsied to confirm the diagnosis because Barrett's metaplasia does possess malignant potential, and careful surveillance endoscopy should be carried out annually.

Hiatal hernia involves a prolapse of a portion of the stomach proximally beyond the diaphragm into the thoracic cavity. These can be of sliding, paraesophageal, or mixed type, with sliding hiatal hernias comprising the vast majority. With a sliding hiatal hernia, the normal squamocolumnar junction (Z-line) is seen 1 to 3 cm above the diaphragmatic hiatus. Having the patient sniff with the endoscope in place will accentuate the position of the diaphragm and help with the diagnosis.

CONCLUSIONS

TNE has been accepted by the otolaryngology community as a well-tolerated office-based procedure that can be easily learned. The procedure can be performed without sedation and with minimal intraprocedural or postprocedural discomfort. The indications for TNE and its use across the otolaryngology community will continue to develop as technology advances and as a greater familiarity with esophageal pathology evolves. Otolaryngology patients have a frequent occurrence of esophagus-related complaints, and TNE is becoming a practical and useful addition to the otolaryngologist's diagnostic repertoire.

Acknowledgment The authors express their appreciation to Ms Seanna Wood from the Medical Media Production Service (MMPS) of the Philadelphia VA Medical Center for her artistic help with the diagram shown in Figure 15–1.

REFERENCES

1. Brampton PA, Reid DP, Johnson RD, et al. A comparison of transnasal and transoral oesophagogastroduodenoscopy. *J Gastroenterol Hepatol.* 1998;13:579–584.
2. Shaker R, Saeian K. Unsedated transnasal laryngo-esophagogastroduodenoscopy: an alternative to conventional endoscopy. *Am J Med.* 2001;111(8A):153S–156S..
3. Bell GD. Premedication and intravenous sedation for upper gastrointestinal endoscopy. *Aliment Pharmacol Ther.* 1990;4:103–122.
4. Scott-Coombes DM, Thompson JN. Hypoxia during upper gastrointestinal endoscopy is caused by sedation. *Endoscopy.* 1993;25:308–309.
5. Lieberman DA, Wuerker CK, Katon RM. Cardiopulmonary risk of esophagogastroduodenoscopy: role of endoscope diameter and systemic sedation. *Gastroenterology.* 1985;88:468–472.
6. Orringer MB. The esophagus: physiology. In: Sabiston DC Jr, ed. *Textbook of Surgery: The Biologic Basis of Modern Surgical Practice.* 14th ed. Philadelphia, PA: WB Saunders Co; 1991:660–663.
7. Belafsky PC. Office endoscopy for the laryngologist/bronchoesophagologist. *Curr Opin Otolaryngol Head Neck Surg.* 2002;10:467–471.
8. Gavaghan M. Anatomy and physiology of the esophagus. *AORNJ.* Feb 1999.
9. Cantanzaro A, Faulx A, Isenberg GA, et al. Prospective evaluation of 4-mm diameter endoscopes for esophagoscopy in sedated and unsedated patients. *Gastrointest Endosc.* 2003;57(3):300–304.
10. Meyer DR. Comparison of oxymetazoline and lidocaine versus cocaine for outpatient dacrocystorhinostomy. *Ophthal Plast Reconstr Surg.* 2000;16:201–205.
11. Postma G, Cohen JT, Belafsky PC, et al. Transnasal esophagoscopy: revisited (over 700 consecutive cases). *Laryngoscope.* 2005;115:321–323.
12. Belafsky PC, Postma GN, Amin MR, et al. Symptoms and findings of laryngopharyngeal reflux. *Ear Nose Throat J.* 2002;81(9 suppl 2):10–13.
13. Postma GN, Belafsky PC, Aviv JE, et al. Laryngopharyngeal reflux testing. *Ear Nose Throat J.* 2002;81(9 suppl 2):14–17.
14. Postma GN, Belafsky PC, Koufman JA. Dilation of an esophageal stricture caused by epidermolysis bullosa. *Ear Nose Throat J.* 2002;81(2):86.
15. Bach KK, Postma GN, Koufman JA. In-office tracheoesophageal puncture using transnasal esophagoscopy. *Laryngoscope.* 2003;113:173–176.
16. Postma GN, Bach KK, Belafsky PC, et al. The role of transnasal esophagoscopy in head and neck oncology. *Laryngoscope.* 2002;112(12):2242–2243.
17. Bach KK, Postma GN, Koufman JA. Evaluation of flaps following pharyngoesophageal reconstruction. *Ear Nose Throat J.* 2002;81(11):766.
18. Belafsky PC, Postma GN, Daniel E, et al. Transnasal esophagoscopy. *Otolaryngol Head Neck Surg.* 2001;125: 588–589.

16

Introduction to the Laboratory Diagnosis of Vocal Disorders

Gwen S. Korovin, MD, FACS
John S. Rubin, MD, FACS, FRCS

As the voice laboratory has evolved over the past thirty years, it has played an ever-increasing role in the diagnosis and treatment of voice disorders. In 1970, only facilities in Syracuse and Chicago, followed by Gainesville and Los Angeles, boasted the presence of laboratories designed solely for the study of voice. We now have nearly 200 voice laboratories throughout the United States and Canada registered with The Voice Foundation (1721 Pine Street, Philadelphia, Pennsylvania 19103).

It is important to remember that voice research did not really begin at that time. We cannot forget the role of the great observations made by many of our predecessors. Interest in the voice dates back as early as the fifth century BC.[1] The first practical observations of the human vocal folds at work can be credited to Manuel García, who in 1854 first used the dental mirror for observations of the vocal folds.[2] Since that time, many investigators have become interested in voice. Individual studies have been carried out in a multitude of laboratories not designed for voice work alone. All have contributed greatly to the field as it is today. They laid the foundation upon which modern voice research has been built. Brewer summarized it well when he stated that "historically the voice came first, then the arts of using it more effectively and only lately the science of dealing with its mechanics."[3] We now have the facilities to deal with the science of voice mechanics in a more highly organized and concise manner. A variety of studies can be done in each of these facilities. Greater collaboration between voice laboratories can occur because of awareness of the research being carried out elsewhere. In this way, we hope to make even greater strides in the study of the voice sciences.

THE VOICE LABORATORY

The analysis of phonation depends on the study of three interrelated systems. These include the respiratory, laryngeal, and articulatory systems. The respiratory system serves as the power source. The laryngeal system serves as the oscillator. The articulatory system functions along with the resonators to shape the sound, thus producing voice. Aerodynamic power from the respiratory system must undergo changes from the laryngeal systems. Adjustments and tuning of the vocal tract are then carried out by the articulatory system.[4-6]

These systems are now being studied in the various laboratories, which exist in many varieties and levels of sophistication. An example of an extensive laboratory is the Wilbur James Gould Recording and Research Center at the Denver Center of the Performing Arts, which is producing a great deal of new and exciting data. Many laboratories are affiliated with otolaryngology residency training programs and/or hospitals and as such are used mainly for teaching purposes and clinical evaluations. These serve to foster interest among residents and students in the field of voice at an early stage in their careers. Many of these also do basic science and/or clinical research, as at the Ames Vocal Dynamics Laboratory at Lenox Hill Hospital in New York City (with which one of the authors [GSK] is connected).

The Role of the Voice Laboratory

The voice laboratory has the capability to provide visual, acoustic, respiratory, aerodynamic, and electrophysiologic information. The laboratory serves as a supplement to the history and physical examination. It should in no way replace this examination, nor should it replace perceptual evaluations of the voice. We should not underestimate the value of the laryngeal mirror examination. It allows us to see the true color and gives an estimate of the true size of the vocal folds. Mirrors that provide three times the magnification of the simple mirror can give even more detail. A majority of lesions can be seen with the mirror. There is minimal anatomic distortion during this examination, although some distortion occurs at the laryngeal entry because of the pulling forward of the tongue.

The laboratory may aid in diagnosis. In most cases, however, vocal disorders are not diagnosed in the voice laboratory. They are diagnosed in the clinical setting, and the diagnosis is supported by the data generated in the laboratory. However, in some cases a lesion that is not readily visible (eg, certain subglottal lesions or glottic scars or partially resolved paralysis of the superior laryngeal nerve) may be uncovered by laboratory assessment. Visual data may provide the diagnosis when the lesion has been missed during the routine examination. In other cases, no lesions or abnormalities are detected on physical examination or during the collection of visual data, but the voice is still disordered. In these cases, the laboratory can help in diagnosis by detecting specific respiratory, aerodynamic, neurologic, or other abnormalities. This is especially true of visual analysis techniques, including the fiberoptic and rigid scopes with the addition of the stroboscope. Videokymography or other high-speed visualization techniques may be used in the clinically advanced or research-oriented center.

The voice laboratory provides objective data that not only serve as support for subjective findings of a physical examination, but also can be used for more accurate assessment of treatment outcome. In patients undergoing a surgical procedure, preoperative and postoperative data can be obtained. In patients going through a voice therapy program, pretherapy and post-therapy data can be documented. These findings can then be used as a guide for any necessary further diagnosis and as an evaluation of the success of the therapy. In these ways the voice laboratory helps the patient, the physician, and the therapist.

The voice laboratory allows for the storage of information. Data may be obtained and retrieved for analysis at a later time. This provides a savings of time that was previously wasted for repetitive data collection. Digitization has proven of particular benefit in this regard. New equipment is being developed continually. If a voice recording is stored, it can be evaluated with new, more advanced equipment in the future. In this way, additional information may be obtained. Also, the recording can be used to compare early data with later data on the same patient.

Voice laboratory data can be helpful in providing information for voice teachers and therapists. These data can be an aid in the treatment regimen, in that physicians and therapists can evaluate how the treatment is progressing. A patient and a voice therapist may perceive a subjective improvement. The voice laboratory information can then be used for objective evidence, and further therapy can then be supported.

The voice laboratory can provide essential information for the patient. The patient and the practitioner may be able to view the results of the study simultaneously. Thus, it acts as an instantaneous form of biofeedback, and holds the promise of playing an even greater role in therapy in the future. The patients can gain better insight regarding their problems and in addition gain understanding of the physiology of their vocal instruments. In this way laboratory data are an effective teaching tool and diagnostic aid.

The voice laboratory provides medical and legal documentation. In our increasingly litigious society, it has become more important to keep a permanent record, which may be needed for legal purposes at a later time. Insurance companies may also require the information.

In this regard, it is helpful to compare voice data or a voice print to an audiogram. It is rare that any otologic treatment is done without an audiogram, and we are working toward a time in which no vocal treatments will be given without some type of "voicegram."

In discussing the role of the voice laboratory, it becomes of great importance to realize that we are treating the whole patient, not just the laboratory results in isolation. We cannot just look at the numbers. We need to look at the entire picture, which includes all the subjective and objective information. (In some ways, the title of this chapter is misleading. Rather than "the laboratory diagnosis of voice disorders," it should more specifically be "the role of the laboratory as an adjunct to the diagnosis of voice disorders.") As stated by Hirano, the purpose of most tests is basically "not to make a diagnosis of the etiologic disease of the voice disorder but to evaluate one or several aspects of the vocal function."[7]

Others have different views of the role of the voice laboratory, but all have a common thread. Gates and Painter see the voice laboratory as a common meeting ground of the four groups of professionals concerned with people with disordered voices: the laryngologist, the speech-language pathologist, the voice teacher, and the clinical voice scientist.[8]

Gould saw research into voice functions as providing an increasingly valuable means to evaluate problems of voice, and objectively measure speech production in the clinical setting.[4] Martin sees the role of the laboratory as assisting the phonosurgeon in diagnosing, evaluating operative results, and developing better phonosurgical procedures.[9] von Leden sees the medical application of these scientific measures as offering substantial clinical benefits for both physician and patient, for their sensitivity often permits the discovery of early changes in the larynx before the eyes and ears of the examiner detect the underlying physiologic or pathologic aberrations.[10]

The point is that the role of the voice laboratory differs depending on the orientation of the particular clinician or scientist. However, the voice laboratory plays an important role for all these people. As Gould stated, "The most important scientific study to the laryngologist derived from research in these areas (ie, respiratory, laryngeal, and articulatory) is that which can be applied directly to patient care."[11] This is the ultimate goal.

How to Set Up a Voice Laboratory

In setting up a voice laboratory, it is most important to determine what your needs are. You must decide what it is that you ultimately want to measure. Will you be doing mostly clinical testing? Will it be primarily a research facility? Will you be doing studies in both these areas? This goal must be set early.

It is most helpful when beginning a new venture to visit other working laboratories. The Voice Foundation keeps a list of essentially all the laboratories and could be helpful in this regard. When visiting, it is advisable to try to learn all you can about the equipment. You probably will not want to reproduce an identical laboratory, as your goals may differ. You must also be aware of how much space you have available. This will help determine which equipment you should choose. Attendance at various voice seminars may be very helpful. The Voice Foundation's annual symposium on care of the professional voice, along with many other voice seminars and workshops throughout the world, can convey valuable, practical information about the working voice laboratory.

It is important to determine the attributes of the planned laboratory personnel—that is, technicians, therapists, physicians, scientists, and so forth—and how much time they will devote to the laboratory. This may play a key role in determining the sophistication of the equipment to be obtained, which will also depend on the patient population available.

Finances are of major importance. Many hospitals and university programs may be able to attract grants and endowments to begin a laboratory. Residency programs may be able to provide funds if the laboratory is to be used for teaching purposes. Although money can be brought in through clinical testing, it may take time to earn back monies that are spent on the laboratory.

TYPES OF ANALYSIS

Visual Analysis

Visual analysis is of great importance in the voice laboratory evaluation. The simple mirror examination done prior to the laboratory studies provides a great deal of information. It is the most widely used method of visualization. The flexible fiberoptic laryngoscope, first introduced by Sawashima and Hirose in 1968, is the next most widely available tool for evaluating the larynx.[12] The fiberoptic scope requires a somewhat powerful light source. A television monitor and recorder can be attached for viewing and recording purposes. Advantages of the flexible scope include visualization of the supraglottic laryngeal tract with relatively minor distortion of the anatomy. Disadvantages include some peripheral distortion and the requirement of a strong light source, particularly if stroboscopy is to be used.

The rigid laryngeal telescope (also commonly referred to as a rigid laryngoscope), first introduced by Andrews and Gould in 1971, allows examination of the vocal folds with better light magnification and resolution.[13] By adjusting the angle of visualization, Gould has shown how subcordal and subglottic changes can be seen more easily.[14] The laryngoscope can be attached to a camera, and movements of the folds can be recorded on CD, DVD, or high-speed film.

The addition of the use of the stroboscope in the clinical setting has been a great technologic advancement. Stroboscopic light allows apparent slow-motion evaluation of vocal fold motion. It gives a clearer, sharper image of the mucosal layer of the vocal fold. The examiner can detect structural or functional changes in the larynx. Minor mucosal changes and early lesions can be diagnosed more easily than with continuous light.

The stroboscope can be used with the flexible fiberoptic scope to give information about vocal fold motion and supraglottic motion during both speech and singing. This provides valuable information to the physician and therapist. When the stroboscope is used with the rigid scope, a closer view of the vocal folds is afforded. Subtle changes of the motion of the glottic and subcordal or subglottic areas can be visualized better.

With any of these methods of visual evaluation, it is important to establish a standardized method of assessment. In one of the author's laboratories (GSK), a form that records the appearance of the vocal folds in full adduction, full abduction, and the paramedian position is used. Symmetry, closure, mobility, amplitude, stiffness, glottal closure, regularity, supraglottal and subglottal movement, and frequency are evaluated. Others use a standardized method proposed by Bless et al that includes an evaluation of fundamental frequency, symmetry of movements, periodicity, glottic closure, amplitude of vibration, mucosal wave, and the presence of nonvibrating portions of the vocal fold.[15] No widespread standard is available at the present time.

Newer methods of high-speed and digital recording have been devised and allow for even more accurate visualization. Some computer equipment can allow frame-by-frame analysis, but this is present in the more research-oriented voice laboratories only. Videokymography, a technique that allows for real-time evaluation of the mucosal wave at a single site on the true vocal fold, is now available commercially. It provides further information on mucosal wave patterns in different pathologic states.[16]

Electroglottography allows further evaluation of the vibratory signal. It traces the opening and closing of the glottis. The traces can be superimposed with the visual images and thus can be correlated. An interesting feature of electroglottography is that not only does it represent an optimal choice for fundamental frequency (F_0) measurement,[6] but it can be used also for measurement of continuous (connected) speech. The technology is still in its infancy, but it is commercially available.[17,18] The technique may be difficult in some subjects because of obesity or other anatomic factors.[6]

Photoglottography, in which the opening and closing of the glottis modulates a beam of light, also provides an electrical signal simple enough for reliable F_0 determination. The technique is somewhat invasive, however.[6]

Acoustic Analysis

The tape recorder remains the most valuable basic tool for the voice laboratory. Analog recordings can be converted to digital, which can then be used for data storage. Digital recording has been replacing the use of the standard analog system. It is arguably more precise and of longer-lasting, higher quality, although some investigators remain concerned about distortion introduced by the digitization and compression process. Data from digital recording are immediately computer-capable, allowing on-line analysis. Alternatively, data can be stored for use at a later date. Digital video computer stroboscopes are now commercially readily available in which both the image and the sound are digitized and stored directly on the hardware or as an individual CD or DVD or on Zip disks.

The stopwatch is another useful and simple tool in the voice laboratory. The maximum phonation time and the "s/z" ratio are both simple measures to obtain, with useful clinical correlations.

The phonetogram is a measure of the maximal phonatory frequency range at varying intensities. This is the range of vocal frequencies encompassing the modal and falsetto registers. Its extension is from the lowest tone sustainable in modal register to the highest tone sustainable in falsetto.[19] It is used commonly in European laboratories. One drawback is that it is time consuming.

Sound spectrographic analysis, the dissection of the acoustic wave into its most basic components, is used widely in the research and clinical laboratory. Sound spectrography resolves a periodic waveform into a series of sine waves of different frequencies, amplitudes, and phase relationships. The fundamental frequency and harmonics can be determined. Different ratios have been established to compare the information obtained. These allow comparison and greater standardization of data. Hundreds of scientific papers have been published on applications of sound spectography. Spectrographic categorizations of hoarse voices were made over 30 years ago.[20]

Although most disorders of the larynx do not, in and of themselves, appear to have significant influence on the mean speaking F_0, F_0 variability and range do seem to reflect tissue changes.[6] Such variability has been evaluated in the voice laboratory.

Many kinds of packaged systems have been developed to aid in the acoustic analysis of the voice.[6] These allow the measurement of fundamental frequency, intensity, and pitch. They are interfaced with microcomputers, allowing analysis and quantification of various acoustic characteristics of phonated speech. More technologically sophisticated packages continue to be under development.

The Visipitch is a self-contained analog fundamental frequency analyzer. It was designed specifically for ease of clinical use. It provides an oscilloscopic display of F_0 and of relative intensity over time. The Visipitch is used regularly in many clinics. It is particularly useful as a feedback tool for the therapist and patient.[6, 21]

In addition, the vocal demodulator that has been developed by Winholtz at the Denver Center has been evaluated for office use and may provide a simple way of measuring fundamental frequency.[22]

Jitter, shimmer, and harmonic-to-noise ratio are other acoustic analyses offered regularly in different commercially available acoustic packages.

Jitter is the name commonly given to frequency (period) perturbation. It is the variability of the F_0. Jitter measurements tend to be concerned with short-term F_0 variation. (In continuous speech, variability is reflected in pitch sigma.) Jitter, then, is a measure of frequency variability not accounted for by voluntary changes in F_0. A considerable body of literature confirms the usefulness of jitter assessment in laryngeal pathology.[6,23]

Measures of amplitude perturbation (shimmer) serve to quantify short-term instability of the vocal signal. Some feel it is as important as jitter in its contribution to perception of hoarseness. Amplitude perturbation is a measure based on the peak amplitude of each phonatory cycle.[24]

Assuming that the pure (average) periodic wave is increasingly contaminated by random noise as hoarseness worsens, this degree of contamination can be expressed as a periodic harmonic-to-noise amplitude ratio. Harmonic-to-noise ratio can be described, relatively simply, as the mean amplitude of the average wave divided by the mean amplitude of the isolated noise components for the train of waves. For convenience, it is expressed in decibels. A characteristic feature of hoarseness is the replacement of harmonics by noise energy (aperiodic sound intensifying at the expense of periodic signal).[6]

Jitter, shimmer, harmonic-to-noise ratio. and mean F_0 are basic tests of acoustic analysis readily available in many commercially available programs. As the algorithms vary between packages, great care must be exercised when comparing results with other packages.

In setting up a laboratory, it is important to evaluate all the different systems available and determine which of these are most appropriate for your individual needs.

Aerodynamic Analysis

The vocal tract is an aerodynamic sound generator and resonator system. The basis for aerodynamic analysis is respiratory analysis. The volume of air that the lungs can hold, the pressures that can be developed, and the characteristics of airflow (the rate of change of the volume) are all critical elements in the production and maintenance of voice. Basic pulmonary function testing, available in most pulmonary laboratories, gives information regarding tidal volume, functional residual capacity, inspiratory capacity, total lung capacity, vital capacity, forced vital capacity, forced expiratory volume, and maximal mid-expiratory volume. Instrumentation is readily commercially available. For example, a flow transducer attached to an anesthetic-type face mask will permit evaluation of airflow.

Studies of airflow efficiency offer valuable information to physicians. Four parameters measured traditionally in the laboratory are subglottal pressure, supraglottal pressure, glottal impedance, and volume velocity of airflow at the glottis. Different calculations can then be done to determine such things as mean flow rate, glottal resistance, and the phonation quotient.

Transglottal airflow can be measured by a newer technique called flow glottography. One method of airflow measurement is the inverse filtering technique. Although inverse filtering was formerly tedious, a simplified method by Rothenberg has made it simpler to use in the clinical research setting.[5] Air volume can be measured with a wet spirometer, a device which has not changed much since its invention over 100 years ago, or a dry spirometer. Two types of portable dry spirometry are in current use: one, a mechanical type, and the other a flow transducer and integrator circuit system. Lung volume changes can be determined by change in the chest wall (rib cage and abdominal size). Articulatory and phonatory volumes can be measured by a pneumotachograph, which can show very small volume changes in time periods involving only a fraction of a second (unlike the spirometer).[6]

Electromyography

Laryngeal electromyography[15] is an objective method available to study the neural function of laryngeal muscle activity. It helps to determine which muscles are in use during different phonatory conditions. Electromyography can be used to follow a patient with laryngeal paralysis. Differentiation between peripheral laryngeal nerve paralysis or paresis, central neurologic disorders, and (by virtue of a normal study) arytenoid fixation or dislocation may be determined. Its importance has increased, proportionate to the number of centers now utilizing it. Laryngeal electromyography is also a useful adjunct in administration of botulinum toxin for various problems. The equipment can be made available as part of a voice laboratory, or it can be used in conjunction with neurologists or physiatrists in their laboratories. Laryngeal electromyography is discussed in detail in another chapter (chapter 18).

COST AND EFFECTIVENESS

Voice laboratories vary from the very rudimentary to the very advanced; the level of sophistication is often dependent on the need. When a voice laboratory is being planned, it is important to determine cost versus effectiveness.

The voice committee of the International Association of Logopedics and Phoniatrics (IALP) sent out a questionnaire in an attempt to determine the most frequently used examinations.[7] The laryngeal mirror, a tape recording, perceptual evaluation, and measures of mean phonation time and fundamental frequency were the most commonly used. The information determined in this study is of great value because these four measures can all be done at low cost in an office setting. They may be all that is necessary for the most rudimentary laboratory. Packaged systems are offered by several companies to provide a means to measure a multitude of functions. A voice laboratory in a hospital setting provides a more central facility that can be used by physicians and therapists in a particular region. It may be easier to fund, as grants and endowments may come from the hospital. Staffing is easier as no one individual is responsible for the entire laboratory and equipment as is the case in the office setting.

In evaluating cost versus effectiveness, it is helpful to keep in mind the words of Ingo Titze, who said, "Many instruments are not necessarily a blessing. A few good instruments usually are."[25] To further evaluate costs versus effectiveness, we must remember that in many ways we are still testing the tests. We know the importance of objective data and documentation. Just as audiograms are an integral part of the otologic evaluation, vocal dynamics evaluation is becoming more of an integral part of the voice evaluation. However, it has not been determined which tests will remain as essential parts of the "voicegram." Vocal testing is undergoing continual changes. We are using many tests in attempts at "cross validation." The question of reliability and reproducibility is slowly being answered. The question of which tests to do in which patients is of continuing importance in our changing economic climate.

THE VOICE TEAM

The treatment of vocal disorders is highly dependent on the voice team. The essential team members include the physician (laryngologist), the therapist (speaking or singing), and the voice scientist. Specialists should familiarize themselves with the voice laboratory and its clinical applications. Only through cooperation and collaboration of the specialists can we truly improve the care of our patients.

Others, including various medical specialists (pulmonologists, endocrinologists, gastroenterologists, gynecologists, neurologists, allergists, maxillofacial specialists, or physical therapists) may also be called in for aid at various times.

Interlaboratory cooperation becomes an integral part of the field of voice as a whole. It is only through the cross-fertilization of different voice specialists and laboratory facilities that we have achieved today's level of sophistication. Teamwork is truly an essential part of the laboratory diagnosis of voice disorders. Herein lies the future of voice science.

REFERENCES

1. von Leden H. The cultural history of the layrnx and voice. In: Gould WJ, Sataloff JR, eds. *Voice Surgery*. St. Louis, MO: Mosby Year Book; 1993:3–65.
2. von Leden H. The cultural history of the human voice. In: Lawrence VL, ed. *Transcripts of the 11th Symposium: Care of the Professional Voice*, part 2. New York, NY: The Voice Foundation; 1982:116–123.
3. Brewer DW. Voice research: the next ten years. *J Voice*. 1989;3(1):7–17.
4. Gould WJ. The clinical voice laboratory: clinical application of voice research. *Ann Otol Rhinol Laryngol*. 1984; 93(4):346–350.
5. Sundberg J. *The Science of the Singing Voice*. DeKalb: Northern Illinois University Press; 1987.
6. Baken RJ. *Clinical Measurement of Speech and Voice*. San Diego, CA: College-Hill Press; 1987.

7. Hirano M. Objective evaluation of the human voice: clinical aspects, *Folia Phoniatr (Basel)*. 1989;41:89–144.

8. Korovin GS. Introduction to the Laboratory Diagnosis of Voice Disorders. In: Rubin JS, Sataloff RT, Korovin GS, Gould WJ, eds. *Diagnosis and Treatment of Voice Disorders*. New York, NY: Igaku-Shoin; 1995:262–268.

9. Martin GF. The contribution of the speech sciences to the development of phonosurgery. In Gould WJ, Sataloff RT, Spiegel JR, eds. *Voice Surgery*. St. Louis, MO: Mosby Year Book; 1993:97–122.

10. von Leden H, Mooie P, Timcke R. Laryngeal vibrations: measuremented the glottic wave. Part III; the pathologic larynx. *Arch Otolaryngol*. 1960;71:16–35.

11. Gould WJ. The clinical voice laboratory: clinical application of voice research. *J Voice*. 1988;1(4):305–309.

12. Sawashima M, Hirose H. New laryngostics technique by use of fibre optics. *J Acoust Soc Am*. 1968;43:168–170.

13. Andrews AN Jr, Gould WJ. Laryngeal and nasal-frigical indirect telescope. *Ann Otol Rhinol Laryngol*. 1977;88:627.

14. Gould WJ. Why is there a need for this conference? In: Cooper JA, ed. *Assessment of Speech and Voice Production: Research and Clinical Applications*. Bethesda, MD: NIDCD Monograph; 1990:1–4.

15. Bless DM, Hirano M, Feder RJ. Videostroboscopic evaluation of the larynx. *Ear Nose Throat J*. 1987;66:289–296.

16. Svec J. On vibration properties of human vocal folds: voice registers bifurcations, resonance characteristics, development and application of videokymography (Ph.D. thesis). Rigksuniversiteit gromingen, the Netherlands; 2000.

17. Fourcin AJ. Voice quality and electrolaryngology. In: Kent R, Ball M, eds. *Voice Quality Measurement*. San Diego, CA: Singular Publications; 1999.

18. Barry WJ, Goldsmith MJ, Fuller HC, Fourcin AJ. Stability of voice frequency measures in speech. *Twelfth Int. Cong Phon Sci (Univ de Provence)*. 1991;2:38–44.

19. Hollien ll, Dew D, Philips P. Phonational frequency ranges of adults. *J Speech Hearing Res*. 1971;14:755–760.

20. Yanagihara N. Significance of harmonic changes and voice components in hoarseness. *J Speech Hearing Res*. 1967;10:531–541.

21. Horii Y. Automatic analysis of voice fundamental frequency and intensity using a *Visipitch*. *J Speech Hearing Res*. 1983;26:467–471.

22. Winholtz WS, Ramig LO. Vocal tremor analysis with the vocal demodulator. *J Speech Hearing Res*. 1992;35:562–579.

23. Kitajima K, Tanabe M, Isshiki N. Pitch perturbation in normal and pathogical voice. *Studia Phonologica*. 1975;9:25–32.

24. Takahashi H, Koike Y. Some perceptual dimensions and acoustical correlates of pathologic voices. *Acta Otolaryngologica*. 1975;338(suppl):1–24.

25. Titze IR. Measurements for the assessment of voice disorders. In: Cooper JA, ed. *Assessment of Speech and Voice Production: Research and Clinical Applications*. Bethesda, MD: NIDCD Monograph; 1990:42–49.

17

Measuring Vocal Fold Function

Raymond H. Colton, PhD
Peak Woo, MD

THE PHYSIOLOGY OF PHONATION

What is commonly known as the voice is the product of the vibratory motion of the vocal folds and the resonant effects of the vocal tract. The vocal folds constitute the major (but not only) source of periodic sound for speech. The vocal folds move to and fro to interrupt the egressive airstream and thus produce an acoustic disturbance. Sound is nothing more than alternating regions of higher-than-normal and lower-than-normal regions of air pressure produced at a rate someone can hear. The exact form of the acoustic disturbance produced by the vocal folds is dependent on the exact pattern of vocal fold movement and its interaction with the airstream.

The shape of the acoustic pulse determines the frequencies present in the complex tone produced by the vocal folds. For example, consider the effect of decreasing the closing time of the vocal folds (top panel of Figure 17–1) on the amplitude of the higher frequencies (bottom panel of Figure 17–1). Physiologically, a decreased closed time could be the result of in-

creased vocal fold tension. The acoustic pulse is generated at the instant of closing[1]: the more rapid closing time results in the increased amplitudes at the higher frequencies.

Increased air turbulence through the glottis may also affect the acoustic pulse produced, primarily by increased noise levels. Increased air turbulence may be produced in a variety of ways including incomplete vocal fold closure, the presence of a mass on one or both vocal folds, and irregularities on the surface of the vocal folds. Such pathologic conditions may also affect the frequency and stability of vibration.

It appears clear that the vibratory motion of the vocal folds and their interaction with the airstream determine the acoustic output of the vocal folds. This acoustic output after modification by the resonators determines the listener's perception of the voice. A pathologic lesion, when it affects the vibratory motion of the vocal folds, affects the acoustic pulse produced and therefore affects the listener's perception of the voice. However, the abnormality may affect some vibratory features more than others. In order to

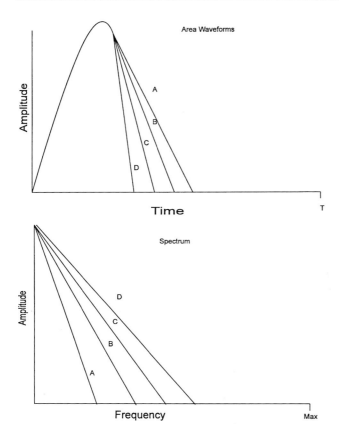

Figure 17–1. The relationship between the shape of the glottal volume velocity waveform and the acoustic properties of the sound. Four glottal pulses, A to D, differing in the abruptness of the change to zero flow at glottal closure, are shown. Shown in the bottom panel are the associated spectra. (Redrawn from Fig. 9–3 Löfqvist.[1])

understand the effect of pathologic lesions on vibratory motion and the production of the acoustic pulse, the vibratory characteristics of the vocal folds should be studied. Part of that study includes careful observation and, where possible, the measurement of vibratory motion and parameters of the acoustic pulse produced. In this chapter, we review the nature of normal vibratory motion, the various ways we have to measure it, and the measurement of its acoustic product.

Physiologic Properties of Phonation

To understand phonatory physiology, one must recognize that two major properties are important to vocal fold vibration. The first is the *myoelastic* properties of the vocal folds and the second is *aerodynamics* of the airstream. This subject is discussed in greater detail in chapter 7.

Myoelastic Properties of the Vocal Folds

The myoelastic properties of the vocal folds include the muscles that make up the vocal folds or affect the size, shape, and tension of the vocal folds together with other nonmuscle tissue present in the vocal folds.

The thyroarytenoid (TA) muscle constitutes the bulk of the vocal folds. Its contraction affects the length, mass, and tension of the vocal folds. Together with the cricothyroid (CT), it can affect the relative stiffness of the various layers of the vocal folds and control the fundamental frequency, intensity, and pulse shape of the vocal fold tone. Additional effects can be produced by the interarytenoid and the lateral cricoarytenoid muscles, which because they are the major adductors of the vocal folds affect the resistance of the vocal folds to opening by the pressures beneath the vocal folds. The posterior cricoarytenoid (PCA), the only abductor of vocal folds, could affect phonation by influencing the degree of glottal opening during phonation.

Muscle tissue and nonmuscle tissue affect the elasticity and stiffness of the vocal folds.[2-5] Elasticity is a mechanical property that restores the shape of the folds after they have been deformed by an external force. Together they determine the exact pattern of vibration and the relative coupling of the various layers of the vocal folds.[6-9] Both properties affect the frequency of vibration of the vocal folds and the intensity of the voice source. Also affected is the shape of the acoustic disturbance that determines the frequency composition of the tone.

Aerodynamic Properties

Air pressure and airflow are the two aerodynamic properties important in vocal fold vibration. Pressure immediately beneath the vocal folds (subglottal pressure) is responsible for blowing the vocal folds open during a cycle of vibration. The magnitude of the subglottal air pressure is dependent on (1) the force of the respiratory system and (2) the magnitude of vocal fold adduction. The latter is reflected in the duration of the closed phase of the vocal folds.

Airflow through the glottis interacts with the vocal folds to produce vibration. The magnitude of the airflow depends on the subglottal air pressure and the magnitude and duration of the glottal opening. Airflow may be laminar or turbulent or both. Turbulent airflows result in the creation of noise or aperiodic vibration.

Vocal Fold Vibration

The vocal folds are a layered structure, with each layer having a differential effect on the movement of the folds depending on the degree of muscle activity, the degree of coupling of the various layers, and the degree of muscle tension. As reported by Hirano,[6,9,10] the vocal fold layers are (1) the epithelium, (2) the lamina propria, and (3) the muscle. The lamina propria consists of the three layers called (1) superficial, (2) intermediate, and (3) deep. Each layer may exhibit different mechanical characteristics. The degree of coupling between the various layers is responsible for the mucosal wave.

The mucosal wave is a wavelike motion along the surface of the vocal folds starting below the folds and progressing to and along the upper surface to the lateral boundaries of the folds. It is similar to the wave created on the surface of a pond when an object is thrown into the water. It probably originates well below the upper surface of the vocal folds,[11] created perhaps by a combination of air pressure increases and the Bernoulli effect. When viewed from above with conventional stroboscopic techniques, it starts at the medial margin of the folds and travels at about a rate of 0.5 to 2 m/s laterally.[12]

Not all phonation produces a mucosal wave, as the wave depends on a loose coupling between the epithelium and the underlying layers of the folds. At higher pitches, the vocal folds are tensed and the coupling between the layers is very high. Thus, usually little or no mucosal wave is visible at higher fundamental frequencies of vocal fold vibration.

Modes of Vibration of the Vocal Folds

There are several modes of vibration of the vocal folds.[13] The most common is that typically heard during speech; its area-versus-time waveform is illustrated in Figure 17–2. Other modes of vibration are described by the terms *creaky voice, falsetto voice, vocal fry, twang,* and *cry.* Each appears to have a different area-versus-time waveform, as illustrated in Figure 17–3. When there is a pathologic lesion on the vocal folds, the mode of vibration may be altered and new modes created. Some of these abnormal modes include breathy voice, hoarse voice, tremor voice, and harsh voice. The specific mode of vibration is determined by many physiologic factors, and it in turn determines the nature of the acoustic pulse created. Although the area-versus-time waveform of the vocal folds is not the acoustic pulse, the two are closely related.[14] Measurements of the area-versus-time waveform of the vocal folds can be used to obtain estimates of the acoustic pulse, and from the acoustic pulse, an analysis of the frequency components of the tone can be made. A listener's perception of a voice is determined by the combination of the fundamental frequency, intensity, and spectrum of the vocal sound.

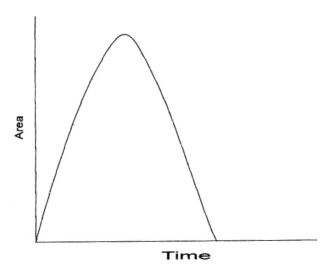

Figure 17–2. Example of an area-versus-time waveform for a normal speaker.

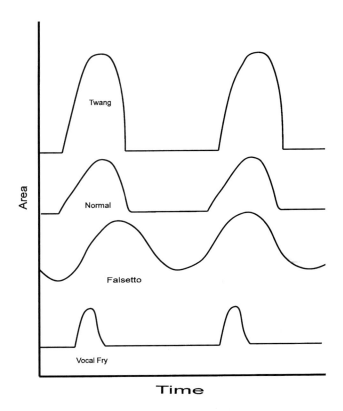

Figure 17–3. Examples of area-versus-time waveforms for various modes of vocal fold vibration.

There are many parameters of the voice one could observe and measure. Some are physiologic, some acoustic, and some perceptual. Although all can be quantified, instruments are readily available to capture and analyze physiologic and acoustic events. These are the focus of this chapter.

WHAT TO MEASURE ABOUT VOCAL FOLD VIBRATION

Myoelastic Properties

Muscle Activity

The measurement of muscle activity is important for several reasons. It provides evidence of (1) innervation of a muscle, that is, whether the muscle is receiving a nerve impulse, (2) muscle tone, that is, whether the muscle is firing to maintain itself in a state of readiness for contraction, (3) abnormal electrical activity in the muscle, that is, whether there are unusual bursts or levels of activity, especially when unexpected, and (4) muscle timing, that is, when the muscle begins and ends its firing. The magnitude of muscle activity is an indirect reflection of the tension exerted in and on the vocal folds.[15-17] Tension is important in controlling the frequency, intensity, and wave shape during phonation. Therefore, EMG studies are important to determine the roles of the various muscles of the larynx on phonation and their effect on the control of frequency, intensity, and waveform. When a muscle abnormality is suspected as a cause of a voice problem, there is also considerable justification for performing an examination of muscle function, yet EMG is not a routine procedure in most offices or clinics. A more complete discussion of EMG techniques and findings is presented in chapter 18.

EMG is performed when there is suspected muscle abnormality, for example, when spasmodic dysphonia (SD), essential tremor, spasticity, myasthenia gravis (MG), or muscle dystonias are present. It has found routine use in the treatment of SD when BOTOX is injected into selected muscles of the larynx. EMG is used to verify the muscle to be injected, study the characteristics of muscle activity, and observe the effects of the BOTOX on muscle activity.[18-22]

EMG may also be used for intraoperative monitoring to differentiate between a true vocal fold paralysis, a fixed arytenoid, posterior glottal stenosis, abnormal reinnervation, and/or paradoxic vocal fold movement.[23-29] The advantage of intraoperative EMG (IEMG) is that it may make it easier to visualize the muscle of interest and it may be of immediate value to the surgeon for planning. In Figure 17–4 is an example

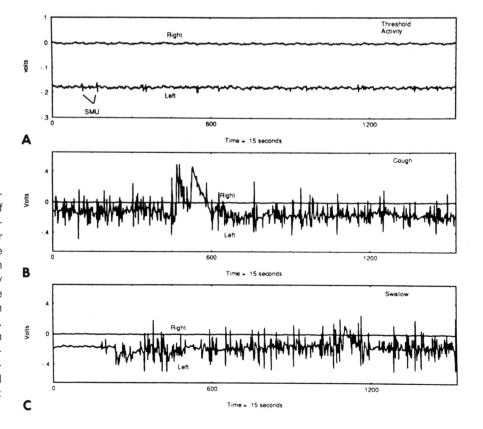

Figure 17–4. A. Fibrillation potentials on the denervated (*right*) side of the TA muscle in a patient with immobile vocal folds. There is little or no recruitment compared with the normal (*left*) side. **B.** Activity when the patient coughed. **C.** Activity when the patient swallowed. Large recruitment potentials are seen from the left side but none from the right. (Reproduced with permission from Woo P, Arandia H. Interoperative laryngeal electromyographic assessment of patients with immobile vocal fold, *Ann Otol Rhinol Laryngol*. 101: 799–806, 1992.)

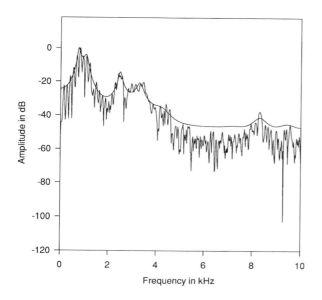

Figure 17–14. FFT of a short segment of a sustained vowel from a normal speaker.

One Third Octave LTAS

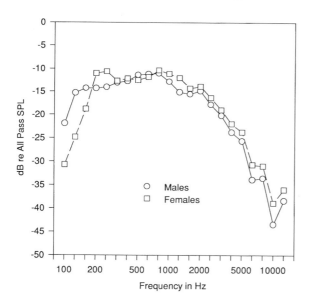

Figure 17–15. LTAS of a paragraph produced by male and female speakers.

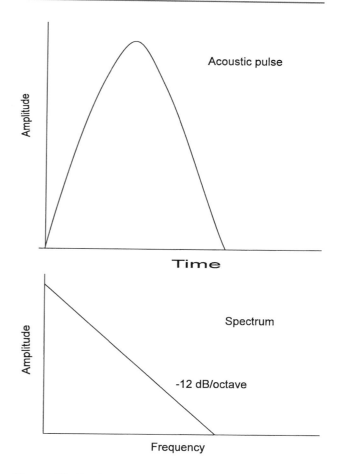

Figure 17–16. Schematic spectrum characteristic of the vocal folds at conversational frequencies.

implemented in the ear, nose, and throat or speech pathology clinic.

Phonation Time

There are several measures in which the maximum duration that a subject can produce on a single breath is recorded. These measures presumably reflect the degree of respiratory control or the efficiency of the conversion of airflow and pressures into sound. Maximum phonation time (MPT) is the duration of phonation an individual can produce on one expiratory breath. It is usually recorded on the vowel /ɑ/ and may be considered an index of phonatory control. Some typical MPTs of normal subjects are presented in Table 17–5. There are also data on MPTs of children and the elderly. A summary of the results for normal speakers as a function of age is shown in Figure 17–17. One of the difficulties with MPT is that a patient may not be able to produce a maximum time, at least not on the first try. Repeated trials are often needed before a reliable estimate of the true MPT is obtained. Kent et al[126] discussed some of the findings of studies in which the performance of subjects on maximum tests of phonation were investigated. Clear instructions,[127] the number of trials,[128] and effects of modeling[129] were considered, and cautions were provided to those interested in obtaining reliable and valid measurement of MPT.

TABLE 17–5. Mean Maximum Phonation Times for 25 Normal-Speaking Men and 25 Normal-Speaking Women

Group	Mean	SD	95% Confidence Interval
Male	34.6	11.75	30.2-39.4
Female	25.7	7.5	22.9-28.7

Source: Adapted from Hirano et al.[145]

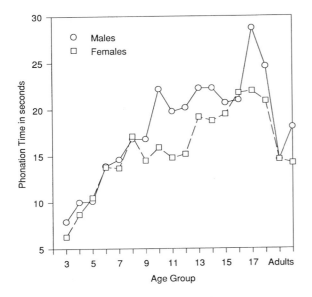

Figure 17–17. Mean MPTs as a function of age. (Data are drawn from references 145 and 146.)

This article also provides an excellent review of the findings relative to MPT and presents considerable data on normal phonation.

The *s/z* ratio is a variant on the concept of maximum phonation time. It is based on the observations by Boone[130] that patients often have a reasonably long production of a voiceless consonant but a much shorter duration of a voice, consonant. Some "normative" data were presented by Eckel and Boone[131] and data in children by Tait, Michel, and Carpenter.[132] The measure has also been used with patients with voice problems.[131,133-135] According to Eckel and Boone, one would expect a normal subject to produce an *s/z* ratio somewhere between 1 and 1.4. Ratios greater than 2.0 are suspect, and such patients should be examined more thoroughly. The *s/z* ratio is meant to be a screening test and does not necessarily have any diagnostic or prognostic value. It may be useful in monitoring the effects of treatment, however.

Phonational and Dynamic Range

Phonational range is the range between the minimum and the maximum frequency an individual can produce, whereas *dynamic range* is the range between the minimum and maximum intensity an individual can produce. Both provide an index of the maximal capabilities of the individual. In Figure 17–18 are some data on phonational ranges of normal speakers. Most normal speakers can produce a phonational range between 2 and 3 octaves, although trained singers can often produce a much greater range. Some data on dynamic ranges of normal speakers are presented in Figure 17–19. Most normal speakers can produce ranges around 40 dB. Typically, the lowest intensity a normal speaker can produce is about 65 dB SPL, and the largest output is 105 to 110 dB SPL. However, the dynamic range depends on the frequency at which it is obtained. If a speaker is asked to maintain approximately the same frequency for both the minimum and the maximum phonations (a task not easily accomplished), the dynamic range may be much less than 40 dB. For example, the subjects whose data are shown in Figure 17–19 were asked to produce their minimum and maximum intensity levels at the 40th percentage point of their phonational range. The mean intensity ranges were 24.50 dB for the male group and 25.52 dB for the female group.

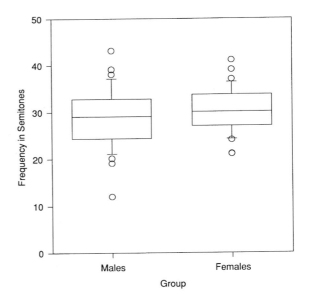

Figure 17–18. Mean phonational ranges, in semitones, of a group of 35 normal-speaking male and 27 normal-speaking female subjects.

Maximum Dynamic Range

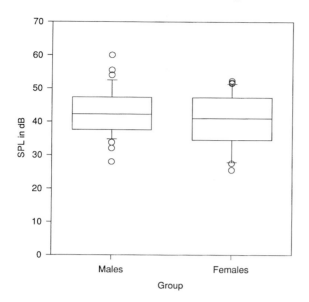

Figure 17–19. Mean dynamic ranges, in decibels, of a group of 35 normal-speaking male and 27 normal-speaking female subjects.

Phonetogram

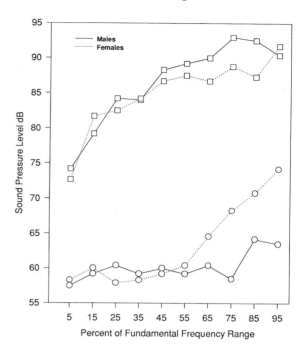

Figure 17–20. Phonetograms of normal male and female speakers. (Redrawn from data reported by Gramming.[137])

There are problems with the measurement of both phonational and dynamic ranges, as was noted for MPT. Is the patient producing the minimum and maximal levels? How many trials are needed before stable data are obtained? We have found it useful to start at a comfortable frequency (or intensity) and then ask the patient to produce higher and higher frequencies (or lower and lower frequencies) until no phonation is produced. It is helpful to present tones from an audio oscillator to the patients so that they can match their production to a target pitch. In some patients, asking them to slowly glide up or down in pitch helps to obtain the end points.

The phonetogram combines the two measurement procedures into a single plot. At selected points along the frequency range of a subject, measurements of the minimum and maximum intensity are obtained. A sample phonetogram of a group of normal subjects is presented in Figure 17–20. The phonetogram has found more extensive use in Europe[136-138] than in the United States. In some cases, the procedure has been automated so that the total time needed for obtaining the data is greatly reduced.[137,139] The phonetogram is not without its problems[140,141] and needs to be carefully interpreted. There is some question if the results obtained and their importance to clinical decisions are worth the time expended.

WHY MEASURE VOCAL FOLD VIBRATION AND ITS ACOUSTIC OUTPUT?

Why should one obtain objective measurements of vocal fold vibration and the acoustic output of phonation? Obviously such information is critical to our understanding of normal voice production, but what value does the expenditure of time, effort, and money have for the diagnosis and treatment of voice problems? There are several reasons to obtain objective data on vocal function in patients. These are (1) the need for objective documentation of the patient's voice, (2) the need for objective data to assess the results of treatment, (3) the need for data to understand the pathologic vibratory process, (4) the potential need for data to support medical decisions in legal proceedings, and (5) the need to determine the minimal set of clinically relevant measurements.

Objective Documentation of a Patient's Voice

Patients and clinicians do not always remember what the patient sounded like before the start of any treatment. Nor do they remember very precisely. Patients may be concerned with a particular aspect of their voice, whereas the clinician reacts to another aspect. Both the patient's and the clinician's impressions of the patient's voice may be vague or use terms that may have multiple meanings. Impressions of a patient's voice are not always reliable indicators of the nature of the voice problem or its severity. Objective data can provide a reliable "picture" of the patient's voice. Such data can be placed into a patient's record, and the tests can be repeated many times to provide indices of any change that has resulted.

Objective data on different aspects of the voice can be obtained. Laryngoscopic observations describe the physical appearance of the vocal folds. Videorecordings of such examinations provide a permanent record. Stroboscopic data can be obtained to describe the vibratory characteristics of the vocal folds, revealing details about vibration that might be invaluable to a proper diagnosis or to developing the best plan of treatment. Airflow and air pressure data can be used to describe the patient's use of these parameters during vocalization. Acoustic data can be used to present a picture of the frequency, intensity, and stability of phonation. The acoustic spectrum provides a picture of the component frequencies in the voice that eventually listeners perceive when listening to the voice. Acoustic data can also be used to assess the capabilities of the system, capabilities that might be important in rendering a prognosis.

One need not try to obtain all possible data but should be selective and sample the relevant physiologic and acoustic features of a patient's voice. Records in the form of pictures, videotapes, graphs, or numbers obtained after the analysis of selected features of the voice may be included in the patient's record, thus providing an objective picture of the patient's voice.

Objective Data Critical for Properly Assessing Treatment Results

Studies in which data are collected on relevant parameters of the voice before and after a course of treatment are invaluable for evaluating the effects of the treatment. Such data should not be simply used to judge the "success" or "failure" of treatment. Rather they should be used to determine what physiologic (or acoustic) features changed in the voice and what such changes may mean to the functioning of the voice. Such data may help to "fine tune" treatment approaches, especially surgical techniques. Such data are invaluable to assess the techniques used in voice therapy.

Objective data may not always support the patient's (or clinician's) perception of the voice change as a result of treatment. In some cases, the patient may obtain relief of a problem that has little to do with the

voice. For example, some patients with voice difficulties complain of difficulty swallowing or liquids aspirating. A surgical procedure may be tried that improves either of these two functions but does little to improve or affect vibratory function. The patient has improved, but the improvement was not with the voice. With voice therapy, a patient may learn to produce voice in a different way that results in a reduction in muscle soreness. Perhaps the muscle soreness was the patient's main concern and the treatment provided the hoped-for relief. However, there may have been little change in the sound of the voice. If there is no change in the voice, one would expect little change in some or all of the measurements obtained before treatment. Patients and clinicians need to be aware of the expected goals of treatment and evaluate objective data on the voice with these goals in mind.

Objective Data Help to Understand the Pathologic Vibratory Process

Proper diagnosis and effective treatment depend on an understanding of the disorder. What is the effect of an observed pathologic condition on vibratory function and how does that affect the production of the pathologic voice? With some abnormalities, the effect may be very subtle. In some patients, there is no observable pathologic lesion, but careful observation and testing may reveal subtle abnormalities in vibratory function. Such abnormalities may be corrected with careful, fine surgery, or with medical management, or may require voice therapy. When the exact nature of the underlying pathophysiology is understood, the likelihood of efficient, effective treatment is greatly increased.

Objective Data for Legal Proceedings

There is a common saying "Ignorance is bliss, but it won't stand up in court." Objective data about a patient's voice, especially before and after treatment, can be critical in justifying treatment decisions in a court of law. Such data provide independent evidence of the exact state of the patient's voice and of the effects of treatment. A simple audiotape recording of a patient's voice, even if unanalyzed, can be an important objective record.

Objective Data to Evaluate Clinically Relevant Measurements

Many potential measurements can be made on the voice. Many have been discussed in this chapter, but the list is by no means complete. Some of these measurements are redundant and may reflect a feature of the voice that has little relationship to the diagnosis or the suggested treatment. Ideally, one would like a small set of measurements that are most relevant to the diagnosis, the prognosis, or both. At the time of the writing of this chapter, there is no such set. Objective data must be collected on many more patients before one could hope to derive the optimum set of measurements one should routinely use in the evaluation of patients with voice problems. Different combinations of measurements may be needed for different needs or patient groups. The set of measurements one requires to obtain a proper diagnosis may not be the same as that one would use to assess the results of treatment. Basic questions about whether such measurements should be solely physiologic or acoustic have not been addressed. Continued research and data collection on normal and pathologic speakers may help to answer these and other questions.

EXAMPLES OF MEASUREMENTS IN PATIENTS WITH PHONATORY DISORDERS

Patients with vocal fold nodules probably constitute the largest number of patients with benign lesions of the vocal folds. In a recent study, systematic ratings of videostroboscopic recordings of 30 patients with nodules were obtained. The patients were all female, and most received voice therapy for treatment of the nodules. The most frequent category for each of eight stroboscopic signs is shown in Figure 17–21. The most frequent glottal configuration (when the vocal folds were most closed) is a posterior chink. The affected fold, that is, the fold or folds with the lesion, had a slightly rough edge, a slightly decreased amplitude, and a slightly decreased lateral extent of the mucosal wave. The other signs were normal. An example of an inverse-filtered airflow and an EGG trace of a nodule patient is shown in Figure 17–22. Relevant acoustic measurements for this patient are reported in Table 17–6.

Acoustic, EGG, or airflow measures of vocal fold function usually cannot guide the physician on treatment or diagnosis. For example, even severe vocal nodules may respond to conservative medical and speech therapy management. Vocal function measurements may reveal high flow rates, low signal-to-noise (S/N) ratios, and other findings of pathologic vibratory function. However, vocal function measures serve as only one criterion to assess the results or progress of treatment. Studies that assess voice results using multidimensional methods include perceptual,

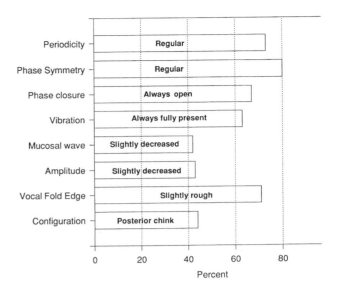

Figure 17–21. Most frequent category for eight stroboscopic signs in 30 patients with vocal fold nodules. (Data are from Colton et al.[147])

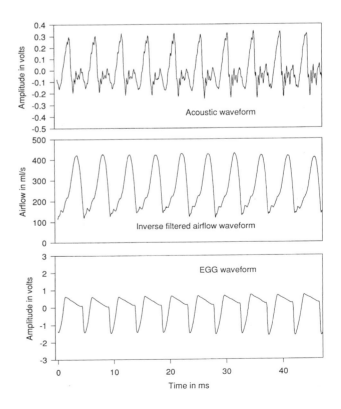

Figure 17–22. Audio trace (*top*), inverse-filtered airflow trace (*middle*), and EGG trace (*bottom*) for a patient with a vocal fold nodule.

TABLE 17–6. Summary of Pre- and Post-treatment Acoustic and Airflow Measurements for a Patient With a Vocal Fold Nodule Shown in Figure 17–22

Measurement	Pretreatment	Post-treatment
Sound pressure level (dB)	77.72	75.3
Fundamental frequency (Hz)	237	248
Phonational range (ST)	23.68	27.75
Dynamic range (DB)	17.25	20.56
Average flow (mL/s)	240.21	317.52
AC flow (mL/s)	204.75	160.25
Leakage flow (mL/s)	157.25	244.46
Open quotient (%)	50.89	63.49
Lung pressure cm H_2O	5.14	5.55
Vocal efficiency	43.66	20.5

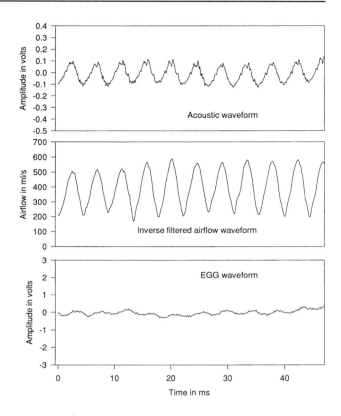

Figure 17–23. Audio trace (*top*), inverse-filtered airflow trace (*middle*), and EGG trace (*bottom*) for a patient with vocal fold paralysis.

videostroboscopic, acoustic, and airflow analysis. It remains to be demonstrated which tests will be most cost-effective and relevant.

Because some vocal fold lesions interfere with the vibratory function of the vocal folds, assessment of mucosal vibratory function by VSL is a cornerstone tool for diagnosis and treatment results. VSL is now routinely used to document the restoration of vocal fold function. To document the restoration of vibratory function, acoustic spectrum analysis and its desired measures in time and frequency domain are useful (ie, S/N ratio, jitter, shimmer, or the ratio of high energy to total energy). Individuals who undergo treatment often show changes in EGG, VSL, and airflow data, and this gives insight on phonatory physiology. However, because of the wide variety of pathologic conditions and the large variations in function, large cohort studies may be necessary before statistical differences between treatment groups can be demonstrated.

An example of an inverse-filtered airflow and an EGG trace of patient with a left vocal fold paralysis is shown in Figure 17–23. Note the large leakage airflow and the small vibratory airflow component. The level of the EGG is very low, making interpretation of the EGG trace almost impossible. A summary of the aerodynamic and acoustic measurements is presented in Table 17–7.

Patients with vocal fold paralysis who seek treatment have three types of complaints: (1) dyspnea with

TABLE 17–7. Summary of Pre- and Post-treatment Acoustic and Airflow Measurements for a Patient With a Vocal Fold Paralysis Shown in Figure 17–23

Measurement	Pretreatment	Post-treatment
Sound pressure level (dB)	73.34	75.64
Fundamental frequency (Hz)	233	227
Phonational range (ST)	20.12	20.61
Dynamic range (dB)	13.04	21.09
Average flow (mL/s)	529.56	175.03
AC flow (mL/s)	201.8	185.11
Leakage flow (mL/s)	423.37	95.03
Open quotient (%)	64.45	58.76
Lung pressure cm H_2O	5.26	8.68
Vocal efficiency	7.72	95.69

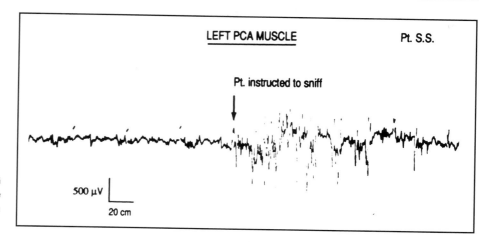

Figure 18–2. A laryngeal EMG recording of the PCA muscle showing a burst of activity on sniffing (maximal stimulation).

brane at the midline, traversing the lumen of the subglottic space and piercing the posterior lamina of the cricoid cartilage to one side or the other of midline.[14] The electrical signal on the far side of the cartilage represents posterior cricoarytenoid muscle. This can be verified by the patient sniffing. In our experience, this approach is most useful in the young patient whose cartilage has not undergone extensive calcification. A tracheal injection of lidocaine is helpful in avoiding airway irritation.

Thyroarytenoid and posterior cricoarytenoid muscle electrodes may also be placed under endoscopic guidance or under direct vision at operative laryngoscopy.[15,16]

PHYSIOLOGY AND PATHOLOGY

An EMG yields a visual signal of electrical activity in muscle, either via oscilloscope, or in all newer systems, a digital trace. In addition, the electrical signal is coupled to a speaker and produces audible output. Different types of potentials have specific acoustic signatures that are readily identified by the experienced examiner, and the audible signal is an important part of the EMG examination. There are four characteristics of electrical activity in muscle: morphology or waveform, amplitude, duration, and frequency. Acoustically, the amplitude of an electrical potential generally corresponds to loudness, and duration and rise time correspond to pitch.[11]

Electrical activity in muscle is the result of changes in the strong negative resting potential of the muscle cell that in turn result from other electrical or chemical signals. Normally, depolarization is the result of neural stimulation via acetylcholine to the motor end plates of a muscle fiber. All muscle fibers innervated by a given motoneuron form a motor unit. The electrical summation of all their potentials forms a motor unit potential (MUP, also called a motor unit action potential, or a muscle action potential), the basic electrophysiologic component of striated muscle.

A useful classification of EMG findings divides electrical activity into three types based on the circumstance in which it appears: insertional, spontaneous, and volitional.[4,11] Upon insertion, irritation by the needle itself may cause a few individual fibers to depolarize, which yields a burst of spike discharges that extinguishes quickly. These may take the form of pseudomyotonic "dive bomber" discharges (discussed below) (Figure 18–3). Any such activity persisting beyond 400 milliseconds from needle movement is considered prolonged and a sign of pathologic muscle membrane instability.

Spontaneous activity in normal muscle at complete rest is minimal, usually limited to subthreshold nonpropagated depolarizations at the end plate that produce extremely brief, irregular, and low amplitude electrical signals. They make a characteristic hissing or white-noise type sound, and have an initial negative deflection (an upward deflection of the trace, by convention). This distinguishes them from fibrillation potentials, which have an initial positive deflection and are pathologic. Measurement of spontaneous activity in laryngeal muscles is difficult because complete silence is rarely achieved. These muscles are continuously active in respiration. Spontaneous activity such as fibrillations and positive sharp waves can be more clearly identified in limb muscles, in which complete relaxation can produce electrical silence. In the larynx, electrical silence in and of itself may suggest pathology.

Volitional activity is examined by having the patient contract the muscle with a needle in place. In the larynx, this consists of an action appropriate for the muscle in question: voicing or a Valsalva maneuver

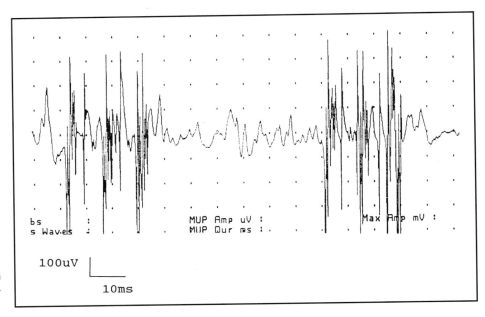

Figure 18–3. A laryngeal EMG recording of the TA muscle showing pseudomyotonic discharges.

for the thyroarytenoid, sniffing for the posterior cricoarytenoid, or a glissando (slide) for the cricothyroid. Contraction results in the appearance of the MUP. Each MUP has its own characteristics and is thus identifiable throughout an examination, but it is possible to make some generalizations.[4,11] The normal MUP is usually bi- or triphasic in shape. Phases are counted by noting the number of times the potential crosses the baseline and adding one. Greater than four phases is considered abnormal and termed "polyphasic." This is reflective of a loss of synchrony among the end plates that make up a motor unit.

The duration and amplitude depend on the muscle studied, and are generally proportional to the muscle size.[4] Faaborg-Andersen[1,2] and Buchtal[3] have described laryngeal MUPs of amplitudes ranging from 224 to 358 microvolts. They also found mean durations of 3.5 milliseconds in the vocalis and 5.3 milliseconds in the cricothyroid. Their data were obtained with concentric needle electrodes. Similar measurements made with monopolar electrodes recorded a mean amplitude of 426 microvolts and duration of 3.5 milliseconds for the vocalis muscle, and 500 microvolts and 4.4 milliseconds for the cricothyroid.[17] MUP duration has been shown to increase with age and with decreasing temperature.[4] Amplitude is also affected by the distance of the needle from the muscle fibers. In order to check this distance, an examiner may measure the rise time of a MUP, the time between the onset of the first negative deflection and its peak. For observations about a given MUP to be valid, its rise time should be less than 200 microseconds.[4,10]

Frequency of MUPs is determined largely by the force of contraction. Besides increasing the frequency of discharge from an individual motor unit, increasing contraction will result in the activation of adjacent motor units. This phenomenon is known as recruitment. At a high level of contraction, multiple motor units will be firing at high frequency, making it impossible to distinguish features of any single MUP either visually or acoustically. This is known as a full interference pattern, and is normally achieved at about 30% of maximum isometric contraction (Figure 18–4).[11] Inability to attain full interference pattern suggests pathology (Figure 18–5).

Like normal findings, abnormalities in EMG may be divided into insertional, spontaneous, and volitional activity.[4,11] Prolonged insertional activity, defined as depolarizations lasting longer than 400 milliseconds, is suggestive of muscle membrane instability, as in polymyositis and other myopathies. Spontaneous firing of individual muscle fibers at rest indicates denervation or myopathy. This may appear either as spike fibrillations or positive sharp waves (PSW), but their significance is the same (Figures 18–6 and 18–7). Both are marked by an initial positive (downward) deflection and fire with a regular periodicity. Higher frequency runs of spike fibrillations and PSWs, usually prompted by needle movement, that wax and wane in amplitude and frequency are called myotonic discharges. The telltale acoustic signal of myotonic discharge has been likened to the sound of a dive bomber or a motocross bike. Myotonic discharges occur in a variety of intrinsic disorders of muscle such as myositis, myotonic dystrophy, glycogen storage diseases, hyperparathyroidism, and so forth. Fasciculation potentials are the result of spontaneous discharge of all or

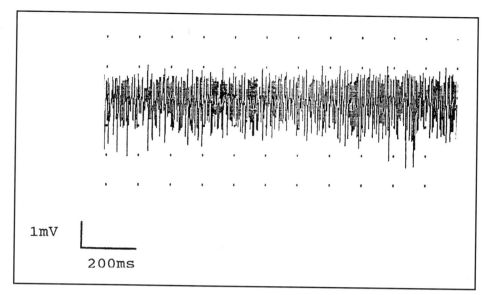

Figure 18–4. A laryngeal EMG recording of the TA muscle during voicing, showing a normal interference pattern.

1mV

200ms

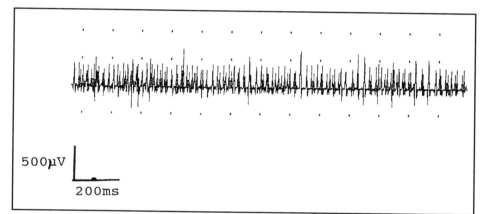

Figure 18–5. A laryngeal EMG recording of the TA muscle during voicing in a patient with vocal fold paresis, showing a decreased interference pattern.

500μV

200ms

part of an entire motor unit, which they resemble, except that they occur singly rather than in trains, and at rest, rather than with movement. They are a typical finding in amyotrophic lateral sclerosis, but can appear in any condition of chronic denervation. MUPs that occur in repetitive runs, but generally constant in duration and amplitude, are termed myokymia, and occur in response to a number of factors that alter the biochemical environment of the nerve, such as demyelination, edema, or toxins. Acoustically, myokymia resembles the sound of marching soldiers. Complex repetitive discharges are abrupt onset and offset, multifiber discharges with bizarre morphologies that are thought to signify chronicity of neuromuscular disease.

Voluntary contraction may yield abnormal MUPs. In general, large amplitude, long duration MUPs suggest neurogenic disease, whereas small amplitude, short MUPs suggest myopathy.[11] There are several ex-

ceptions to this, like early reinnervation potentials and potentials of chronic severe myopathy. Forceful contraction that fails to produce a full interference pattern suggests denervation, as discussed above.

As is evident, the spectrum of abnormal findings in EMG is broad, and reflects the disordered physiology of the disease under investigation. Most findings can occur in a variety of conditions; none is pathognomonic. Whether they carry significance depends on the frequency with which they occur and their clinical context. There are few lists of strict diagnostic criteria for specific diseases in the EMG literature for this reason. The beginning electromyographer may find this frustrating, but with experience, EMG becomes a useful and thought-provoking means of evaluating laryngeal function.

As laryngeal EMG is often applied to conditions of nerve injury, let us examine such a situation as an example of the mutability of electrical findings over time

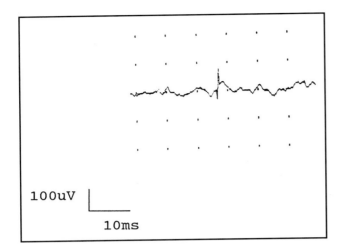

Figure 18–6. A laryngeal EMG recording of the TA muscle in a patient with vocal fold paralysis, showing an example of a fibrillation potential suggestive of denervation.

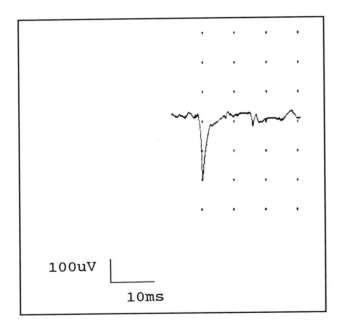

Figure 18–7. A laryngeal EMG recording of the TA muscle in a patient with vocal fold paralysis, showing an example of a positive sharp wave, suggestive of a denervating process.

and the integration of electrical and clinical observations. (The sequence of electrical changes in vocal fold denervation have been well demonstrated in a canine model.[18-20])

Initially, following a nerve injury, no electrical signals can travel to the distal end of any of the compromised axons to prompt release of neurotransmitter. Therefore, no depolarization of the affected motor units occurs. In cases of extreme injury, such as a nerve

section, in which all axons are interrupted, there can be electrical silence both at rest and with efforts at movement. Alternatively, the injury may be incomplete and some motor units may remain intact. In this case, the examiner asks the patient to activate the muscle—for example, to phonate, in the case of the thyroarytenoid. A nerve injury severe enough to cause symptomatic vocal fold paresis would almost certainly disrupt enough motor units to impair recruitment and cause an incomplete interference pattern at maximal effort. Because of the appearance of the trace of this phenomenon, it is referred to as a "picket-fence" pattern (see Figure 18–5).

If the site of nerve injury is unknown, comparison of findings in the cricothyroid and the thyroarytenoid muscle can be helpful. Signs of denervation in both point toward the jugular foramen and the central nervous system, whereas abnormal findings restricted to the thyroarytenoid direct workup along the course of the recurrent laryngeal nerve.

Over time, the resting potential of a muscle cell that receives no neural input falls to near the depolarization threshold.[11] From time to time, it crosses this threshold and the cell fires, repolarizes, and then repeats the cycle. On EMG, this manifests as fibrillation potentials or PSWs—single positive spikes that occur with some regularity (see Figures 18–6 and 18–7). There is some variability in how long a muscle must be denervated to produce fibrillations; three weeks is widely quoted in the literature, but it may take up to five weeks.[4,10,11,18] Because of the change in muscle cell resting potential, prolonged insertional activity may also occur, as cells are more likely to depolarize with irritation.[11] In fact, prolonged insertional activity usually precedes the appearance of fibrillations. If no neural ingrowth occurs, fibrillation potentials will persist until the muscle atrophies and is replaced by connective tissue.

If reinnervation occurs, early nerve fibers grow in irregularly to encounter atrophied muscle fibers and disordered neuromuscular junctions.[4,11] The result is motor unit weakness and asynchrony, and thus MUPs of early reinnervation are typically low in amplitude, polyphasic, and prolonged (Figure 18–8). Yet, they provide clear evidence that neural regeneration is occurring. With time, synchronicity improves, although nearly never to preinjury levels. Therefore, the MUP of late reinnervation still tends to be polyphasic and prolonged, although perhaps less so than before. Because the late-reinnervation motor unit generally incorporates many more muscle fibers than a normal, preinjury motor unit, its MUP demonstrates high amplitude—the so-called giant wave.

Because EMG evidence of reinnervation appears before clinical return of function, EMG can have prognostic value. Yet, reinnervation is not synonymous with return

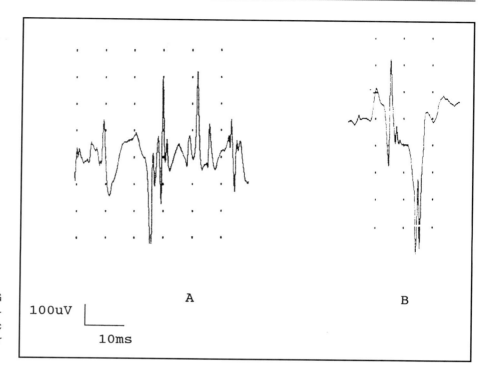

Figure 18–8. A laryngeal EMG recording of the TA muscle showing two examples of polyphasic potentials suggestive of a repair process.

of function. The recurrent laryngeal nerve contains fibers for both vocal fold abduction and adduction, and these fibers do not necessarily find their way back to the appropriate motor units. Anomalous regrowth may result in an immobile, albeit reinnervated, vocal fold. EMG findings in this circumstance are not spurious, although they may appear to be. The clinically important phenomenon of synkinesis in the larynx, although appreciated as early as 1963,[20] is often overlooked, although it has implications for voice function and treatment.[21]

In order to make sense of the various electrical findings of denervation, the examiner must first have an idea of the age of the nerve injury. For instance, fibrillation potentials carry different significance at one month following injury than they do one year later. Second, the examiner must combine the EMG examination findings with those of the laryngoscopic examination. Finally, comparison with previous EMGs is often useful to see if reinnervation is ongoing or has reached a plateau.

CLINICAL APPLICATIONS OF LARYNGEAL ELECTROMYOGRAPHY

Laryngeal EMG is useful in separating mechanical from neurogenic causes of vocal fold immobility (Table 18–1).[16,20-24] EMG has been found to be more reliable than computed tomography scanning (CT) for this purpose,[23] and offers a safer and less costly alternative to operative endoscopy. Conditions such as cricoarytenoid arthritis and or arytenoid dislocation

TABLE 18–1. Common Clinical Uses of EMG

1. Differentiating laryngeal paralysis from mechanical fixation
2. Estimating the degree and prognosis of paralysis or paresis
3. Diagnosing neurologic disease (eg, myasthenia gravis, amyotrophic lateral sclerosis, myopathy)
4. Determining the site of neurologic lesion
5. Evaluating laryngeal synkinesis and other phenomena of misdirected reinnervation
6. Intraoperative nerve monitoring
7. Therapeutic injection of laryngeal muscles
8. Biofeedback in speech and swallowing disorders

generally yield near-normal EMGs, although Yin and coauthors have cautioned that patterns of myopathy or neuropathy may occur in long-standing arytenoid dislocation, and have emphasized the importance of testing multiple sites within the muscle.[25] Neurogenic vocal fold immobility, on the other hand, can show a wide variety of abnormal electrical activity, as described above.

In cases of denervation, comparison of findings in muscles innervated by the superior laryngeal nerve (cricothyroid) and the recurrent laryngeal nerve (thyroarytenoid) can indicate the site of lesion.[26] Abnormal findings in both muscles suggest an injury proximal to the branching of the superior nerve form the main trunk of the vagus, whereas abnormalities isolated to the thyroarytenoid direct investigation into lower neck and the mediastinum.

With respect to prognosticating return of vocal fold function, researchers have reported rates of 69% to 90% correct prediction of return of motion.[27-30] These results are difficult to interpret and reconcile with each other because much depends on the criteria used in each study. In general, though, the preservation of normal-morphology MUPs, suggesting incomplete nerve injury, is a positive sign and a good argument for early EMG examination following neural injury.[19,30] Polyphasic MUPs are more problematic, but also generally improve chances of return of function. However, the absence of motor unit potentials, either normal or polyphasic, and the presence of fibrillations and PSWs, are reliable indicators of poor prognosis.[27,30]

Setting strict criteria for reinnervation can create the impression that it is an all-or-none phenomenon, whereas it more likely occurs on a continuum that includes misdirected growth resulting in synkinetic muscular activity.[21,31-34] Some studies have dismissed immobile vocal folds that demonstrate electrical signs of reinnervation as false positives, whereas, these are probably more appropriately considered cases of dysfunctional reinnervations. Such reinnervation is not merely a matter of classic synkinesis, but represents a variety of phenomena of misdirected and inadequate nerve regrowth.[35,36] Even with persistent vocal fold immobility, voice quality can be near normal because of restoration of muscle tone.[21] In summary, EMG evidence of reinnervation is not synonymous with return of vocal fold motion, but may suggest voice improvement. In prognosticating return of function to a denervated vocal fold, as in other aspects of clinical EMG, serial examinations and clinical correlation are helpful.

More widespread use of laryngeal EMG has created a new appreciation for the entity of laryngeal nerve paresis including superior laryngeal nerve palsy.[37-41] Both conditions may cause subtle glottic insufficiency, and EMG can help distinguish between that caused by these neurologic factors and from glottic insufficiency caused by other factors such as atrophy, sulcus vocalis, and postsurgical scarring.

Laryngeal EMG is an essential tool in the investigation of disorders of vocal fold mobility associated with a wide variety of systemic neurologic conditions, including hereditary sensory and motor neuropathy,[42] postpolio syndrome,[43,44] the Parkinson-plus syndromes,[45,46] and in distinguishing upper from lower motor neuron lesions.[47] With multiple muscle samples, the diagnosis of bulbar palsy (anterior horn cell disease), primary lateral sclerosis, Arnold-Chiari malformation, or syringomyelia can be entertained.[10] When there is regular, slow, repetitive firing of MUPs in the larynx, with synchronous firing of muscles in the palate and pharynx, the diagnosis of myoclonus is easily made (Figure 18–9). A regular 4- to 8-Hz repetitive signal can suggest essential tremor. Once again, evaluation of extralaryngeal muscles may be useful. In some patients, the amplitude and numbers of potentials decrease with repetitive function or repetitive stimulation. This is suggestive of myasthenia gravis (Figure 18–10).

Patients with spasmodic dysphonia have been studied extensively, and certain EMG characteristics have helped differentiate spasmodic dysphonia from other disorders. An effective method is to synchronize the EMG with the voice spectrogram and measure the delay from the onset of electrical activity to the onset of sound. It is characteristically delayed in patients with spasmodic dysphonia by 500 milliseconds to 1 second (normal: 0 to 200 milliseconds) (Figure 18–11).[10,48]

EMG can be used for intraoperative monitoring of the recurrent laryngeal nerve during surgeries that place this structure at risk. Hooked-wire electrodes can be placed into the thyroarytenoid-vocalis muscle complex endoscopically, or surface electrodes can be placed on top of the postcricoid area or attached to the endotracheal tube at the level of the vocal folds in order to provide warning when the recurrent nerve is stimulated.[6,49,50] Surgeons should be aware that anesthetic agents, including paralytics and local agents, can inhibit electrical activity in muscle.

EMG has proved to be the ideal method of guiding therapeutic injection of botulinum toxin. A hollow needle can be used as a monopolar electrode to inject toxin where the electrical signal is crisp, loud, and high-pitched, indicating that motor end plates, and therefore nerve terminals, are nearby.[51] Because botulinum toxin acts at nerve terminals to prevent the release of acetylcholine, this method serves to minimize the dose needed for a therapeutic effect and increases accuracy of placement, thereby reducing diffusion and unintended effects.

Finally, surface EMG is an evolving tool in biofeedback therapy of both speech and swallowing disorders.[8,9]

CONCLUSION

In the years since the seminal work of Faaborg-Andersen and Buchtal, electromyography (EMG) has become a useful tool for the laryngologist. It is valuable in making distinctions between mechanical limitation and denervation in the immobile vocal fold. In the case

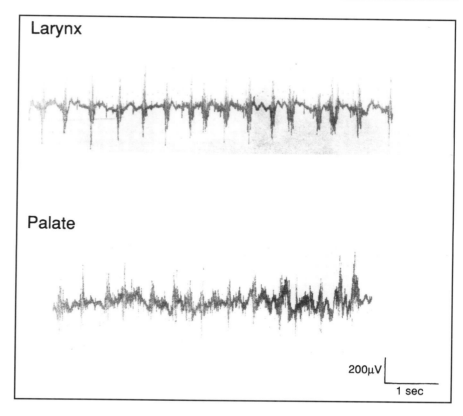

Larynx

Palate

200μV

1 sec

Figure 18–9. A simultaneous recording of the EMG of the TA muscle and palate showing a synchronous myoclonic electrical pattern.

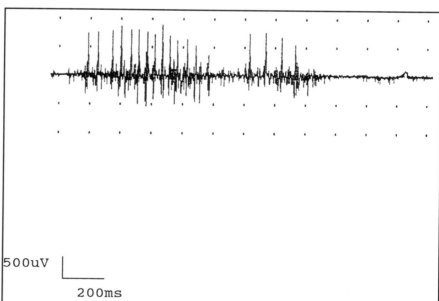

500uV

200ms

Figure 18–10. A laryngeal EMG recording of the TA muscle showing decreasing amplitude and numbers of potentials with continued function, suggestive of myasthenia gravis.

of denervation, it can point to the site of lesion and provide prognostic information that guides treatment. EMG is an integral part of the investigation of neurologic disorders affecting the larynx. Intraoperatively, it can be used to monitor the recurrent laryn-

geal nerves during procedures that put these structures at risk. EMG is the standard method of directing therapeutic injection of botulinum toxin, and has been used in biofeedback therapy for speech and swallowing disorders

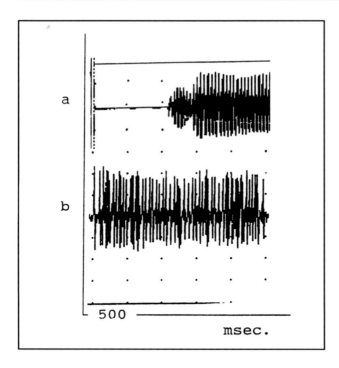

Figure 18–11. (A) Voice spectrogram and (B) electromyogram of patient with spasmodic dysphonia, showing a greater than 1-second delay between the onset of electrical activity and the onset of voice.

Although EMG yields measurable data, it is in essence a qualitative test. The comparison with endoscopy and imaging studies made by Woodson is apt.[52] EMG diagnosis of neuromuscular disease is based on patterns of abnormalities and change over time, and, like the other tests, requires clinical correlation.

The most important contribution of EMG to laryngology has been to catalyze interest in mechanisms of neural control of the larynx. The resulting refinement of electrodiagnostic approaches to the larynx, including quantitative and single-fiber EMG and evoked potential testing, should, with time, yield as much insight into these mechanisms as we now have into the structure and function of vocal fold mucosa.

REFERENCES

1. Faaborg-Andersen K. Electromyographic investigation of intrinsic laryngeal muscles in humans. *Acta Physiol.* 1957;41(suppl 140):1–149.
2. Faaborg-Andersen K, Buchtal F. Action potentials from internal laryngeal muscles during phonation. *Nature.* 1956;177:340–341.
3. Buchtal F. Electromyography of intrinsic laryngeal muscles. *J Exp Physiol.* 1959;44:137–148.
4. Aminoff MJ. Clinical electromyography. In: Aminoff MJ, ed. *Electrodiagnosis in Clinical Neurology.* 4th ed. Philadelphia, PA: Churchill Livingstone; 1999:223–252.
5. Fujita M, Ludlow CL, Woodson GE, et al. A new surface electrode for recording from the posterior cricoarytenoid muscle. *Laryngoscope.* 1989;99:316–320.
6. Khan A, Pearlman RC, Bianchi DA, Hauck KW. Experience with two types of electromyography monitoring electrodes during thyroid surgery. *Am J Otolaryngol.* 1997;18:99–102.
7. Guindi GM, Higenbottam TW, Payne JK. A new method for laryngeal electromyography. *Clin Otolaryngol.* 1981; 6:271–278.
8. Andrews S, Warner J, Stewart R. EMG biofeedback in the treatment of hyperfunctional dysphonia. *Br J Disord Commun.* 1986;21:353–369.
9. Hillel AD, Robinson LR, Waugh P. Laryngeal electromyography for the diagnosis and management of swallowing disorders. *Otolaryngol Head Neck Surg.* 1997;116:344–348.
10. Lovelace RE, Blitzer A, Ludlow C. Clinical laryngeal electromyography. In: Blitzer A, Brin MF, Sasaki CT, et al, eds. *Neurologic Disorders of the Larynx.* New York, NY: Thieme Medical Publishers; 1992:66–82.
11. Campbell WW. Needle electrode examination. In: Campbell WW, ed. *Essentials of Electrodiagnostic Medicine.* Baltimore, MD: Williams & Wilkins; 1999:93–116.
12. Hirano M, Ohala J. Use of hooked-wire electrodes for electromyography of the intrinsic laryngeal muscles. *J Speech Hearing Res.* 1969;12:362–373.
13. Blitzer A, Brin MF, Stewart C, Fahn S. Abductor laryngeal dystonia: a series treated with botulinum toxin. *Laryngoscope.* 1992;102:163–167.
14. Mu LC, Yang SL. A new method of needle-electrode placement in the posterior cricoarytenoid muscle for electromyography. *Laryngoscope.* 1990;100:1127–1131.
15. Thumfart WF. Electromyography of the larynx and related technics. *Acta Otorhinolaryngol Belg.* 1986;40:358–376.
16. Woo P, Arandia H. Intraoperative laryngeal electromyographic assessment of patients with immobile vocal fold. *Ann Otol Rhinol Laryngol.* 1992;101:799–806.
17. Rodriquez AA, Myers BR, Ford CN. Laryngeal electromyography in the diagnosis of laryngeal nerve injuries. *Arch Phys Med Rehabil.* 1990;71:587–590.
18. Shindo ML, Herzon GD, Hanson DG, Cain DJ, Sahgal V. Effects of denervation on laryngeal muscles: a canine model. *Laryngoscope.* 1992;102:663–669.
19. Mu L, Yang S. An experimental study on the laryngeal electromyography and visual observations in varying types of surgical injuries to the unilateral recurrent laryngeal nerve in the neck. *Laryngoscope.* 1991;101:699–708.
20. Siribodhi C, Sundmaker W, Adkins JP, Bonner FJ. Electromyographic studies of laryngeal paralysis and regeneration of laryngeal motor nerves in dogs. *Laryngoscope.* 1963;73:148–163.
21. Blitzer A, Jahn AF, Keidar A. Semon's law revisited: an electromyographic analysis of laryngeal synkinesis. *Ann Otol Rhinol Laryngol.* 1996;105:764–769.

22. Rontal E, Rontal M, Silverman B, Kileny PR. The clinical differentiation between vocal fold paralysis and vocal cord fixation using electromyography. *Laryngoscope.* 1993;103:133–137.

23. Sataloff RT, Bough ID, Spiegel JR. Arytenoid dislocation: diagnosis and treatment. *Laryngoscope.* 1994;104:1353–1361.

24. Hoffman HT, Brunberg JA, Winter P, Sullivan MJ, Kileny PR. Arytenoid subluxation: diagnosis and treatment. *Ann Otol Rhinol Laryngol.* 1991;100:1–9.

25. Yin SS, Qiu WW, Stucker FJ. Value of electromyography in differential diagnosis of laryngeal joint injuries after intubation. *Ann Otol Rhinol Laryngol.* 1996;105:446–451.

26. Quiney RE. Laryngeal electromyography: a useful technique for the investigation of vocal cord palsy. *Clin Otolaryngol.* 1989;14:305–316.

27. Min YB, Finnegan EM, Hoffman HT, Luschei ES, McCullough TM. A preliminary study of the prognostic role of electromyography in laryngeal paralysis. *Otolaryngol Head Neck Surg.* 1994;111:770–775.

28. Hirano M, Nosoe I, Shin T, Maeyama T. Electromyography for laryngeal paralysis. In: Hirano M, Kirchner J, Bless D, eds. *Neurolaryngology: Recent Advances.* Boston, MA: College Hill; 1987:232–248.

29. Thumfart W. Electromyography of the larynx. In: Samii M, Gannetta PJ, eds. *The Cranial Nerves.* Berlin, Germany: Springer Verlag; 1981:597–606.

30. Parnes SM, Satya-Murti S. Predictive value of laryngeal electromyography in patients with vocal cord paralysis of neurogenic origin. *Laryngoscope.* 1985;95:1323–1326.

31. Crumley RL. Laryngeal synkinesis: its significance to the laryngologist. *Ann Otol Rhinol Laryngol.* 1989;98:87–92.

32. Crumley RL. Laryngeal synkinesis revisited. *Ann Otol Rhinol Laryngol.* 2000;109:365–371.

33. Nahm I, Shin T, Watanabe H, et al., Misdirected regeneration of the injured recurrent laryngeal nerve in the cat. *Am J Otolaryngol.* 1993;14:43–48.

34. Hiroto I, Hirano M, Tomita H. Electromyographic investigation of human vocal cord paralysis. *Ann Otol Rhinol Laryngol.* 1968;77:296–304.

35. Zealear DL, Billante CR. Neurophysiology of vocal fold paralysis. *Otolaryngol Clin North Am.* 2004;37:1–24.

36. Maronian RC, Robinson L, Waugh P, Hillel AD. A new electromyographic definition of laryngeal synkinesis. *Ann Otol Rhinol Larngol.* 2004;113:877–886.

37. Simpson DM, Sternman D, Graves-Wright J, Sanders I. Vocal cord paralysis: clinical and electrophysiologic features. *Muscle Nerve.* 1993;16:952–957.

38. Koufman JA, Postma GN, Cummins MM, Blalock PD. Vocal fold paresis. *Otolaryngol Head Neck Surg.* 2000;122:537–541.

39. Dursun G, Sataloff RT, Spiegel JR, Mandel S, Heuer RJ, Rosen DC. Superior laryngeal nerve paresis and paralysis. *J Voice.* 1996;10:206–211.

40. Dray TG, Robinson LR, Hillel AD. Idiopathic bilateral vocal fold weakness. *Laryngoscope.* 1999;109:995–1002.

41. Tanaka S, Hirano M, Chijiwa K. Some aspects of vocal fold bowing. *Ann Otol Rhinol Laryngol.* 1994;103:357–362.

42. Dray TG, Robinson LR, Hillel AD. Laryngeal electromyographic findings in Charcot-Marie-Tooth disease type II. *Arch Neurol.* 1999;56:863–865.

43. Robinson LR, Hillel AD, Waugh PF. New laryngeal muscle weakness in post-polio syndrome. *Laryngoscope.* 1998;108:732–734.

44. Driscoll BP, Gracco C, Coelho C, et al. Laryngeal function in postpolio patients. *Laryngoscope.* 1995;105:35–41.

45. Guindi GM, Bannister R, Gibson WP, Payne JK. Laryngeal electromyography in multiple system atrophy with autonomic failure. *J Neurol Neurosurg Psychiatry.* 1981;44:49–53.

46. Isozaki E, Osanai R, Horiguchi S, Hayashida T, Hirose K, Tanabe H. Laryngeal electromyography with separated surface electrodes in patients with multiple system atrophy presenting with vocal cord paralysis. *J Neurol.* 1994;241:551–556.

47. Palmer JB, Holloway AM, Tanaka E. Detecting lower motor neuron dysfunction of the pharynx and larynx with electromyography. *Arch Phys Med Rehabil.* 1991;72:214–218.

48. Blitzer A, Lovelace RE, Brin MF, Fahn S, Fink ME. Electromyographic findings in focal laryngeal dystonia (spasmodic dysphonia). *Ann Otol Rhinol Laryngol.* 1985;94:591–594.

49. Lipton RJ, McCaffrey TV, Litchy WJ. Intraoperative electrophysiologic monitoring of laryngeal muscle during thyroid surgery. *Laryngoscope.* 1988;98:1292–1296.

50. Mermelstein M, Nonweiler R, Rubinstein EH. Intraoperative identification of laryngeal nerves with laryngeal electromyography. *Laryngoscope.* 1996;106:752–756.

51. Brin MF, Blitzer A, Stewart C, Fahn S. Treatment of spasmodic dysphonia (laryngeal dystonia) with local injections of botulinum toxin: review and technical aspects. In: Blitzer A, Brin MF, Sasaki CT, Fahn S, Harris KS, eds. *Neurologic Disorders of the Larynx.* New York, NY: Thieme Medical Publishers; 1992:214–228.

52. Woodson GE. Clinical value of laryngeal EMG is dependent on experience of the clinician. *Arch Otolaryngol Head Neck Surg.* 1998;124:476.

19

Laryngeal Photography and Videography

Eiji Yanagisawa, MD, FACS
Brian P. Driscoll, MD, FACS
H. Steven Sims, MD

The Spanish-born singing teacher Manuel García is credited with the first successful visualization of the intact larynx. In 1854, using a dental mirror, with a hand-held mirror for reflecting sunlight, he was able to visualize the movements of his own vocal folds.[1] The first successful photographs of the larynx were taken by Thomas French of New York in 1882. Using a box camera with an attached laryngeal mirror and a device to concentrate sunlight (Figure 19–1A), he was able to produce surprisingly good quality black-and-white photographs (Figure 19–1B).[2,3]

Since the early photographs of the larynx by French, many other methods of laryngeal documentation have been described. These include: (1) indirect laryngoscopic photography,[4,5] (2) direct laryngoscopic photography,[4,6-9] (3) fiberscopic photography,[10-28] (4) telescopic photography,[19,21-24,26-48] and (5) microscopic photography.[5,29,49-58] Although many have contributed to the evolution and refinement of laryngeal documentation, several authors merit special mention.

In 1941, P. Holinger, J. D. Brubaker, and J. E. Brubaker introduced the Holinger and Brubaker 35 mm camera.[6,8] This camera, although expensive and bulky, set a new standard for laryngeal photography. Most would agree that the clarity, color, and brilliance of these photographs have not been surpassed even by today's standards. This system is no longer used.

In 1954, Yutaka Tsuiki of Tohoku University, Japan, was the first to "televise" the larynx. He used a "tele-endoscope" attached to a large television camera. He predicted the importance of video recording the larynx as a method of documentation and teaching.[59]

In 1963, Oscar Kleinsasser of Cologne adapted the Zeiss otologic microscope for laryngoscopic use by utilizing a 400-mm objective lens.[51-53] Later with the use of a photoadapter, beam splitter, and single lens reflex (SLR) camera, he produced extremely high-quality pictures of the larynx.[52]

In 1968, Sawashima and Hirose of Tokyo introduced the flexible laryngoscope.[14] This instrument is

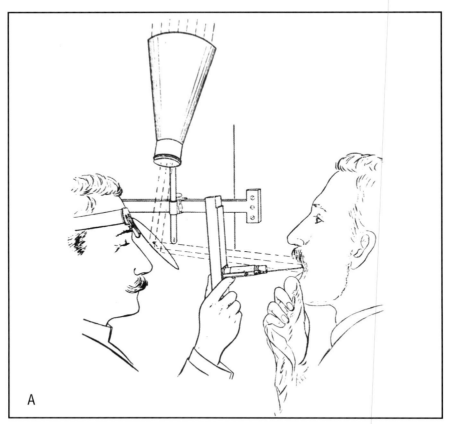

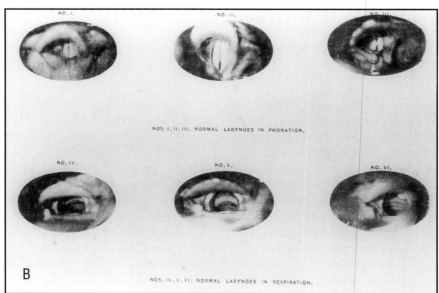

Figure 19–1. A. Dr. French's method of laryngeal documentation used in 1882. He used a sunlight concentrator as a light source. The light was then reflected off a forehead reflector onto a laryngeal mirror. **B.** Sample photographs taken by Dr. French.

now standard equipment for the practicing otolaryngologist. The quality of photodocumentation through this instrument, although acceptable, is not of high resolution. The advent of modern telescopes such as the

the following: (1) use an extra-light-sensitive video camera (low lux), (2) increase the video camera sensitivity by using the gain control switch, (3) advance the tip of the fiberscope very close to the vocal folds, (4) change the image size by using a zoom adapter for a micro CCD camera, or (5) use a fiberscope with a large diameter such as the Olympus ENF-L3 (4.2 mm) (Figure 19–13B). The image and color quality can also be improved during printing using adjustment control of the color video printer.

Telescopic Videolaryngoscopy

Telescopic videolaryngoscopy[23,26,28,62-66] is performed using much the same technique as the fiberscopic method, except that the telescope is passed through the mouth and the camera is connected to a telescope instead of a fiberscope. This method gives a brilliant picture and is particularly well-suited for diagnosing subtle changes in laryngeal structure.

The necessary equipment includes a single- or three-chip CCD miniature camera or a video camera, and a rigid telescope such as the (1) Karl Storz 8706CL, (2) Kay Elemetrics 9105, (3) Nagashima SFT-1, (4) Wolf Stuckrad, or (5) Karl Storz 8702D. These telescopes are attached to the CCD camera via a special adapter if the CCD camera does not have a built-in adapter. The 70 degree telescopes such as the Nagashima SFT-1, Karl Storz 8706CL, and Kay Elemetrics 9105 permit excellent visualization of the anterior commissure and posterior portions of the larynx, which makes them especially useful for laryngostroboscopy.

The examination is performed in the following manner: (1) the patient's soft palate and posterior tongue are anesthetized with 4% Xylocaine (lidocaine), (2) the scope is dipped in warm water or sprayed with defogger, (3) the patient's tongue is grasped by the examiner with one hand while the scope is inserted with the other hand, keeping the glossoepiglottic fold in the midline while advancing the scope, ensuring optimal (midline) orientation of the larynx (Figure 19–14A), and (4) video recording is begun when the vocal folds are in clear focus.

The major benefit of this system is the superior optics offered by the telescope. This provides (1) a wide-angle view of the larynx with a large, clear image and (2) a close-up view of the larynx to detect subtle anatomic lesions. The larger diameter of the scope also allows for increased light transmission and a much brighter and clearer stroboscopic image. The disadvantages of this technique include the following: (1) children and some adults with hyperactive gag reflexes may be unable to tolerate the examination, (2) fogging of the scope requires cleaning and reinsertion,

and (3) voice and vocal mechanics may be distorted.

The authors prefer the telescopic examination because of the superior image produced (Figure 19–14B): the image is larger, brighter, and sharper than that of the fiberscope. This translates to increased diagnostic capabilities for subtle laryngeal changes. In the authors' hands, this technique has a 90% success rate.

Microscopic Videolaryngoscopy

This technique is similar to that described for microscopic still photography in the office using the Zeiss operating microscope. The only difference is that a video camera hookup is used instead of an SLR camera. This technique (as one might expect) is time-consuming and awkward. The authors have abandoned this technique in favor of the techniques described above.

Videography in the Operating Room

Telescopic Videolaryngoscopy

In the operating room, telescopic videolaryngoscopy[62,64-66] is accomplished with the use of the straight-forward Hopkins rigid telescope 8700A, a miniature CCD camera (Figure 19–15A), and a xenon light source. In this setting, the miniature CCD camera is more useful and convenient than the home video camera. After the laryngoscope is suspended, the telescope is placed through the laryngoscope and the image is centered. The advantage of this system is the splendid image quality (Figure 19–15B). With the use of a color video printer, still images can be obtained easily during or after the procedure. The major disadvantages are that (1) it requires interruption of the surgical procedure and (2) it is difficult to document surgical technique.

The senior author always passes the 0° telescope for documentation prior to microlaryngoscopic surgery as he believes telescopic videolaryngoscopy provides the best possible laryngeal images. In selected cases, he uses the other angled telescopes (30°, 70°, 90°, 120°). The 30° and 70° telescopes allow excellent visualization of the anterior commissure. The 70° and 90° telescopes are useful for evaluation and documentation of laryngeal ventricles. The inferior border of the true vocal fold lesion can be readily identified with the 70° or 120° telescopes. The involvement of the anterior commissure by an anterior lesion of the vocal fold can be precisely identified with the 30° and 70° telescopes in most cases.

Telescopic video documentation of subglottic lesions in a tracheotomized patient can be performed through

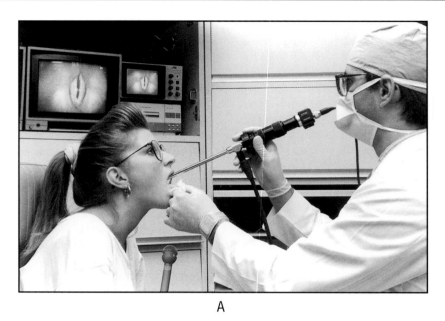

A

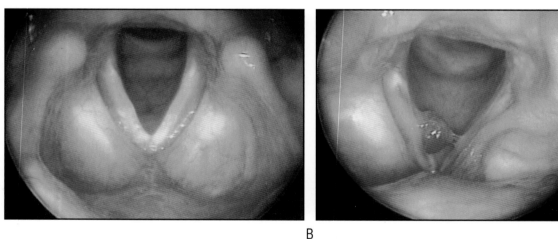

B

Figure 19–14. A. Method of telescopic videolaryngoscopy in the office using the 70 degree Nagashima SFT-1 telescope attached to the miniature CCD camera, Elmo EC-202 with Nagashima videoadapter. **B.** Images of a normal larynx (*left*) and a laryngeal polyp (*right*) taken with this method. The images were produced with a Sony UP-5100 video printer.

a tracheotomy opening using the Hopkins 4-mm 70° telescope.

Microscopic Videolaryngoscopy

Microscopic videolaryngoscopy[26] remains the single most convenient and effective method to teach and document microsurgery of the larynx. This is the authors' preferred method of operative documentation.[26]

The equipment used includes: (1) a photographic laryngoscope such as the Dedo or Ossoff (these laryngoscopes have two channels that house large-bore fiberoptic cables); (2) a light source, such as the Pilling 2X; (3) the (Zeiss) operating microscope with a straight eyepiece and 400-mm objective lens (Figure 19–16A); (4) a beam splitter; (5) a photoadapter, such as the Zeiss or Telestill photoadapter; (6) a miniature CCD camera or pickup tube camera (Figure 19–16A); (7) a video recorder; and (8) a color TV monitor. With their small size and weight, the miniature CCD cameras interfere minimally with the operative procedure. However, the more expensive and bulkier three-tube cameras, such as the Hitachi DK5050 or Ikegami ITC-350 M, produce video images of excellent quality (Figure

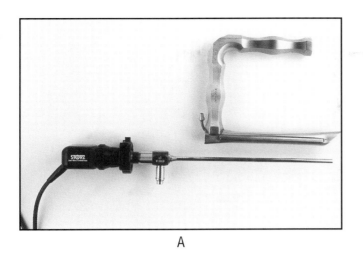

A

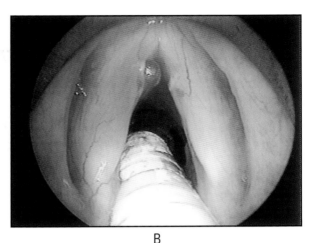

B

Figure 19–15. A. Telescopic videolaryngoscopy in the operating room using the Dedo laryngoscope and the Karl Storz Supercam CCD miniature camera attached to the 8700A 0 degree telescope. **B.** Image of a laryngeal polyp taken with this system. The image was produced with a Sony UP-5100 video printer.

19–16A and B). For those seeking the highest-quality images, the three-tube cameras have been replaced with the newer three-chip cameras, such as the Sony DXC-750 ($16,000) and Hitachi, Ikegami, or Stryker three-chip camera. Sony introduced a moderately priced three-chip CCD camera, Sony DXC 960 MD (approximately $6,000) in 1993.

Some of the multiple advantages of this system are: (1) minimal interference with the operative procedure, (2) live viewing by an unlimited audience, (3) equipment that is readily available in most medical centers, (4) variability of magnification, facilitating precise documentation of small lesions, (5) pediatric and adult use, (6) video documentation for teaching surgical techniques, and (7) the capability of producing instant color prints of publication quality when a color video printer is used. Among the disadvantages are: (1) the depth of field is shallower, (2) instrumentation is more difficult, as the microscope is between the surgeon and the patient, (3) at times surgery must be carried out through one eyepiece because of the small proximal opening of the laryngoscope, and (4) refocusing at various magnifications may be necessary.

Kantor-Berci Telescopic Videomicrolaryngoscope

In 1990, Kantor, Berci, Partlow et al introduced a new approach to microlaryngeal surgery and its documentation.[39] Their method is akin to performing endoscopic sinus surgery. Using a specially designed microlaryngoscope that houses a rigid telescope with attached camera, they are able to both video-record and perform the operation while viewing a high-resolution TV screen (Figure 19–17A and B). The required equipment includes: (1) a Kantor-Berci videomicrolaryngoscope (Karl Storz 8590 VJ) (an improved model is now available) and Lewy (or other) laryngoscope holder; (2) a Karl Storz Supercam micro CCD video camera; (3) a xenon light source (Karl Storz 615, or 487C); (4) a large, high-resolution TV monitor and recorder; and (5) a color video printer (Sony UP-5100).

Some of the advantages of the Kantor-Berci system include the following: (1) it gives a clear, sharp image with excellent depth of field, (2) it facilitates instrumentation of the larynx, as the microscope is not between the surgeon and patient, and (3) it provides superior documentation. Some disadvantages are that: (1) the equipment is costly, (2) specialized equipment such as the angled forceps are needed, (3) it requires a dedicated video camera, (4) refocusing may be necessary (Supercam camera) when the zoom lens is used, (5) there is some image distortion, and (6) depth perception may be impaired because the system creates a monocular image.

In a series of patients, the senior author (EY) has compared this technique with the standard microscope technique at the same setting. While the Kantor-Berci system is an effective means of documenting laryngeal surgery and offers superior visualization of the anterior larynx with an excellent depth of field, the microscopic system has the advantage of variable magnification with a depth of field that is generally better than expected, and permits true binocular vision.

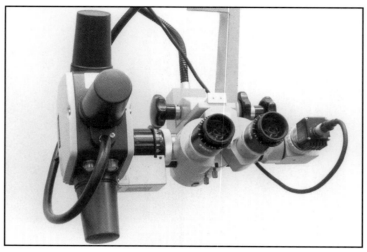

A

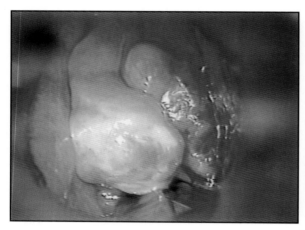
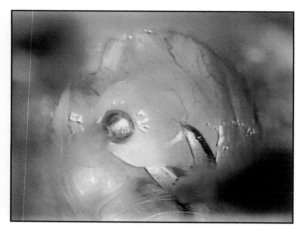

B

Figure 19–16. A. Techniques for microscopic videography. Coupled to the left of the Zeiss microscope is the Hitachi three-tube camera attached to a beam splitter. By comparison, coupled to the right of the scope is the Elmo EC-202 mini CCD camera attached to the Zeiss photoadapter. **B.** Images taken with this technique demonstrating obstructive laryngeal polyps (*left*) and excision of a polyp with scissors (*right*). Images were produced with a Sony UP-5100 video printer.

Video Image Transfer to Print and Slide

Video images can be transferred to either prints or slides, in color or black and white. This can be accomplished in several ways.

Production of Prints

This can be accomplished instantaneously while videotaping, or at a later viewing through the use of the video printers (Figure 19–18A-C).[26,41] The authors initially used the Sony UP-5000 (Figure 19–18A) but currently prefer the Sony UP-5100 or UP-5500 color video printer, which produces a superior high-resolution image. However, this unit is quite expensive ($7,000 to $8,000). The more affordable Sony CVP G700 ($1,500) or Sony DPM 1000 ($400) (Figure 19–18B), which produces very acceptable images, may be used. However, the time required to produce a print is longer with less expensive printers. Black-and-white prints for publication can also be made by photographing the color video printouts using black-and-white film (such as ASA 400 Tri-X or T-Max). Prints can also be made using a computer, as described in the following digital imaging section.

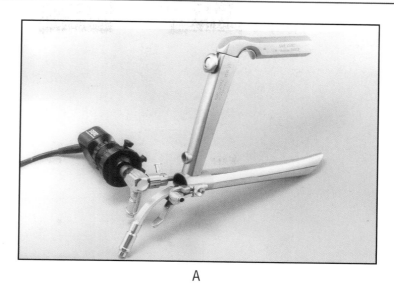

A

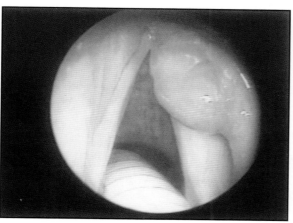

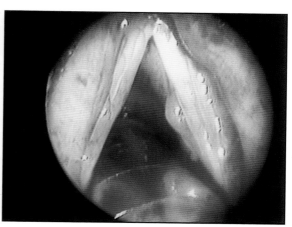

B

Figure 19–17. A. Kantor-Berci's video microlaryngoscopic technique. Karl Storz Supercam CCD miniature camera is attached to the specially designed telescope (Karl Storz 8575A) and inserted into the built-in channel on the left side of the Kantor-Berci video microlaryngoscope (Karl Storz 8590B). **B.** Images taken with this technique showing a false vocal fold polyp (*left*) and laryngeal polyp (*right*). Images were produced with a Sony UP-5100 video printer.

Production of Slides

There are several methods of producing slides from video images. The first is to photograph the video image on the TV screen (TV screen photography) (Figure 19–18 D-F).[26,62-64,67] The equipment necessary is: (1) a 35-mm SLR camera, (2) Ektachrome Daylight ASA 400 color film, (3) a 50-mm macrolens, (4) a tripod, and (5) an orange-colored filter (Kodak CC40R or Tiffen CC40) when using color film. The camera is placed on the tripod (Figure 19–18D), and the laryngeal image on the TV screen is brought into focus. The shutter speed should be one-half per second or slower (thus the need for the tripod) to cut out interference (raster)

lines. For best results the room should be dark to avoid glare on the TV screen, and the video player should be in the play mode. In the pause mode, unwanted horizontal lines may be seen either at the top or bottom of the screen. Each photograph is usually bracketed (–1, 0, +1) using the exposure compensation dial on the camera. This is the least expensive method of producing quite satisfactory results.

The second method of slide production is to copy the color video printouts using color slide film (Ektachrome ASA 320 Tungsten film).

The third method is to use a video/slide making system such as Sony Slidemaker MD, which receives RGB video signals from a color printer (Sony UP

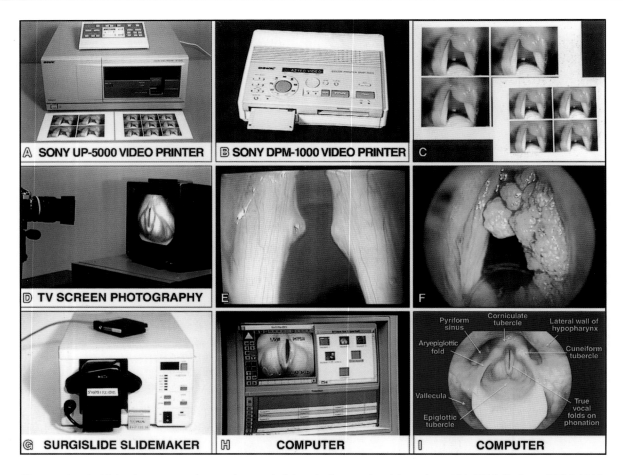

Figure 19–18. Video image transfer to prints and slides. **A.** Sony color video printer UP-5000. **B.** Sony DPM-1000 color video printer. **C.** Color video prints produced by Sony UP-5100 and by Sony CVP-G700. **D.** TV screen photography. **E.** Image of laryngeal nodules produced by TV screen photography. **F.** Image of transglottic laryngeal carcinoma produced by TV screen photography. **G.** Stryker Surgislide slide maker. **H.** Digitized laryngeal image on the computer screen, which can be annotated. Prints are made using a digital color printer. **I.** Annotated image of the normal larynx produced by a digital color printer Sony UP-5500.

5100/5500) and allows one to photograph the desired image with its attached 35-mm camera (ISO 100 or Polachrome ISO 40 color slide film).

The fourth method is by the use of the Stryker Surgislide Slidemaker (Figure 19–18G). This is a relatively new analog image capture device for the production of 35-mm slides from either a video camera during videography or a prerecorded video image later. The recommended film is ASA 100 Professional Daylight Ektachrome. A 35-mm automatic SLR camera is attached to the front of the image capture device. This system produces excellent color slides. The advantage of the Stryker Slidemaker is the ability to capture images directly onto 35-mm slide film without the need for additional hardware or software. However, the disadvantage is its high cost (approximately $9,000).

Documentation by Digital Imaging

Digital imaging is the newest technology for permanently recording images without film.

There are a number of advantages to digital imaging: (1) the image is produced immediately and thus can be "re-shot" if needed, (2) the image can be transferred via modem to other computers for immediate consultation, (3) the image does not degrade with time, (4) various types of editing of the image are possible, (5) images taken over time can be displayed on one screen, (6) storage and retrieval of images is much simpler, and (7) photographic quality resolution is possible (though expensive). Disadvantages include the initial start-up expense and the time needed to master the system.[68]

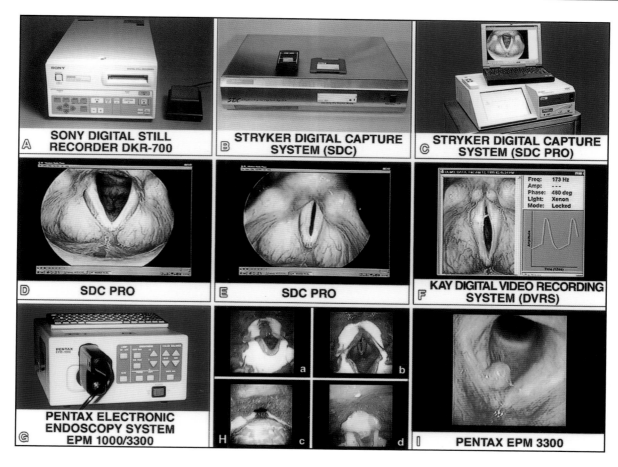

Figure 19–19. Documentation by digital imaging. **A.** Sony digital still recorder DKR-700. **B.** Stryker Digital Capture System SDC. It captures still images only. **C.** Stryker Digital Capture System SDC Pro. It captures both still and motion images. **D.** Computer still image of the larynx on inspiration captured by Stryker SDC Pro. **E.** Computer still image of the larynx on phonation captured by Stryker SDC Pro. **F.** Still computer image of stroboscopic view of the vocal folds on phonation captured by Kay digital video recording system. Note on-screen display of an EGG waveform. **G.** Pentax electronic endoscopy system EPM 1000 (a newer smaller version of EPM 3300). This is an excellent device to capture still images in single and multiple image formats. **H.** Still images of swallowed milk in various stages taken with Pentax EPM 3300. **I.** Computer still image of the laryngeal polyp captured by Pentax EPM 3300.

The image can be digitized from a video camera, a digital camera (still or video), a videotape, a slide, a print, or a negative.

Laryngeal documentation can be accomplished by digitizing images from prerecorded videotape (Figure 19–18H and I). Video recording has been the senior author's method for many years. Software is available that can capture video images either as still frames or as full-motion video. These digitized images may be made into composite pictures, labeled, and saved as a computer file. The image may be printed with a digital printer. The authors use the Sony UP-5500 digital color video printer, which utilizes a dye sublimation printing process. This printer produces high-quality photo-realistic prints suitable for publication (Figure

19–18I), although the printer is quite expensive (approximately $9,000). Less expensive digital color printers are available. Color slides may be obtained by photographing these computer prints. Alternatively, the computer file may be transferred to photo prints or 35-mm slides by a computer service bureau, usually via high-capacity removable storage devices such as Zip disks, optical drives, or compact disks (CDs).

More recently, still digital image capture devices such as the Sony DKR-700 Digital Still Recorder, the Stryker Digital Capture System SDC, and the Stryker Digital Capture System SDC Pro have become available and can be used for laryngeal imaging. The digital recording systems such as the Kay Digital video recording system (DVRS) and the Pentax Electronics video recording system are useful for digital imaging of the larynx.

Sony Digital Still Recorder

The Sony DKR-700 (Figure 19–19A) is a compact digital still recorder. It captures the images and stores them on convenient high capacity 2.5 inch Sony MD data disks. The images can be easily retrieved, sorted, and annotated. It can store 100 noncompressed images on a MD data disk. The advantages of Sony DKR-700 include its compatibility with popular software programs. A disadvantage of the Sony DKR-700 is its long capture time (approximately 28 seconds). This means that during these 28 seconds, the surgeon cannot take another picture. This is unacceptable for laryngeal documentation unless the capture time is shortened in future versions of this product.

Stryker Digital Capture System SDC

The Stryker SDC (Figure 19–19B) is a device which instantly transports surgical images to a high-density computer disk. Software is available which allows for annotation and enhancement of the images. This system is simple to operate. No adjustments are necessary. Images can be saved as a standard bit-map file, which means that they are uncompressed. Image capture time is very fast (about one second) and the system is quite acceptable for laryngeal documentation. The cost of this system is approximately $10,000.

Stryker Digital Capture System SDC Pro

The Stryker SDC Pro (Figure 19–19C-E) capture device is a newer version of the Stryker SDC and can be used to record still images or video segments. Housed within the device are a central processing unit (CPU) and hard drive that can capture digital images or streaming video onto a writeable CD (compact disk). The CD system included within the Stryker SDC Pro digital capture device is the CDWriter Plus 9100 series.

The CD has become the standard for data storage, accessible using either a Macintosh or Windows based operating system. A single CD may hold approximately 650 images captured in bit-map (BMP) format, or approximately 12,000 images in compressed Joint Photographic Expert Group (JPEG) format. Alternatively, a single CD may record up to 20 minutes of continuous video, and a CD may contain a mixture of both still images and video. Capture is nearly immediate without hardware delay.

Advantages to the new Stryker SDC Pro system include the ability to capture not only still images but also streaming video. Although the Zip format used for the Stryker SDC is a popular medium for storage, the CD is a more universally accepted medium for data storage and retrieval. The Stryker SDC Pro allows for the import of images and video into popular software applications for digital annotation, such as Microsoft PowerPoint.

The Stryker SDC Pro system is an excellent technique for documentation of still and motion images of the larynx. The main disadvantages of this system is its high cost (approximately $13,000).

Kay Digital Video Recording System (DVRS)

The Kay digital video recording system (DVRS) (Figure 19–19F) is a newer version of its previous 9100 Stroboscopy Recording System based on VHS or S-VHS videotape recorders. Unlike its predecessor, the DVRS records video images directly to computer storage media. It captures both full-motion video and high-resolution still images. Audio and video are captured together. Image retrieval is easy. It allows instantaneous review of the data, and allows on-screen display of important information such as an EGG waveform (Figure 19–19F).

Pentax Electronic Endoscopy System EPM 1000/3300

The Pentax electronic videoendoscopic system (Figure 19–19G-I) is a highly integrated digital imaging system, utilizing the Pentax EPM 3300 (the EPM 1000 is a smaller unit used for laryngoscopic imaging) and a flexible electronic videolaryngoscope. It was primarily developed for the evaluation of gastrointestinal disorders. However, more recently it has been used for evaluation of the larynx and pharynx. It is useful for the study of swallowing disorders (Figure 19–19H). The Pentax flexible electrolaryngoscope, which has a CCD chip at the tip of the endoscope, provides remarkably clear images of the larynx and hypopharynx (Figure 19–19I). Images of various stages of swallowing of milk taken with the Pentax system are shown in Figure 19–19H.

The Pentax electronic videoendoscopy system has an excellent image capture device. It captures instantaneously. Images can be obtained in single, four, or nine-in-one formats and can be videoprinted right after the examination. The main disadvantage is its cost.

So far, all chip-tip camera flexible endoscopes have had their camera systems combined with their light sources. Therefore, despite their excellent image quality, they cannot be connected to a stroboscope. Recently, Olympus has developed a prototype chip-tip laryngoscope that works with any light source (including a stroboscope) and shows great promise for advancing diagnostic laryngeal imaging (Robert T. Sataloff, MD, personal communication, August 2000).

CONCLUSION

Laryngeal documentation can be accomplished by videography, still photography, and digital imaging. Various methods of these modalities in the office and in the operating room setting are described.

Still photography remains a valuable method of laryngeal documentation for those who own or are familiar with still photographic equipment. The photographic images obtained through the telescope are clearly superior to those captured through the fiberscope. The main disadvantage of still photography is that one cannot see the results until the films are developed.

At the beginning of this new century (2000), videography is the most versatile and useful means of laryngeal documentation because it permits excellent demonstration of anatomy, pathology, and physiology with simultaneous voice recording. It also serves as an important source for digital imaging. With the use of a color video printer, high-resolution video prints of laryngeal pathology can be obtained instantaneously for medical records and educational purposes. The image can also be replayed immediately after the procedure and shown to the patient.

Videography of the larynx in the office can be accomplished by using a flexible fiberscope or a rigid telescope. Fiberscopic documentation results in images with less resolution but permits examination of laryngeal motion and can be performed in children and adults with hyperactive gag reflexes. Telescopic documentation provides superior structural images with high resolution.

Videography of the larynx in the operating room can be accomplished by means of microscopic, telescopic, and direct laryngoscopic videolaryngoscopy. Microscopic video documentation is currently the preferred method of documenting laryngeal pathology and teaching microlaryngeal surgery. Telescopic videography through the laryngoscope using a (0°, 30°, 70°, 90°, or 120°) telescope produces the clearest images of the larynx.

Digital imaging is the newest technology for permanently recording images. Digital imaging of the larynx can be accomplished by transferring video images from a prerecorded videotape into a computer. High-quality color prints can be produced utilizing a dye sublimation digital color printer. Digital imaging of the larynx can now be accomplished without film or videotape by utilizing a newer digital image capture device such as the Stryker Digital Capture System. This device captures laryngeal still images from a video camera and quickly transports them to a computer disk from which slides and prints can be generated. The newer digital capture systems record both still and motion images.

Advantages of digital imaging include: (1) safe, long-term storage without image degradation, (2) easy computer manipulation and retrieval, and (3) production of superior quality images using a digital printer. Disadvantages are the high cost of the system and the constantly evolving technologic improvements, which make the systems obsolete quickly and make upgrades necessary.

As this new technology improves and the cost of digital imaging decreases, the use of digital imaging of the larynx will likely become widespread.

REFERENCES

1. Garcia M. Observations on the human voice. *Proc R Soc Lond.* 1855;7:399–420.
2. French TR. On photographing the larynx. *Trans Am Laryngol.* 1882;4:32–35.
3. French TR. On a perfected method of photographing the larynx. *NY Med J.* 1884;4:655–656.
4. Ferguson GB, Crowder WJ. A simple method of laryngeal and other cavity photography. *Arch Otolaryngol.* 1970;92:201–203.
5. Padovan IF, Christman NT, Hamilton LH, et al. Indirect microlaryngoscopy. *Laryngoscope.* 1973;83:2035–2041.
6. Holinger PH. Photography of the larynx, trachea, bronchi and esophagus. *Trans Am Acad Ophthalmol Otolaryngol.* 1942;46:153–156.
7. Holinger PH, Tardy ME. Photography in otorhinolaryngology and bronchoesophagology. In: English GM, ed. *Otolaryngology.* Vol 5. Philadelphia, PA: Lippincott; 1986: chap 22.
8. Holinger PH, Brubaker JD, Brubaker JE: Open tube, proximal illumination mirror and direct laryngeal photography. *Can J Otolaryngol.* 1975;4:781–785.
9. Rosnagle R, Smith HW. Hand-held fundus camera for endoscopic photography. *Trans Am Acad Ophthalmol Otolaryngol.* 1972;76:1024–1025.
10. Brewer DW, McCall G. Visible laryngeal changes during voice study. *Ann Otol Rhinol Laryngol.* 1974;83:423–427.
11. Davidson TM, Bone RC, Nahum AM. Flexible fiberoptic laryngo-bronchoscopy. *Laryngoscope.* 1974;84:1876–1882.
12. Hirano M. *Clinical Evaluation of Voice (Disorders of Human Communication, 5).* New York, NY: Springer-Verlag Wien; 1981.
13. Inoue T. Examination of child larynx by flexible fiberoptic laryngoscope. *Int J Pediatr Otorhinolaryngol.* 1983;5:317–323.

14. Sawashima M, Hirose H. New laryngoscopic technique by use of fiberoptics. *J Acoust Soc Am.* 1968;43:168–169.

15. Selkin SG. Flexible fiberoptics for laryngeal photography. *Laryngoscope.* 1983;93:657–658.

16. Selkin SG. The otolaryngologist and flexible fiberoptics—photographic considerations. *J Otolaryngol.* 1983; 12:223–227.

17. Silberman HD, Wilf H, Tucker JA. Flexible fiberoptic nasopharyngolaryngoscope. *Ann Otol Rhinol Laryngol.* 1976;85:640–645.

18. Yamashita K. Endonasal flexible fiberoptic endoscopy. *Rhinology.* 1983;21:233–237.

19. Yamashita K. *Diagnostic and Therapeutic ENT Endoscopy.* Tokyo, Japan: Medical View; 1988.

20. Yamashita K, Mertens J, Rudert H. Die flexible Fiberendoskopie in der HNO-Heildunde. *HNO.* 1984;32:378–384.

21. Yamashita K, Oku T, Tanaka H, et al. VTR endoscopy. *J Otolaryngol Jp.* 1977;80:1208–1209.

22. Yanagisawa E. Videolaryngoscopy using a low cost home video system color camera. *J Biol Photogr.* 1984; 52:9–14.

23. Yanagisawa E. Videolaryngoscopy. In: Lee KJ, Stewart CH, eds. *Ambulatory Surgery and Office Procedures in Head and Neck Surgery.* Orlando, FL: Grune & Stratton; 1986:chap 6.

24. Yanagisawa E, Carlson RD. Physical diagnosis of the hypopharynx and the larynx with and without imaging. In: Lee KJ, ed. *Textbook of Otolaryngology and Head and Neck Surgery.* New York, NY: Elsevier; 1989:chap 37.

25. Yanagisawa E, Yamashita K. Fiberoptic nasopharyngolaryngoscopy. In: Lee KJ, Stewart CH, eds. *Amburatory Surgery and Office Procedures in Head and Neck Surgery.* Orlando, FL: Grune & Stratton; 1986:31–40.

26. Yanagisawa E, Yanagisawa R. Laryngeal photography. *Otolaryngol Clin North Am.* 1991;24:999–1022.

27. Yanagisawa E, Carlson RD, Strothers G. Videography of the larynx—fiberscope or telescope? In: Clement PAR, ed. *Recent Advances in ENT—Endoscopy.* Brussels, Belgium: Scientific Society for Medical Information; 1985:175–183.

28. Yanagisawa E, Owens TW, Strothers G, et al. Videolaryngoscopy—a comparison of fiberscopic and telescopic documentation. *Ann Otol Rhinol Laryngol.* 1983;92:430–436.

29. Alberti PW. Still photography of the larynx—an overview. *Can J Otolaryngol.* 1975;4:759–765.

30. Albrecht R. Zur Photographie des Kehlkopfes. *HNO.* 1956;5:196–199.

31. Andrew AH. Laryngeal telescope. *Trans Am Acad Ophthalmol Otolaryngol.* 1962;66:268.

32. Benjamin B. Technique of laryngeal photography. *Ann Otol Rhinol Laryngol.* 1984;93:(suppl 109).

33. Benjamin B. *Diagnostic Laryngology—Adults and Children.* Philadelphia, PA: Saunders; 1990.

34. Berci G. *Endoscopy.* New York, NY: Appleton-Century-Crofts; 1976.

35. Berci G, Caldwell FH. A device to facilitate photography during indirect laryngoscopy. *Med Biol Illus.* 1963;13:169–176.

36. Berci G, Calcaterra T, Ward PH. Advances in endoscopic techniques for examination of the larynx and nasopharynx. *Can J Otolaryngol.* 1975;4:786–792.

37. Gould WJ. The Gould laryngoscope. *Trans Am Acad Ophthalmol Otolaryngol.* 1973;77:139–141.

38. Hahn C, Kitzing P. Indirect endoscopic photography of the larynx—a comparison between two newly constructed laryngoscopes. *J Audiov Media Med.* 1978;1:121–130.

39. Kantor E, Berci G, Partlow E, et al. A completely new approach to microlaryngeal surgery. *Laryngoscope.* 1991; 101:678–679.

40. Konrad HR, Hopla DM, Bussen J, et al. Use of video tape in diagnosis and treatment of cancer of larynx. *Ann Otol Rhinol Laryngol.* 1981;90:398–400.

41. Mambrino L, Yanagisawa E, Yanagisawa K, et al. Endoscopic ENT photography—a comparison of pictures by standard color films and newer color video printers. *Laryngoscope.* 1991;101:1229–1232.

42. Muller-Hermann F, Pedersen P. Modern endoscopic and microscopic photography in otolaryngology. *Ann Otol Rhinol Laryngol.* 1984;93:399.

43. Oeken FW, Brandt RH. Lupenkontrolle endolaryngealer Operationen Modifikation der Schwenklupenhalterung nach Brunings. *HNO.* 1967;15:210–211.

44. Steiner W, Jaumann MP. Moderne otorhinolaryngologische Endoskopie beim Kind. *Padiat Prax.* 1978;20:429–435.

45. Stuckrad H, Lakatos I. Uber ein neues Lupenlaryngoskop (Epipharyngoskop). *Laryngol Rhinol Otol.* 1975; 54:336–340.

46. Ward PH, Berci G, Calcaterra TC. Advances in endoscopic examination of the respiratory system. *Ann Otol Rhinol Laryngol.* 1974;83:754–760.

47. Yanagisawa E. Office telescopic photography of the larynx. *Ann Otol Rhinol Laryngol.* 1982;91:354–358.

48. Yanagisawa E, Casuccio JR, Suzuki M. Video laryngoscopy using a rigid telescope and video home system color camera—a useful office procedure. *Ann Otol Rhinol Laryngol.* 1981;90:346–350.

49. Jako GJ. Laryngoscope for microscopic observations, surgery and photography. *Arch Otolaryngol.* 1970;91:196–199.

50. Jako GJ, Strong S. Laryngeal photography. *Arch Otolaryngol.* 1972;96:268–271.

51. Kleinsasser O. Entwicklung und Methoden der Kehlkopffotografie (Mit Beschreibung eines neuen einfachen Fotolaryngoskopes). *HNO.* 1963;1:171–176.

52. Kleinsasser O. *Microlaryngoscopy and Endolaryngeal Microsurgery.* Philadelphia, PA: Saunders; 1968.

53. Kleinsasser O. *Tumors of the Larynx and Hypopharynx.* New York, NY: Thieme; 1988:124–130.

54. Olofsson J, Ohlsson T. Techniques in microlaryngoscopic photography. *Can J Otolaryngol.* 1975;4:770–780.

55. Scalo AN, Shipman WF, Tabb HG. Microscopic suspension laryngoscopy. *Ann Otol Rhinol Laryngol.* 1960;69:1134–1138.

56. Strong MS. Laryngeal photography. *Can J Otolaryngol.* 1975;4:766–769.

57. Tardy ME, Tenta LT. Laryngeal photography and television. *Otolaryngol Clin North Am*. 1970;3:483–492.

58. Yanagisawa E, Eibling DE, Suzuki M. A simple method of laryngeal photography through the operating microscope—"Macrolens technique." *Ann Otol Rhinol Laryngol*. 1980;89:547–550.

59. Tsuiki Y. *Laryngeal Examination*. Tokyo, Japan. Kanehara Shuppan; 1956.

60. Benjamin B. Art and science of laryngeal photography. (Eighteenth Daniel C. Baker, Jr, Memorial Lecture). *Ann Otol Rhinol Laryngol*. 1993;102:271–282.

61. Yanagisawa E, Carlson RD. Videophotolaryngography using a new low cost video printer. *Ann Otol Rhinol Laryngol*. 1985;94:584–587.

62. Yanagisawa E. Documentation. In: Ferlito A, ed. *Neoplasms of the Larynx*. Edinburgh, Scotland: Churchill Livingstone; 1993:chap 21.

63. Yanagisawa E, Weaver EM. Videolaryngoscopy: equipment and documentation. In: Blitzer A, et al, eds. *Office-Based Surgery in Otolaryngology*. New York, NY: Thieme; 1998:chap 25.

64. Yanagisawa E. Videography and laryngeal photography. In: Ferlito A, ed. *Diseases of the Larynx*. London, England: Arnold, 2000:chap 7.

65. Yanagisawa E, Horowitz JB, Yanagisawa K, et al. Comparison of new telescopic video microlaryngoscopic and standard microlaryngoscopic techniques. *Ann Otol Rhinol Laryngol*. 1992;101:51–60.

66. Yanagisawa K, Yanagisawa E. Current diagnosis and office practice—technique of endoscopic imaging of the larynx. *Curr Op Otolaryngol Head Neck Surg*. 1996;4:147–153.

67. Yanagisawa K, Shi J, Yanagisawa E. Color photography of video images of otolaryngological structures using a 35 mm SLR camera. *Laryngoscope*. 1987;97:992–993.

68. Stone JL, Peterson RL, Wolf JE. Digital imaging techniques in dermatology. *J Am Acad Dermatol*. 1990;23:913–917.

20

3D Laryngeal CT Scan for Voice Disorders
Virtual endoscopy—Virtual dissection

Jean Abitbol, MD
Albert Castro, MD,
Rodolphe Gombergh, MD
Patrick Abitbol, MD

HISTORY

X-ray

Radiology developed as a result of both the understanding of electricity and the ability to create a vacuum lamp. Sir Wilhelm Croobes, a physician and a president of the Royal Society of Medicine in London, performed the first experiment to create the cathodic-ray tube in 1856. He found that a few particles of gas remain in the vacuum tube when used as a vehicle of electricity. The molecules of radiation matter in front of the cathode that escape and bombard the surfaces they meet are the cathodic rays.

It was the experiment known as the "Shadow of the Maltese Cross" in which Professor W. Goodspeed, from the University of Pennsylvania in Philadelphia, and the English photographer, William Jennings, performed the first "ray photography" with a Crookes tube.[1-3] This experiment took place in 1890 and is considered the embryology of radiology.[4] William C. Roentgen, considered the "father of radiology" performed the first x-ray for medical purposes in 1895 when he x-rayed his wife's hand. He gave his name to the process of x-ray of the photonic emission. The medical applications of Roentgen rays (x-rays) began in 1896 and W.C. Roentgen was awarded the Nobel prize in 1901 for his pioneering work.[5-7]

By the end of the 19th century, Otto Glasser reported on the works of 23 pioneers in radiology in the United States alone.[8] For example, in Chicago, in 1896, the surgeon James Burry successfully x-rayed his hands, assisted by an engineer, Charles Ezra Scribner. At the 1896 Medical Society of Philadelphia meeting, Henry Ware Cattell presented the first communication on radiology. Following this meeting, W.W. Keen and E.P. Davies published "Medical Applications of X-rays or Roentgen Rays" in the *American Journal of Medical Sciences,* in March of 1896. Thus, the principles and applications of x-rays were established.

Kymography

Kymography was first described by Kaestle, Riedor, and Rosenthal in 1909, in Munich. They used a number of plates running at a speed of 5 cm/sec producing an illusion of a movement: it was also called the radiocinema. Thus, the roentgen cinema developed, and allowed the study of the movements of organs inside the body with x-rays.[9] HP Mosher, in 1927, studied the movements of the tongue, the epiglottis, and the hyoïd bone during speech and swallowing, which was the first cineradiograph of the vocal tract.[10] In September 1945, G. Henny, and B. Boone, published in the *American Journal of Roentgenology,* "electrokymography for heart." They studied the parallelism between the electrocardiogram (ECG) and the radiographic movements, while recording their data.[11]

Tomography

The radiograph is a projection of an organ on a film called summation. Tomography is a slice by slice image of the organ. Laryngeal radiotomography, developed by André Bocage in 1921, was the first to "image slice" the body with slice-thickness from 1 mm to 10 mm. The principle was to move synchronously the plate and the tube, with the patient being immobile, so the synchronous motion of these parameters would print a specific and precise area of the organ to study.

In 1935, Georges Massiot and his son, Jean, made the first recorded tomography collecting all their data on film.[12-14] Until the early 1960s, the radiograph was merely a view of one plane. Tomography of the lungs or the larynx was interesting and very useful for diagnosis, but it had shortcomings. The density of the tissue was useful in distinguishing a tumor from normal tissue.

Air is used as a differentiating contrast medium within soft tissues when processing radiographs of the vocal tract.[15] However, the overlapping cervical spine disturbs the anterior-posterior views. To try to avoid this disturbance, high-kilovolt (120 kV) filtered radiographs and tomographs have been used with a copper filter placed in front of the x-ray tube to enhance the air-soft tissue interface by obscuring bone shad-

ows.[16,17] There are series of anterior-posterior views at 5 mm intervals from the cervical spine to the thyroid cartilage. The images may be acquired during respiration or sustained phonation on /i/. The radiation exposure will be very high if multiple slices are taken. The most helpful tomography of the larynx is the anterior-posterior view or frontal view avoiding the cervical spine shadow. The lateral plane yields very little additional information. Tomography shows the laryngeal surface and is useful in examination of any soft tissue, benign or malignant mass, laryngocele, or thickening of the mucosa. However, the anterior commissure, the posterior wall of the glottic space, the cricoarytenoid and cricothyroid joints are poorly visualized. This new technology using multiple and complex movements of the x-ray tube and the receptor improved very satisfactorily the imaging quality.[18]

Conventional and Numerized Radiology

Today, conventional diagnostic x-ray technology utilizes a numerized technique, both direct and indirect.

The direct technique uses an x-ray tube instead of a film as its receptor. This receptor sends the data to a computer, and the result is an image summation. It is then possible to analyze, to magnify, and to distinguish bone from soft tissue, but it is limited to one plane. The indirect technique instead of a receptor uses a support which can be digitalized in a computer and analyzed in the same way as the direct technique.

Computerized Tomography Scanning: CT Scan

In 1967, Hounsfield studied a new concept with the EMI corporation, the analysis of x-ray data with appropriate software.[19] This idea occurred to him when he was asked by EMI to perform research on the shape of blood cells. He studied all angles of these structures, first in two dimensions and later in three dimensions, and found the computer to be crucial in his work. Hounsfield had the idea to take multiple radiographs, with frames being computerized with a specific program. This process was the birth of computerized tomography. Hounsfield published his first manuscript on this subject "Computerized Transverse Axial Scanning" in 1973 in the *British Journal of Radiology* with J. Ambrose, who developed the clinical applications. Cormach and Hounsfield received the Nobel prize in 1979 for this discovery.

Initially, axial transverse tomography was the only possible connection to the computer. Thus, it was named computed tomography (CT). In 1990, spiral CT was available with one detector, in 1993 it was used with two detectors, and in 1999, it was a technique utilizing multiple detectors. At the same time, important computer advances occurred. In 1995, the first work-station with multiplane imaging became available; and in 1999, volume-rendering and transparency techniques became practical.

Magnetic Resonance Imaging: MRI

In 1946, 51 years after Roentgen created the x-ray, Edward Purcell and Felix Bloch developed magnetic resonance imaging (MRI), and in 1952 were awarded the Nobel prize for their work. They analyzed the behavior of the body's own protons on a magnetic field (instead of using x-rays, which bombard the body and the plate), after having been excited by a magnetic system. The protons are oriented with an accurate spin. The first MRI was performed in New York by Demadiour in 1977[20] with the capability of distinguishing tumor mass from normal tissue by analysis of the tissue density. This imaging is often called "protonic imaging" because it uses the variations of the magnetic field or gradient. The x-rays are called "calcic imaging" because they use the photonic transmission of x-rays that are strongly absorbed by the human body because of its high percentage of calcium. MRI is capable of multiplanar, high-resolution imaging and may be superior or more accurate for soft tissue definition compared to the CT scan.[21-23] There is no exposure to irradiation with MRI; however, artifacts are numerous because of the respiratory movements, the pulsatile flow of the carotid and other arteries. These artifacts may be reduced by using fast-spin echo techniques. The sections may be 3 to 5 mm, parallel to the vocal folds and perpendicular to the vocal folds. Fatty tissue yields a high signal and gives a very satisfactory anatomic analysis of the paraglottic space. The ossified cartilage will give a bright signal, the non-ossified cartilage, a low signal. MRI must never be used if a patient has surgical clips (after thyroid surgery), pacemakers, or cochlear implants.

Other Techniques

Xeroradiography

Xeroradiography is performed with wider latitude of exposure with edge enhancement; thus, images have a higher resolution with a better contrast.[24] It has provided a large amount of information on laryngeal cartilages, on the soft tissues, and a precise analysis of the ventricles. It has proven accurate when looking for foreign bodies and in distinguishing a subglottic mass not always visible on stroboscopy. It is also a technique that the author (JA) has used to analyze vocal

tract behavior during sustained vowels "a," "i," "u." Today, xeroradiography is no longer available because of the high exposure to radiation required, which, compared to numerized radiology and CT scan, is 5 times higher.[24,25]

Fluoroscopy—Laryngography

Fluoroscopy is rarely used to study the larynx, partly because of the high radiation exposure. Pharyngolaryngography with barium contrast was commonly used for the visualization of the posterior wall of the tongue, the vallecula, the piriform sinuses, and the posterior wall of the hypopharynx, in the 1980s.[26]

Positron Emission Tomography: PET Scan

Positron emission tomography or PET scan is a relatively new and interesting imaging technique based on the difference in the uptake and metabolism of glucose, H_2O_3, or fluorine-18-FDG. PET scans should prove very useful in future laryngeal research for voice fatigue and can be compared with the other techniques.[27]

ANATOMY RELATED TO RADIOGRAPHY

Phylogenetically, the larynx is an organ which functions as a constrictor-dilator mechanism in the airway. From amphibians to mammals, the larynx develops as a complex structure of cartilages, muscles, and mucosa primarily from branchial arches in utero. At 6 weeks, the epiglottis is seen at the base of the third and fourth pharyngeal arches. At 8 weeks, the thyroid, the cricoid, and the arytenoid cartilages are formed. Around 10 to 12 weeks, the vocal folds are individualized. At 7 months, the larynx is anatomically and functionally a sketch of an adult larynx. An understanding of the skeletal elements and articulations of the vocal tract is necessary to avoid misdiagnosis when interpreting imaging of the larynx.

Cartilages of the Larynx

The cartilages of the larynx, including the thyroid, cricoid, arytenoid, and corniculates consist of three components: nonossified hyaline cartilage, a cortical bone marrow cavity containing fatty tissue, and scattered bony trabeculae. Enchondral (such as thyroid cartilage) ossification starts around 30 years of age. The ossification process follows specific patterns in each cartilage.[28,29] The epiglottis and the arytenoids are composed of yellow fibrocartilage that does not usually ossify. However, in our series, on helical CT scan at around 70 years of age, the authors have seen numerous ossified arytenoids.[30,31] On CT scan, ossified cartilage shows a high-alternating, outer and inner cortex, and a central, low-alternating medullary space. Nonossified hyaline cartilage and nonossified fibroelastic cartilages have the same attenuation values of soft tissue.[32-38]

The angle of the two laminae of the thyroid or "shield of the folds" is approximately 110° in children, 120° in females, and 90° in males.[39]

The cricoarytenoid joint depends on the articular surface, as described by Lampert in 1926.[40] The facets of the cricoid are cylindrically curved with an axis sharply inclined horizontally. The angles between the horizontal plane and the cricoarytenoid joint axis are primate specific: 25° for the Mycetes, 55° for the *Macacas*, and 55° to 60° for *Homo sapiens*. These facets do not exist in nonprimates.[41,42]

The cricoid cartilage is a complete ring with a height of 2.5 cm at the posterior arch and 0.75 cm at the anterior arch.

The arytenoids measure around 1.2 cm in height and are mobile and symmetric. The corniculate cartilages are at the apices of the arytenoids. The virtual dissection used in helical CT scanning by the authors shows the facet of the arytenoids.

The cricothyroid joint lies between the convex articular facet of the thyroid inferior horn and the flat articular facet of the posterolateral surface of the cricoid cartilage.

The cricoarytenoid joint is a saddle-shaped synovial joint with a strong capsular ligament. The arytenoid joints have complex sliding, rocking, and tilting movements described for decades by the observations gained through indirect and direct laryngoscopy but never by a CT scan "virtual arthroscopy" in vivo. Because of their low mass, they allow abduction-adduction in less than 0.1 second. This joint is critical for understanding not only the function of the laryngeal framework but also the source of most laryngeal pathologies.[43,44]

Soft Tissues of the Larynx

Radiography depends on tissue density in the larynx.

1. The mucosa of the larynx shows no enhancement except with a specific algorithm with the vocal-scan (the technique utilized by the authors to generate the images illustrated in this chapter)
2. Muscular tissue has no relevant enhancement in the conventional CT scan but does with the vocal-scan
3. Connective tissue is usually not seen except with the vocal-scan, which has a cross-sectional imaging capacity that is ideally suited to differentiate

the different compartments of the larynx and hypopharynx. The paraglottic space is symmetric between the mucosa and the laryngeal framework, and extends into the aryepiglottic folds. The supraglottic region (ventricles, false vocal folds) is adjacent to the pre-epiglottic space. The aryepiglottic folds separate the endolarynx (anteromedially) from the piriform sinuses (posteromedially). At the glottic level the medial boundary is the conus elasticus of the vocal ligament to the upper edge of the cricoid cartilage and joins the cricothyroid membrane anteriorly. The cricothyroid membrane posterolaterally forms the lateral boundary of the paraglottic space.[45,46] Also, at the glottic level, the thyroarytenoid muscle forms the bulk and shape of the vocal fold, which also occupies most of the volume of the paraglottic space.[47]

Dynamic Aspects of the Larynx

For the first time, laryngeal movements were observed and analyzed radiographically by the authors using three-dimensional (3D) CT, which allows observations of the movements of cartilages and joints. The anatomy of the soft tissues is well known and does not need any further explanation to understand the "virtual dissection."

The first roentgenologic laryngeal closure study was published in 1940 by Lindsay demonstrating the behavior of a laryngocele during phonation.[48] These tomograms also showed that the laryngeal airway is closed by apposition of both the vocal folds and the vestibular folds. The first observation by the way of laryngeal cineradiography during breathing was published by Ardran, Kemp, and Manen in 1953.[49] They noted that the larynx falls slightly on inspiration and rises on expiration and that the lumen widens on inspiration and narrows during expiration. These findings were confirmed in 1956 by Fink.[50] The first functional tomographies were produced 10 years later in 1966, by Ardran et al. They studied the role of the epiglottis, the cricoid, and the arytenoid cartilages and the ventricles during breathing and phonating.[51,52] R. Fink, in a retrospective on the human larynx, emphasized the role of the cricoarytenoid joint.[53,54] The vocal scan brings us a better understanding of the dynamic and functional aspects of this joint and the cricothyroid joint. It demonstrates the movements of the cricoarytenoid joint laterally, anteriorly, and posteriorly.

In the movie *Voice Performers and Voice Fatigue* by the author Jean Abitbol, in 1988, a parallel study between xerography and the flexible laryngoscope gave a satisfactory analysis of the physiology of the larynx during phonation.[55]

CLINICAL AND MULTIMEDIA EVALUATION OF LARYNGEAL DISEASES

Laryngeal diseases usually have a typical clinical history and generally do not require extensive imaging. The laryngologist can assess the laryngeal mass with his or her simple clinical examination, videolaryngoscopy, or videolaryngostroboscopy. The numerous techniques of laryngeal evaluation, developed in the last two decades, have provided an accurate approach of the diagnosis of laryngeal pathologies. The "good morning doctor" from the patient can provide diagnostic guidance by analysis of his or her maximum phonation time and voice characteristics. Listening to the patient's voice is the indispensable first step.

Manuel García developed the first method of indirect laryngoscopy in 1854. This examination is still routinely used, as it provides assessment of the real color of the mucosa and gives information in three dimensions.[56] The stroboscopic light became the second fundamental step in laryngeal examination. To be able to see the vocal folds in slow motion has brought forth a new harvest of unknown diagnoses and misdiagnoses. Video or computerized stroboscopy of the larynx may be stored on tape or DVD and can be compared with other examinations. Photographs of the larynx provide objective data that are helpful when comparing the laryngeal imaging before and after treatment.

Objective acoustic measures such as spectrographic analysis, fundamental F_0 measurements, formants, shimmer, and jitter during speech and singing are also valuable.

Electromyography has become a valuable clinical tool in the evaluation of vocal fold paresis or immobility, and allows for accurate location of the branch of the recurrent nerve or the superior laryngeal nerve that is impaired.[57]

Nowadays, radiology of the larynx is not only used to confirm pathology but also assists in diagnosis as with the 3D CT scan to visualize a "virtual dissection." The data gained from both clinical videolaryngoscopy and imaging provide a better understanding of the disease and lead to a better strategy for therapy.

CT SCAN

How Does a CT Scan Work? What Was the Basis for Development of the Vocal Scan?

Basics of Helical CT Scan

Principles. As previously discussed, x-rays are photons with a wavelength from 10^{-4} nm to 10^2 nm, are produced by the tube, and require an important power supply.

The x-ray tube moves with a circular movement and x-ray data are gathered by a detector. The table on which the patient lies moves horizontally. This dual movement creates a helical figure in a virtual cylinder.

Projections of data collected are digitized. This revolutionary method was a major radiologic advance in the ability to assess density of the mass. Hounsfield had the ingenious idea to detect x-rays with a crystal, thus producing a visible light spectrum. The CT scan improved resolution dramatically by permitting smaller, more discrete image slices. The detectors are crystals, which increase the sensitivity, and thus, the different densities may be analyzed by the computer. Data analysis was made possible once the computer became available. Algorithms then allowed reconstruction imaging.

Acquisition

- The slice-thickness is defined by the collimation of x-rays (Figures 20–1 through 20–5).
- The flux of photons depends on the power supply of the tube (120 kV usually, at 15 mA). The flux is limited by the heat effect.
- The speed of the table on which the patient lies going in to the gantry is measured in mm/sec. It is related to the collimation.
- $$\text{Pitch} = \frac{\text{Table incrementation during each gantry rotation}}{\text{Collimation}}$$
- The time of the spiral is linked to the volume acquisition and the slice-thickness.

Reconstruction

Algorithms that improve resolution are used. Here a 360° rotation technique is used. There are two rotations of the tube (720°). Then, the image parameters are calculated for a 360° reconstruction essentially doubling the amount of information in the computer from which the image is resolved, thereby enhancing detail. Table speed, related to "pitch" is also important. The more rapidly the table is moving, the more the thickness slices increase.

Applications for Acquisition

The gantry angles used in helical CT scanning are almost the same as those used in conventional CT. For the helical CT scan of the larynx, the gantry angles are parallel to the vocal folds during abduction and adduction.

Inaccurate gantry angle may cause a misdiagnosis with an artificial thickening of the anterior commissure, and the interposed laryngeal ventricle may disturb the evaluation of the paraglottic space.[58,59]

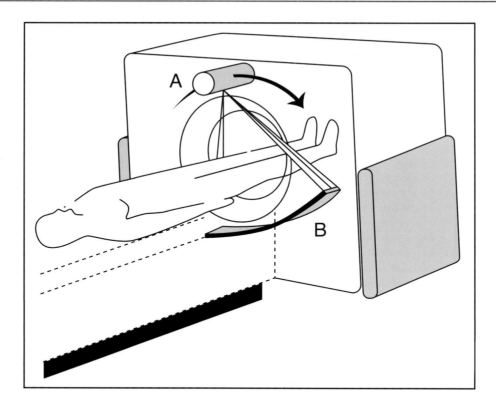

Figure 20–1. X-ray tube with a double detector: **A.** X-ray tube. **B.** Double detector.

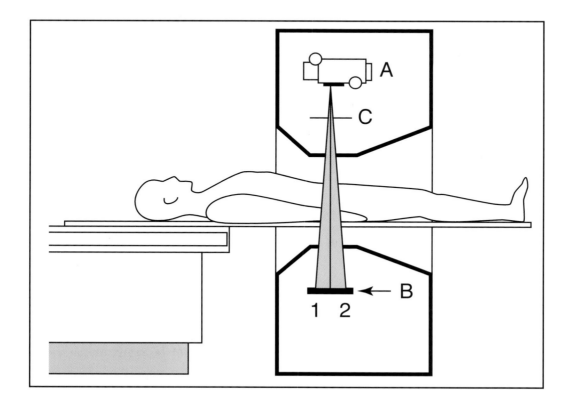

Figure 20–2. **A.** X-ray tube; **B.** Double detector. **C.** Collimation.

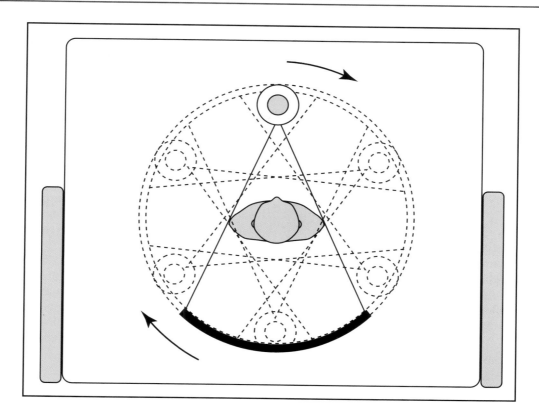

Figure 20–3. Acquisition. X-ray tube and detectors move simultaneously. The patient is inside the gantry.

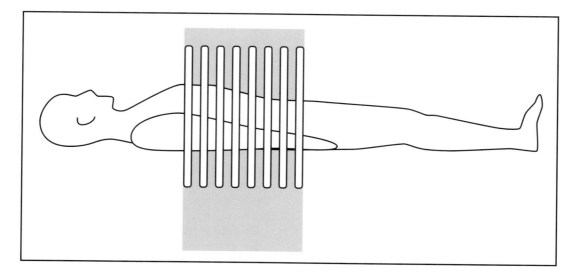

Figure 20–4. Conventional CT scan: slice by slice requiring 30 minutes for acquisition. Each slice needs 6 to 10 seconds with a relapse time of 10 to 20 seconds.

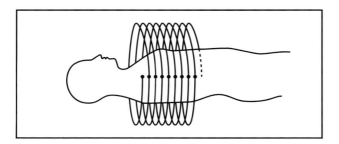

Figure 20–5. Helical CT scan—The spiral technique allows a 20-second acquisition time.

However, misdiagnoses decrease with the practical application of the 3D CT scan with sagittal, coronal, and 120° planes that the authors use, the ability to retrospectively study the images, along with the collaboration of a radiologist and a laryngologist, but a zero risk of misdiagnosis never exists.

Contrast. The rapid acquisition of the helical CT has dramatically decreased the use of intravenous contrast. The contrast dose is reduced by at least one-third for better enhancement of the main vessels and of the soft tissues (thyroarytenoid muscle, cricothyroid membrane).[60]

Approximately, 150 ml of intravenous contrast is required if there is an angulation of the gantry and 100 ml if not. Prior to the scan 46 mg of contrast medium at a rate of 1 ml/sec are injected and followed by infusion at a rate of 0.5 ml/sec.

Slice-Thickness/Collimation. The best image quality, as illustrated in this chapter, is obtained when the interval of reconstruction is equal to the slice-thickness with overlapping slices.[61]

For example, an acquisition set obtained with a 3 mm collimation can be reconstructed into images of 3 mm (same slice-thickness) in 1 mm increments only resulting in 2 mm overlap of adjacent images.

Pitch. It is proportional to collimation. Increasing the pitch will decrease the longitudinal resolution; that is why a pitch of 1 seems to be the optimal level for preserving the Z-axis resolution. It allows multiplane reconstruction for the arytenoids and the laryngeal joints.

Power Supply. The tube current is a critical factor in helical CT: 200–250 amps and 120 kV are used. If the power supply is not adequate, increased noise, poor contrast enhancement, and grainy images will result.

Applications for Reconstruction

Reconstruction. Accurate and adequate algorithms are necessary for high-quality reconstruction, which depends on slice-thickness, slice overlapping, and contrast resolution.

Slice-thickness is used for a volumetric acquisition and, retrospectively, a reconstruction. Because data acquisition is volumetric, the scanning time of the patient is not increased and the slice-thickness used during the scanning does not have to be equal to the slice-thickness used for reconstruction. To improve the images, the reconstruction can also be obtained with slice overlapping. For laryngeal pathology, we use a 0.6 mm reconstruction interval made with 1 mm collimation through the laryngeal framework. This technique has been performed in the temporal bone.[62] The 3D information displayed is used for diagnosis and aids in planning phonosurgery. To ensure better quality of the images and, thus, more accurate diagnosis, the larynx must be studied with at least two helical acquisitions.[63]

Principles of the CT Scan

Technology with very powerful computers bring us to the third dimension: "virtual endoscopy," and "transparent body."

Evaluation of the tissue density is possible and from this point, the quality of the structures are more precise. To render homage to Hounsfield the units of density in CT were named Hu (Hounsfield unit), the scale is from -1000 to +1000 (Figure 20–6).

Air = –1000 Hu;

Water = 0 Hu; and

Bone = +1000 Hu.

There exist 2000 levels of shades in black and white from –1000 Hu to +1000 Hu. To distinguish the different structures' density and, thus, the different type of tissue, a color is applied on the Hu scale for better definition and imaging.

The color chosen to analyze our frames in 3D CT scan has proven to be indispensable. It should be recalled that the human eye can distinguish only 20 levels of gray but 250,000 colors. It is necessary to adapt the image to the location to be explored. The image is distinguished by two parameters: the width and the density of the window. The more the window is decreased, the more density differentiation is appreciated. Therefore, the threshold of the window must be equal to the average tissue density to be imaged (Figure 20–6). The screen is coupled with a color laser

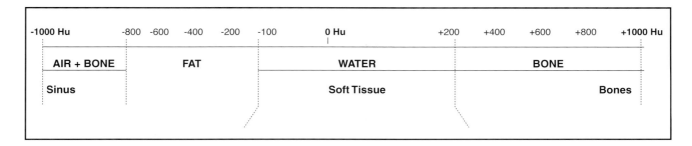

Figure 20–6. Hounsfield units: Density of the tissue in Hu.

printer to obtain a hard copy and recorded on CD-ROM or a DVD. With this machine, it is possible to do a fly-through, and the CT scan has proven irreplaceable in the diagnosis of deep lesions, which are hard to see. Thus, CT and MR imaging are more useful in these cases.[64-69]

The laryngeal joints are very well observed with the 3D CT scan.

CT is very helpful in cricoarytenoid joint injury when preparing the surgical strategy.

Angiography is helpful in conjunction with 3D CT for providing a better understanding of the laryngeal physiology and pathologies such as angiomas and paragangliomas.[70]

Vocal Scan

Helical computer-assisted tomography scanning or helical CT scan has been improved by the advances in computer technology. Planes are stored to create the 3D imaging. The program with an accurate workstation can perform reformations/reconstructions. All the planes may be used. For the vocal scan, the authors have determined specific parameters, including orientation of the plane, measurement of tissue density in Hounsfield units (Hu), the time exposure, and the "shadow" work.

Acquisition

Technical advances have not only improved image quality in the last two decades, but also the way in which such images are obtained.

Conventional CT Scanners. Conventional CT scanners need sophisticated cables to couple the x-ray and detector assembly to the reconstruction process. It also needs high voltage. The protocol for individual scans was performed with a 2-second scan time separated by a 6-second interscan delay. This delay allows time to re-orient the source-detector assembly within

the gantry, time for table movement, and a short breath for the patient.[71]

The patient lies on a sliding table. The table moves into a gantry, a central circular aperture housing the x-ray source and detectors. The slices are parallel to the vocal folds. The imaging procedure is performed from the inferior maxilla to the sixth cervical vertebra. The more detail needed, the thinner the slices must be and the longer the imaging time required. With the conventional CT scan, most images are 1 to 2 mm thickness-slices, every 3 to 5 mm. The patient moves the prescribed distance through the gantry for each slice; the table moves 3 mm, one image shot, 3 mm, another image is shot with a total imaging time of approximately 20 to 30 minutes.

Vocal Scan. The authors use a spiral CT scanner. The procedure is much faster, requiring only 20 seconds exposure time. The spiral CT scanner moves the subject continuously in a circle and creates a volume acquisition imaging. These data are collected and stored. The first step is a multiplanar study (coronal, sagittal, and axial). Then the analysis begins for three-dimensional imaging. The images are colored regarding the tissue density. We have 2000 levels of gray or 2000 Hu, which are converted to color. The advantages are enormous: rapid acquisition time, few motion artifact, a color and 3D picture, and animation.[72,73]

Intravenous contrast may be required for some purpose (laryngeal arteries) or presurgical mapping of a hemorrhagic mass (angioma). Data are recorded in the computer with an adequate program capable of analyzing every detail, both from the technical point of view (scale of density rendering) and the anatomic point of view (for example, if the focus of analysis is on the joints or on the vocal ligament), which are intimately linked. The laryngologist must work with and interpret the images with the radiologist at the workstation to change some parameters of contrast if the pathology being evaluated is not visible on the first images. The Hu must be chosen to identify the specific lesion; protocols have been developed accordingly.

One of the successes of the helical CT scan from the very beginning was the ability to analyze the anterior commissure that was previously impossible to see with computed tomography. The anterior commissure was found to have a mean width of 1 to 1.6 mm in normal subjects.[74]

Vocal Scan Reconstruction

The helical CT reconstruction requires multiple angles for the same structures to be analyzed. With the helical CT, there is a 360° view with a complete gantry rotation. During the procedure, the patient moves continuously through the gantry.

Mathematical interpolation with specific parameters allows the reconstruction through the computer. Parameters include collimation, table speed or incrementation, and image reconstruction intervals. Although the slice-thickness of collimation is preset before the scan, the computer can generate overlapping images. If a 2-mm collimation is used, slices may be reconstructed every 1 mm. For example, in laryngeal imaging a 1-cm collimation with a 20-sec helical exposure, covering 20 cm of tissue along the z-axis has a pitch of 1.

Advantages of Helical CT Scan

The advantages of helical CT technology are numerous.[75-78]

1. The procedure is fast; in a single 20-second interval an entire vocal tract is helically scanned and ready to be reconstructed in 3D.
2. Helical CT is able to eliminate respiratory artifacts and is able to reconstruct overlapping images at arbitrary intervals on the workstation. The 3D CT scan gives a very high-quality image with the reconstruction, not only of the image but also of a virtual mobility between two scanning points. For example, aperture and closure of the glottis can be generated from helical acquisitions; this has dramatically improved the scope of analysis for the vocal tract (and also for the entire body).
3. Helical CT has the ability to shift the location of slice reconstruction and create new images, retrospectively, with the image and the laryngologist in front of the screen of the workstation.
4. In some instances, helical CT scan has replaced the conventional CT in laryngeal imaging as numerized radiology did for conventional radiology. Improved vascular identification allows easier separa-

tion of mass lesions from vessels. The contrast enhancement is tremendously improved by the choice of the filter with reconstruction having the same advantages observed in thoracic or color imaging.

Limits of Helical CT Scan

The limits of the helical CT are few as described below:

- The chainsaw artifact: a few slices are missing; this problem is solved by overlapping imaging.
- The lego effect is caused by squared edges of each slice at the convexity. This artifact is corrected by using a smoothing algorithm during the 3D reconstruction or by using a thinner slice-thickness during scanning (1 mm).
- The threshold selection is a crucial factor. 3D images depend both on the algorithm and the threshold chosen during reconstruction.
- Artifacts related to metallic objects (dental crowns, bridges, surgical clips, and prostheses and cochlear implants).
- Volume rendering will create an artificially smooth surface of the endolaryngeal structures.

Image quality also depends on the power source. A high power is needed, especially in large patients, in which the images may be excessively grainy. Refinements in detection technology, higher-heat-capacity of x-rays tubes, and improvements in new workstations will advance the possibilities in achieving optimal images.

Although helical CT allows a rapid acquisition and reduces artifact such as respiratory misregistration, the swallowing artifacts may still cause degradation of images in the vocal tract study. A near perfect acquisition technique is needed.[79]

Virtual Endoscopy and Virtual Dissection

The postprocessing of helical CT data allows creation of a reconstruction from axial slices into a high-quality picture of variable orientation. The virtual endoscopy was described for the first time in 1994 by Vining et al.[80,81] They used an accurate three-dimensional software, the voxel viewer, and a silicon graphics machine. Computer simulations allow creation of virtual endoscopy. A "virtual dissection" from the lumen of the larynx and trachea to the vessels and muscles is performed via the applications of acquisitions and reconstructions. In other words, 3D imaging is accurately created, recorded, and printed.[82-85]

Previously, diagnosis of airway disease was only possible by invasive endoscopy, considered the gold

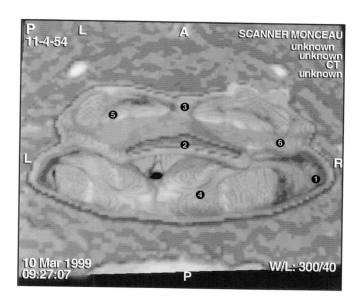

Figure 20–13. Virtual endoscopy of the larynx from a superior view with a Valsalva maneuver. 1. Piriform sinus. 2. Epiglottis. 3. Glossoepiglottic fold. 4. Aryepiglottic fold. 5. Valleculae. 6. Pharyngoepiglottic fold.

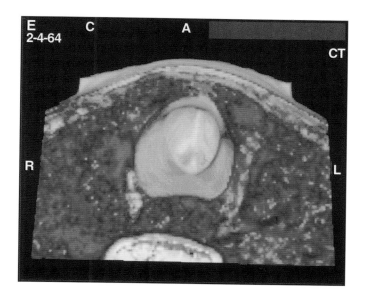

Figure 20–14. Inferior view of the vocal folds seen on virtual endoscopy but not seen by the consultation scope.

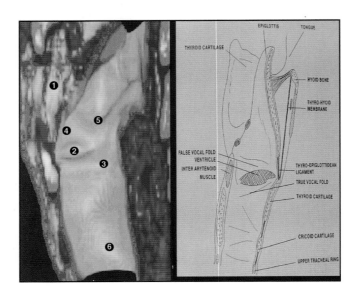

Figure 20–15. Lateral and internal views of the larynx: virtual endoscopy.1. Hyo-thyro epiglottic space (fat pad). 2. Ventricle 3. Vocal fold. 4. False vocal fold. 5. Piriform sinus. 6. Trachea.

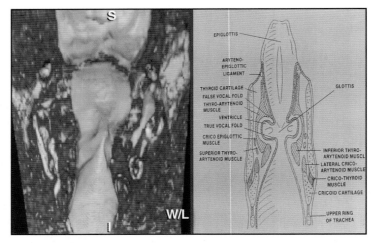

Figure 20–16. Lateral and internal views of the larynx: virtual endoscopy.

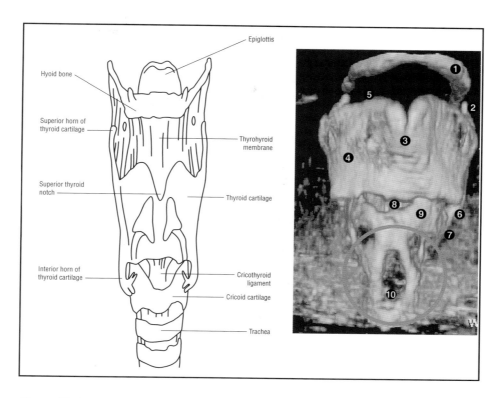

Figure 20–17. Framework of the larynx (can be used to observe a tracheostomy scar): anterior view (post tracheotomy). 1. Hyoid bone. 2. Sup. horn of thyroid cartilage. 3. Laryngeal prominence. 4. Thyroid cartilage. 5. Oblique line. 6. Inf. horn of thyroid cartilage. 7. Cricothyroid joint. 8. C-T ligament. 9. Cricoid cartilage. 10. Old tracheostomy.

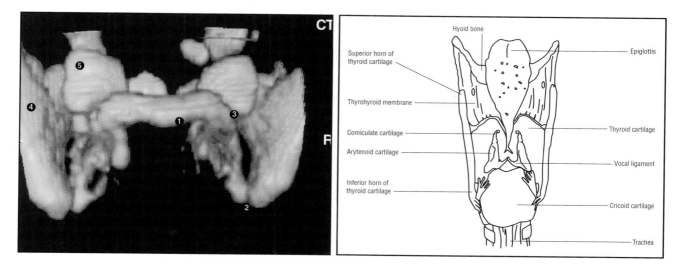

Figure 20–18. Cricoarytenoid joint during slow inspiration: posterior view. 1. Cricoid cartilage. 2. Cricothyroid joint. 3. Cricoarytenoid joint. 4. Thyroid cartilage. 5. Arytenoids.

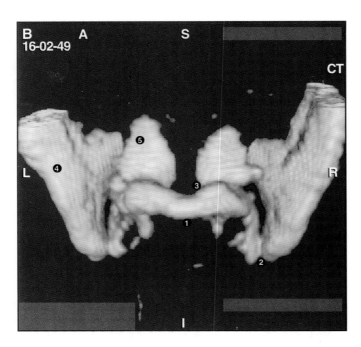

Figure 20–19. Cricoarytenoid joint during phonation with a sustained vowel /i/: posterior view. 1. Cricoid cartilage. 2. Cricothyroid joint. 3. Cricoarytenoid joint. 4. Thyroid cartilage. 5. Arytenoids.

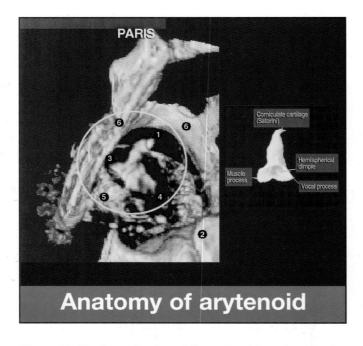

Figure 20–20. Accurate view of the arytenoids: anterosuperior view. 1. Corniculate cartilage. 2. Vertebral body. 3. Muscular process. 4. Vocal process. 5. Cricoid cartilage. 6. Thyroid cartilage.

Developing measures to assess voice quality and its health impact has been difficult. Most of the present measurements deal with objective specifics of voice production; the mechanics of voice production, such as posture, support, and resonance; or specific physiologic actions such as vocal fold vibration. Although these measures have great value and are critical for improved understanding and training of the voice, they fail to measure either the importance of voice production and the impact of voice disorders on the overall quality of life of the voice user or the effects from an intervention or treatment. Even with objective tests, there are no generally agreed-on gold standards of measurement. Furthermore, different objective tests have been designed for different measures of function, such as fundamental frequency, frequency range, airflow parameters, perturbation, or vocal fold vibration. Variation also occurs among clinicians in the performance and interpretation of these tests. These limitations have prevented valid comparisons of the impact of an intervention in different environments or comparisons of two different interventions.

Although it would be expected that improvements in objective tests would correlate with improvements in outcome, severity of disease as measured by these tests does not necessarily measure its impact on an individual. Minimal variations in pitch would likely have a much greater impact on a performing vocalist than a person who has minimal voice demands. A cured small laryngeal cancer may prevent a singer or other professional speaker from performing. Its impact on his or her quality of life would be expected to be greater and likely to be represented poorly by objective tests.

With the development of general quality of life surveys such as the SF-36, the clinician can assess the impact of disease or treatment on quality of life. Furthermore, comparisons can be made between patients and others without the disorder or between patients with two or more different disorders. One of our studies showed that there are significant differences in perception of quality of life between dysphonic (disordered voice) patients and unaffected average people in the United States.[7] When evaluating the specific domains of the SF-36, we found that the domains of "role function emotion" and "role function physical" were significantly different between dysphonic and nondysphonic people. These two domains deal with the ability to perform work and other daily tasks as a result of the physical or emotional impact of their disorder. As voice problems might be expected to have an impact on work and other daily activities, this finding is not unexpected. The "social functioning" score was also worse in dysphonic patients. Because "physical functioning," "vitality," and "mental health" scores were also worse for dysphonic patients than for normals, it can be seen that these voice disorders affect a broader sense of well-being than the specific symptoms. Other studies have also found that voice disorders significantly influence patients' health-related quality of life and have an impact on daily activities.[9,10] Objective tests of voice function or standard questionnaires would not be expected to measure these quality of life impacts.

THE VOICE HANDICAP INDEX

Traditionally, outcomes for patients with voice disorders have been measured with a clinical or biomedical frame of reference. The variables used to indicate a favorable or unfavorable treatment outcome do not rely on attitudinal input from the patients. In an effort to shift the focus from the clinicians' judgments to patients' self-perceptions of their voice disorders, we developed the Voice Handicap Index (VHI)[8] (Figure 21–1.) The VHI consists of 30 statements that reflect the variety of experiences that a patient with a voice disorder may encounter. Patients note the frequency of each experience on a 5-point equally appearing scale (never—0, almost never—1, sometimes—2, almost always—3, always—4), with a maximuml total score of 120. The VHI is able not only to measure the physical effects of their voice problem but also the functional and emotional aspects, or subscales. The VHI is scored for each of the three individual subscales and a total score. Therefore, it can serve as an independent, objective measure of the impact on quality of life of voice dysfunction.

Our studies show that impact of a disordered voice on the quality of life is substantial even when compared to other chronic diseases such as angina, sciatica, chronic sinusitis, or back pain, particularly in the areas of social functioning and role playing.[7] Overall, however, other chronic diseases tend to produce worse scores than dysphonia.

Because the SF-36 is scaled for the individual domains, and not for a total score, direct overall total comparisons to the VHI cannot be made. Nonetheless, by evaluating the individual domains, a comparison of quality of life impact of various disorders can be made between the SF-36 and VHI. For example, when attempting to correlate the VHI with the SF-36, strong correlations were found between the total VHI scores and the individual subscales to the SF-36 domains of social functioning, role functioning (emotional and physical), and mental health. The greatest disability of voice patients is in the functional areas, as was validated by our study in assessing the relationship of the VHI to the SF-36.[7] Because patients with voice disor-

VOICE HANDICAP INDEX (VHI)

3622008629

Today's Date ☐☐ - ☐☐ - ☐☐

First Name

Last Name

MRN

Birth Date
Month - Day - Year

Age
○ Male
○ Female

Provider

Date of Operation
Month - Day - Year

Type of Visit:
○ New Visit   ○ Pre-Treatment   ○ Pre-Surgical Treatment
○ Return Visit   ○ Post Medical Treatment   ○ Post Surgical Treatment

Diagnosis:
○ Functional Dysphonia
○ Spasmodic Dysphonia
○ Other Neurogenic Dysphonia
○ Bowing/ Presbylarynges
○ Benign Masses (polyp/ nodule/ MRC)

○ Edidermoid Cyst/ Sulcus
○ Vocal Fold Paralysis
  ○ a) unilateral
  ○ b) bilateral
  ○ c) SLN

○ Reflux Laryngitis
○ Leukoplakia
○ Benign Laryngeal Tumor
○ Malignant Laryngeal Tumor
○ Other (Describe)

Instructions: These are statements that many people have used to describe their voices and the effects of their voices on their lives. Check the response that indicates how frequently you have the same experience.

	Never	Almost Never	Sometimes	Almost Always	Always
F1. My voice makes it difficult for people to hear me.	O	O	O	O	O
P2. I run out of air when I talk.	O	O	O	O	O
F3. People have difficulty understanding me in a noisy room.	O	O	O	O	O
P4. The sound of my voice varies throughout the day.	O	O	O	O	O
F5. My family has difficulty hearing me when I call them throughout the house.	O	O	O	O	O
F6. I use the phone less often than I would like.	O	O	O	O	O
E7. I'm tense when talking with others because of my voice.	O	O	O	O	O
F8. I tend to avoid groups of people because of my voice.	O	O	O	O	O
E9. People seem irritated with my voice.	O	O	O	O	O
P10. People ask "What's wrong with your voice?"	O	O	O	O	O
F11. I speak with friends, neighbors, or relatives less often because of my voice.	O	O	O	O	O
F12. People ask me to repeat myself when speaking face-to-face.	O	O	O	O	O
P13. My voice sounds creaky and dry.	O	O	O	O	O
P14. I feel as though I have to strain to produce voice.	O	O	O	O	O
E15. I find other people don't understand my voice problem.	O	O	O	O	O

Figure 21–1. The Voice Handicap Index. *(continued)*

7177008628

	Never	Almost Never	Sometimes	Almost Always	Always
F16. My voice difficulties restrict my personal and social life.	0	0	0	0	0
P17. The clarity of my voice is unpredictable.	0	0	0	0	0
P18. I try to change my voice to sound different.	0	0	0	0	0
F19. I feel left out of conversations because of my voice.	0	0	0	0	0
P20. I use a great deal of effort to speak.	0	0	0	0	0
P21. My voice is worse in the evening.	0	0	0	0	0
F22. My voice problem causes me to lose income.	0	0	0	0	0
E23. My voice problem upsets me.	0	0	0	0	0
E24. I am less outgoing because of my voice problem.	0	0	0	0	0
E25. My voice makes me handicapped.	0	0	0	0	0
P26. My voice "gives out" on me in the middle of speaking.	0	0	0	0	0
E27. I feel annoyed when people ask me to repeat.	0	0	0	0	0
E28. I feel embarrassed when people ask me to repeat.	0	0	0	0	0
E29. My voice makes me feel incompetent.	0	0	0	0	0
E30. I'm ashamed of my voice problem.	0	0	0	0	0

P Scale ☐☐

F Scale ☐☐

E Scale ☐☐

Total Scale ☐☐☐

Please circle the word that matches how you feel your voice is today.

Normal   Mild   Moderate   Severe

Figure 21–1. *(continued)*

ders generally do not have significant changes in bodily pain, general health, vitality, and general physical functioning, the VHI would not be expected to be very sensitive to changes in these domains of the SF-36.

Patients with vocal fold paralysis had worse scores in many of the domains of the SF-36 than other dysphonic patients, particularly in the domains of role playing, emotional and physical functioning.[7] This is likely caused by the impact of vocal fold paralysis on lifting and straining and other daily activities. In general, patients with paralysis appear to be more disabled and have poorer overall quality of life than the other categories of patients with dysphonia, as measured by both the SF-36 and VHI. When evaluated with the VHI, patients with vocal fold edema had better scores for the total, functional, and physical scores than the patients with vocal fold masses (eg, nodules or polyps). Individuals with vocal fold paralysis in general had worse scores than individuals with other voice disorders as measured by the VHI.[7]

In a subsequent as yet unpublished study, we attempted to compare the VHI and its three subscales to various objective tests. We were able to show that the functional subscale of the VHI correlated well with both signal-to-noise ratio (SNR) and maximum phonatory time (MPT). Other measures, such as jitter, shimmer, fundamental frequency, semitones, and airflow volume had little correlation with the patients' perception of the quality of life impact of their voice disorder as measured by the VHI. Although these specific measures did not correlate with the VHI, as the voices of patients worsened, as measured by the objective laboratory parameters, a corresponding change in the VHI scores occurred. Objective laboratory measures and the VHI cannot be seen as interchangeable. There are corresponding appropriate changes in both with worsening voice, but strong correlations only in SNR and MPT. This suggests that the tests may measure different parameters of voice. It also may suggest that the objective laboratory tests now used may measure specific parameters of voice, but not the global impact of a voice disorder on the patient's emotional, functional, and physical perception of health.

Several studies have evaluated the success of treatment of voice disorders on the patient-perceived quality of life using the VHI.[11,12] One important aspect of these assessments is that both medical and surgical treatment have been shown to have a positive impact on VHI scores and quality of life for a diverse group of voice disorders including cysts/polyps, spasmodic dysphonia, vocal fold paralysis, and muscular tension dysphonia.[11,12] Although the VHI is broadly scaled, in clinical practice it may be somewhat cumbersome to use, due to the 30-item scale. A 10-item scale, Voice Handicap Index-10, has recently been validated.[13]

There is also growing evidence that VHI scores may be different between singers and nonsingers, with a low VHI score still representing a significant handicap to a singer with a voice problem.[14]

The VHI, therefore, is a statistically validated, objective test that can be used to measure the emotional, physical, functional, and total quality of life impact of a voice disorder. It can be used to measure the response to treatment or nontreatment, to perform research related to voice, or to evaluate patients in different clinical environments. In the absence of definitive, established gold standards for measuring voice, the VHI may serve as the template for assessing voice outcome. Finally, the VHI can be used along with other objective tools or tests to assess the characteristics of an individual's voice and the impact of those characteristics on quality of voice and quality of life.

OTHER VOICE OUTCOMES MEASUREMENT TOOLS

A number of other voice outcomes measurement tools have been developed. One of the more widely used is the GRBAS, developed by the Japan Society of Logopaedics.[15] The GRBAS is not a true outcomes tool, but rather a composite of a judged perception of voice quality with the individual components being overall grade of hoarseness (G), roughness (R), breathiness (B), aesthenic (A), and strained (S). It has, however, seemed to correlate with other patient-centered measures of severity. Similarly, the Dysphonia Severity Index was developed to describe perceived voice quality based on objective measures.[16]

Because voice disorders may also have a different impact on children than on adults, a pediatric voice quality-of-life instrument has been validated, and it has shown that in children voice-related quality of life is affected by clinical conditions such as a tracheotomy.[17] Another tool that has been developed is the Voice Related Quality of Life (V-RQOL),[18] which is similar to the VHI-10. In 2002, the United States Agency for Health Research and Quality published an evidence-based review, *Criteria for Determining Disability in Speech Language Disorders,* of the above tools; only the VHI "met our criteria for reliability, validity and availability of normative data."[19]

SUMMARY

The future challenges related to outcomes research in voice will revolve around the application of these

hearsals. It may also be caused by other forms of voice abuse and by mucosal irritation produced by allergy, smoke inhalation, and other causes. Mucous stranding between the anterior and middle thirds of the vocal folds is seen commonly in inflammatory laryngitis. Laryngitis sicca is associated with dehydration, dry atmosphere, mouth breathing, and antihistamine therapy. Deficiency of mucosal lubrication causes irritation and coughing and results in mild inflammation. If no pressing professional need for performance exists, inflammatory conditions of the larynx are best treated with relative voice rest in addition to other modalities. However, in some instances, speaking and singing may be permitted. The patient should be instructed to avoid all forms of irritation and to rest the voice at all times except during warm-up and performance. Corticosteroids and other medications discussed later may be helpful. If mucosal secretions are copious, low-dose antihistamine therapy may be beneficial, but it must be prescribed with caution and should generally be avoided. Copious, thin secretions are better than scant, thick secretions or excessive dryness. The patient with laryngitis must be kept well hydrated to maintain the desired character of mucosal lubrication. The patient should be instructed to "pee pale," consuming enough water to keep urine diluted. Psychologic support is crucial. For example, it is often helpful for the physician to intercede on a singer's behalf and to convey "doctor's orders" directly to agents or theater management. Such mitigation of exogenous stress can be highly therapeutic.

Infectious laryngitis may be caused by bacteria or viruses. Subglottic involvement frequently indicates a more severe infection, which may be difficult to control in a short period of time. Indiscriminate use of antibiotics must be avoided; however, when the physician is in doubt as to the cause and when a major voice commitment is imminent, vigorous antibiotic treatment is warranted. In this circumstance, the damage caused by allowing progression of a curable condition is greater than the damage that might result from a course of therapy for an unproven microorganism while culture results are pending. When a major concert or speech is not imminent, indications for therapy are the same as for the nonsinger or nonprofessional speaker.

Voice rest (absolute or relative) is an important therapeutic consideration in any case of laryngitis. When no professional commitments are pending, a short course of absolute voice rest may be considered, as it is the safest and most conservative therapeutic intervention. This means absolute silence and communication with a writing pad. The patient must be instructed not to whisper, as this may be an even more traumatic vo-

cal activity than speaking softly. Whistling through the lips also involves vocal fold activity and should not be permitted. So does the playing of many musical wind instruments. Absolute voice rest is *necessary* only for serious vocal fold injury such as hemorrhage or mucosal disruption. Even then, it is virtually never indicated for more than seven to ten days. Three days are often sufficient. Some excellent laryngologists do not believe voice rest should be used at all. However, absolute voice rest for a few days may be helpful in patients with laryngitis, especially those gregarious, verbal singers who find it difficult to moderate their voice use to comply with relative voice rest instructions. In many instances, considerations of finances and reputation mitigate against a recommendation of voice rest. In advising performers to minimize vocal use, Punt counseled, "Don't say a single word for which you are not being paid."[4] This admonition frequently guides the ailing singer or speaker away from preperformance conversations and backstage greetings and allows a successful series of performances. Patients should also be instructed to speak softly and as infrequently as possible, often at a slightly higher pitch than usual; to avoid excessive telephone use; and to speak with abdominal support as they would in singing. This is relative voice rest, and it is helpful in most cases. An urgent session with a speech-language pathologist is extremely helpful for discussing vocal hygiene and in providing guidelines to prevent voice abuse. Nevertheless, the patient must be aware that some risk is associated with performing with laryngitis even when performance is possible. Inflammation of the vocal folds is associated with increased capillary fragility and increased risk of vocal fold injury or hemorrhage. Many factors must be considered in determining whether a given speech or concert is important enough to justify the potential consequences.

Steam inhalations deliver moisture and heat to the vocal folds and tracheobronchial tree and may be useful. Some people use nasal irrigations although these have little proven value. Gargling has no proven efficacy, but it is probably harmful only if it involves loud, abusive vocalization as part of the gargling process. Some physicians and patients believe it to be helpful "moistening the throat," and it may have some relaxing or placebo effect. Ultrasonic treatments, local massage, psychotherapy, and biofeedback directed at relieving anxiety and decreasing muscle tension may be helpful adjuncts to a broader therapeutic program. However, psychotherapy and biofeedback, in particular, must be expertly supervised if used at all.

Voice lessons given by an expert teacher are invaluable. When technical dysfunction is suggested, the singer or actor should be referred to his/her teacher.

Even when an obvious organic abnormality is present, referral to a voice teacher is appropriate, especially for younger actors and singers. Numerous "tricks of the trade" permit a voice professional to overcome some of the impairments of mild illness safely. If a singer plans to proceed with a performance during an illness, he or she should not cancel voice lessons as part of the relative voice rest regimen; rather, a short lesson to ensure optimal technique is extremely useful.

Sinusitis

Chronic inflammation of the mucosa lining the sinus cavities commonly produces thick secretions known as postnasal drip. Postnasal drip can be particularly problematic because it causes excessive phlegm, which interferes with phonation, and because it leads to frequent throat clearing, which may inflame the vocal folds. Sometimes chronic sinusitis is caused by allergies and can be treated with medications. However, many medications used for this condition cause side effects that are unacceptable in professional voice users, particularly mucosal drying. When medication management is not satisfactory, functional endoscopic sinus surgery may be appropriate.[5] Acute purulent sinusitis is a different matter. It requires aggressive treatment with antibiotics, sometimes surgical drainage, treatment of underlying conditions (such as dental abscess), and occasionally surgery.[5]

Lower Respiratory Tract Infection

Lower respiratory tract infection may be almost as disruptive to a voice as upper respiratory tract infection. Bronchitis, pneumonitis, pneumonia, and especially reactive airway disease impair the power source of the voice and lead to vocal strain, and sometimes injury. Lower respiratory tract infections should be treated aggressively, pulmonary function tests should be considered, and bronchodilators (preferably oral) should be used as necessary. Coughing is also a very traumatic vocal activity, and careful attention should be paid to cough suppression. If extensive voice use is anticipated, nonnarcotic antitussive agents are preferable because narcotics may dull the sensorium and lead to potentially damaging voice technique.

Tonsillitis

Tonsillitis also impairs the voice through alterations of the resonator system and through technical changes secondary to pain. Although there is a tendency to avoid tonsillectomy, especially in professional voice users, the operation should not be withheld when clear indications for tonsillectomy are present. These include, for example, documented severe bacterial tonsillitis six times per year. However, patients must be warned that tonsillectomy may alter the sound of the voice, even through there is no change at the vocal fold (oscillator) level.

Other Infections

Autoimmune deficiency syndrome (AIDS) is becoming more and more common. This lethal disease may present as hoarseness and xerostomia. Unexplained oral candidiasis, *Candida* infections of the tracheobronchial tree, and respiratory infections with other unusual pathogens should raise a physician's suspicions. However, it should also be remembered that infections with *Haemophilus influenzae*, *Streptococcus pneumoniae*, and common viruses are the most frequent pathogens in AIDS patients, just as they are in patients without AIDS. This disease should be considered in patients with frequent infections.

The laryngologist must also be alert for numerous other acute and chronic conditions that may cause laryngeal abnormalities, or even vocal fold masses that may be mistaken for malignancy and biopsied unnecessarily. Tuberculosis is being seen more often in modern practice. Although laryngeal lesions used to be associated with extensive pulmonary infection, they are now usually associated with much less virulent disease, often only a mild cough. Laryngeal lesions are usually localized.[6,7]

Sarcoidosis, a granulomatous disease, demonstrates laryngeal symptoms in 3% to 5% of cases.[8] Non-caseating granulomas are found in the larynx, and the false vocal folds are involved frequently, producing airway obstruction rather than dysphonia. Less common diseases, including leprosy,[9,10] syphilis,[11] scleroderma,[12] typhoid,[13] typhus,[13] and other conditions, may produce laryngeal lesions that may mimic neoplasms and lead the laryngologist to obtain unnecessary biopsy of lesions that can be cured medically.

Confusing lesions may also be caused by a variety of mycotic infections, including histoplasmosis,[14-16] coccidiomycosis,[17] cryptococcosis,[18] blastomycosis,[19,20] actinomycosis,[21,22] candidiasis,[23] aspergillosis,[24-26] mucormycosis,[27] rhinosporidiosis,[28] and sporotrichosis.[29] Parasitic diseases may also produce laryngeal masses. The most prominent example is leishmaniasis.[30] More detailed information about most of the conditions discussed above is available in an excellent text by Michaels.[31] Some viral conditions may also cause laryngeal structural abnormalies, most notably papillomas. However, herpes virus, variola, and other organisms have also been implicated in laryngeal infection.

SYSTEMIC CONDITIONS

Aging

This subject is so important that it has been covered extensively in other literature.[32] Many characteristics associated with vocal aging are actually deficits in conditioning, rather than irreversible aging changes. For example, in singers, such problems as a "wobble," pitch inaccuracies (singing flat), and inability to sing softly are rarely caused by irreversible aging changes, and these problems can usually be managed easily through voice therapy and training.

Hearing Loss

Hearing loss is often overlooked as a source of vocal problems. Auditory feedback is fundamental to speaking and singing. Interference with this control mechanism may result in altered vocal production, particularly if the person is unaware of the hearing loss. Distortion, particularly pitch distortion (diplacusis) may also pose serious problems for the singer. This appears to cause not only aesthetic difficulties in matching pitch, but also vocal strain, which accompanies pitch shifts.[33] In-depth discussion is not presented here as this subject is discussed in other literature.[2]

Respiratory Dysfunction

The importance of "the breath" has been well recognized in the field of voice pedagogy. Respiratory disorders are discussed at length in other literature.[34] Even a mild degree of obstructive pulmonary disease can result in substantial voice problems. Unrecognized exercise-induced asthma is especially problematic in singers and actors, because bronchospasm may be precipitated by the exercise and airway drying that occurs during voice performance. In such cases, the bronchospastic obstruction on exhalation impairs support. This commonly results in compensatory hyperfunction.

Treatment requires skilled management and collaboration with a pulmonologist and a voice team.[35] Whenever possible, patients should be managed primarily with oral medications; the use of inhalers should be minimized. Steroid inhalers should be avoided altogether whenever possible. It is particularly important to recognize that asthma can be induced by the exercise of phonation itself,[36] and in many cases a high index of suspicion and methacholine challenge test are needed to avoid missing this important diagnosis.

Allergy

Even mild allergies are more incapacitating to professional voice users than to others. This subject can be reviewed elsewhere.[37] Briefly, patients with mild intermittent allergies can usually be managed with antihistamines although they should never be tried for the first time immediately prior to a voice performance. Because antihistamines commonly produce unacceptable side effects, trial and error may be needed in order to find a medication with an acceptable balance between effect and side effect for any individual patient, especially a voice professional. Patients with allergy-related voice disturbances may find hyposensitization a more effective approach than antihistamine use, if they are candidates for such treatment. For voice patients with unexpected allergic symptoms immediately prior to an important voice commitment, corticosteroids should be used rather than antihistamines, in order to minimize the risks of side effects (such as drying and thickening of secretions) that might make voice performance difficult or impossible. Allergies commonly cause voice problems by altering the mucosa and secretions and causing nasal obstruction. Management will not be covered in depth in this brief chapter. However, it should be recognized that many of the medicines commonly used to treat allergies have side effects deleterious to voice function, particularly dryness and thickening of secretions. Consequently, when voice disturbance is causally related to these conditions, more definitive treatment through allergic immunotherapy should be considered. This is especially important to professional voice users.

Gastroesophageal Reflux Laryngitis

Gastroesophageal reflux laryngitis is extremely common among voice patients, especially singers.[38] This is a condition in which the sphincter between the stomach and esophagus is inefficient, and acidic stomach secretions reflux (reach the laryngeal tissues), causing inflammation. The most typical symptoms are hoarseness in the morning, prolonged vocal warm-up time, halitosis and a bitter taste in the morning, a feeling of a "lump in the throat," frequent throat clearing, chronic irritative cough, and frequent tracheitis or tracheobronchitis. Any or all of these symptoms may be present. Heartburn is not common in these patients, so the diagnosis is often missed. Prolonged reflux also is associated with the development of Barrett esophagus, esophageal carcinoma, and laryngeal carcinoma.[38]

Physical examination usually reveals erythema (redness) of the arytenoid mucosa. A barium swallow radiographic study with water siphonage may provide additional information but is not needed routinely. However, if a patient complies strictly with treatment recommendations and does not show marked improvement within a month, or if there is a reason to suspect more serious pathology, complete evaluation by a gastroenterologist should be carried out. This is often advisable in patients who are over 40 years of age or who have had reflux symptoms for more than five years. Twenty-four hour pH impedance monitoring of the esophagus is often effective in establishing a diagnosis. The results are correlated with a diary of the patient's activities and symptoms. Bulimia should also be considered in the differential diagnosis when symptoms are refractory to treatment and other physical and psychologic signs are suggestive.

The mainstays of treatment for reflux laryngitis are elevation of the head of the bed (not just sleeping on pillows), antacids, H$_2$ blockers and/or proton pump inhibitors, and avoidance of eating for three to four hours before going to sleep. This is often difficult for singers and actors because of their performance schedule, but if they are counseled about minor changes in eating habits (such as eating larger meals at breakfast and lunch), they usually can comply. Avoidance of alcohol, caffeine, and specific foods is beneficial. Medications that decrease or block acid production may be necessary. It must be recognized that control of acidity is not the same as control of reflux. In many cases, reflux is provoked during singing because of the increased abdominal pressure associated with support. In these instances, it often causes excessive phlegm and throat clearing during the first ten or fifteen minutes of a performance or lesson, as well as other common reflux laryngitis symptoms even when acidity has been neutralized effectively. Laparoscopic Nissen fundoplication has proven extremely effective and should be considered a reasonable alternative to lifelong medication in this relatively young patient population.[38]

Endocrine Dysfunction

Endocrine (hormonal) problems warrant special attention. The human voice is extremely sensitive to endocrinologic changes. Many of these are reflected in alterations of fluid content of the lamina propria just beneath the laryngeal mucosa. This causes alterations in the bulk and shape of the vocal folds and results in voice change. Hypothyroidism is a well-recognized cause of such voice disorders, although the mechanism is not fully understood.[39-42] Hoarseness, vocal fatigue, muffling of the voice, loss of range, and a sensation of a lump in the throat may be present even with mild hypothyroidism. Even when thyroid function tests results are within the low-normal range, this diagnosis should be entertained, especially if thyroid-stimulating hormone levels are in the high-normal range or are elevated. Thyrotoxicosis may result in similar voice disturbances.[43]

Voice changes associated with sex hormones are encountered commonly in clinical practice and have been investigated more thoroughly than have other hormonal changes. Although a correlation appears to exist between sex hormone levels and depth of male voices (higher testosterone and lower estradiol levels in basses than in tenors),[44] the most important hormonal considerations in males occur during the maturation process.

When castrato singers were in vogue, castration at about age 7 or 8 resulted in failure of laryngeal growth during puberty, and voices that stayed in the soprano or alto range and boasted a unique quality of sound.[45] Failure of a male voice to change at puberty is uncommon today and is often psychogenic in etiology.[1] However, hormonal deficiencies such as those seen in cryptorchidism, delayed sexual development, Klinefelter's syndrome, or Fröhlich's syndrome may be responsible. In these cases, the persistently high voice may be the complaint that causes the patient to seek medical attention.

Voice problems related to sex hormones are most common in female singers.[46] Although vocal changes associated with the normal menstrual cycle may be difficult to quantify with current experimental techniques, unquestionably they occur.[2,46-50] Most of the ill effects are seen in the immediate premenstrual period and are known as laryngopathia premenstrualis. This common condition is caused by physiologic, anatomic, and psychologic alterations secondary to endocrine changes. The vocal dysfunction is characterized by decreased vocal efficiency, loss of the highest notes in the voice, vocal fatigue, slight hoarseness, and some muffling of the voice. It is often more apparent to the singer than to the listener. Submucosal hemorrhages in the larynx are more common in the premenstrual period.[48] In many European opera houses, singers used to be excused from singing during the premenstrual and early menstrual days ("grace days"). This practice is not followed in the United States and is no longer in vogue in most European countries. Premenstrual changes cause significant vocal symptoms in approximately one-third of singers. Although ovulation inhibitors have been shown to mitigate some of these symptoms,[49] in some women (about 5%),[51] birth control pills may deleteriously alter voice range and character even after only a few months of therapy.[52-55] When oral contraceptives are used, the voice should

67. Rosen DC, Sataloff RT. *Psychology of Voice Disorders.* San Diego, CA: Singular Publishing Group; 1997:1–261.

68. Sataloff RT. Vocal fold scar. In: Sataloff RT. *Professional Voice: The Science and Art of Clinical Care.* 3rd ed. San Diego, CA: Plural Publishing Inc; 2005:1309–1314.

69. Sataloff RT, Spiegel JR, Hawkshaw M, Rosen DC. Vocal fold hemorrhage. In: Sataloff RT. *Professional Voice: The Science and Art of Clinical Care.* 3rd ed. San Diego, CA: Plural Publishing Inc; 2005:1291–1308.

70. Hochman I, Sataloff RT, Hillman R, Zeitels S. Ectasias and varicies of the vocal fold: clearing the striking zone. *Ann Otol Rhinol Laryngol.* 1999;108(1):10–16.

71. Zeitels SM. Phonomicrosurgical techniques. In: Sataloff RT. *Professional Voice: The Science and Art of Clinical Care.* 3rd ed. San Diego, CA: Plural Publishing Inc; 2005:647–658.

72. Zeitels SM, Sataloff RT. Phonomicrosurgical resection of glottal papillomatosis. *J Voice.* 1999;13(1):123–127.

73. Wellens W, Snoeck R, Desloovere C, et al. Treatment of severe laryngeal papillomatosis with intralesional injections of Cidofovir [(S)-1-(3-hydroxy-phosphonyl-methoxypropyl) cytosine, HPMPC, Vistide®]. In: McCafferty G, Coman W, Carroll R, eds. Sydney; 1997. Bologna, Italy: Monduzzi Editor; 1997:455–549.

74. Anderson, TD, Sataloff RT. Laryngeal cancer. In: Sataloff RT. *Professional Voice: The Science and Art of Clinical Care.* 3rd ed. San Diego, CA: Plural Publishing Inc; 2005: 1375–1392.

75. Wolman L, Drake CS, Young A. The larynx in rheumatoid arthritis. *J Laryngol.* 1965;79:403–404.

76. Bridger MWM, Jahn AF, van Nostrand AWP. Laryngeal rheumatoid arthritis. *Laryngoscope.* 1980;90:296–303.

77. Virchow R. Seltene Gichtablagerungen. *Virchows Arch Pathol.* 1868;44:137–138.

78. Marion RB, Alperin JE, Maloney WH. Gouty tophus of the true vocal cord. *Arch Otolaryngol.* 1972;96:161–162.

79. Stark DB, New GB. Amyloid tumors of the larynx, trachea or bronchi; report of 15 cases. *Ann Otol Rhinol Laryngol.* 1949;58:117–134.

80. Michaels L, Hyams VJ. Amyloid in localized deposits and plasmacytomas of the respiratory tract. *J Pathol.* 1979;128:29–38.

81. Urbach E, Wiethe C. Lipoidosis cutis et mucosae. *Virchows Arch Pathol Anat.* 1929;273:285–319.

82. Sataloff RT, Hawkshaw M, Ressue J. Granular cell tumor of the larynx. *Ear Nose Throat J.* 1998;77(8):582–584.

83. Charow A, Pass F, Ruben R. Pemphigus of the upper respiratory tract. *Arch Otolaryngol.* 1971;93:209–210.

84. Heuer RJ, Rulnick RK, Horman M, Perez KS, Emerich KA, Sataloff RT. Voice therapy. In: Sataloff RT. *Professional Voice: The Science and Art of Clinical Care.* 3rd ed. San Diego, CA: Plural Publishing Inc; 2005:961–986.

85. Sataloff RT, Baroody MM, Emerich KA, Carroll JM. Singing voice specialist. In: Sataloff RT. *Professional Voice: The Science and Art of Clinical Care.* 3rd ed. San Diego, CA: Plural Publishing Inc; 2005:1021–1040.

86. Freed SL, Raphael BN, Sataloff RT. The role of the acting voice trainer in medical care of professional voice users. In: Sataloff RT. *Professional Voice: The Science and Art of Clinical Care.* 3rd ed. San Diego, CA: Plural Publishing Inc; 2005:1051–1060.

87. Sataloff RT. Voice surgery. In: Sataloff RT. *Professional Voice: The Science and Art of Clinical Care.* 3rd ed. San Diego, CA: Plural Publishing Inc; 2005:1137–1214.

88. Sataloff RT, Spiegel JR, Heuer RJ, et al. Laryngeal mini-microflap: a new technique and reassessment of the microflap saga. *J Voice.* 1995;9(2):198–204.

89. Abitbol, J. Limitations of the laser in microsurgery of the larynx. In: Lawrence VL, ed. *Transactions of the Twelfth Symposium: Care of the Professional Voice.* New York, NY: The Voice Foundation; 1984.

90. Tapia RG, Pardo J, Marigil M, Pacio A. Effects of the laser upon Reinke's space and the neural system of the vocalis muscle. In: Lawrence VL, ed. *Transactions of the Twelfth Symposium: Care of the Professional Voice.* New York, NY: The Voice Foundation; 1984:289–291.

91. Sataloff RT, Feldman M, Darby KS, Carroll LM, Spiegel JR. Arytenoid dislocation. *J Voice.* 1988;1(4):368–377.

92. Sataloff RT, Bough ID, Spiegel JR. Arytenoid dislocation: diagnosis and treatment. *Laryngoscope.* 1994; 104(10):1353–1361.

93. Ford CN. Bless DM. Collagen injected in the scarred vocal fold. *J Voice.* 1988;1(1):116–118.

94. Sataloff RT, Spiegel JR, Hawkshaw M, Rosen DC, Heuer RJ. Autologous fat implantation for vocal fold scar. *J Voice.* 1997;11(2):238–246.

24

Congenital Anomalies of the Larynx

Ted L. Tewfik, MD, FRCSC
Steven E. Sobol, MD, FRCSC
Khalil Al Macki, MD

Congenital anomalies of the larynx are a common reason for consultation in pediatric otolaryngology. Symptoms of congenital laryngeal anomalies frequently present at birth but may be delayed. The clinical findings range from subtle changes in feeding or speech, to life-threatening respiratory obstruction.

Stridor is a sign of upper respiratory obstruction. Generally, inspiratory stridor suggests obstruction above the glottis and expiratory stridor indicates a lesion in the lower trachea. Biphasic stridor suggests a glottic or subglottic obstruction.

Anomalies of the larynx are the major cause of neonatal stridor, accounting for 60% of such cases,[1] and must be differentiated from tracheal anomalies, bronchial or other acquired lesions. [2]

In this chapter, we review the common congenital anomalies of the larynx in terms of their epidemiology, etiology, clinical presentation, diagnosis, and management.

LARYNGOMALACIA

Epidemiology

Laryngomalacia is the most common congenital anomaly of the larynx, accounting for 60% of all cases.[3] Male infants are affected twice as commonly as females.[4]

Etiology and Pathogenesis

The exact cause of laryngomalacia is not known. Theories include abnormal development of the cartilaginous structures and immaturity of neuromuscular control.[5]

The epiglottis derives from the third and fourth branchial arches. Overgrowth of the third arch portion of the epiglottis results in elongation and lateral extension of the mature structure, which may be seen in patients with laryngomalacia.[3] There is some evidence that the laryngeal cartilages are intrinsically weaker in patients with laryngomalacia.[6] Other histological studies, however, have shown no difference between children with and without laryngomalacia.[7]

Immature neuromuscular control may be responsible for the arytenoid prolapse seen in laryngomalacia.[8] This theory is supported by the finding that children with laryngomalacia have an increased incidence of hypotonia, associated with gastrointestinal reflux (GER), obstructive sleep apnea, and failure to thrive.[9] However, there is no increase in the incidence of laryngomalacia in premature infants who are generally hypotonic.[10]

In a recent prospective study, Gianonni et al[11] observed GER in 64% of patients with laryngomalacia. They concluded also that GER was significantly associated with severe symptoms and a complicated clinical course. Fetal warfarin syndrome (FWS), or warfarin embryopathy, a rare condition that results from maternal ingestion of warfarin during pregnancy, has been associated with various congenital anomalies including laryngomalacia.[12]

Clinical Presentation

The most common symptoms of laryngomalacia include noisy respiration and inspiratory stridor, accentuated by supine positioning, feeding, and agitation and relieved by neck extension and prone positioning. Symptoms are usually absent at birth, begin within the first few weeks of life, increase over several months, and resolve by 18 months to two years of age. Less commonly, the child may experience feeding difficulties but rarely failure to thrive. Respiratory distress and cyanosis are also rare.

On examination, the child with laryngomalacia is usually within the normal range of growth, appears healthy, and does not exhibit signs of respiratory distress (nasal flaring, supraclavicular or intercostal indrawing, and/or cyanosis). The cry is normal and strong. Head and neck examination is usually normal.

Flexible endoscopy may reveal several characteristic abnormalities, such as[13]:

1. Elongation and lateral extension of the epiglottis (omega-shaped), which falls posteroinferiorly on inspiration
2. Redundant, bulky arytenoids, which prolapse anteromedially on inspiration
3. Shortening of the aryepiglottic folds, resulting in tethering the arytenoids to the epiglottis
4. Inward collapse of the aryepiglottic folds (with the cuneiform cartilages) on inspiration.

Expiration results in the expulsion of these supraglottic structures with unimpeded flow of air. The vocal folds usually can be visualized and have normal structure and function in patients with laryngomalacia[10] (Figure 24–1).

Shah and Wetmore[14] proposed a classification for laryngomalacia based on the clinical presentation and anatomical site of collapse. The severity of the *s*tridor, *w*eight gain, *a*ge of presentation, and the *n*eurological status (SWAN) represent the clinical factors.

The adoption of similar classifications should facilitate documentation and statistical analyses of management and outcome in future reports (Table 24–1).

Diagnosis

In cases of mild to moderate stridor, the classic history and endoscopic examination are usually sufficient to establish a diagnosis of laryngomalacia.

Radiographic studies may suggest a diagnosis of laryngomalacia and should be performed to rule out coexisting anomalies of the airway (tracheomalacia, innominate artery compression, or vascular rings of the trachea).[4,15] In a recent study, Masters et al demonstrated a strong association between congenital malacia and other anomalies such as congenital heart dis-

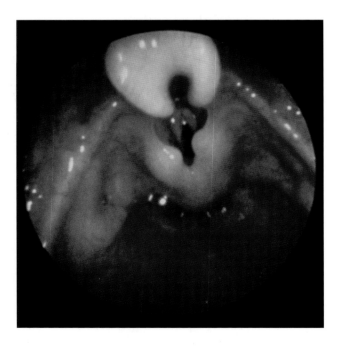

Figure 24–1. Laryngomalacia: Omega-shaped epiglottis and short epiglottic folds. (Courtesy of Dr. J. Paul Willging of Cincinnati)

Table 24–1. Types of Laryngomalacia.[14]

Type I	Inward collapse of A/E folds, corniculate and cuneiform cartilages. Obstruction occurs as these cartilages are drawn inward during inspiration.
Type II	A long tubular epiglottis (exaggerated omega-shaped) curls on itself and contributes to the obstruction.
Type III	Anterior, medial collapse of the corniculate and cuneiform cartilages to occlude the laryngeal inlet during inspiration.
Type IV	Posterior inspiratory displacement of the epiglottis against the posterior pharyngeal wall, or inferior collapse of the vocal folds.
Type V	Short A/E folds.

orders (13.7%), tracheo-esophageal fistula (9.6%), and various syndromes (8%).[16] Even though understanding of these disorders is still in its infancy, physicians should maintain a high level of awareness for malacial lesions and consider the possibility of concomitant anomalies, even when one symptom predominates or occurs alone.[16] Inspiratory plain films of the neck may show inferior and medial displacement of the epiglottis and arytenoids. Fluoroscopy may reveal supraglottic collapse and hypopharyngeal dilatation.

Microlaryngoscopy and rigid bronchoscopy under general anesthesia should be performed when the child is experiencing respiratory distress or there is suggestion of coexisting anomalies on radiologic imaging.[17]

Multiple authors have reported on the effects of acid and pepsin on the larynx and tracheobronchial tree. Persistent edema in patients with GER is a common finding in infants with laryngomalacia.[18] A band of inflammation beneath the epithelium associated with the presence of intra-epithelial eosinophils appear to be a histological indication for concurrent reflux in laryngomalacia.[19] Bronchoalveolar lavage (BAL) findings obtained in infants with laryngomalacia demonstrated that these patients have episodes of microaspiration by calculating the amount of lipids in the alveolar macrophages.[20]

Management

The majority of patients with laryngomalacia can be managed by observation given that the condition is generally self-resolving by 12 to 18 months of age.

Medical management of documented esophageal reflux disease should be employed, as this is known to contribute to laryngomalacia.[21] The therapy includes positioning measures and medications (see Table 24–2).

Surgical management is indicated for patients failing to thrive and patients with respiratory complications.

1. Tracheotomy is indicated for acute respiratory distress and should be left in place until the supraglottic pathology resolves with age.[4]
2. Supraglottoplasty avoids the need for tracheotomy. In this procedure, the laryngeal inlet is widened by removing a wedge of the aryepiglottic folds bilaterally, trimming the epiglottis, removing the corniculate and cuneiform cartilages and redundant arytenoid mucosa. The procedure is usually performed using laser surgery. Patients are extubated the day after surgery.[10] Relief of respiratory symptoms occurs in more than 80% of cases.[22] Complications of the bilateral procedure include the development of posterior supraglottic stenosis, which may be prevented by unilateral endoscopic supraglottoplasty [23] (see Figures 24–2 and 24–3). In our opinion, it is always advisable to avoid excessive excision and reassess the patient if symptoms persist.

Complications

Although some studies have quoted a high percentage of respiratory distress in patients with laryngomalacia,[24,25] the condition resolves without complications in the vast majority of patients.[15] Complications, in rare cases, include chest deformities, attacks of cyanosis, obstructive apnea, pulmonary hypertension, right heart failure, and failure to thrive.

VOCAL FOLD PARALYSIS

Epidemiology

According to Cotton and Prescott,[26] vocal fold paralysis is the second most common congenital anomaly of the larynx. It represents 15% of all congenital laryngeal anomalies; however other authors list its incidence around 10%.[27] There is no gender difference in the prevalence of this anomaly. Paralysis may be either bi-

Table 24–2. Commonly Used Medications for the Treatment of GER[21]

Drug (Generic) (Trade name)	Dosage	Class
Cimetidine (Tagamet)	*Neonate:* 5–10 mg/kg/day po in div. doses q8-12h *Infant:* 10–20 mg/kg/day po in div. doses q6-12h *Child:* 20–40 mg/kg/day po in div. doses q6h	H-2 receptor antagonist
Ranitidine (Zantac)	*Child & infant > 1 month old:* 5–10 mg/kg/day po in 2–3 div. doses	H-2 receptor antagonist
Famotidine (Pepcid)	1–2 mg/kg/day po in 2 div. doses	H-2 receptor antagonist
Omeprazole (Prilosec)	*Infant:* 0.5 mg/kg po q24h *Child:* 0.7–3.3 mg/kg po q24h	H+/K+ ATPase inhibitor
Cisapride (Propulsid)	*Neonate & Infant :* 0.1 mg/kg/dose po 8h *Child:* 0.1–0.2 mg/kg/dose po q6-8h	Prokinetic agent
Metoclopramide (Reglan)	*Neonates, infants, & children:* 0.4–0.8 mg/kg/day in 4 div. doses	Prokinetic agent

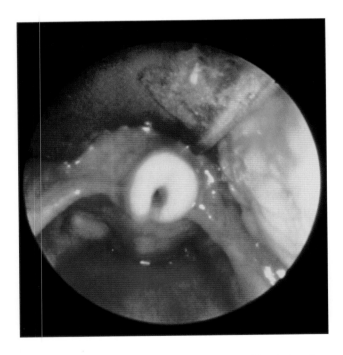

Figure 24–2. Laryngomalacia associated with obstructive sleep apnea. (Courtesy of Dr. J. Paul Willging of Cincinnati)

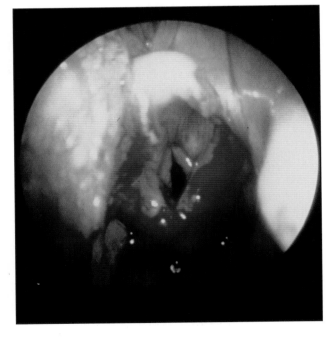

Figure 24–3. Same patient in Figure 24–2, after supraglottoplasty. (Courtesy of Dr. J. Paul Willging of Cincinnati)

lateral or unilateral. Approximately half of all cases of bilateral vocal fold paralysis are congenital.[28, 29]

Etiology and Pathogenesis

Overall, the most common cause of bilateral vocal fold paralysis is Arnold-Chiari malformation, followed by birth trauma causing excessive strain on the cervical spine., One third of all cases are idiopathic.[29-31] Birth-trauma-induced vocal fold paralysis, which may be bilateral or unilateral, is responsible for approximately 20% of cases, usually following high forceps or abnormally presenting deliveries. Fifty percent of patients with bilateral vocal fold paralysis have associated anomalies. Other acquired cases of bilateral vocal fold paralysis may be secondary to central neuromuscular immaturity, cerebral palsy, hydrocephalus, myelomeningocele, spina bifida, hypoxia, hemorrhage, or infection.[32]

Central nervous system defect is usually responsible for bilateral vocal fold paralysis, whereas unilateral disease is usually secondary to peripheral nerve pathology.[30] The most common cause of unilateral vocal fold paralysis is iatrogenic following cardiac surgery.[30, 31] Blunt trauma causing traction injuries to the recurrent laryngeal nerve may be responsible for a number of cases. Lesions in the mediastinum, such as tumors or vascular malformations, may be the cause of certain cases of unilateral vocal fold paralysis.[32,33]

Clinical Presentation

Bilateral vocal fold paralysis presents in children with near-normal phonation and progressive airway obstruction, manifesting as biphasic or inspiratory stridor at rest, which is exacerbated by agitation. Respiratory compromise becomes more pronounced with age as the oxygen requirements increase.[34] Obstruction can progress to a state of respiratory distress requiring airway intervention. Aspiration is common with bilateral vocal fold paralysis, often resulting in recurrent chest infections.

Unilateral vocal fold paralysis may present during the first few weeks of life or may go unnoticed due to the paucity of respiratory symptoms. The most common symptoms are a hoarse, breathy cry, which may be aggravated by agitation. Feeding difficulties and signs of aspiration may also be present in children with unilateral vocal fold paralysis.

Head and neck examination may reveal the presence of other cranial nerve deficits. A full examination should be performed to rule out associated anomalies in patients with vocal fold paralysis.

Diagnosis

Bilateral vocal fold paralysis is suggested by a history of early inspiratory stridor associated with signs of respiratory distress and abnormal voice or cry.[35] If the child is stable, flexible endoscopy may be performed to allow dynamic visualization of vocal fold movement. The limitations of this diagnostic modality, however, are the inability to palpate the cricoarytenoid joint and visualize the rest of the upper airway. Rigid laryngobronchoscopy should be done to confirm the diagnosis and to assess the airway for other anomalies. If the diagnosis is uncertain, the procedure should be repeated one week later to confirm the diagnosis.

Flexible endoscopic examination is usually sufficient to establish a diagnosis of unilateral vocal fold paralysis. In the presence of respiratory distress, rigid bronchoscopy should also be done to rule out the presence of concurrent airway anomalies.

Radiographic imaging for patients with vocal fold paralysis can be used for both diagnosis and to rule out concurrent pathology. Ultrasound of the larynx can be used to assess vocal fold function in patients unable to tolerate endoscopy or as a noninvasive follow-up study in patients with known paralysis.[36] Patients with bilateral vocal fold paralysis should have imaging of the central nervous system to rule out abnormalities or injuries. Patients with unilateral vocal fold paralysis should have radiographic studies (CT mediastinum and neck) to rule out other lesions compromising the function of the recurrent laryngeal nerve.

Laryngeal electromyography (EMG) is now used in the evaluation and management of vocal fold mobility disorders and to differentiate vocal fold fixation from paralysis.[37]

Management

Patients with bilateral vocal fold paralysis may need urgent airway intervention, which is usually achievable by endotracheal intubation. Tracheotomy is necessary to relieve the obstruction and should remain in place for 2 years to allow spontaneous recovery, which occurs completely in more than half of patients. For patients with bilateral vocal fold paralysis, supportive measures are also necessary to ensure that adequate nutrition is received while aspiration is prevented.

If recovery does not occur, consideration should be given to vocal fold lateralization procedures in an effort to decannulate the patient. Arytenoidectomy produces reliable results in maintaining a patent airway and achieving decannulation. Transverse laser cordotomy has had early success in allowing decannulation in older children and adults. To prevent the complications of long-term tracheotomy, some authors advocate early lateralization procedures in patients with bilateral vocal fold paralysis.[38-40]

The majority of cases of unilateral vocal fold paralysis can be managed by observation, ensuring that respiratory and feeding difficulties do not develop. Upright positioning is usually sufficient to alleviate aspiration difficulties. Rarely, intubation may be necessary to acquire a stable airway in distressed patients.

CONGENTICAL SUBGLOTTIC STENOSIS

Epidemiology

Congenital subglottic stenosis is defined as subglottic narrowing in the absence of endotracheal intubation or any other apparent cause.[34] It is the third most common congenital anomaly of the larynx.[4,26] It is the most common laryngeal anomaly to require tracheotomy in infants.[41] Males are affected twice as commonly as females.

Etiology and Pathogenesis

Incomplete recanalization of the laryngotracheal tube during the third month of gestation leads to different degrees of congenital subglottic stenosis. At the extreme spectrum of this condition is complete laryngeal atresia (see below), which results from complete failure to recanalize the lumen in the tenth week of gestation.[42]

Classification

Congenital subglottic stenosis can be classified according to the gross and histological characteristics of the obstruction.[4] Membranous congenital subglottic stenosis is the result of circumferential submucosal hypertrophy with excess fibrous connective tissue and mucous glands,[43] On examination, it usually appears as circumferential, soft-tissue thickening, which is compressible. It is the most common and mildest form of congenital subglottic stenosis.

Cartilaginous subglottic stenosis is the result of abnormal development of the cricoid cartilage and usually appears as an elliptically shaped narrow lumen of the subglottis.[43,44] The defect is usually lateral thickening of the cricoid cartilage but, in some cases, may also be due to anteroposterior narrowing.

Holinger[45] described different types of cricoid cartilage abnormalities associated with congenital subglottic stenosis. They include elliptical-shaped cricoid, subglottic laryngeal cleft, flattened cricoid, large anterior lamina, and generalized thickening, as well as a rare anterior submucous cleft.

Clinical Presentation

The manifestations of congenital subglottic stenosis usually appear in the first few months of life. The stenosis is not evident until the child develops an acute inflammatory process, which further compromises the subglottic space.[46] The clinical presentation during this period does not differ from that of infectious laryngotracheobronchitis (croup). Biphasic stridor with or without respiratory distress is the most common presenting symptom. The child may have a barking cough, but the cry is usually normal. Suspicion of congenital subglottic stenosis should be aroused when these symptoms recur or are prolonged

beyond the normal duration of infectious croup despite adequate medical therapy.[17,47] Another clinical scenario that should arouse suspicion of congenital stenosis is in asymptomatic children who are difficult to intubate, or decannulate. Children with Down syndrome are at increased risk of having congenital subglottic stenosis and may present in this fashion.[48]

On examination, the child with congenital subglottic stenosis may or may not be in significant respiratory distress (nasal flaring, supraclavicular or intercostal indrawing, cyanosis). Head and neck examination is usually normal.

Flexible endoscopy does not adequately assess the subglottis but is important to rule out vocal fold paralysis and other glottic and or supraglottic anomalies. Myer, O'Connor, and Cotton[49] proposed a practical grading system for subglottic stenosis as follows:

> Grade I up to 50% narrowing,
>
> Grade II from 51% to 70% stenosis, and
>
> Grade III more than 70% with any detectable lumen.

An airway with no lumen is assigned to grade IV. This grading is useful especially when tracheal reconstruction is contemplated.

Diagnosis

Congenital subglottic stenosis is usually suggested by a history of recurrent episodes of croup. Rigid bronchoscopy under general anesthesia should be done to confirm the diagnosis, plan future management, and assess the airway for other anomalies. The stenosis should be evaluated in terms of its length and diameter, which may be adequately assessed by passing a scope or endotracheal tube of known outer diameter through the stenosis. The largest tube or scope to pass through the airway is a good measure of the lumen diameter.[49] A diagnosis of congenital subglottic stenosis is made when the lumen diameter is less than 4 mm in a term infant or 3 mm in a preterm infant. The findings at endoscopy characteristically are less severe than in children with acquired subglottic stenosis.

Radiographic evaluation may help to assess the subglottic airway prior to bronchoscopy or when the diagnosis is unclear. Plain lateral or anteroposterior (AP) x-rays will show a characteristic narrowing at the level of the subglottis.[50]

Management

Most cases of congenital subglottic stenosis will resolve spontaneously with growth of the child and can be managed conservatively. During episodes of acute laryngo-tracheobronchitis, patients with congenital subglottic stenosis should be managed aggressively to avoid intubation, as this increases trauma to the airway.[46] Less than half of all children with congenital subglottic stenosis will require surgical airway intervention.[51]

Endotracheal intubation and tracheotomy may be required in patients who have significant airway compromise. Most children who require tracheotomy can be decannulated by 3 to 4 years of age when the subglottic space matures to a sufficient diameter.

Laryngotracheoplasty is not usually necessary but may be required to reconstruct the airway in patients who cannot be decannulated. In neonates who fail extubation, anterior cricoid split should be considered when the pathology is anterior glottic or subglottic, The patient weight should be more than 1500 grams.[49,52,53] A vertical split is carried through the lower thyroid cartilage, the cricoid cartilage, and the first two tracheal rings.[31] An endotracheal tube is used as a stent for approximately 7 days before extubation.[54] In properly selected patients, the anterior cricoid split results in less hospitalization, morbidity, and mortality when compared to tracheotomy.[53] Medical treatment of gastroesophageal reflux, and use of antibiotics and steroids during the intubation period, should be routine in patients undergoing open procedures.

An anatomical study showed that thyroid alar cartilage (TAC) could be used for anterior grafting in laryngotracheoplasty in premature and newborn babies. Its indications should be limited to grade II and a few grade III of the Myer subglottic stenosis classification without glottic or tracheal extension.[55]

Monnier et al published their experience with partial cricotracheal resection (PCTR) for severe subglottic stenosis. They described a high rate of successful decannulation rate.[56]

Laser ablation has a limited role in the management of congenital subglottic stenosis and is usually reserved for soft lesions less than 5 mm in thickness.

SUBGLOTTIC HEMANGIOMA

Epidemiology

Subglottic hemangiomas account for 1.5% of all congenital anomalies of the larynx.[3,4]. Females are affected twice as commonly as males.[57]

Etiology and Pathogenesis

Subglottic hemangiomas result from vascular malformations derived from mesenchymal rests of vaso-active tissue in the subglottis.[1] Histologically, the majority of these lesions are composed of capillarylike vessels as opposed to the cavernous hemangiomas, which present often in older patients.[58]

Clinical Presentation

The child with a subglottic hemangioma is usually asymptomatic at birth. As the lesion rapidly increases in size from 2 to 12 months of age, the baby develops progressive respiratory distress, which is at first intermittent and then continuous. The symptoms are similar to those of infectious croup, presenting with biphasic stridor, barking cough, normal or hoarse cry, and failure to thrive. Some patients may develop airway obstruction significant enough to necessitate intervention. After the first year of life, most patients experience progressive resolution of their symptoms, as the lesion regresses spontaneously by 5 years of age.[57,59,60]

On examination, the child with a subglottic hemangioma may or may not be in significant respiratory distress (nasal flaring, supraclavicular or intercostal indrawing, and/or cyanosis). Head and neck examination is usually normal. Cutaneous hemangiomas are present in half of these patients.[4]

Flexible endoscopy does not demonstrate the lesion but is necessary to rule out other laryngeal anomalies (Figure 24–4).

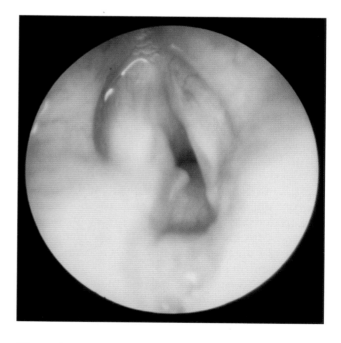

Figure 24–4. Posterior subglottic hemangioma. (Courtesy of Dr. J. Paul Willging of Cincinnati)

Diagnosis

Rigid bronchoscopy under general anesthesia is necessary to establish diagnosis of subglottic hemangiomas. The lesion usually presents as a smooth, compressible submucosal mass located posterolaterally in the subglottis.[61] It may be unilateral or bilateral and may extend to the upper trachea. It is usually sessile, pink-blue in color, and easily compressible. When the diagnosis is unclear, biopsy of the lesion should be undertaken with caution due to the risk of significant hemorrhage.[57]

Plain x-rays of the neck may aid in making the diagnosis prior to endoscopy. AP views will show an asymmetric narrowing of the subglottis, and lateral views will demonstrate posterior subglottic soft-tissue density.

Management

Observation is usually sufficient for subglottic hemangiomas that do not cause significant airway obstruction. However, a substantial number of patients will require surgical intervention to relieve airway obstruction at some point during the acute growth phase.

Surgical approaches in patients with subglottic hemangiomas can be classified as open or endoscopic. The goal is to establish an adequate airway. It should be emphasized that all surgical interventions in cases of subglottic hemangiomas should be as conservative as possible, to avoid iatrogenic subglottic stenosis.[62]

Open surgical procedures may be necessary to establish an airway in the acute setting or, rarely, can be employed to resect lesions not amenable to endoscopic approaches.[63] Tracheotomy is usually necessary to secure the airway, and should be left in place until the lesion regresses spontaneously, usually by 5 years of age.

Steroid injection into small- or moderate-size hemangiomas may precipitate involution secondary to suppression of estradiol stimulation of the lesion and increased responsiveness to vasoconstrictors.[64] Steroids, which have been found to decrease the size and increase the rate of involution of hemangiomas, may be considered as adjuvant therapy in certain cases.[65,66] However, for the majority of subglottic hematomas, the use of systemic steroid therapy is not sufficient as a sole treatment option.

Other endoscopic surgical techniques that have been described include carbon dioxide laser ablation,[4] electrocautery,[67] intralesional interferon,[68] or sclerosing agent injection. Of these, endoscopic laser ablation is most frequently successful for the treatment of small, unilateral lesions.[61,69] Hemangiomas can recur

in certain cases where the lesion extends beyond the submucosa and goes undetected at the time of surgery.

External beam irradiation and radioactive gold implants have a 93% success rate at curing subglottic hemangiomas,[58] but are not used due to the increased risk of thyroid cancer.[70] Finally, selective embolization of large laryngeal hemangiomas may be used in cases refractory to other therapies.[71]

Hughes et al[72] studied the safety and efficacy of individualized management to determine the various strategies in avoiding tracheostomy. They concluded that morbidity and the need for tracheostomy in cases of congenital subglottic hemangioma can be minimized using a combination of therapeutic modalities. Treatment should be individualized according to the severity of the symptoms and the morphology of the lesion.

In a study of 46 consecutive patients over 26 years, Nicolai et al[73] found that, compared to steroids and tracheostomy, a significant reduction in morbidity and speech developmental delay, and an improved quality of life, were achieved with carbon dioxide (CO_2) laser resection. This approach was superior to the Neodym-YAG laser

LARYNGEAL WEBS

Epidemiology

Laryngeal webs are rare congenital anomalies of the larynx.

Etiology and Pathogenesis

Incomplete recanalization of the laryngotracheal tube during the third month of gestation leads to different degrees of laryngeal webs. The extreme of this situation is complete laryngeal atresia (see below). The most common site of development of laryngeal webs is at the anterior part of the vocal folds, although they may be present as posterior interarytenoid, subglottic, or supraglottic webs.[74,75]

Clinical Presentation

Laryngeal webs may present with symptoms ranging from mild dysphonia to significant airway obstruction, depending on the size and location of the web. Stridor is rare except in cases of posterior interarytenoid webs . These cases typically present with airway obstruction in the presence of a normal voice or

or 5p14.3) or rarely due to interstitial deletion. An attempt to localize the developmental field affected in cri-du-chat syndrome was made by Kjaer and Niebuhr from Denmark.[94] They found that specific malformations occurred in the bony contours of the sella tursica and the clivus in cri-du-chat patients with terminal deletions. These specific regions develop around the notochord where the neurons to the larynx have migrated ventrally.

The frequency of the syndrome is 1 in 50,000 births. Approximately 1% of profoundly retarded patients are diagnosed with cri-du-chat syndrome. Affected individuals exhibit microcephaly, hypotonia, and cardiovascular defects. The characteristic mewy cry (cat cry) is present only during infancy. The high-pitched stridor is the result of interarytenoid muscle paralysis in an elongated larynx with a floppy epiglottis. Faces of these patients are round with hypertelorism and broad nasal root.[95,96]

Arthrogryposis multiplex congenita is associated with multiple joint disorders and central nervous system abnormalities. Laryngeal manifestations include bilateral vocal fold paralysis, hypertrophy of the cricopharyngeus, and supraglottic redundancy similar to laryngomalacia. These children almost always require tracheotomy, and their prognosis is poor.[97]

Plott syndrome, an X-linked disorder, is associated with laryngeal adductor paralysis.[98]

Table 24–3 includes other syndromes and conditions associated with laryngeal and or tracheal anomalies.

CONCLUSION

In this chapter, we presented an overview of the different congenital anomalies of the larynx. The most common anomaly is laryngomalacia. It accounts for approximately 60% of all cases. Symptoms include inspiratory stridor that is accentuated by supine position, feeding, and agitation. The child with laryngomalacia is usually healthy and has a normal cry. Flexible laryngoscopy is essential to make the diagnosis. Omega-shaped epiglottis, redundant bulky arytenoids, and short aryepiglottic folds are characteristic signs. The majority of patients can be managed conservatively, and the condition usually resolves by 12 to 18 months.

Vocal fold paralysis accounts for 15% of congenital anomalies of the larynx. The most common cause of bilateral vocal fold paralysis is Arnold-Chiari malformation. Birth trauma accounts for 20% of all cases. Aspiration is common in bilateral paralysis. CT scan is essential to rule out lesions compromising the recurrent laryngeal nerve. The majority of unilateral vocal fold paralysis are managed by observation; however, tracheotomy is necessary in cases of bilateral paralysis.

Congenital subglottic stenosis is the most common laryngeal anomaly to require tracheotomy in infants. Biphasic stridor is the most common symptom. A diagnosis of the condition is made when the luminal diameter is less than 4 mm in the full-term infant. Most cases resolve spontaneously, and laryngotracheoplasty is required in patients who cannot be decannulated.

Subglottic hemangioma constitutes 1.5% of all congenital anomalies of the larynx. The symptoms include biphasic stridor and barking cough with or without failure to thrive. Most cases resolute gradually in 4 to 5 years. Rigid endocopy is essential to make the diagnosis. If the airway obstruction is significant, a surgical procedure may be needed. The treatment has to be individualized depending on the clinical picture.

Laryngeal webs are rare laryngeal anomalies. Symptoms vary according to the size and location of the web. Treatment options also will depend on airway status and the morphology of the lesion.

The chapter also includes other less common congenital laryngeal anomalies such as laryngotracheoesophageal clefts (LTEC), laryngeal atresia, cysts, and lymphangiomas as well as a comprehensive table of congenital syndromes and conditions associated with laryngeal anomalies.

Acknowledgment The authors would like to thank Dr. J. Paul Willging of Cincinnati for contributing the photographs to this chapter.

REFERENCES

1. Batsakis JG. *Tumors of the Head and Neck–Clinical and Pathological Considerations.* 2nd ed. Baltimore, MD: Williams & Wilkins; 1979:220–221.
2. Leung AK, Cho H. Diagnosis of stridor in children. *Am Fam Physician.* 1999;60:2289–2296.
3. Holinger PH, Brown WT. Congenital webs, cysts, laryngoceles and other anomalies of the larynx. *Ann Otol Rhinol Laryngol.* 1967;76:744–752.
4. Willging JP, Cotton RT. Congenital Anomalies of the Larynx. In: Tewfik TL, Der Kaloustian VM, eds. *Congenital Anomalies of the Ear, Nose, and Throat.* New York, NY: Oxford University Press; 1997:383.
5. Belmont JR, Grundfast K. Congenital laryngeal stridor (laryngomalacia): etiologic factors and associated disorders. *Ann Otol Rhinol Laryngol.* 1984;93:430–437.
6. Shulman JB, Hollister DW, Thibeault DW, Krugman ME. Familial laryngomalacia: a case report. *Laryngoscope.* 1976;86:84–91.
7. Keleman G. Congenital laryngeal stridor. *Arch Otolaryngol.* 1953;58:245–248.

Table 24–3. Syndromes and Conditions Associated with Congenital Anomalies of the Larynx[99] (continues)

Syndrome or Condition	MIM No. POSSUM No.[A]	Inheritance[B]	Ear, Nose, and Throat Manifestations	Other Manifestations
Adducted thumb syndrome, Christian syndrome or craniosynostosis, arthrogryposis, cleft palate	*201550 3591	AR	Myopathic face, micrognathia, cleft palate, low-set ears, abnormal fissures, telecanthus, shape of ears, torticollis, laryngomalacia, dysphagia	Craniosynostosis, microcephaly, downward slanting palpebral fissures, telcanthus, ophthalmoplegia, pectus excavatum, adducted thumbs, contractures, mental retardation, seizures, hypotonia, early death
Agnathia, synotia, microstoma or otocephaly syndrome	202650 3478	sporadic	Absence of mandible, micrognathia, small nostrils, choanal atresia, microstomia, aglossia, blind mouth, cleft palate, low-set ears, ears fused in the midline, middle ear anomalies, bilobed epiglottis, rudimentary vocal folds, webbed neck	Epicanthal folds, epibulbar dermoids, abnormal rib number, vertebral anomalies, dextrocardia, situs inversus, hypoplastic lungs, renal agenesis, cardiac defects, holoprosencephaly, lethal
Atelosteogenesis, type 3	4761		Midface hypoplasia, microstomia, micrognathia, cleft palate, flat nasal bridge, anteverted nostrils, low-set ears, helix hypoplastia, stenosis of the external auditory canal, laryngomalacia	Prominent forehead, hypertelorism, long clavicles, atlantoaxial instability, scoliosis, cleft of vertebral bodies, multiple joint dislocations, rhizomelic short/bowed limbs
Bilateral ptosis, vocal fold paralysis	4792	AD	Vocal fold paralysis, abnormal cry	Failure to thrive, normal intelligence, ptosis
Chondrodysplasia punctata, X-linked recessive	*302950 3737	XLR	Small nose, broad nasal bridge, anteverted nostrils, deafness, short neck, laryngeal abnormality	Cicatricial alopecia, ichthyosis, coarse hair, frontal bossing, short stature, MR (del Xp22)
Chromosome 5, partial del 5p or Cri-du-chat syndrome	3073		High, shrill mewing cry, broad cheeks, cleft lip/palate, micrognathia, broad nasal bridge, small posteriorly angulated ears, preauricular tags, laryngeal abnormality	Microcephaly, round face, hypertelorism, hypotonia, heart defects, cryptorchidism, epicanthic folds, moderate to severe MR
Chromosome 7, partial dup 7q	3076		Micrognathia, beaked nose, everted lips, cleft palate, macroglossia, anteverted or bat ears, short neck, hearing abnormality, laryngeal abnormality	Short stature, macrocephaly or hydrocephalus, frontal bossing, hypertelorism, cryptorchidism, single palmar crease, MR
Craniofacial digital genital anomalies	4163		Narrow face, pointed chin, microstomia, micrognathia, anteverted ears, abnormal cry, laryngeal abnormality	Hypotelorism, cryptophthalmos (not obligatory), ambiguous genitalia, hypospadias, cryptorchidism, anal stenosis or atresia, thymic aplasia, hypotonia, MR

8. Martin JA. Congenital laryngeal stridor. *J Laryngol Otol.* 1963;77:290–294.

9. Grundfast KM, Harley E. Vocal cord paralysis. *Otolaryngol Clin North Am.* 1989;22:569–597.

10. Zalzal GH, Anon JB, Cotton RT. Epiglottoplasty for the treatment of laryngomalacia. *Ann Otol Rhinol Laryngol.* 1987;96:72–76.

11. Gianonni C, Sulek M, Friedman EM, Duncan NO III. Gastroesophageal reflux association with laryngomalacia: a prospective study. *Int J Pediatr Otorhinolaryngol.* 1998;43:11–20.

12. Hou JW. Fetal warfarin syndrome *Chang Gung Med J.* 2004;27(9):691–695.

13. Chen JC, Holinger LD. Congenital laryngeal lesions: pathology study using serial macrosections and review of the literature. *Pediatr Pathol.* 1994;14:301–325.

14. Shah UK, Wetmore RF. Laryngomalacia: a proposed classification form. *Int J Pediatr Otorhinolaryngol.* 1998;46:21–26.

15. Friedman EM, Williams M, Healy GB, McGill TG. Pediatric endoscopy: a review of 616 cases. *Ann Otol Rhinol Laryngol.* 198493:517–519.

16. Masters IB, Chang AB, Patterson L, et al. Series of laryngomalacia, tracheomalacia, and bronchomalacia disorders and their associations with other conditions in children. *Pediatr Pulmonol.* 2002;34:189–195

17. Holinger PH. Clinical aspects of congenital anomalies of the larynx, trachea, bronchi and esophagus. *J Laryngol Otol.* 1961;75:1–44.

18. Matthews BL, Little JP, McGuirt WF Jr, Koufman JA. Reflux in infants with laryngomalacia: results of 24-hour double-probe pH monitoring. *Otolaryngol Head Neck Surg.* 1999;120: 860–864.

19. Iyer VK, Pearman K, Raafat F. Laryngeal mucosal histology in laryngomalacia: the evidence for gastro-oesophageal reflux laryngitis. *Int J Pediatr Otorhinolaryngol.* 1999;49:225–230.

20. Midulla F, Guidi R, Tancredi G, et al. Microaspiration in infants with laryngomalacia *Laryngoscope.* 2004;114:1592–1596.

21. Clinical Pharmacology. In: Gold Standard Multimedia. Available at http://www.gsm.com), Accesssed July 31, 2000.

22. Sichel JY, Dangoor E, Eliashar R, Halperin D. Management of congenital laryngeal malformations. *Am J Otolaryngol.* 2000;21:22–30.

23. Kelly SM, Gray SD. Unilateral endoscopic supraglottoplasty for severe laryngomalacia. *Arch Otolaryngol Head Neck Surg.* 1995;121:1351–1354.

24. Fearon B, Ellis D. The management of long term airway problems in infants and children. *Ann Otol Rhinol Laryngol.* 1971;80:669–677–677.

25. Friedman EM, Vastola P, McGill TJ, Healy GB. Chronic pediatric stridor: etiology and outcome. *Laryngoscope.* 1990;100:277–280.

26. Cotton RT, Prescott AJ. Congenital anomalies of the larynx. In: Cotton RT, Myers CM III, eds. *A Practical Approach to Pediatric Otolaryngology.* Philadelphia, PA: Lippincott-Raven; 1988:497–513.

27. Hughes CA, Dunham ME. Congenital anomalies of the larynx and trachea. In: Wetmore RF, Munz HR, McGill TJ, eds. *Pediatric Otolaryngology.* New York, NY: Thieme Publications; 2000:778.

28. Holinger LD. Etiology of stridor in the neonate, infant and child. *Ann Otol Rhinol Laryngol.* 1980;89:397–400.

29. Cohen SR, Geller KA, Birns JW, Thompson JW. Laryngeal paralysis in children: long-term retrospective study. *Ann Otol Rhinol Laryngol.* 1982;9:417–424.

30. Gentile RD, Miller RH, Woodson GE. Vocal cord paralysis in children 1 year of age or younger. *Ann Otol Rhinol Laryngol.* 1986;95:622–625.

31. Rosin DF, Handler SD, Potsic WP, et al. Vocal cord paralysis in children. *Laryngoscope.* 1990;100:1174–1179.

32. Holinger LD, Holinger PC, Holinger PH, Etiology of bilateral abductor vocal cord paralysis: a review of 389 cases. *Ann Otol Rhinol Laryngol.* 1976;85:428–436.

33. Ferguson CF. Congenital abnormalities of the infant larynx. *Otolaryngol Clin North Am.* 1970;3:185–200.

34. McGill TJ, Healy GB. Congenital and acquired lesions of the infant larynx. A refresher survey. *Clin Pediatr* (Phila). 1978;17:584–589.

35. Takamatsu I. Bilateral vocal cord paralysis in children. *Nippon Jibiinkoka Gakkai Kacho* [Journal of the Oto-rhino-laryngological Society of Japan]. 1996;99:91–102.

36. Friedman EM. Role of ultrasound in the assessment of vocal cord functions in infants and children. *Ann Otol Rhinol Laryngol.* 1997;106:199–209.

37. Jacobs IN, Finkel RS. Laryngeal electromyography in the management of vocal cord mobility problems in children. *Laryngoscope.* 2002;112:1243–1248.

38. Bower CM, Choi SS, Cotton RT. Arytenoidectomy in children. *Ann Otol Rhinol Laryngol.* 1994;103:271–278.

39. Kirchner FR. Endoscopic lateralization of the vocal cord in abductor paralysis of the larynx. *Laryngoscope.* 1979; 89:1779–1783.

40. Narcy P, Contencin P, Viala P. Surgical treatment of laryngeal paralysis in infants and children. *Ann Otol Rhinol Laryngol.* 1990;99:124–128.

41. Tucker GF, Osoff RH, Newman AN, Holinger LD. Histopathology of congenital subglottic stenosis. *Laryngoscope.* 1979;89:866–877.

42. Tucker JA, O'Rahilly R. Observations on the embryology of the human larynx. *Ann Otol Rhinol Laryngol.* 1972; 81:520–523.

43. Smith RJ, Catlin FI. Congenital anomalies of the larynx. *Am J Dis Child.* 1984;138:35–39.

44. Holinger LD, Oppenheimer RW. Congenital subglottic stenosis: the elliptical cricoid cartilage. *Ann Otol Rhinol Laryngol.* 1989;98:702–706.

45. Holinger LD. Histopathology of subglottic stenosis. *Ann Otol Rhinol Laryngol.* 1999;108:101–111.

46. Healy GB. Subglottic stenosis. *Otolaryngol Clin North Am.* 1989;22:599–606.

47. Fearon B, Crysdale WS, Bird R. Subglottic stenosis of the larynx in the infant and child: methods of management. *Ann Otol Rhinol Laryngol.* 1978;87:645–648.

48. Bertrand P, Navarro H, Caussade S, Holmgren N, Sanchez I. Airway anomalies in children with Down

syndrome: endoscopic findings. *Pediatr Pulmonol.* 2003;36:137–141.

49. Myer CM III, O'Connor DM, Cotton RT.. Proposed grading system for subglottic stenosis based on endotracheal tube sizes. *Ann Otol Rhinol Laryngol.* 1994;103:319–323.

50. Dunbar JS. Upper respiratory tract obstruction in infants and children. *Am J Roentgenol Radium Ther Nucl Med.* 1970;109:227–246.

51. Holinger PH, Kutnick SL, Schild JA, Holinger LD. Subglottic stenosis in infants and children. *Ann Otol Rhinol Laryngol.* 1976;85:591–599.

52. Holinger LD, Stankiewicz JA, Livingstone GL. Anterior cricoid split: the Chicago experience with an alternative to tracheotomy. *Laryngoscope.* 1987;97:19–24.

53. Rosenfeld RM, Bluestone CD. Does early expansion surgery have a role in the management of congenital subglottic stenosis? *Laryngoscope.* 1993;103:286–290.

54. Cotton RT. Prevention and management of laryngeal stenosis in infants and children. *J Pediatr Surg.* 1985;20:845–851.

55. Fayoux P, Devisme L, Merrot O, Chevalier D. Thyroid alar cartilage graft in laryngoplasty: anatomical study in premature and newborn babies. *Int J Pediatr Otorhinolaryngol.* 2002;66:259–263.

56. Monnier P, Lang F, Savary M. Partial cricotracheal resection for pediatric subglottic stenosis: a single institution's experience in 60 cases. *Eur Arch Otorhinolaryngol.* 2003;260:295–297.

57. Benjamin B, Carter P. Congenital laryngeal hemangioma. *Ann Otol Rhinol Laryngol.* 1983;92:448–455.

58. Brodsky L, Yoshpe N, Ruben RJ: Clinical-pathological correlates of congenital subglottic hemangiomas. *Ann Otol Rhinol Laryngol* Suppl. 1983;105:4–18.

59. Pitanguy I, Caldeira AM, Calixto CA, Alexandrino A. Clinical evaluation and surgical treatment of hemangiomata. *Head Neck Surg.* 1984;7:47–59.

60. Riding K. Subglottic hemangioma: a practical approach. *J Otolaryngol.* 1992;21:419–421.

61. Healy GB, Fearon B, French R, McGill T. Treatment of subglottic hemangioma with carbon dioxide laser. *Laryngoscope.* 1980;90:809–813.

62. Cotton RT, Tewfik TL. Laryngeal stenosis following carbon dioxide laser in subglottic hemangioma. Report of three cases. *Ann Otol Rhinol Laryngol.* 1985;94:494–497.

63. Seid AB, Pransky SM, Kearns DB. The open surgical approach to subglottic hemangioma. *Int J Pediatr Otorhinolaryngol.* 1993;26:95–96.

64. Hawkins DB, Crockett DM, Kahlstrom EJ, MacLaughlin EF. Corticosteroid mangement of airway hemangiomas: long-term follow-up. *Laryngoscope.* 1984;94:633–637.

65. Cohen SR, Wang CI: Steroid treatment of hemangioma of the head and neck in children. *Ann Otol Rhinol Laryngol.* 1972;81:584–590.

66. Hoeve LJ, Kuppers GL, Verwoerd CD. Management of infantile subglottic hemangioma: laser vaporization, submucous resection, intubation, or intralesional steroids? *Int J Pediatr Otorhinolaryngol.* 1997;42:179–186.

67. Davidoff AM, Filston HC. Treatment of infantile subglottic hemangioma with electrocautery. *J Pediatr Surg.* 1992;27:436–439.

68. Ohlms LA, Jones DT, McGill TJ, Healy GB. Interferon alfa-2a therapy for airway hemangiomas. *Ann Otol Rhinol Laryngol.* 1994;103:1–8.

69. Healy G. Treatment of subglottic hemangioma with the carbon dioxide laser. *Laryngoscope.* 1980;90:809–813.

70. Fisher JM. Cancer in the irradiated thyroid. [Letter.] *N Engl J Med.* 1975;292:975–977.

71. Konior RJ, Holinger LD, Russell EJ. Superselective embolization of laryngeal hemangioma. *Laryngoscope.* 1988;98:830–834.

72. Hughes CA, Rezaee A, Ludemann JP, Holinger LD. Management of congenital subglottic hemangioma. *J Otolaryngol.* 1999;28:223–228.

73. Nicolai T, Fischer-Truestedt C, Reiter K, Grantzow R. Subglottic hemangioma: a comparison of CO_2 laser, Neodym-Yag laser, and tracheostomy. *Pediatr Pulmonol.* 2005;39:233–237.

74. Cohen SR. Congenital glottic webs in children. A retrospective review of 51 patients. *Ann Otol Rhinol Laryngol* Suppl. 1985;121:2–16.

75. McHugh H, Loch J. Congenital webs of the larynx. *Laryngoscope.* 1942;52:43.

76. Benjamin B, Mair EA. Congenital interarytenoid web. *Arch Otolaryngol Head Neck Surg.* 1991;117:1118–1122.

77. Benjamin B. Congenital laryngeal webs. *Ann Otol Rhinol Laryngol.* 1983;92:317–326.

78. Unal M: The successful management of congenital laryngeal web with endoscopic lysis and topical mitomycin-C. *Int J Pediatr Otorhinolaryngol.* 2004;68:231–235.

79. Evans JN. Management of the cleft larynx and tracheoesophageal clefts. *Ann Otol Rhinol Laryngol.* 1985;94:627–630.

80. Benjamin B, Inglis A. Minor congenital laryngeal clefts: diagnosis and classification. *Ann Otol Rhinol Laryngol.* 1989;98:417–420.

81. Moungthong G, and Holinger LD. Laryngotracheoesophageal clefts. *Ann Otol Rhinol Laryngol.* 1997;106:1002–1011.

82. Gatti WM, MacDonald E, Orfei E. Congenital laryngeal atresia. *Laryngoscope.* 1987;97:966–969.

83. Okada T, Ohnuma N, Tanabe M, et al. Long-term survival in a patient with congenital laryngeal atresia and multiple malformations. *Pediatr Surg Int.* 1998;13:521–523.

84. Kanamori Y, Kitano Y, Hashizume K, et al. A case of laryngeal atresia (congenital high airway obstruction syndrome) with chromosome 5p deletion syndrome rescued by ex utero intrapartum treatment. *J Pediatr Surg.* 2004;39:E25–E28.

85. Kalache KD, Franz M, Chaoui R, Bollmann R. Ultrasound measurements of the diameter of the fetal trachea, larynx and pharynx throughout gestation: applicability to prenatal diagnosis of obstructive anomalies of the upper respiratory digestive tract. *Prenat Diagn.* 1999;19:211–218..

cedure is applicable to all cases. Surgical options include Gelfoam injection, fat injection, collagen injection, thyroplasty (vocal fold medialization or lateralization), arytenoidectomy, partial cordotomy, and reinnervation techniques (ansa hypoglossi, ansa-strap-nerve muscle pedicle implantation).

Laryngocele

A laryngocele is an abnormal dilatation of the saccule filled with air. It is rarely seen in the pediatric population. Anatomically it is divided into three groups depending on the extension of the cyst: (1) *Internal laryngocele:* located in the anterior ventricle and with extension superiorly and posteriorly to the false vocal fold, but remaining within the laryngeal framework; (2) *External laryngocele:* dilated cyst piercing through the thyrohyoid membrane with cephalad extension; (3) *Combined laryngocele:* has both internal and external components. Diagnosis is confirmed with endoscopy, and computerized tomography can be helpful. The most common surgical treatment includes endoscopic marsupialization or an external approach through a laryngofissure for complete removal.

Laryngeal Web

A laryngeal web is a membrane of variable thickness that is formed during the embryogenesis of laryngotracheal groove (Figure 25–1). A majority of laryngeal webs (75%) are located anteriorly at the level of the true vocal folds with a posterior glottic opening.[4] Webs are associated with hoarseness and a weak or absent cry. Cohen and colleagues (1982) reported the largest series of congenital glottic web, 51 patients over a 30-year period.[11] In this series, hoarseness was the most

common presentation, and tracheotomy was required in 38% of cases with thick webs.

Treatment depends on the degree of the airway compromise, consistency, and thickness. A thin glottic web can be lysed endoscopically (scissors, or surgical laser) without the need for stenting. The authors have employed topical application of Mitomycin-C successfully to decrease the degree of scar formation and restenosis postoperatively. The management of thick glottic web is more challenging. The surgical method utilized (endoscopic, laryngofissure with stenting, temporary tracheotomy) and time of surgery should be individualized.

Ductal Cysts

Ductal cysts or retention cysts may occur anywhere in the larynx (Figure 25–2). Patients often present with hoarseness and weak cry. The etiology is unknown, but is thought to be caused by local irritation causing obstruction of the submucosal glands and their dilated collecting ducts. They may also present in the subglottic area secondary to intubation trauma. Surgical treatment includes endoscopic removal with forceps or laser.

Saccular Cysts

Saccular cysts arise as a result of obstruction of the saccular orifice. They are fluid-filled and lack communi-

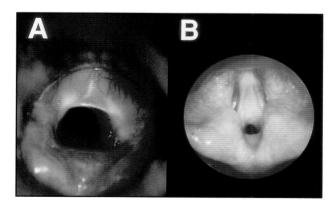

Figure 25–1. A. Thin glottic web. **B.** Thick glottic web.

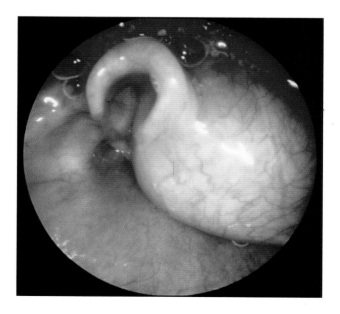

Figure 25–2. Supraglottic congenital laryngeal cyst.

cation with the airway. Airway obstruction may occur intermittently as the cyst impedes upon the airway lumen, or may be continuous with ongoing inspiratory stridor. Saccular cysts are divided into two groups: (1) *Anterior saccular cysts:* located between the false and true vocal folds; (2) *Lateral saccular cysts:* extending into the false vocal fold and aryepiglottic fold. Diagnosis is made by flexible fiberoptic laryngoscopy or direct laryngoscopy. Initial treatment is usually by surgical laser vaporization of the cyst and its contents or by resection with "cold" instruments. Endoscopic or external excision may be required in recurrent cases.

Laryngeal Hemangioma

Laryngeal hemangioma most commonly presents in the subglottic area. Cutaneous hemangiomas are found in 50% of patients with airway hemangiomas.[13] The most common presenting symptoms include progressive biphasic stridor, barking cough, and hoarseness. The natural history is one of growth over the first 6 to 18 months of life, followed by gradual regression. Diagnosis is confirmed by endoscopy, and biopsy is generally not indicated because of the risk of bleeding. Treatment is based on the symptoms and includes observation, steroids (systemic or injection), surgical laser excision, open surgical excision, systemic interferon, and in some cases, tracheotomy.[13-15]

Laryngeal Cleft

A laryngeal cleft is caused by the failure of closure of the tracheoesophageal septum at approximately 35 days' gestation. Laryngeal clefts are divided into four types depending on their extent: *Type I* is confined to the interarytenoid space above the level of the vocal folds; *Type II* represents a partial cricoid cleft; *Types III and IV* transverse the cricoid completely and extend through various levels of the trachea down to the carina (Figure 25–3). Alternative classifications are also used (see chapter 24).

It is a rare anomaly, most commonly presenting with stridor and/or aspiration. Respiratory distress and cyanosis are usually precipitated by feeding. Diagnosis is confirmed with endoscopy, but barium swallow is also an important diagnostic tool. The first line of management for a small laryngeal cleft is thickening of the feeding. Small clefts with persistent aspiration can be repaired endoscopically or through a laryngofissure. Laryngeal clefts with extension to the trachea usually require a combination of transcervical and thoracotomy approach, and large clefts may require emergency management.

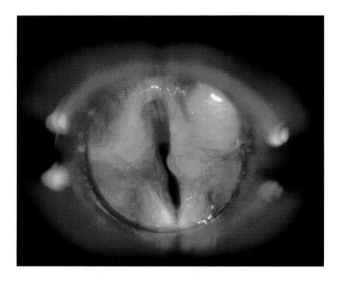

Figure 25–3. Interarytenoid laryngeal cleft.

ACQUIRED VOICE DISORDERS

Vocal Fold Nodules

The most common cause of voice disorders in children is vocal fold nodules. It is estimated that more than one million children in the United States have vocal fold nodules, with the lesion being more common in boys than girls.[2] Nodules are often associated with behavioral problems, family conflict, or aggressive behavior. Vocal fold nodules occur from overuse and/or misuse of the larynx causing mechanical trauma of the vocal fold mucosa at the point of maximum impact. Patients present with hoarseness, throat clearing, or cough. There is no dependable correlation between the size of the nodule and the degree of dysphonia.[16] They are often bilateral and located at the junction of the anterior one-third and the posterior two-thirds of the vocal fold. Nodules may appear rounded or fusiform. A fusiform or spindle-shaped thickening is more commonly seen in children, whereas discrete nodules are more common in adults (Figure 25–4).

The diagnosis of vocal fold nodules is made by flexible or rigid laryngoscopy, and videostroboscopy should be performed to help differentiate nodules from cysts and other lesions. Treatment modalities depend on the age of the patient, symptoms, level of cooperation to undergo voice therapy, and the size and firmness of the nodules. It is difficult to assess the success rate of the different treatment modalities because of questions regarding accuracy of diagnosis and the lack of controlled studies and adequate follow-up. However, treatment in a young cooperative

common in children. Optimal management requires psychotherapy or psychologic counseling in conjunction with speech therapy.[32]

INFLAMMATORY LESIONS AND VOICE DISORDERS

Any inflammatory or infectious process can cause edema and erythema of the laryngeal mucosa. Depending on the etiology, systemic manifestation may be mild and voice changes with dysphonia may present as the only sign. Bacterial and viral infections are the most common form of inflammatory processes affecting the larynx. Fungal laryngitis can be seen in immunocompromised children or those on long-term inhaled steroids. The spectrum of disease and management are similar in children and adults and are covered elsewhere throughout this book.

LARYNGEAL NEOPLASM AND VOICE DISORDERS

Malignant tumors of the pediatric larynx are rare. The most common neoplasm in the pediatric age group is rhabdomyosarcoma. Other malignancies involving the larynx have also been reported, including squamous carcinoma, neuroectodermal tumor of infancy, lymphoma, and mucoepidermoid carcinoma.[33-35] Benign neoplasms include neurofibromas, hamartomas, adenomas, and chondromas. Hoarseness is the most common initial presentation of any laryngeal neoplasm. Respiratory distress and stridor are later manifestations as the tumor grows. Because of low suspicion, there is usually a delay in the diagnosis. Because of the aggressive nature of laryngeal malignancy in children, management often includes the combination of surgery, radiation, and chemotherapy, depending on the tumor histology and the stage of the disease.[34,35]

REFERENCES

1. Wilson DK. *Voice Problems of Children.* 3rd ed. Baltimore, MD: Williams & Wilkins; 1987.
2. Choi SS, Cotton RT. Surgical management of voice disorders. *Pediatr Clin North Am.* 1989;36:1535–1549.
3. Zajac DJ, Farkas Z. Dindzans LJ, et al. Aerodynamic and laryngographic assessment of pediatric vocal function. *Pediatr Pulmonol.* 1993;15:44–51.
4. Morrison M, Rammage L. *The Management of Voice Disorders.* London, England: Chapman and Hall Medical; 1994.
5. Hirano M, Bless DM. Videostroboscopic examination of the larynx. London: Whurr; 1993.
6. Pengilly AJ. Pediatric voice disorders. In: Cotton RT, Myer CM, III eds. In: *Practical Pediatric Otolaryngology.* Philadelphia, PA: Lippincott-Raven; 1999:75–95.
7. Aronson AE. *Clinical Voice Disorders, an Interdisciplinary Approach.* New York, NY: Thieme-Stratton; 1980:57–61.
8. Maddern BR, Campbell TF, Stool S. Pediatric voice disorders. *Otolaryngol Clin North Am.* 1991;24:1125–1140.
9. Scott-Brown WG. *Scott-Brown's Otolaryngology,* 5th ed. Evans JNG, ed. Vol 6. *Paediatric Otolaryngology.* London, England: Butterworth; 1987:412–419.
10. Friedman EM, Vastola AP, McGill TJ, et al. Chronic pediatric stridor: etiology and outcome. *Laryngoscope.* 1990;100:277–280.
11. Cohen SR, Geller KA, Birns JW, et al. Laryngeal paralysis in children: a long-term retrospective study. *Ann Otol Rhinol Laryngol.* 1982;91:417–424.
12. Emery PJ, Fearon B. Vocal cord palsy in pediatric practice: a review of 71 cases. *Int J Pediatr Otorhinolaryngol.* 1984;8:147–154.
13. Froehlich P, Stamm D, Floret D, et al. Management of subglottic hemangioma. *Clin Otolaryngol.* 1995;4:336–339.
14. Seid AB, Ransky SM, Kearns DB. The open surgical approach to subglottic hemangioma. *Int J Pediatr Otorhinolaryngol.* 1993;22:85–90.
15. MacArthur CJ, Senders CW, Katz J. The use of interferon Alpha-2A for life-threatening hemangioma. *Arch Otolaryngol Head Neck Surg.* 1995;121:690–693.
16. von Leden H. Vocal nodules in children. *Ear Nose Throat J.* 1985;64:29–41.
17. Quick CA, Krzyzed RA, Watts SL, et al. Relationship between condylomata and laryngeal papillomata: clinical and molecular virological evidence. *Ann Otol.* 1980;89:467–471.
18. Kashima HK, Kessis T, Mounts P, et al: Polymerase chain reaction identification of human papillomavirus DNA in CO_2 laser plume from recurrent respiratory papillomatosis. *Otolaryngol Head Neck Surg.* 1991;104:191–195.
19. Leventhal B, Kashima HK, Mounts P, et al. Long-term response of recurrent respiratory papillomatosis to treatment of lymphoblastoid interferon alpha-n1. *N Engl J Med.* 1991;325:613–617.
20. Healy GB, Gelber RD, Trowbridge AL, Grundfast KM, Ruben RJ, Price KN. Treatment of recurrent respiratory papillomatosis with human leukocyte interferon—results of a multicenter randomized clinical trial. *N Engl J Med.* 1988;319:401–407.
21. Lundquist PG, Haglund S, Carlson B, et al. Interferon therapy in juvenile laryngeal papillomatosis. *Otolaryngol Head Neck Surg.* 1984;92:386–391.
22. Benjamin B, Croxson G. Vocal nodules in children. *Ann Otol Rhinol Laryngol.* 1987;96:530–531.
23. Irving RM, Baily CM, Evans JNG. Posterior glottic stenosis in children. *Int J Pediatr Otorhinolaryngol.* 1993;28:11–23.
24. Holinger LD, Tucker GF. Jr Trauma. In: *Otolaryngology—Head and Neck Surgery.* 2nd ed. St. Louis, MO: Mosby-Year Book; 1993:2331–2338.

25. Brown PM, Schaefer SD. Laryngeal and esophageal trauma. In: *Otolaryngology—Head and Neck Surgery.* 2nd ed. St. Louis, MO: Mosby-Year Book; 1993:1864–1874.

26. Zhar RIS, Smith RJH. Vocal fold paralysis in infants twelve months of age and younger. *Otolaryngol Head Neck Surg.* 1996;114:18–21.

27. Cohen SR, Thompson JW, Geller KA, et al. Voice change in the pediatric patient. *Ann Otol Rhinol Laryngol.* 1983; 92:437–443.

28. Scott-Brown WG. Scott-Brown's Otolaryngology. 5th ed. Stell PM, ed. Vol 5. *Laryngology.* London, England: Butterworth; 1987:119–144.

29. Plott D. Congenital laryngeal abductor paralysis due to nucleus ambiguus dysgenesis in three brothers. *N Engl J Med.* 1964;271:593–596.

30. Jones KI. *Smith's Recognizable Patterns of Human Malformation.* 4th ed. Philadephia, PA: Saunders Publishing; 1988:40–114.

31. Froese AP, Sims P. Functional dysphonia in adolescence: two case reports, *Can J Psychiatry.* 1987;32:389–391.

32. Morrison MD, Nichol H, Rammage LA. Diagnostic criteria in functional dysphonia. *Laryngoscope.* 1986;94:1–5.

33. Ohlms LA, McGill T, Healy GB. Malignant laryngeal tumors in children: a 15-year experience with four patients. *Ann Otol Rhinol Laryngol.* 1994;103:686–688.

34. Gindhart TD, Johnston WH, Chism SE, et al.Carcinoma of the larynx in childhood. *Cancer.* 1980;46:1683–1687.

35. Mitchell DB, Humphreys S, Kearns DB. Mucoepidermoid carcinoma of the larynx in a child. *Int J Pediatr Otorhinolaryngol.* 1988;15:211–215.

26

Pediatric Laryngology: Office-Based Evaluation of Children with Dysphonia

Christopher J. Hartnick MD, MS Epi

Evaluation of a child with a vocal disorder represents a potentially challenging and time-consuming undertaking. The previous chapter, "Voice Disorders in the Pediatric Population," by Drs. Rahbar and Healy focused on the variety of pediatric laryngologic disorders a practitioner might encounter. This chapter focuses not on the diagnoses but rather on how technology and laryngologic techniques used with adults have influenced the field of pediatric laryngology, providing more detailed means of diagnosing pediatric vocal disorders. With new tools available both for diagnosis and treatment, the field has begun the evolution experienced earlier in its adult counterpart where laryngology consisted of treating laryngeal cancer and airway lesions and evolved toward comprehensive care of the voice as well as the airway. As we move toward such an evolution in pediatric laryngology, we need to understand anatomic and structural development as it relates to evaluating a child's voice. We also have to keep in mind that children are not "small adults" and that their

care has to make sense with where they are developmentally and emotionally and with the knowledge that their desires and motivations (as well those of their parents) may well change as they mature and develop.

THE HUMAN VOCAL FOLD: A PRIMER ON MODERN UNDERSTANDING OF ITS HISTOPATHOLOGY

Most modern otolaryngologic textbooks address the issue of laryngeal growth and maturation. The larynx itself changes in position and structure throughout childhood. The larynx descends in the neck in relationship to the cervical vertebrae from infancy where the inferior aspect of the cricoid approximates the fourth cervical vertebra (C4) to the mature position (C6–C7) by mid-adolescence. At birth, the vocal process of the arytenoids comprises 75% of the vocal fold length; by 3 years of age, the membranous aspect of the vocal fold is dominant.[1] That being said, knowledge of the development and maturation of the human vocal fold itself has been difficult to glean from the literature. The "modern" description of the microanatomy of the human vocal folds has been properly attributed to Dr. Hirano with his seminal work in 1975 entitled *Phonosurgery. Basic and Clinical Investigations.*[2] Hirano and his colleagues examined the developing larynges and characterized the growth of the human vocal cord with time. Hirano also focused closely on the histologic structure of the human vocal fold and described its laminar structure in detail. Hirano divided the layers into a surface epithelial layer followed by a trilaminar lamina propria structure (superficial lamina propria (SLP), middle lamina propria (MLP), and deep layer of the lamina propria (DLP).[2-4] He further divided these structures into the "cover," which included the epithelium and the SLP and the "body," which included the vocalis muscle, and the "transition zone," which included the MLP and DLP. In Hirano's model, the SLP is distinguished by a relative paucity of elastin and collagen fibers and is noted to be loose and pliant. The MLP contains an abundance of elastin fibers; the DLP contains fewer elastin fibers and a predominance of collagen fibers (primarily types 1, 2, and 3). The "vocal ligament" is defined as the combination of the MLP and DLP; the fibers of this ligament are oriented in a longitudinal fashion parallel to the thyroarytenoid muscle. This definition has been supported in ensuing anatomic and mechanical models of the vocal folds (Table 26–1).

In histopathologic examination of newborn vocal folds, Tucker et al have commented on the general similarities between neonatal epithelium and that described for the adult.[9] They noted distinct ciliary distribution patterns that change over time and with maturation. With regard to the lamina propria in particular, Sato et al have reported that there exists a uniform, nonlayered lamina propria with no vocal ligament.[10] The maculae flavae (the regions at the anterior and posterior ends of the membranous vocal folds) are thought to be responsible for the development of the vocal ligament[11] and are composed of fibroblasts, ground substance, elastin fibers, reticular fibers, and collagenous fibers.[11] Hirano also supported the notion that there is no defined layered structure and no vocal ligament seen in the true vocal fold in the newborn.[12] Ishii et al performed scanning electron microscopy on pediatric cadaveric larynges and noted the development of superficial and deep structures by 10 years of age and a defined, layered lamina propria structure by 17 years of age.[13] Ishii et al noted no discernable SLP at ages 3 or 5 but identified an SLP structure by age 12.

Recent studies have questioned the exact timepoints in the development of these microlayer structures within the developing vocal fold. Hartnick et al examined 34 archived human larynges from children ages 0 to 18 years and described the following changes over time.[14] At birth and shortly thereafter, there exists a relative hypercellular monolayer of cells throughout the lamina propria. By 2 months of age, the first signs of differentiation into a bilaminar structure of distinct cellular population densities appear. Between 11 months and 5 years, two distinct patterns are seen: (1) this bilaminar structure and (2) a lamina propria in which exists a third more hypocellular region immediately adjacent to the vocalis muscle (this region is similar to the superficial hypocellular region found just deep to the surface epithelium). By 7 years of age, all of the specimens exhibit this transition between the middle and the deeper layers according to differential density of cell populations. A lamina propria structure defined by differential fiber composition (elastin and collagen fibers) is not present until 13 years of age and then is present throughout adolescence (Figures 26–1 and 26–2) More work with greater numbers of specimens is needed to pin down moments of development and to begun to answer the important questions of cell-signaling that prompt these periods of maturation.

Table 26–1. Different Systems of Defining the Cover/Body of the Lamina Propria of the Vocal Fold

	Cover	Body	Transition
Hirano[2,3,4]	Epithelium, SLP	Vocalis muscle	MLP, DLP
Titze[7]	Epithelium, SLP, MLP	DLP, Vocalis Muscle	
Hammond[5]	Epithelium, SLP, MLP	MLP, DLP, Vocalis Muscle	
Dikkers[6]	Epithelium, SLP	Conus Elasticus, Vocalis Muscle	

Note: Varying descriptions and definitions of the layered structure of the human vocal fold as seen in the published English literature. SLP = superficial layer of the lamina propria, MLP = middle layer of the lamina propria, DLP = deep layer of the lamina propria.

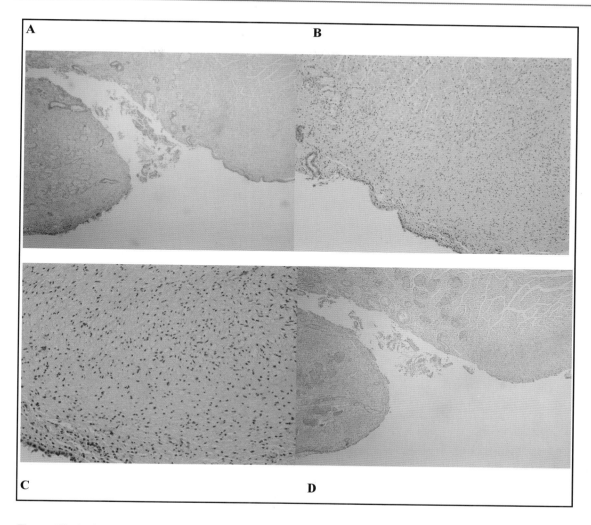

Figure 26–1. 4-micrometer section of 2-day-old female true vocal cord: **A.** 4× magnification using Hematoxylin and Eosin stain. **B.** 10× magnification using Hematoxylin and Eosin stain. **C.** 20× magnification using Hematoxylin and Eosin stain. **D.** 4× magnification using Alcion Blue stain. Note the staining of the mucin glands with the Alcion Blue stain demonstrating adequate positive contols.

FROM ANATOMY TO FUNCTION: VIEWING THE PEDIATRIC LARYNX "IN VIVO"

To understand a vocal disorder as completely as possible, the vocal folds must be visualized *during* this disorder and, therefore, "in live action." Adult laryngology has made strides toward developing a comprehensive office-based evaluation of phonologic disorders by means of technologic advances in the ability to transmit adequate light through steadily shrinking endoscopes, which permit either direct visualization of the larynx in motion or the illusion of a larynx in slow motion, as made possible by either rigid or flexible digital stroboscopy. The challenge in pediatric laryngology lies in adopting these forms of technology to children with small noses, small mouths, and who, more often than not, exhibit far less cooperation during the examination than do adults. Nevertheless, with the aid of improved technology, we have come far from the days when Kirstein reported, over a century ago, that transoral mirror laryngoscopy was problematic in children and, therefore, predicted that transoral direct laryngoscopy would represent the best means of evaluation of young children with laryngeal problems:[15] "In all probability autoscopy (direct laryngoscopy) will assume an important role in the examination of children, *on an equal footing* with laryngoscopy (transoral mirror examination); but in *preference to* laryngoscopy in very

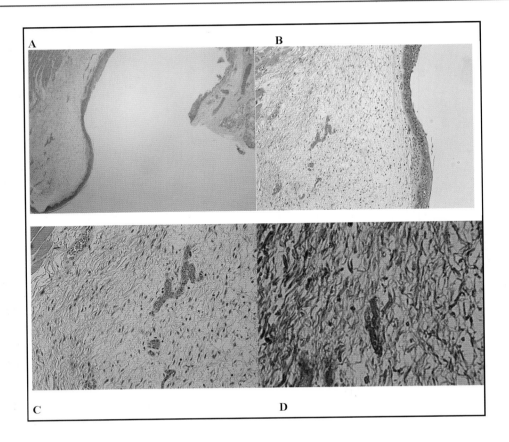

Figure 26–2. 4-micrometer section of 13-year-old female: **A.** 4 × magnification using Hematoxylin and Eosin staining. **B.** 10 × magnification using Hematoxylin and Eosin staining. **C.** 20 × magnification using Hematoxylin and Eosin staining. **D.** 20 × magnification using Trichrome staining.

young children. Even infants can be examined with the autoscope (direct laryngoscope) . . . ."

The application of stroboscopy to the evaluation of patients with voice disorders allowed the refinement of diagnoses as well as more precise pre- and postoperative evaluation and planning either in terms of surgical or speech therapy strategies. Peroral laryngostroboscopy is performed by means of a standard rigid Hopkins rod angled telescope. Through this technique, highly accurate images of the vocal folds can be obtained as the glottis cycles during respiration and then in phonation. At least one company to date now produces rigid endoscopes with smaller diameters to allow better tolerance in the pediatric populations. The limitations of this technique arise from the need for substantial cooperation during a peroral examination. With the tongue protruding, the head extended, and the neck flexed, it is difficult to simulate the conditions associated with conversational phonation. Alternatively, the flexible stroboscope allows a more normal head position as well as more ease in speech during the ex-

amination. Other advantages of flexible laryngostroboscopy include a greater tolerance of passage of the scope through a transnasal rather than a peroral route in some patients (especially children) because of a diminished need for a hyperactive gag reflex. These advantages are particularly important when analyzing the young child with a voice disorder as this examination has traditionally remained a challenging problem. The disadvantages of this technique are a product of the limitations of chip size and include less detail of the microvascular anatomy and mucosal pliability (as compared to the view obtained from rigid stroboscopy). Defects of glottal closure are readily apparent.

A range of flexible and rigid scopes designed to evaluate a child's larynx are available. The smaller endoscopes allow visualization of even a newborn's larynx although without the addition of stroboscopy. For younger children, this is not a tremendous limitation because children will not be able to consistently trigger the stroboscope. For children under 3, small endoscopes of 2.3 mm are routinely used as the larger 4.0-mm scopes are too large to pass through a young child's nasal chamber. At birth to 2 months of age, the median right anterior mucosal width of the nares (the distance from the inferior aspect of the middle turbinate to the septum on CT imaging) has been reported as 2.91 ± 0.94 mm, which explains the need for the smaller diameter nasal endoscopes.[16] Although the growth of the nasal choanae has been well documented,[17-19] there is a relative paucity of information regarding the actual growth and dimensions of the anterior and middle regions of the normal healthy infant's nose. This limits a better understanding of the optimal diameter endoscope that should be used for a given child, and future research is needed. The present endoscopes of 3.8 mm and the newer 3.2-mm endoscopes being developed come closer to the size at which a more comfortable endoscopy can be performed, and the coupling of stroboscopy to these scopes, presents an impressive technological discovery that should allow more refined clinical investigations and diagnoses (Table 26–2).

Some portion of the pediatric population with vocal disorders will not tolerate any form of office-based laryngeal examination. These patients can still have acoustic analysis, recently, recent efforts have been made to provide normative pediatric data as a reference mark. Moreover, in these cases, there is still a role for suspension laryngoscopy in the operating room when a diagnosis is needed prior to planning further treatment and potential therapy.

OUTCOME MEASURES AVAILABLE TO ADDESS THE PEDIATRIC VOICE

Validated instruments measuring health status and health-related (and voice-related) quality of life (HRQOL) have begun to emerge as another important tool with which to measure the impact of a vocal disorder on a patient and to measure the effect of therapy or surgical manipulation on these disorders. Several instruments have been designed with the purpose of measuring HRQOL relative to voice and vocal issues. The Voice Handicap Index has been validated as a 10-item instrument designed to measure the emotional, physical , and functional aspects of adult voice disorders by specifically recording the patient's perception of his or her vocal handicap.[20] The Voice-Related Quality of Life Measure (V-RQOL) is another 10-item instrument that was designed and validated as a self-administered instrument for adult populations with voice disorders to measure both social-emotional and physical-functioning aspects of voice problems.[21] Finally, the Voice Outcomes Survey was designed and validated as a 5-item instrument to measure clinical change in adults with unilateral vocal fold paralysis who would be undergoing surgery.[22]

Although meaningful data have been published with regard to strategies of obtaining voice samples and performing voice analysis in children,[23,24] there has been little work exploring V-RQOL in the pediatric population. The majority of instruments validated to explore issues related to V-RQOL in adults [20-22] have not been validated either for direct child's response or for parent-proxy application. The two exceptions to date are the modified Voice Outcomes Survey (VOS), also known as the Pediatric Voice Outcomes Survey (PVOS), and the Pediatric Voice-Related Quality of Life Instrument.[25] The PVOS was validated by examining a specific population of children with and without tracheotomies. The survey was shown to be internally consistent as well as "to be able to support a proposed interpretation of scores based upon theoretical implications within the constructs" (a concept known as discriminant validity).[25] To broaden the applicability of the PVOS to children with a full spectrum of vocal disorders, normative scores were identified for a pediatric otolaryngologic population who presented without voice concerns.[26] The PVOS was shown to be a brief, valid and reliable instrument that was simple to administer and to complete and was responsive to

Table 26–2. Rigid and Flexible Videostroboscopes for Pediatric Voice Evaluation

Flexible Rhinostroboscope			
Company	Rhino-stroboscope	Outer Diameter	Degree
KayPentax, Lincoln Park, NJ	VNL-1170K	3.6 mm	
Olympus America Inc., Melville, NY		XP3.2 mm	
Rigid Hopkins Rod Stroboscope			
Company	Rigid endoscope	Outer Diameter	Degree
Karl Storz Endoscopy, Culver City, CA	8712-E	5 mm	120
Karl Storz Endoscopy, Culver City, CA	8712-CA	5 mm	70

changes in voice-related quality of life. The brevity of the instrument, however, hindered the ability of the PVOS to reflect specific subdomains such as social-emotional concerns associated with voice problems. Moreover, the VOS itself was designed specifically to document global changes in voice pre and postoperatively; it was not designed to be sensitive enough to track potentially more subtle changes in vocal function over time following less dramatic interventions. To this end, the VR-QOL instrument was converted from its adult application to allow for parent-proxy administration to measure two subdomains of VR-QOL, namely "physical-functioning" and "social-emotional" subdomains[27] (Figure 26–3).

CONTROVERSIES IN PEDIATRIC LARYNGOLOGY: WHAT TO DO WITH VOCAL FOLD NODULES

As mentioned in the first paragraph of this chapter, the purpose of this chapter is not to cover the full spectrum of pediatric voice disorders as this has been covered in other chapters. However, one particular disorder, dysphonia secondary to vocal fold nodules and cysts warrants attention, first because it is one of the more common etiologies for dysphonia and, second, because the diagnosis is sometimes difficult to make and the treatment options reflect the particular problems faced by the practitioner who cares for children with vocal disorders.

Vocal fold nodules are considered to result from phonatory trauma and consist of subepithelial fibrovascular depositions along the membranous vocal fold.[3,4,28] The etiology of vocal fold nodules may well be multifactorial and include genetic predisposition, behavioral factors, as well as environmental factors such as exposure to laryngopharygeal reflux.[28] Vocal fold nodules are the most common cause of hoarseness in children occurring in 6 to 23% of pediatric patients.[28,29]

Diagnosis of vocal fold nodules depends on accurate flexible fiberoptic laryngoscopy; stroboscopy may be limited due to the patient's age and compliance. For this reason alone, differentiation from other vocal fold pathologies, such as a vocal fold polyp as well as the deeper situated vocal fold cyst, may be difficult to accomplish by office-based examination of the child (Figures 26–4). Diagnosis may be aided by the use of computer-assisted voice analysis, as suggested by Campisi et al, where elevated frequency perturbation measurements may be evident in children with vocal fold nodules.[23] Children with vocal fold nodules may also have relatively poor voice-related quality of life as measured either by the PVOS or the PV-RQOL instruments.

Treatment of pediatric vocal fold nodules remains controversial. The mainstay of treatment is voice therapy; however, the efficacy of this therapy is anecdotal and randomized trials have yet to be performed. Surgery for removal of pediatric vocal fold nodules is performed in only extreme cases after voice therapy has had no effect, when the child is significantly incapacitated by his or her voice, and in the rare case where the child is compliant to and will tolerate postoperative voice rest and therapy.[30] The proper duration of postoperative voice rest also is controversial. Children and their families need to be carefully counseled and educated as to the environmental and behavioral factors that can influence vocal fold nodule formation. If laryngopharyngeal reflux is suspected, it can be treated medically. There is the real risk of vocal fold re-formation if the nodules are removed and the underlying vocal behavioral characteristics that predisposed to the original nodule formation persist.

CONCLUSION

The study of pediatric voice disorders is a new and exciting field with much work to be done both in the field of developmental as well as molecular biology, as well as in the clinical arena where improved technology promises better and more accurate diagnoses and, therefore, identification of more refined and effective treatment plans. Cofactors such as genetic, environmental, and behavioral characteristics that predispose to vocal pathology need further investigation to more clearly understand their role in the genesis of pediatric vocal disorders.

REFERENCES

1. Cummings CW, Fredrickson JM, Harker LA, et al. *Otolaryngology-Head and Neck Surgery.* St. Louis, MO: Mosby; 1998.
2. Hirano M. Phonosurgery. Basic and clinical investigations. *Otologia (Fukuoka).* 1975;21(supp 1):239–260.
3. Hirano M. Structure and vibratory behavior of the vocal folds. In: Sawashima M, Franklin S, eds. *Dynamic Aspects of Speech Production.* Tokyo: University of Tokyo Press; 1977:13–30.
4. Hirano M. Structure of the vocal fold in normal and disease states: anatomical and physical studies. *ASHA Reports.* 1981;11:11–30.
5. Hammond TH, Gray SD, Butler J, Zhou R, Hammond E. Age- and gender-related elastin distribution changes in human vocal folds. *Otolaryngol Head Neck Surg.* 1998;119:314–322.

Q1) In general, how would you say your child's speaking voice is:
- Excellent
- Good
- Adequate
- Poor or inadequate
- My child has no voice

The following items ask about activities that your child might do in a given day.

Q2) To what extent does your child's voice limit his or her ability to be understood in a noisy area?
- Limited a lot
- Limited a little
- Not limited at all

Q3) During the past 2 weeks, to what extent has your child's voice interfered with his or her normal social activities or with his or her school?
- Not at all
- Slightly
- Moderately
- Quite a bit
- Extremely

Q4) Do you find your child "straining" when he or she speaks because of his or her voice problem?
- Not at all
- A Little bit
- Moderately
- Quite a bit
- Extremely

```
if vox2 = 1 then vox2a = 25;
if vox2 = 2 then vox2a = 18.75;
if vox2 = 3 then vox2a = 12.5;
if vox2 = 4 then vox2a = 6.25;
if vox2 = 5 then vox2a = 0;

if vox3 = 1 then vox3a = 0;
if vox3 = 2 then vox3a = 12.5;
if vox3 = 3 then vox3a = 25;

if vox4 = 1 then vox4a = 25;
if vox4 = 2 then vox4a = 18.75;
if vox4 = 3 then vox4a = 12.5;
if vox4 = 4 then vox4a = 6.25;
if vox4 = 5 then vox4a = 0;

if vox6 = 1 then vox6a = 25;
if vox6 = 2 then vox6a = 18.75;
if vox6 = 3 then vox6a = 12.5;
if vox6 = 4 then vox6a = 6.25;
if vox6 = 5 then vox6a = 0;


sumvox = vox2a + vox3a + vox4a + vox6a
```

Figure 26–3. Pediatric Voice Outcomes Survey and Pediatric Voice-Related Quality of Life Instrument *(continues)*

PV-RQOL Instrument

Please answer these questions based upon what your child's voice (your own voice if you are the teenage respondent) has been like over the past 2 weeks. Considering both how severe the problem is when you get, and how frequently it happens, please rate each item below on how "bad" it is (that is, the amount of each problem that you have). Use the following rating scale:

1 = none, not a problem
2 = a small amount
3 = A moderate amount
4 = A lot
5 = Problem is "as bad as it can be"
6 = Not applicable

Because of my voice	How much of a problem is this?
Q11) My child has trouble speaking loudly or being heard in noisy situations	1 2 3 4 5 6
Q12) My child runs out of air and needs to take frequent breaths when talking	1 2 3 4 5 6
Q13) My child sometimes does not know what will come out when s/he begins speaking	1 2 3 4 5 6
Q14) My child is sometimes anxious or frustrated (because of his or her voice)	1 2 3 4 5 6
Q15) My child sometimes gets depressed (because of his or her voice)	1 2 3 4 5 6
Q16) My child has trouble using the telephone or speaking with friends In person (because of his or her voice)	1 2 3 4 5 6
Q17) My child has trouble doing his or job schoolwork (because of his or her voice)	1 2 3 4 5 6
Q18) My child avoids going out socially (because of his or her voice)	1 2 3 4 5 6
Q19) My child has to repeat himself/herself to be understood	1 2 3 4 5 6
Q20) My child has become less outgoing (because of his or her voice)	1 2 3 4 5 6

```
if quest11 = 1 then vox11a = 10;
if quest11 = 2 then vox11a = 7.5;
if quest11 = 3 then vox11a = 5;
if quest11 = 4 then vox11a = 2.5;
if quest11 = 5 then vox11a = 0;

if quest12 = 1 then vox12a = 10;
if quest12 = 2 then vox12a = 7.5;
if quest12 = 3 then vox12a = 5;
if quest12 = 4 then vox12a = 2.5;
if quest12 = 5 then vox12a = 0;

if quest13 = 1 then vox13a = 10;
if quest13 = 2 then vox13a = 7.5;
if quest13 = 3 then vox13a = 5;
if quest13 = 4 then vox13a = 2.5;
if quest13 = 5 then vox13a = 0;

if quest14 = 1 then vox14a = 10;
if quest14 = 2 then vox14a = 7.5;
if quest14 = 3 then vox14a = 5;
if quest14 = 4 then vox14a = 2.5;
if quest14 = 5 then vox14a = 0;
```

Figure 26–3. *(continued)*

```
if quest15 = 1 then vox15a = 10;
if quest15 = 2 then vox15a = 7.5;
if quest15 = 3 then vox15a = 5;
if quest15 = 4 then vox15a = 2.5;
if quest15 = 5 then vox15a = 0;

if quest16 = 1 then vox16a = 10;
if quest16 = 2 then vox16a = 7.5;
if quest16 = 3 then vox16a = 5;
if quest16 = 4 then vox16a = 2.5;
if quest16 = 5 then vox16a = 0;

if quest17 = 1 then vox17a = 10;
if quest17 = 2 then vox17a = 7.5;
if quest17 = 3 then vox17a = 5;
if quest17 = 4 then vox17a = 2.5;
if quest17 = 5 then vox17a = 0;

if quest18 = 1 then vox18a = 10;
if quest18 = 2 then vox18a = 7.5;
if quest18 = 3 then vox18a = 5;
if quest18 = 4 then vox18a = 2.5;
if quest18 = 5 then vox18a = 0;

if quest19 = 1 then vox19a = 10;
if quest19 = 2 then vox19a = 7.5;
if quest19 = 3 then vox19a = 5;
if quest19 = 4 then vox19a = 2.5;
if quest19 = 5 then vox19a = 0;

if quest20 = 1 then vox20a = 10;
if quest20 = 2 then vox20a = 7.5;
if quest20 = 3 then vox20a = 5;
if quest20 = 4 then vox20a = 2.5;
if quest20 = 5 then vox20a = 0;
* to fit VRQOL for transformation to a 0 to 100 scale without using
published algorithm;

sumvrqol = vox11a + vox12a + vox13a + vox14a + vox15a
+ vox16a + vox17a + vox18a + vox19a + vox20a;
* transformed VRQOL score without using published transformation
metric;

socemot = vox14a + vox15a + vox18a +vox20a;
phyfunct = vox10a + vox12a + vox13a + vox16a + vox17a + vox19a
```

Figure 26–3. *(continued)*

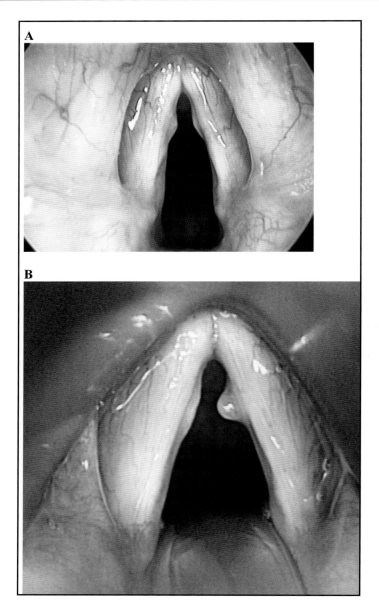

Figure 26–4. Endoscopic view of **A.** Pediatric vocal fold nodules and **B.** Pediatric vocal fold cysts.

6. Dikkers F. *Benign Lesions of the Vocal Folds—Clinical and Histopathological Apects.* Groningen, The Netherlands: Rijksuniversiteit Groningen; 1994.

7. Titze IR. *Principles of Sound Production.* Englewood Cliffs, N.J.: Prentice-Hall Inc., 1994.

8. Sato K, Sakaguchi S, Kurita S, Hirano M. A morphological study of aged larynges. *Larynx Jpn.* 1992:84–94.

9. Tucker J, Vidic B, Tucker GF, Stead J. Survey of the development of laryngeal epithelium. *Ann Otol Rhinol Laryngol.* 1976;85(5 suppl 30):1–16.

10. Sato K, Hirano M, Nakashima T. Fine structure of the human newborn and infant vocal fold mucosae. *Ann Otol Rhinol Laryngol.* 2001;10:417–424.

11. Sato K, Hirano M. Histologic investigation of the macula flava of the human newborn vocal fold. *Ann Otol Rhinol Laryngol.* 1995;104:556–562.

12. Hirano M, Kurita S, Nakashima T. Growth, development, and aging of human vocal folds. In: Titze, IR, Scherer, RC, eds. *Vocal Fold Physiology.* San Diego, CA: College Hill Press; 1983:23–43.

13. Ishii K, Yamashita K, Akita M, Hirose H. Age-related development of the arrangement of connective tissue fibers in the lamina propria of the human vocal fold. *Ann Otol Rhinol Laryngol.* 2000;109:1055–1064.
14. Hartnick CJ, Rehbar R, Prasad V. Development and maturation of the pediatric human vocal fold lamina propria. *Laryngoscope.* 2005;115:4–15.
15. Kirstein A. *Comparison Between Autoscopy and Laryngoscopy: Examination of Children.* Philadelphia, PA: F.A. Davis Co., 1897:44–46.
16. Contencin P, Gumpert L, Sleiman J, et al. Nasal fossae dimensions in the neonate and young infant: a computed tomographic scan study. *Arch Otolaryngol Head Neck Surg.* 1999;125:777–781.
17. Crockett DM, Healy GB, McGill TJ, Friedman EM. Computed tomography in the evaluation of choanal atresia in infants and children. *Laryngoscope.* 1987; 97:174–183.
18. Sweeney KD, Deskin RW, Hokanson JA, Thompson CP, Yoo JK. Establishment of normal values of nasal choanal size in children: comparison of nasal choanal size in children with and without symptoms of nasal obstruction. *Int J Pediatr Otorhinolaryngol.* 1997;39:51–57.
19. Slovis TL, Renfro B, Watts FB, Kuhns LR, Belenky W, Spoylar J. Choanal atresia: precise CT evaluation. *Radiology.* 1985;155:345–348.
20. Jacobson B, Johnson A, Grywalsky C. The Voice Handicap Index (VHI): development and validation. *J Voice.* 1998;12:54–55.
21. Hogikyan ND, Wodchis WP, Terrell JE, Bradford CR, Esclamado RM. Voice-related quality of life (V-RQOL) following type I thyroplasty for unilateral vocal fold paralysis. *J Voice.* 2000;14:378–386.
22. Gliklich RE, Glovsky RM, Montgomery WW. Validation of a voice outcome survey for unilateral vocal cord paralysis. *Otolaryngol Head Neck Surg.* 1999;120:153–158.
23. Campisi P, Tewfik TL, Manoukian JJ, Schloss MD, Pelland-Blais E, Sadeghi N. Computer-assisted voice analysis: establishing a pediatric database. *Arch Otolaryngol Head Neck Surg.* 2002;128:156–160.
24. Cheyne HA, Nuss RC, Hillman RE. Electroglottography in the pediatric population. *Arch Otolaryngol Head Neck Surg.* 1999;125:1105–1108.
25. Hartnick C. Validation of a pediatric voice quality of life instrument: the Pediatric Voice Outcome Survey (PVOS). *Arch Otolaryngol Head Neck Surg.* 2002;128:919–922.
26. Hartnick CJ, Volk M, Cunningham M. Establishing normative voice-related quality of life scores within the pediatric otolaryngology population. *Arch Otolaryngol Head Neck Surg.* 2003;129:1090–1093.
27. Boseley M, Cunningham M, Volk M, Hartnick C. Validation of the Pediatric Voice-Related Quality of Life Instrument (PV-RQOL). *Arch Otolaryngol Head Neck Surg.* 2005; In Press.
28. Gray SD, Smith ME, Schneider H. Voice disorders in children. *Pediatr Clin North Am.* 1996;43:1357–1384.
29. Maddern BR, Campbell TF, Stool S. Pediatric voice disorders. *Otolaryngol Clin North Am.* 1991;24:1125–1140.
30. Wohl DL. Nonsurgical management of pediatric vocal fold nodules. *Arch Otolaryngol Head Neck Surg.* 2005;131: 68–70; discussion 71–72.

27

The Larynx:
A Hormonal Target

Jean Abitbol, MD
Patrick Abitbol, MD

Endocrinology is a science, which started with voice. In 400 BC, Aristotle described the effect of castration on the songbird. Galen was the first to describe and to name the thyroid gland. It was another 1,500 years before Leonardo da Vinci began the study of the numerous endocrine organs. *De Humanis Corporis Fabrica,*[1] published in 1543, provided the first text on human anatomy and endocrine glands. The word "hormone" comes from the Greek *hormao,* which means to arouse.

Endocrinology is the study of the relationship between two cells via a molecule: the hormone. This molecule stimulates, via the bloodstream, a response in a distant organ. The methods of communication by messenger molecules from one cell to another are called:

- *Autocrine:* the molecule that has an impact on the cell where it has been synthesized

- *Paracrine:* the molecule that has an impact on the cells adjacent to the cell that has synthesized the molecule

- *Endocrine:* the molecule enters the bloodstream without any excretory channel

All hormonal activity needs a target organ or target cells with specific receptors. If their actions are limited in time, they may have an irreversible impact.

The mediators between the central nervous system and the glands are the suprachiasmic nuclei and the hypothalamus with its indispensable partner, the pituitary gland. Hence, any information processed will have a wide range of responses adapted to physical and psychologic stimuli.[2] The principles of hormonal action are based on the understanding of the genome, and the concept of receptors, which can be located on the cell membrane or its nucleus.

GENOME

The primary function of the gene is to produce a specific protein. The hormones act as commander. The genome for a haploid eukaryotic cell consists of approximately 100,000 genes. The action of a hormone is mediated by specific receptors: either on the membrane of the cell, and/or on the nucleus. The expression of the gene depends on the receptors or more precisely, on the number of activated receptors.[3]

TWO KINDS OF RECEPTORS

Membrane receptors are not liposoluble. Leutinizing hormone (LH), follicle stimulating hormone (FSH), thyroid stimulating hormone (TSH), growth factors, and insulin activate them. These hormones stimulate a specific receptor, which follows a complex biomechanical chain of events leading to the formation of the mRNA via the transcription factor.[4]

Nuclear receptors. In order to act directly on the nucleus, hormones must be liposoluble to cross the cell membrane. They include steroid hormones, sex hormones, thyroid hormones, and active vitamin metabolites such as retinoids, vitamin A metabolites, and vitamin D. These hormones go through the cell membrane and activate directly the intracellular receptors in the nucleus. From then on, the hormone–gene journey is the same as for membrane receptors. It leads to the formation of the mRNA via the transcription factor.

ENDOCRINE ORGAN

There are 8 endocrine glands:

1. The *pituitary gland* is located in the sella turcica inside the sphenoid bone. It is divided in two parts: the anterior part or adenohypophysis that secretes FSH, LH, adrenocorticotrophic hormone (ACTH), growth hormone (GH), and the posterior part, which is a transmitter and a reserve for neurohormones.
2. The *pineal gland,* located at the junction of the cerebrum, the brainstem and the cerebellum, is fixed on the roof of the third ventricle. It is an appendage of the brain and secretes melatonin. It is an evolutionary relic of fish.
3. The *thyroid gland* is located in front of the trachea between the second and the fifth cartilage rings. It secretes the thyroxin hormones: T_3 and T_4.
4. The *parathyroid glands,* located at the posterior aspect of the thyroid gland, are 4 in number. They secrete parathormone.
5. The *adrenal gland* with the adrenal cortex and the adrenal medulla is located above the kidney. The adrenal cortex secretes mineralocorticoids, glucocorticoids, and androgens. The adrenal medulla, like the paraganglia, secretes catecholamines (adrenaline and noradrenaline) and dopamines.
6. The *thymus* is located in the upper part of the thorax, posterior to the sternum. It secretes the hormone thymosin.
7. The *pancreas* secretes glucagon and insulin.
8a. The *testicles* secrete androgens and 25% of the total daily production of 17β-estradiol (the remainder being derived by conversion of both testicular and adrenal androgens in peripheral tissues).
8b. The *ovaries* secrete estrogen (E), progesterone (P), and the androgen dehydroepiandrosterone (DHEA).

The endocrine organs without glands are:

- The cerebrum for endorphins. The suprachiasmic nucleus (SCN), the gyrus, the hypothalamus, the posterior part of the hypophysis for endorphins, catecholamines, dopamines, and cytokines
- The epithelium of the digestive tract: the gastric epithelium for gastrin, secretin
- The kidney, the placenta, and heart: for renin–angiotensin

THE LARYNX IS A HORMONAL TARGET

The voice is at the crux of the psyche and the hormonal world. Voice mutation is controlled by sex hormones. The voice is changed by the hypothalamic–pituitary axis through its endocrine impact and, during everyday life, because of the hormones of the cerebrum. Emotional stress and the psyche may also provide the hormonal trigger to induce a change in voice production.

The common denominators of endocrine effects on laryngeal structures are numerous: The actions of estrogens and progesterone produce changes in the extravascular spaces and modification of glandular secretions; by the action of progesterone, there is modification of nerve transmission speed; by the action of androgen, hypertrophy or atrophy of striated muscles occurs as well as calcification of cartilages. The thyroid hormones also affect dynamic function of the vocal folds.

Sex Hormones and the Larynx

Does voice have a chromosomal sex? The voice changes with advancing years, with the scars of life, with its physical and emotional conditions, but the essential element that remains constant is that voice has a sex chromosome: XY for males, XX for females. However, this issue is not as clear-cut as it may appear. Consider the principal effects caused by the three main sex hormones, estrogen, progesterone, and androgens.

Estrogen

Estrogens are present in women and at very low levels in men. They have a hypertrophic and proliferative effect on mucosa. They reduce the desquamating effect of the superficial layers and cause differentiation and complete maturation of fat cells. The degree of cytoplasmic acidophilia and of nuclear pyknosis, as noted in gynecologic cervical smears and in smears from the vocal folds, is a measure of this maturational effect. Estrogens have no effect on striated muscles. Their effects on cerebral tissue are well known. Among other things, they are theorized to reduce the risk of contracting Alzheimer's disease.[5]

Progesterone

As its name implies, this hormone promotes gestation and, thus, is only present in adult women with ovulatory cycles. The central action of estrogen is the modification of steroid hormone activity by affecting receptor concentration. Estrogen increases target tissue responsiveness to itself, to progesterone, and to androgens by increasing the concentration of its own receptors and that of the intracellular progesterone and androgen receptors. The effects of progesterone can be felt only if there has previously been estrogenic influence of the tissues.[6,7] The progesterone receptor is induced both by estrogen and progestin. Estrogen exerts its influence on the progesterone receptor gene.[8] Apparently, this is the only known case of hormonal harmony in the human organism, wherein the influence of estrogens is a prerequisite to allow the action of progesterone to take place, as only estrogens will trigger the possibility of action and of growth in the receptor sites of progesterone. Progesterone has an antiproliferative effect on mucosa and accelerates desquamation. Hence, there is no satisfactory cellular differentiation. In the authors' study on uterine cervical and vocal fold smears, the pathologist is not able to distinguish between the two samples. Basophil cells have been observed on both slides. Therefore, there is a menstrual-like cycle on the vocal fold epithelium. Furthermore, one can observe a drying-out of the mucosa with a reduction in secretions of the glandular epithelium. Progesterone has a diuretic effect by its action on sodium metabolism, which is opposed to that of aldosterone. Estrogen increases capillary permeability and allows the passage of intracapillary fluids to the interstitial space. Progesterone decreases capillary permeability, thus trapping the extracellular fluid out of the capillaries and causing tissue congestion. This congestion is quite apparent in the breasts, in the lower abdominal and pelvic tissues, as well as in the vocal folds, where it causes premenstrual dysphonia.

Some synthetic progestins, such as the derivatives of nortestosterone, have an androgenic effect caused by active metabolites. They have a masculinizing effect on the female voice. They should never be prescribed in voice professionals if there is any therapeutic alternative, as discussed below.

Androgens

Testosterone is the essential male hormone, secreted by the testis.[9] In women, androgens are secreted principally by the adrenal cortex and formed as derivatives of aldosterone, but they are also secreted by the *theca interna* of the ovaries. Studies have shown that androgens cause an increase in the female libido.[10-11] Furthermore, there is a masculinizing action when the concentration of testosterone is greater than 150 micrograms/dl.[12] Androgens are essential for male sexuality, but they cause in women an often irreversible masculinizing effect at doses greater than 200 micrograms/dl. Man is the only primate with adrenal glands that secrete an important amount of dehydroepiandrosterone (DHEA), that is converted to androstenedione. In skin, these androgens cause acne, seborrhea, and hirsutism. In mucosa, they cause a loss of hydration with a reduction in glandular secretions. In muscles, they cause a hypertrophy of striated muscles with a reduction in the fat cells in skeletal muscles. There is also a reduction in the whole body fatty mass.[13] Anabolic steroids increase the volume and the power of the muscular mass, and may lead to definitive male voice, which may be an irreversible effect.

Puberty

The influence of sex hormones at puberty is modulated through the hypothalamus–pituitary axis. Puberty usually lasts from 2 to 5 years, and occurs between the ages of 12 to 17.

The passage from childhood to adulthood is marked by appearance of secondary sexual characteristics, as well as the physical and physiologic changes that are peculiar to each sex. The hypothalamo–hypophyseal pituitary axis and its testicular or ovarian response determine and influence the physical, psychic, and emotional sexuality of the person. In the Western world, the average age at which puberty begins is around 12 years for girls and 13 years for boys. In the girl, estrogen and progesterone secretion will lead to a woman's voice. In the boy, testosterone will yield a man's voice: a fundamental frequency one-third lower than a child's voice for the woman and an octave lower for the man; the pulmonary capacity, the cardiovascular apparatus, the level of hemoglobin, and the striated muscle mass all increase in man. Androgens are the most important hormones responsible for the passage of the boy-child voice to the man's voice, and their impact is irreversible. The thyroid prominence or Adam's apple appears, the vocal folds lengthen and become rounded, and the epithelium thickens with the formation of three distinct layers. The laryngeal mucus becomes more viscous. The arytenoids become bigger. The thyroarytenoid ligaments become thicker and more powerful. The anterior portion of the cricothyroid muscle broadens, becomes more resistant, and its contraction will permit a head voice. Closure of the cricothyroid space induces a forward tilt of the thyroid cartilage. The anterior commissure is thus brought downward and backward, thereby shifting the glottic plane from the horizontal. The horizontal projection of the vocal fold is therefore shortened, which may contribute to the ability to produce high notes.

The Castrato: A Pure Example of the Impact of Sex Hormone on Voice

In the fifteenth century the Roman Catholic Church wanted to have high-pitched, feminine voices in the chapel choirs, but without any women. The ecclesiastic world followed scrupulously the maxim of St Paul, *"mulliers in ecclesiae taceant"* or *"women should not be heard in the Church."*[14] Castration, to keep the beauty of the feminine voice, was an eccentricity of the Church at that time, for which voice was more important than virility. To allow the castrato to have a feminine voice, the castration had to be performed before any sign of puberty, before any secretion of testosterone. Even at that time, the importance of the definitive and indelible hormonal influence of testosterone had been recognized. The castrato has a powerful crystalline voice with an exceptional register. It is an ambiguous voice. The voice comes from a body born XY, but one that has never been clothed by testosterone, and, hence, this voice does not have a male print.

Castrati had the external skeletal envelope of a male with a lung capacity of 5 liters. They also possessed the muscular abdominal and pelvic girdle necessary to sustain a male voice. This is caused by growth hormones, adrenal hormones, and thyroid hormones. Their resonating chambers were defined by a male-type bony architecture. However, the vocalis muscle is highly sensitive to the impact of male hormones, and in particular to the lack of androgens. They, therefore, keep their childlike characteristics. Vocal folds having kept a childlike configuration and being made to vibrate in a female register by the power of a man in a

male skeletal environment define the quality of the voice. However, this is not the whole story. As in any musical instrument, there must exist a harmony between the two vocal folds vibrating one against the other, the power of the pulmonary bellows producing the sound energy, and the resonating chambers that allow the amplification and the coloring of the voice. This harmony is especially tenuous in the creation of an operatic castrato voice. This is why during the Renaissance many were called, but few chosen. According to written reports and to the one wax cylinder recording made in 1904, the castrato had a voice, with a range of 3 to 4 octaves. He could hold a note for some 120 seconds and could work his voice for up to 8 hours per day.[14]

THE FEMALE VOICE

In females, voice breaks are much less apparent. The female voice is not a childlike voice: it is 3 tones lower and has 5 to 12 formants, as opposed to the pediatric voice, which only has 3 to 6 formants. In females, there is little development of the thyroid cartilage or of the cricothyroid membrane. The vocal muscle thickens slightly, but remains very supple and quite narrow. The squamous mucosa also differentiates into three distinct layers on the free edge of the vocal folds. The sub- and supraglottic glandular mucosa becomes hormone-dependent to estrogens and progesterone. The ovaries start to work. The first menstrual cycles appear, at first rather irregularly and then regularly. The hormonal rhythm is also modulated through the hypothalamo–hypophyseal axis by the action of FSH and LH on the ovary. Menstrual cycles will continue for the next 40 years. For each cycle, the follicular and the luteal phases are distinguishable and linked together by ovulation.[15] During the follicular phase, the secretion of estrogens increases progressively, activated by FSH between day 4 and day 8, and reaching a peak on day 13 of the cycle. LH reaches its peak on day 14, leading to ovulation. The egg is snapped up by the fallopian tube. The luteal phase allows the creation of a new endocrine gland: the corpus luteum, that secretes progesterone and estrogen.

The exocervical squamous mucosa has three layers: the lamina propria, and the chorion, with a basal and a parabasal membrane. The junction between the different cells is relatively large in the first part of the cycle and less so in the second phase. This intercellular space is therefore hormone-dependent (Figure 27–1). Its important effect on the human voice is discussed in the section on premenstrual voice syndrome. The en-

ACOUSTIC ANALYSIS

- Narrow register
- Lack of high harmonics
- Loss of intensity
- Loss of high pitch
- Maximum Phonation Time (MPT)
- Jitter and Shimmer

STROBOSCOPY

- Microvarices, dilatation of capillaries, varicoses
- Asymmetrical vibration: lack of amplitude
- Ephemeral nodules: hour-glass shape
- Thickness of mucus: "sticky"
- Edema of arytenoids and posterior wall: reflux
- Posterior linkage
- Slight edema on the middle third of the vocal fold

Figure 27–6. Voice parameters during PMVS.

Physiologically and anatomically:

The *vascular signs* of patients with a premenstrual voice syndrome:

- 70% demonstrated premenstrual dilation of microvarices, with reactive edema: microvarices (Figure 27–7), microhemorrhage (Figure 27–8), or multiple vascular lesions (Figure 27–9);
- 10% demonstrated a submucosal vocal fold hematoma (Figure 27–10). These hematomas often result in a normal, but easily fatigued, speaking voice. Singing may be impossible.[53]

The *mucosal signs* have been noted in all patients who complain of premenstrual dysphonia. These include:

- Edema of the vocal mucosa
- Thickened and diminished glandular secretions, which lead to dryness of the larynx

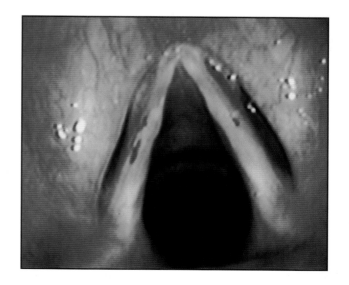

Figure 27–7. Microvarices.

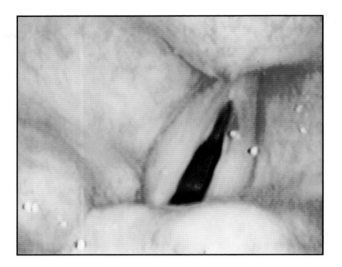

Figure 27–8. Microvarices + microhemorrhage.

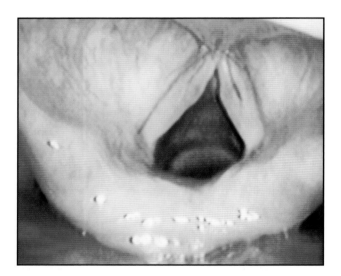

Figure 27–9. Microvarices, + edema + hemorrhage.

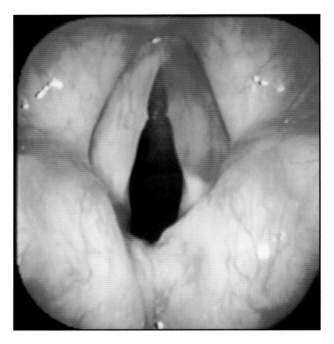

Figure 27–10. Hemorrhage.

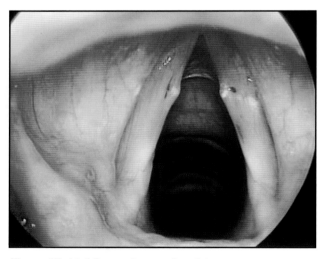

Figure 27–11. Microvarices and nodules.

- Abnormal videostroboscopic findings, including impaired mucosal amplitude and asymmetric vocal fold vibrations, as well as vocal fold nodules without or with microvarices (Figure 27–11). These nodules are bilateral and symmetric and are usually almost asymptomatic. They are located on the middle third of the vocal folds and lead to a lowering of the register by about 2 to 3 tones, giving a "blues" voice.

Muscular signs were noted in 60% of PMVS patients, including:

- Decreased muscular tone;
- Diminished power of contraction of the vocal muscle after a 10 second sustained phonation of the vowel /i/;

- Vocal fold closure achieved with the participation of the false folds in high pitch;
- Gap between the free edges during phonation and a posterior chink.

Inflammatory signs:

- 3% had a very inflamed nasopharyngeal mucosa;
- 2% had an allergic-type tracheitis with bronchospasm.[53]

In the author's experience (JA), in a study of female patients of childbearing age not taking oral contraceptives, it was noted that about 33% of women suffered from a vocal premenstrual syndrome.

Multifactorial elements explain the PMVS: the effects of estrogen and progesterone on the vocal fold mucosa, on the vocal ligament, on the blood vessels, on the lubrication, and on the psychologic state may explain the premenstrual voice syndrome. The involvement of aldosterone has often been raised, but is controversial.[57-58] Progesterone and estrogens have a synergistic effect.[59] Attempted explanations of the rheologic effects on tissues have included the progesterone/aldosterone ratio and the progesterone/estrogen ratio,[60,61] but there is currently no definitive conclusion. Objectively, one can note:

- A loss of tone in all striated muscles (the vocal muscles, the abdominal musculature, and the intercostal muscles, resulting in reduced pulmonary effort);
- Relaxation of the cardia muscles constituting the angle of Hiss, leading to episodes of gastroesophageal reflux. Acid reflux may cause posterior laryngitis with edema of the posterior third of the vocal folds and a reduced mobility of the edematous cricoarytenoid joints;
- Edema in the interstitial tissues and in Reinke's space. This edema is normally reversible, but less so in smokers, who, after some years, develop Reinke's edema or pseudomyxedema that leads to a masculine voice caused by vocal fold thickening (Figure 27–12). It may occur in women from the age of 35 on, but never after menopause. A woman who has not suffered from pseudomyxedema before her menopause will rarely suffer from it during the menopause;

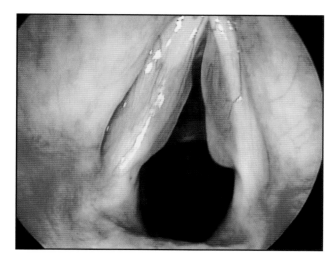

Figure 27–12. Reinke's edema + microvarices, increase during PMVS.

- Dilation of the microvarices that may be complicated by small ruptures leading to a hematoma. This explains why vocal professionals should abstain from taking aspirin or NSAIDs at this time. Overuse of these drugs increases the risk of such complications, especially in the "emotionally stressed" performer, who is over-rehearsing or overperforming.

The respiratory, and nasopharyngeal mucosa are also subject to allergic inflammatory effects. During the premenstrual period, a tenfold increase in allergic response is noted in 2% of patients. Hence, the estrogen-progesterone effect leads to a thickening of laryngeal mucus, frequent throat clearing and a reduction of hydration of the free edges of the vocal folds. Vocal lubrication is reduced and vocal fatigue becomes apparent after about 25 to 30 minutes of phonation.

Treatment of the Premenstrual Voice Syndrome

Generally, hormonal treatment is not necessary for premenstrual voice syndrome; natural remedies are usually satisfactory (Figure 27–13). In light of what we now understand about edema, insulin impairment, neurotransmitter disturbance, low levels of serotonin, and endorphin deficiency, it is clear that multifactorial treatment is appropriate. This therapy is individualized for each woman. In our practice, we have noted good results with natural remedies, including multivitamins and minerals such as: vitamins A, B6, B5, C, and E, and minerals including Mg, Cu, P, Fe, Ca, and Zn. These remedies are combined with vascular therapy and antiedema drugs, such as bromelaines from pineapples; prostaglandin inhibitors, such as mefenamic acid; and with antireflux treatment. This treatment is prescribed for 10 days per month: 8 days before the menses and 2 days during the menses. Also, during this period, we suggest the following diet: low protein, vegetables (carrots), fibers, olive oil, and no alcohol. Great care must be taken never to prescribe progesterone with potential androgenic metabolites, as this may lead to a permanently masculine voice.

Complications of premenstrual voice syndrome may occur. The most significant is recurrent vocal fold hemorrhage, which leads to hemorrhagic masses. Surgery may be necessary in such cases. (Figures 27–14 to 27–18: on the same patient, we see in Figures 27–14 and 27–15, laryngoscopic examination; Figures 27–16 and 27–17, laser phonosurgery; and Figure 27–18, results two months after laser surgery.)

Timing of Phonosurgery in Women

Finally, one must also consider the risk of trauma by endotracheal intubation for any surgery performed during the premenstrual period. Procedures on voice

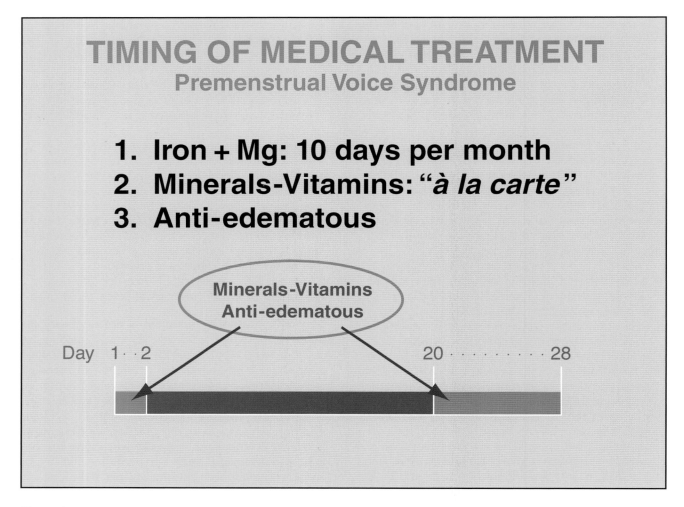

Figure 27–13. Timing of medical treatment: premenstrual voice syndrome.

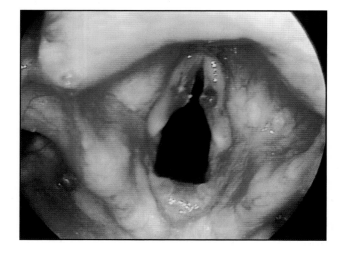

Figure 27–14. Complications of PMVS (1): hemorrhagic nodules during breathing.

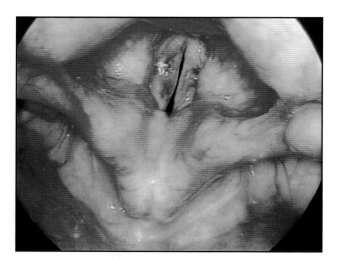

Figure 27–15. Complications of PMVS (2): during phonation.

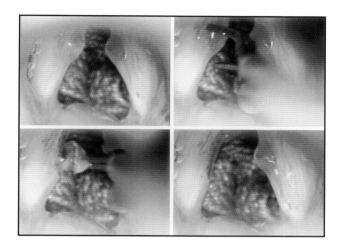

Figure 27–16. Complications of PMVS (3): laser surgery, left side.

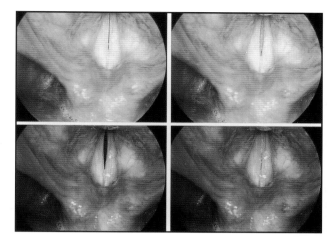

Figure 27–18. Complications of PMVS (5): two months after surgery.

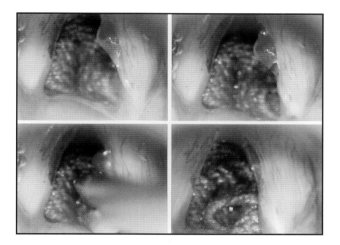

Figure 27–17. Complications of PMVS (4): laser surgery, right side.

professionals, requiring general anesthesia, must be performed with great care to avoid any direct trauma by the endotracheal tube during intubation and/or trauma caused by rotating the head during surgery. Such care will minimize the risks of postintubation granulomas and submucosal hematomas of the vocal folds. Blood vessels are very fragile during this period of the cycle. Without question, if surgery is emergent, it must be done; however, if there is no emergency, when the patient has premenstrual voice syndrome, surgery should be postponed. The author (JA) prescribes prephonosurgery medical treatment for 2 months with minerals, vitamins, antiedema, and antireflux medications. In voice professionals, even if they do not have clinical signs of PMVS, the authors prescribe the same treatment. Other surgeons may reschedule the surgery for a different point in the menstrual cycle. In addition to the risks noted above, premenstrual changes may lead to excessive removal of the lesion because of edema of the vocal fold, which distorts the limits of the lesion. The healing process may be impaired or prolonged. Phonosurgery should be performed ideally between day 5 and day 20 after menses.

The Perimenopausal Female

Perimenopausal symptoms are well recognized. Hot flashes are the most common symptom. Irregular cycles, anxiety, irritability, fatigue, inappropriate emotional response, insomnia, drying of the throat, drying and thinning of the gastrointestinal tract, vaginal dryness, dizziness, muscle weakness, and weight changes are some of the perimenopausal symptoms. Osteoporosis and cardiopulmonary changes, such as palpitations, high blood pressure, and shortness of breath occur and must be treated. The impact on the voice is very unpredictable and may take more than 15 years following the onset of the perimenopausal symptoms just described.

The Menopausal Voice Syndrome

During menopause, the hormonal climate is greatly altered and may result in changes in the voice. The menses become irregular and vary in quantity as progesterone's influence is reduced premenopause. The disappearance of ovarian follicles leads to the end of menstruation and of progesterone secretion.[62,63] The hypothalamic–hypophyseal axis is greatly altered and there is an increase in FSH and LH secretions that stimulate the ovaries. The ovaries become a unique endocrine organ, as their secretions change, consisting not only of estrogens but also of male hormones. Henceforth, androgens are free to act and their effects are numerous.[64-68] Androgens act on the cerebral cortex, especially the left hemisphere; on the genital organs (uterus, ovaries, breasts); on sebaceous glands; on striated muscles, and on the vocal muscles and the vocal mucosa. This has been demonstrated by comparing smears of the vocal folds and cervical smears (Figure 27–19), which exhibit a striking parallelism, in that there is relative mucosal atrophy with basophils, but there also appears to be muscular atrophy that worsens with age and with diminished use of the voice (Figure 27–20). Glandular cells usually located only above and under the vocal folds become more sparse. Hence, there is reduced hydration of the free edges of the vocal folds,[69] resulting in dryness during phonation, leading rapidly to vocal fatigue and to dysphonia. This vocal syndrome is progressive and is especially noticeable in voice professionals: including but not limited to popular singers, opera singers, comedians, barristers, hostesses, and schoolteachers. This gradual deterioration is noticed in high notes and in soft singing. Many women consult physicians more often because they are worried about general menopausal symptoms than because of actual vocal symptoms.

The menopausal voice syndrome presents the following clinical signs:

- During dynamic vocal assessment, acoustically, there is a slight loss in speed of staccato tones at the extremes of range, a loss of intensity, a narrowed range, and a loss of formants in the high tones (hardly noticeable in the day-to-day spoken voice). Anatomically, the vocal folds show a thinner mucosa and a reduced vibratory amplitude;
- Vocal fold cytology is consistent with cervical cytology revealing an atrophic mucosa with basophils present and a reduction in glandular cells in the mucosa of the ventricular band;
- Unilateral or bilateral vocalis muscle atrophy (Figure 27–21);
- Thinning of the vocal fold mucosa with a reduction in amplitude during phonation and asymmetry of the vocal folds noted during stroboscopy;
- The mucosa loses its pearly-white appearance and becomes dull, sometimes with microvarices becoming visible during the premenopausal phase;
- The cricoarytenoid joints move normally, but this diminishes after the age of 65 years, with a loss of the suppleness of the ligaments and with arthrosis;
- The electroglottograph signal is less strong and irregular, bearing witness to the reduced resistance of the vocal fold vibrations;
- The spectral acoustic analysis of the voice shows a 20% to 30% power reduction in the speaking voice, the projected voice, and the singing voice and a narrowed range with the loss of some frequencies.

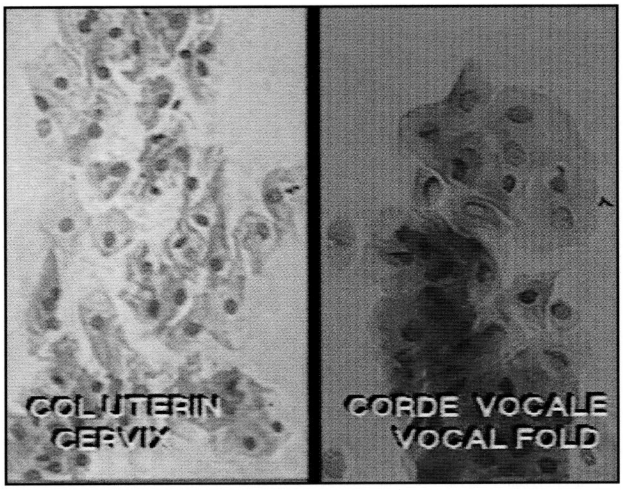

Figure 27–19. Smear test at menopause: the parallelism is amazing.

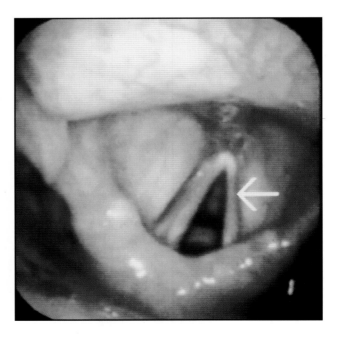

Figure 27–20. Atrophic changes of the right vocal fold.

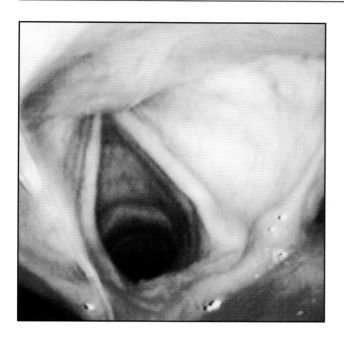

Figure 27–21. Atrophic changes of both vocal folds.

This seems to vary with individual cases. The vocal "athletes" such as singers and actors may find that two or three tones are altered, but for them, this may be of dramatic importance. The timbre appears to be flat and colorless, as some harmonics have been lost. A loss of melody may be noted in the spoken and the speaking voice.

The authors consider menopausal patients to fit into two broad types: the "Modigliani" types, rather thin and slender, with little adipose tissue, and the "Rubens" types, with a rounded figure.

Since 1978, MacDonald et al[70] demonstrated that estrogen synthesis can take place in fat cells in men and in women. The relationship between obesity and the increase in estrone secretion with reference to the subject's age has also been proven. Cytochrome P450 is responsible for this biosynthesis of estrone from androgens in the fat cells,[16,71-73] and the gene involved is Cyp19. Transcription of P450 aromatase in fat cells increases with age (Figure 27–22).

Androstenedione and other androgen derivatives are transformed to estrogens in lipocytes. More re-

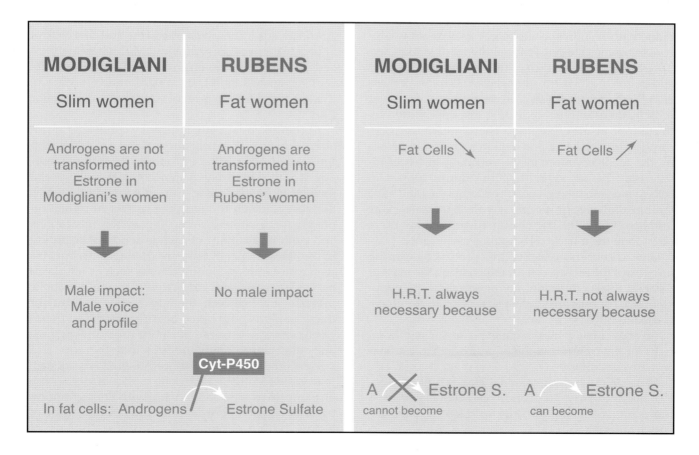

Figure 27–22. Physiopathology of the impact of fat cells in menopausal women.

cently, it has been shown that this transformation not only takes place in the lipocytes, but also in the cells of the stroma, in contact with and surrounding the fat cells. These cells can therefore be considered to be "pre-lipocytes." This action is increased by the influence of glucocorticoids.[74-76] Hence, the major site for estrogen synthesis in the menopausal woman is the lipocyte, and the same applies for the obese man.[77-81] It seems to be why an obese tenor has a low testosterone level, as the testosterone is trapped by the adipose tissues and undergoes transformation. In contrast, the deep bass with a slim body has a higher testosterone level, as there is no mass of adipose tissue to lead to estrone metabolism. As we grow older, the lean muscle mass diminishes and the fat mass increases, with a new body cell distribution. Glucocorticoids contribute to the increase in the fat mass, thus showing that great care must be taken when prescribing steroids to a menopausal patient.[82]

Estrone is an estrogen with a weaker action on the target organs than estradiol. Its synthesis in the fat cells is multifactorial. It is stimulated by glucocorticoids, by cAMP (cyclic adenosine monophosphate) and its derivatives but is inhibited by many growth factors.[82] The lipocytes also possess a cellular membrane with insulin specific receptors that allow glucose entry into the cells, thus allowing oxidation and lipogenesis. Maintenance of this property allows the absorption of glucose by the specific receptors of these cells. In the middle of the cell membranes of striated muscle, there is a loss of insulin response with a reduction of insulin receptors. These muscle cells become insulin resistant and insulin secretion increases by the feedback mechanism, resulting in hyper-insulinism. This secondary hyperinsulinism allows fat cells to increase their glucose uptake, as they still have their insulin-specific receptors with an increase in the number of fat cells. The obese patient becomes more obese, and the muscle cells become even leaner.

Glucocorticoids accelerate this process by causing atrophy of the muscle cells and increasing the mass of fat cells, thus contributing to the secondary hyperinsulinism. Fat cells are specific target organs for glucocorticoids.[68,83,84]

An obese menopausal woman possesses significant risks for the transformation of androgens to estrones and estrone sulfate.[85]

More precisely,[86] the adrenal glands will produce 95% and the ovary, 5% of androstenedione. Estrone is indirectly and predominantly secreted by the adrenals at an average of 3,000 μg per day. Conversion occurs in peripheral tissues; adipose tissue is active in aromatization:

- if obese, 3,000 μg, 7% become estrone (200 μg per day) and
- if slender, 3,000 μg, only 1.5% is active in aromatization

The "Rubens" type is certainly much less dependent on hormone replacement therapy than the "Modigliani" type, but needs close attention.

The "Modigliani" patient has little adipose mass, and hence androgens are only slightly transformed to estrones or estrone sulfate, if at all.[87-89] The androgenic action is strong and is often triggered rapidly. In these cases, the authors feel that hormonal replacement therapy for voice professionals is essential[90-92] unless it is contraindicated medically.

Hormone replacement therapy therefore needs careful control, because of the risk of a secondary hyperestrogenemia.[85] As the fat cell mass increases, the level of endogenous estrogens also increases. If the hormone replacement dose remains high, it may result in a classical hyperestrogenemia syndrome (tense feeling in the breasts, flatulence, edema, and irritability). Each case must be given individual attention.

Treatment of the Menopausal Voice Syndrome

At menopause, alternative medicine and diet control appear to help reduce symptoms. Multivitamins, minerals, and good hydration are advised: vitamins A, B6, B5, C, E, and vitamin D, as well as minerals Mg, Cu, Zn, P, Fe, and Ca are prescribed by the senior author (JA).

Antireflux treatment is usually advisable in an obese woman. The drugs prescribed are taken continuously for 3 months. Hormone replacement therapy is individualized. A gynecologist with special interest in endocrinology, or an endocrinologist, is the best clinician to judge the correct hormone replacement treatment according to the indications and contraindications of each individual, including in the assessment not only vocal symptoms, but also the more common manifestations such as hot flashes, osteoporosis, and cardiovascular and metabolic impairment.[93] Speech therapy is also helpful for many patients with voice disturbance.[94] The therapeutic synergy between hormone replacement therapy, alternative medicine and diet therapy, and voice therapy in selected cases yields a very satisfactory voice result.[95-96] Hormone replacement therapy also improves the quality of life with the prevention or delay of osteoporosis, of cardiovascular risks, of certain central nervous system (CNS) diseases, of dermatologic aging changes, and with the maintenance of an active libido.

Sex Hormone Medication and Voice Disorders

Anabolic steroids may result in a masculine voice. In some athletes, anabolic steroids have been used to enhance athletic performance and appearance. The tragedy in women was that these drugs were often given around the immediate postpubertal period. Their voices became deeper and never returned to normal. Although the peripubescent voice *may* be particularly sensitive, permanent androgenic voice virilization can occur in women of any age.[97] Altered vocal parameters are observed after 2 to 4 months on androgen-containing drugs, and sometimes sooner. The pitch drops by as much as 3 to 6 tones; the register narrows from 2 octaves to 1 octave and attaining high notes becomes very difficult.[98,99]

Treatment is first to stop all androgenic hormones. Unfortunately, most of the vocal changes are usually irreversible. Surgery of the laryngeal framework or endoscopic laser surgery may be indicated in certain instances to return the voice to a feminine range. Other surgical techniques to give a higher pitch have also been described by the senior author (JA).[100-102]

Most current contraceptive pills do not affect the voice permanently. Some of the "older birth control pills," prescribed 20 years ago, contained synthetic progesterone components with androgenic side effects and these may still be encountered occasionally in some countries.

As previously stated, the castrato has a feminine voice, and was never exposed to testosterone. The child has a feminine voice, range, and also was never exposed to testosterone. During the childbearing years, a female voice professional must never take male hormones or hormones with androgenic metabolites such as certain progesterones, if she wants to maintain her feminine voice. The menopausal woman will keep her feminine voice if physiologic androgens are not allowed a "free reign" when estrogens and progesterones disappear. Androgens are the only hormones capable of producing a male voice. Hence, early treatment at the first sign of menopause or, in certain cases, perimenopause, is critically important.

In Summary

The voice of a woman changes with the cycle of life and with the aging process. It is constantly under hormonal influence. Before puberty, there is no progesterone. The voice is childlike, supple, and with no vocal fold edema. During the childbearing years, progesterone is produced. About one-third of women suffer from a vocal premenstrual syndrome associated with vocal fatigue and decreased range. At menopause, there is no production of progesterone,

there are few estrogens, and androgens appear. In a "Rubens" type female, the fat cells will metabolize the androgens to estrones. In a "Modigliani" type of physiognomy, the androgen impact will predominate. Hormone replacement therapy is often indispensable in voice professionals to avoid the development of a male voice and presbyphonia.[103,104]

LARYNGOPATHIA GRAVIDARUM

In the author's experience, 15% of women exhibit a vocal change during the last 5 months of pregnancy, almost always associated with rhinitis. In a 1942 study, Schemer reported approximately 20% of women exhibit voice changes during the last trimester of pregnancy.[96] The symptoms are the same as in the PMVS because of a progesterone environment.

INTERSEXUALITY, HYPOPHYSEAL DISORDERS

Chromosomal Abnormalities

Turner's syndrome[105,106] and Klinefelter's syndrome[107] are typical examples of intersexuality and voice disorders. Some groups of hermaphrodites have both ovaries and testicles, but this is rare. The voice is then under the sole control of the testosterone level, above 200 µg/dl, and because of its concentration, the voice has masculine characteristics. In this population with ovaries and testicles, or in transsexuals, the speaking voice may be transformed artificially by phonosurgery in male to female and by androgen therapy and/or surgery in female to male individuals.

Gonadotrophic Disorders

Gonadotrophic Adenoma

In Men. A lack of LH secretion (because of a physical compression of the cells by the adenoma so that the hormones are not able to be released into the bloodstream), will result in a lack of testosterone. This leads to decreased libido with asthenia. Intensity of the voice is weak, the range becomes narrow, the pitch does not change, the voice has fewer harmonics, and the timbre is thin.

In Women. The voice does not change, but there is an indirect consequence on the voice, a reduced muscular tone in the vocal folds, resulting from the impact of other hormones such as ACTH or TSH.

Hypergonadotrophic Disorders

In Men. High FSH levels are almost always associated with testicular deficiency. Hypoandrogenous symptoms appear such as gynecomastia, defects of spermatogenesis, and a higher or falsetto voice.

The testicle is smaller than normal by approximately 40%.[107] Klinefelter's syndrome XXY is the most common etiology. This genetic disease is associated with structural abnormalities of the long bones, excessive growth, and very high levels of FSH and LH.

The testosterone/estradiol ratio is elevated, because the testicle is an important secretor of estradiol.

- The larynx is lengthened, with long, thin vocal folds. The arytenoids are less mobile.
- The voice has a narrow range with loss of timbre as well as power.

Similar symptoms are observed in mosaic patients 46 XY/XXY and also in 46 XX patients of the male morphotype.[108]

Noonan's syndrome[109] is very rare. Here, LH and FSH levels are high and the testicular secretion is low. There is mental retardation and cryptorchidism. It is an autosomal dominant syndrome 46 XY. As there is a similarity in physical profile with Turner's syndrome with webbed neck, short stature, it is also known as the male Turner's syndrome. Voice is affected because of a depressed nasal bridge, a high arched palate, dental malocclusion, pectus excavatum, and hypotonia. The voice has female characteristics, with vocal atonia, a narrow register, and a shift of the register in the high tones.

Infection with the mumps virus may lead to testicular failure. Usually, it is a failure of spermatogenesis, but sometimes the testosterone producing Leydig cells may also be damaged.[110] There is lack of testosterone and the voice is like a pseudo "castrato."

These symptoms may also appear in males with diminished blood flow to the testicles, with bilateral testicular torsion, following chemotherapy or irradiation, and before puberty.

If similar problems occur after puberty, the voice lacks strength, but the timbre remains masculine.

The most severe testicular deficiency is caused by pathology of both testicles. Occasionally, it may be caused by a problem with gonadotrophins, receptors, or antibodies.

In Women. The FSH level is greater than twice normal during the follicular phase. There is a hypo-estrogenic syndrome with amenorrhea. When these symptoms appear before 40 years of age, they indicate an early menopause or a premature ovarian deficiency.[111]

LH is also high. There is no progesterone, and a very low level of estrogens.

The pathognomonic signs are hot flashes with insomnia, and vaginal dryness. In these women, menopause appears before menarche!

The vocal symptoms are similar to those of menopause, but more dramatic. Similar problems may be observed after irradiation or chemotherapy.

Autoimmune diseases may also be involved. Antibodies to both the FSH receptors and the LH receptors have been found in patients suffering from lupus erythematosus.[112]

Hypogonadotrophic Disorders

In Men. Lack of testosterone with low or normal levels of FSH and LH indicate abnormal hypothalamic function resulting in alterations in quantity and rhythm of the gonadotropin-releasing-hormone (GnRH) production. The voice is less powerful, higher pitched, and weak, similar to a senile voice. This is caused by a decrease in bulk of the vocal muscle, yielding a high voice, and a thinning of the epithelium causing a loss of vibratory amplitude and, hence, of vocal power.

In Women. These patients frequently suffer from insomnia, chronic illness or excess emotional stress, indulge in excessive physical exercise like athletes, and have difficulty maintaining their ideal weight. Basically, they have suffered from a major physical or psychologic upheaval.

Maintaining a balance of hypothalamic secretions with the environment is fundamental. It may be destabilized by external or internal factors. For example, stage fright may induce in a voice professional many responses, some positive and some negative. She may lose her vocal timbre because of an adrenalin-induced vasoconstriction; she may become amenorrheic through inhibition of FSH and LH secretion; she may also give a "once-in-a-lifetime" great performance because of the effect of endorphins from the hypothalamus.

In the polycystic ovarian syndrome (PCOS), androgen excess is typical, with amenorrhea or oligomenorrhea usually starting at adolescence. This leads to an irreversible masculinization of the voice.[113,114]

Growth Hormone

Growth Hormone Insufficiency

The body appearance is abnormal in this condition. The bones are small; there is a protuberant forehead, with very small hands and feet, and a small skull. The skin is thin. Some males may have a microphallus. The striated muscles are small and slim. However, the fat/muscle-mass ratio and the weight-to-height ratio tend to be normal during prepuberty.

The voice in childhood and in male adults is rather peculiar; the resonance cavities are abnormal. The sinus cavities and the nasal fossae are small. Dental eruption is delayed and permanent teeth are irregularly positioned. Bone aging is also very delayed. The lungs are also small.

The thyroid cartilage stays immature for a long time. The vocal fold epithelium is thin, and the amplitude of vibrations during phonation is diminished. The vocal fold muscle is thin and short. The voice is high pitched, but intensity is satisfactory. The register is appropriate. In males, a childlike vocal characteristic occurs, while in women, there is an almost-normal female voice. However, both show a lack of harmonics with a pediatric formants structure.[115,116]

Growth Hormone Excess

Hypersomatotropism and acromegaly are the common conditions resulting from excess of GH. There is an increase in connective tissue throughout the entire body as a result of this excess of secretion. There are transformations of the skin and the connective tissue, as well as facial tissue swelling and acromegaly[117,118] The patient may be recognized by a weak feeling of the handshake or an increase in heel pad thickness, with hypertrophy of distal bones (hands and feet). Gigantism throughout the skeleton (costal bones, inferior and superior maxillary, frontal bone protuberance, vertebral bones, and joints) is observed.

Women grow excess hair and have excessive perspiration because of sebaceous gland hypertrophy.

There is substantial androgenlike effect *except* on striated muscles and gonadal development at puberty. Cartilage growth is prolonged. Body proportions are eunuchlike. The liver, kidneys, thyroid gland, and other internal organs are all increased in size. There is often thickening of the heart's ventricular walls and the cardiac septum, which results in hypertension.

Other abnormalities include:

1. The resonance cavity abnormalities:
   - the skin of the face and the lips are thickened
   - the sinus cavities enlarge
   - there is often prognathism
   - the soft palate and uvula are enlarged and thickened
   - the nasal and oropharyngeal tissues are very thick and less flexible
   - respiratory function is decreased (weak)[118]

2. Laryngeal anomalies (observations based on personal [JA] experience):
   - the epiglottis is enlarged
   - the thyroid cartilage is increased in size
   - the mobility of the cricoarytenoid joint is impaired
   - the laryngeal mucosa is thickened: the vocal folds have a very thick epithelium with essentially normal vibration, and elongated thyroarytenoid muscle
   - the voice is deep, of low intensity, and often a narrowed range, but the harmonics and formants are within normal limits

THYROID DISORDERS

Mechanisms of Thyroid Hormone Action

Thyroid gland function has many physiologic effects on fetal growth, maintainance of body weight, the basal metabolic rate, and particularly on cellular differentiation and development. The syndrome of cretinism illustrates the impact of thyroid hormone during development, and suggests that there is a multifactorial effect during the production of other hormones. The thyroid gland plays a crucial role during puberty. It influences the range of the voice and influences the growth parameters. In adulthood, it will affect the metabolic parameters. Basal metabolic rate is increased in hyperthyroidism and decreased in hypothyroidism.

Innervation of the thyroid gland is provided by the sympathetic and parasympathetic nervous systems. The adrenergic nerve fibers and the sympathetic nerve fibers originate from the superior cervical ganglia. The acetylcholinesterase-positive fibers, the parasympathetic fibers, come from the jugular ganglia. Both the cholinergic and the adrenergic fibers are localized around the blood vessels, between the thyroid follicles.

This close association between the thyroid follicles, the thyroid vessels (with their laryngeal branches), and the sympathetic and parasympathetic systems probably partially explains the direct impact on psycho-emotional status and on T_3 and T_4 production.[119,120] The author (JA) has noted that thyroid inflammation comes and goes at times of stress, and in some premenstrual syndromes.

Hyperthyroidism

Hyperthyroidism, of which Graves' disease is the most common kind, is caused by overproduction of thyroid hormone. It is considered to be of an autoimmune etiology and its main symptoms are goiter, weight loss, tremor, agitation, diarrhea, sweating, and an ophthalmopathy. The ophthalmic manifestations such as exophthalmus, extraocular muscle hypertrophy, orbital edema, and an exposed cornea may be serious; this infiltrative ophthalmopathy is still not very well understood because it is independent of the thyroid hormone level in the plasma.

Voice disorders are poorly defined and are especially caused by muscular hyperstimulation by the elevated levels of thyroxin. Anxiety increases and the voice becomes hoarse and tremulous. The vocal folds appear hypervascularized and hyperkinetic.[121] Laryngopharyngeal-esophageal reflux associated with gastric hypermotility causes posterior edema of the larynx, often with a chronic cough and dysphonia. An increase in the respiratory rate, and a reduction in vital capacity have been seen.

Hyperthyroidism is very frequently associated with a hypervascular thyroid. In such cases, it has been the author's (JA) observation that the vocal folds look hypoxic. A "laryngeal artery steal syndrome" could explain this aspect: the blood being diverted by the goiter; however, this is only a clinical hypothesis, and an empiric deduction. The vocal fold muscles are weak and vocal fatigue occurs. Examination of the vocal folds also often shows a glottic chink during phonation with a loss of amplitude in the vibrations of the epithelium resulting in a hoarse and breathy voice. High pitches are very hard to maintain; low pitches are weak but possible. Similar observations have been made after total thyroidectomies where the laryngeal arteries have been ligated (personal observations).

Hypothyroidism

Hypothyroidism is caused by a lack of thyroxin production. If congenital and untreated, it will lead to cretinism and a small larynx.[122,123] Hearing is decreased. Speech is slow, hesitant, and movements are clumsy. Examination of the larynx shows muscle stiffness. The vocal folds are rarely hypertrophied, but the epithelium is dry and has a narrow amplitude during vibration. There is mucosal edema. The cricoarytenoid joint may be stiff and pain may occur during speaking. The vocal folds are pale; and in some patients, there may be Reinke's edema. There is voice fatigue, hoarseness, and weak intensity. The range is narrow and confined to low tones. The maximum phonation time (MPT) is reduced.

Respiration is altered, with characteristics of dyspnea and shortness of breath, nasal congestion, and a low oxygen saturation, which is often associated with sleep apnea. Sleep apnea is common because of enlargement of the tongue, hypertrophy of oropharyngeal muscles with interstitial edema and muscle fiber enlargement, respiratory muscle weakness, and depression of the respiratory center.[124]

PINEAL GLAND

The pineal gland is an endocrine gland in mammals, while in fish, it is photoreceptive. It is a small, unpaired central structure, an appendage of the brain. The pineal weight is around 130 mg. Its role in reptiles and birds is mixed: photoreceptor and secretory function. The principal cellular component is the pinealocyte. In human, both photoreceptive function and pinealocyte secretion exist. The gland, richly vascularized, is chiefly innervated by sympathetic nerve fibers from the superior cervical ganglion. Pineal denervation abolishes the rhythmic synthesis of melatonin and the light-dark control of its production.[125] The main role of this gland is to organize the body rhythms and the light-dark cycles by inducing the secretion of the pineal hormone melatonin. The retina and the gut also secrete melatonin. Melatonin is secreted by the influences of the SCN (suprachiasmic nucleus), the body clock synchronized with the retina. It is synthesized during the dark phase of the day. It affects the central nervous system. Melatonin influences the GnRH secretion. It has an effect, as in all other striated muscles, on the quality of the voice through its influence on the CNS at different times of the day and night, as is well known by voice professionals traveling with jet lag.

PARATHYROID DISORDERS

Hypoparathyroidism

Hypoparathyroidism causes hypocalcemia. It stops or slows down the calcification of the larynx and may cause osteomalacia. Hypocalcemia may cause muscle cramps, hyperexcitability and spasmodic contractions. It may also lead to lethal complications such as laryngospasm or a heart attack. Stridor, arrhythmia, and muscle fatigue with spastic muscle contraction are typical of hypocalcemia. It may also lead to paresthesias, circumoral tingling, and, ultimately, tetany. Chvostek's sign will help in the diagnosis, as will Trousseau's sign (a compression of the vessels of the upper arm gives a tetanic state). Voice fatigue, hoarseness, and, rarely, aphonia are observed. Videolaryngoscopy shows the development of vocal fold tetany when the subject is asked to phonate the vowel \ɑ\. During times of emotional stress, these symptoms are aggravated because the patient "consumes" more and more calcium when stressed, and also because of decreased blood supply caused by the vasoconstriction.

In actors and other voice professionals, these signs must be looked for to avoid and prevent serious consequences before going onstage and treated by giving calcium replacement therapy and vitamin D.

Hyperparathyroidism

Hyperparathyroidism causes hypercalcemia, with gastrointestinal, renal, musculoskeletal, and central nervous systems symptoms.

Muscle weakness and hyporeflexia are observed as are dysphonia and aphonia.

ADRENAL DISORDERS

Adrenal Insufficiency

Adrenal insufficiency was the first endocrine disorder described as an endocrine disease by Addison, and was named Addison's syndrome by Trousseau in 1856.[126-128] Addison's disease is a deficiency of the adrenal cortex with hypoproduction of cortisol and aldosterone. Weakness, muscular hypofunction, a weak larynx, and dysphonia are observed.[129] The adrenal cortex controls the tone of striated muscles by controlling the supply of energy to the muscle cells.

In adrenal insufficiency, the subject appears weak, always tired, and the muscular toxins cannot be eliminated. The voice is normal for about 10 minutes and then, suddenly, it breaks, with a husky voice leading to aphonia. The vocal folds vibrate normally for a few minutes and then stop, almost like an intermittent claudication. The vocal fold muscles soon become pathologic. Shouting and singing become almost impossible and the range becomes very narrow. It is easier for the patient to speak in a reclined position than in a standing position.

Congenital Adrenal Hyperplasia

Excess adrenal androgen produces abnormalities. In females, there is an androgenic effect, and in males, a hyperandrogenic effect.[130] The voice is stronger, the male voice is powerful with a wide range, and the female voice is more often a contralto with powerful musculature. The child with signs of virilization, also called "Hercules child," may be caused by hyperproduction of hormones of the adrenal cortex.

The hypersecretion of adrenalin acts as an antidote to muscle fatigue.

DIABETES MELLITUS

Diabetes mellitus is an endocrine disease of the pancreas. More than 10 million people in the United States and 14 million in Europe are diabetic. This pathology is a defect in the metabolic pathways of glucose.

Coronary artery disease and eye problems such as diabetic retinopathy with microaneurysms, conjunctival and irideal hemorrhages resulting from glycogen deposits, depigmentation, and neovascularization are the most dramatic complications. Neural pathology may present as an acute or chronic peripheral neuropathy, involving the limbs as well as the cranial nerves in the head and neck. The autonomic nervous system may also be affected.

As far as voice disturbance is concerned, involvement of the spinal cervical nerves is the most commonly observed mononeuropathy. It causes vocal fatigue because of pain, sensory loss, and weakness of the cervical muscles by an alteration of sympathetic and parasympathetic function. Occasionally, involvement of the third, fifth, sixth, seventh, eighth, and twelfth cranial nerves has been described.[131,132]

The dysphonia can be associated with dysphagia and aspiration. Vocal fold paralysis may rarely be seen with a peripheral lesion of the vagus nerve or a nuclear or supranuclear lesion.[129] Thus, in cases of vocal fold paralysis or paresis, a test of carbohydrate metabolism (glucose) should be done to rule out diabetes. Diabetes may also cause capillary pathology, and poor oxygenation of the vocal fold muscles, with vocal fatigue.

Voice disorders may also occur because of hearing loss caused by diabetes. Thus, in these patients, when there is dysphonia, an audiogram should be performed. In infectious laryngitis with reflux, the management of diabetes is critically important.

CUSHING'S SYNDROME

Harvey Cushing was the first to incorporate the following symptoms into one specific disease: obesity, diabetes, hirsutism, and adrenal hyperplasia.[133] Cushing's syndrome is a symptom complex that reflects excessive tissue exposure to cortisol. The etiologies are usually characterized by excessive ACTH production from a corticotrophic adenoma. Pseudo-Cushing's syndrome can result from long-term steroid therapy.

The typical patient presents with symptoms of virilization, hypokalemia, and high cortisol excretion.

The physical examination reveals hypertension, obesity, abnormal fat distribution (moon face), decreased proximal muscle strength, and menstrual irregularity in women.[134,135]

In our experience, the male voice is not affected. The singing voice is usually normal. In women, it will depend on the influence of the secretion of the dehydro-epiandrosterone from the adrenal gland. Nevertheless, the disease increases weakness of the voice and a loss of high notes.

CONCLUSION

This chapter would not be complete without mention of an article in *Nature* by Bennett et al in 1995. They reported that in man, the cerebral projection of speech was not only on the left hemisphere but also on the right side, the side of emotions.[136]

The vocal imprint is characteristic to each individual. It reveals personality and translates emotions. The voice evolves with age and is hormone dependent. The human voice is fluid, both charming and sensual. It bears the scars of life, as well as its joys and pleasures. Nevertheless, the human voice remains intangible, and a fertile field for future research in the cycle of life.

REFERENCES

1. Vesalius A. *De Humanis Corporis Fabrica.* Base; 1543.
2. Harris GW. Neural control of the pituitary gland. *Physiol Rev.* 1948;28:139–179.
3. Darnell J, Lodish H, Baltimore D. *Molecular Cell Biology.* New York, NY: Scientific American Books; 1990.
4. Gammelhoft S, Kahn CR. Hormone signaling via membrane receptors. In: De Groot LJ, ed. *Endocrinology.* Philadelphia, PA: WB Saunders; 1995:49.
5. Asthana S, Craft S, Baker LD, et al. Cognitive and neuroendocrine response to transdermal estrogen in postmenopausal women with Alzheimer's disease: results of a placebo-controlled, double-blind, pilot study. *Psychoneuroendocrinology.* 1999;24(6):657–677.
6. Kerr JB, Sharpe RM. Follicle stimulating hormone induction of Leydig cell maturation. *Endocrinology.* 1985;116:2592–2604.
7. Grossmann A, Kruxeman A, Perry L, et al. A new hypothalamic hormone, CRF, specifically stimulates the release of adrenocorticotrophin and cortisol in man. *Lancet.* 1982;1:921–922.
8. Chauchereau A, Savouret J-F, Milgrom E. Control of biosynthesis and post-transcriptional modification of the progesterone receptor. *Biol Reprod.* 1992;46:174.
9. De Kretser DM, Kerr JB. The cytology of the testis. In: Knobil E. Neill J, eds. *The Physiology of Reproduction.* New York, NY: Raven; 1988;837–932.
10. Sherwin BB, Gelfand MM, Brender W. Androgen enhances sexual motivation in females: a prospective, cross-over study of sex steroid administration in the surgical menopause. *Psychosom Med.* 1985;17:339–351.
11. Persky H, Driesbach L, Miller WR. The relation of plasma androgen levels to sexual behaviors and attitudes of women. *Psychosom Med.* 1982;44:305–319.
12. Longcope C. Adrenal and gonadal androgen secretion in normal female. *Clin Endocrinol Metab.* 1986;15:213–228.
13. Moltz L, Schwartz U. Gonadal and adrenal androgen secretion in hirsute females. *Clin Endocrinol Metab.* 1986;15:229–245.
14. Bouvier RF. *Le Chanteur des Rois.* Paris: Albin Michel; 1943;12–31.
15. Gougeon A. Dynamics of follicular growth in the human: a model from preliminary results. *Human Reproduction I.* 1986;81–87.
16. MacDonald PC, Dombroski RA, Casey ML. Recurrent secretion of progesterone in large amounts: an endocrine/metabolic disorder unique to young women? *Endocr Rev.* 1991;12:372–401.
17. Harada N. A unique aromatas (P450arom) mRNA formed by alternative use of tissue specific exons I in human skin fibroblasts. *Biochem Biophys Res Commun.* 1992;189:1001–1007.
18. Friedrich G, Lichtenegger R. Surgical anatomy of the larynx. *J Voice.* 1997;11(3):345–355.
19. Barnhart KT, Freeman EW, Sondheimer SJ. A clinician's guide to the premenstrual syndrome. *Med Clin North Am.* 1995;79:1457–1472.
20. Richardson JT. The premenstrual syndrome: a brief history. *Soc Sci Med.* 1995;41:761–767.
21. Smith S. The premenstrual syndrome; diagnosis and management. *Fertil Steril.* 1989;53:527–543.
22. Facchinetti F, et al. Oestradiol/progesterone imbalance and the premenstrual syndrome. *Lancet.* 1983;2:1302.
23. Munday MR, Brush MG, Taylor RW. Correlations between progesterone, oestradiol and aldosterone levels in the premenstrual syndrome. *Clin Endocrinol.* 1981;14:1–9.
24. Rubinow DR, Roy-Byrne P. Premenstrual syndrome: overfire from a methodological perspective. *Am J Psychiatr.* 1984;141:163–172.
25. Brayshaw ND, Brayshaw DD. Thyroid hypofunction in premenstrual syndrome. *New Engl J Med.* 1986;315:1486–1487.
26. Aganoff JA, Boyle GJ. Aerobic exercise, mood states and menstrual cycle symptoms. *J Psychosom Res.* 1994;38:183–192.
27. Choi PY, Salmon P. Symptom changes across the menstrual cycle in competitive sportswomen, exercisers and sedentary women. *Br J Clin Psychol.* 1995;34:447–460.
28. Steege JF, Blumenthal J. The effects of aerobic exercise on premenstrual symptoms in middle-aged women: a preliminary study. *J Psychosom Res.* 1993;37(2):127–133.
29. Weyerer S, Kupfer B. Physical exercise and psychological health. *Sports Med.* 1994;17:108–116.
30. Byrne A, Byrne DG. The effects of exercise on depression, anxiety and other mood states: a review. *J Psychosom Res.* 1993;37:565–574.
31. Dua J, Hargreaves L. Effect of aerobic exercise on negative affect, positive affect, stress, and depression. *Percept Mot Skill.* 1992;75:355–361.

32. Lafontaine TP, et al. Aerobic exercise and mood: a brief review, 1985–1990. *Sports Med.* 1992;13:160–170.

33. Longcope C, et al. The effect of a low fat diet on oestrogen metabolism. *J Clin Endocrinol Metab.* 1987;64:1246–1250.

34. Hodgen GD. The dominant ovarian follicle. *Fertil Steril.* 1982;38:281–300.

35. Chihal HJ. *Premenstrual Syndrome: A Clinic Manual.* 2nd ed. Dallas, TX: Essential Medical Information Systems; 1990:18–47.

36. Jones MM. The premenstrual syndrome; part 1. *Br J Sex Med.* 1983;10:9–11.

37. Abraham GE. Nutritional factors in the etiology of the premenstrual tension syndromes. *J Reprod Med.* 1983; 28:446–464.

38. Mortola. The premenstrual syndrome. *Reprod Endocrinol Surg Tech.* 1995;2:1635–1647.

39. Frable M. Hoarseness, a symptom of premenstrual tension. *Arch Otolaryngol.* 1962;75:80–82.

40. Lewis PD, Harrison MJG. Involuntary movement in patients taking oral contraceptives. *Br Med J.* 1969;4:404–405.

41. Riddoch D. Jefferson M. Bickerstaff ER. Chorea and the oral contraceptives. *Br Med J.* 1971;4:217–218.

42. Cogen PH, Zimmerman EA. Ovarian steroid hormones and cerebral function. *Adv Neurol.* 1979;26:123–133.

43. Gordon JH, Borison RL, Diamond BI. Modulation of dopamine receptor sensitivity by estrogen. *Biol Psychiatry.* 1980;15:389–396.

44. Miller NH, Gould WJ. Fluctuating sensorineural hearing impairment associated with the menstrual cycle. *J Aud Res.* 1967;7:373–385.

45. Procacci P, Zoppi M, Maresca M, Romano S. Studies on the pain threshold in man. In: Bonica JJ, ed. *Advances in Neurology. International Symposium on Pain.* Vol. 4. New York, NY: Raven Press; 1974:107–113.

46. Meiri H. Is synaptic transmission modulated by progesterone? *Brain Res.* 1986;385:193–196.

47. Rosner JM, Nagle CA, de Laborde NP, et al. Plasma levels of norepinephrine during the periovulatory period and after LH-RH stimulation in women. *Am J Obstet Gynecol.* 1976;124;567–572.

48. Coffey CE, Ross DR, Ferren EL, Bragdon AC, Hurwitz BJ, Olanow CW. The effect of lithium on the on-off phenomenon in Parkinsonism. *Adv Neurol.* 1983;37:61–73.

49. Wyke BD. Laryngeal myotatic reflexes and phonation. *Folia Phoniatr.* 1974;26:249–264.

50. Newman SR, Butler J, Hammond EH, Gray SD. Preliminary report on hormone receptors in the human fold. *J Voice.* 2000;14:72–81.

51. Higgins MB, Saxman JH. Variation in vocal frequency perturbation across the menstrual cycle. *J Voice.* 1989;3: 233–243.

52. Abitbol J, de Brux J, Millot G, et al. Does a hormonal vocal cord cycle exist in women? Study of vocal premenstrual syndrome in voice performers by videostroboscopy-glottography and cytology on 38 women. *J Voice.* 1989;3:157–162.

53. Abitbol J. *The Female Voice* [movie 22 min]. San Diego, CA: Singular Publishing Group; 1997.

54. Silverman EM, Zimmer CH. Effect of the menstrual cycle on voice quality. *Arch Otolaryngol.* 1978;104:7–10.

55. Montagnani CF, Arena B, Maffulli N. Estradiol and progesterone during exercise in healthy untrained women. *Med Sci Sports Exerc.* 1992;24:764–768.

56. Edman CD, MacDonald PC. The role of extraglandular estrogens in women in health and disease. In: James VHT, Serio M, Giusti G, eds. *The Endocrine Function of the Human Ovary.* New York, NY: Academic Press; 1976:135–140.

57. Meisfelt RL. The structure and function of steroid receptor proteins. *Crit Rev Biochem Mol Biol.* 1989;24:101–117.

58. Munday MR, Brush MG, Taylor RW. Progesterone, aldosterone levels in premenstrual syndrome. *J Endocrinol.* 1977;73:21–22.

59. Mortola JF, Girton L. Fischer U. Successful treatment of severe premenstrual syndrome by use of gonadotrophin-releasing hormone agonist and estrogen/progestin. *J Clin Endocrinol Metab.* 1991;71:252–260.

60. Taylor AE, Schneyer A, Sluss P, Crawley WF Jr. Ovarian failure, resistance and activation. In: Adashi EY, Leung CK, eds. *The Ovary.* New York, NY: Raven Press; 1993.

61. O'Brien PM, Selby C, Symonds EM. Progesterone, fluids and electrolytes in premenstrual syndrome. *Br Med J.* 1981;280:1161–1163.

62. Adashi EY. The climateric ovary: an androgen-producing gland. *Reprod Endocrinol Surg Tech.* 1995;2:1745–1757.

63. Applegarth LD. Emotional implications. *Reprod Endocrinol Surg Tech.* 1995;2:1953–1968.

64. Chang RJ, Judd HL. The ovary after menopause. *Clin Obstet Gynecol.* 1981;24:181.

65. Chodzko-Zajko WJ, Ringer RL. Physiological aspects of aging. *J Voice.* 1987;1:18–26.

66. Fedor-Feyberg P. The influence of estrogens on the wellbeing and mental performances in climateric and postmenopausal women. *Acta Obstet Gynecol Scand.* 1979;64:1–6.

67. Grodin JM, Siiteri PK, MacDonald PC. Source of estrogen production in postmenopausal women. *J Clin Endocrinol Metab.* 1973;36:207–214.

68. Hemsell DL, Grodin JM, Brenner PF, Siiteri PKK, MacDonald PC. Plasma precursors of estrogens II. Correlations of the extent of conversion of plasma androstenedione to estrone with age. *J Clin Endocrinol Metab.* 1974; 38:476–479.

69. Buchsbaum HJ. *The Menopause.* New York, NY: Springer-Verlag; 1987.

70. MacDonald PC, Edman CD, Hernsell DI, Porter JC, Citeri PK. Effect of obesity on conversion of plasma androstenedione to estrone in post-menopausal women with and without endometrial cancer. *Am J Obstet Gynecol.* 1978;130:448–452.

71. Inkster SE, Brodie AMH. Expression of aromatase cytochrome P-450 in premenopausal and postmenopausal human ovaries and immunocytochemical study. *J Clin Endocrinol Metab.* 1991;73:717.

72. Sasano H, Okamoto M, Mason JL, et al. Immunolocalization of aromataze, 17α-hydroxylase and side-chain-cleavage P-450 in the human ovary. *J Reprod Fertil.* 1989; 85:163–169.

73. Zhao Y, Nichols JE, Buln SE, Mendelson CR, Simpson ER. Aromatase P450 gene expression in human adipose tissue. *J Biol Chem.* 1995;270:16449–16457.

74. Edman CD, MacDonald PC. The role of extraglandular estrogens in women in health and disease. In: James VHT, Serio M, Giusti G, eds. *The Endocrine Function of the Human Ovary.* New York, NY: Academic Press; 1976:135–140.

75. Evans DJ, Hoffmann RG, Kalkhoff RK, Kissebah AH. Relationship of androgenic activity to body fat topography, fat cell morphology, and metabolic aberrations in premenopausal women. *J Clin Endocrinol Metab.* 1983;57:304–310.

76. Hauner H, Schmid P, Pfeiffer EF. Glucocorticoids and insulin promote the differentiation of human adipocyte precursor cells into fat cells. *J Clin Endocrinol Metab.* 1987;64:832–835.

77. Nagamani M, Hannigan EV, Dinh VT, Stuart CA. Hyperinsulinemia and stromal luteinization of the ovaries in postmenopausal women with endometrial cancer. *J Clin Endocrinol Metab.* 1988;67:144.

78. Perel E, Killinger DW. The interconversion and aromatization of androgens by human adipose tissue. *J Steroid Biochem.* 1979;10:623–627.

79. Roncari DAK. Hormonal influences on the replication and maturation of adipocyte precursors. *Int J Obesity.* 1981;5:547–552.

80. Schneider J, Bradlow HL, Strain G, Levin J, Anderson K, Fishman J. Effects of obesity on estradiol metabolism: decreased formation of non-uterotropic metabolites. *J Clin Endocrinol Metab.* 1983;56:973–978.

81. Bulun SE, Mahendroo MS, Simpson ER. Aromatase gene expression in adipose tissue: relationship to breast cancer. *J Steroid Biochem Molec Biol.* 1994;49:319–326.

82. Struhle U, Boshart M, Klock G. Stewart F, Schultz G. Glucocorticoid and progesterone specific effects are determined by differential expression of the respective hormone receptors. *Nature* (London). 1989;339:6329–6332.

83. Mattingly RF, Huang WY. Steroidogenesis of the menopausal and post-menopausal ovary. *Am J Obstet Gynecol.* 1969;103:679–693.

84. Exton JH. Regulation of gluconeogenesis by glucocorticoids. In: Baxter JD, Rousseau GG, eds. *Glucocorticoid Hormone Action.* Berlin: Springer Verlag; 1979:535–546.

85. Odell WD. The menopause and hormonal replacement: In: DeGroot L, ed. *Endocrinology.* Philadelphia, PA: WB Saunders; 1995;2129–2137.

86. Emperaire JC. Gynécologie *Endocrinienne du Praticien.* Paris: Editions Frison-Roche; 1995.

87. Tsai-Morris CH, Aquilana DR, Dufau ML. Cellular localization of rat testicular aromatase activity during development. *Endocrinology.* 1985;116:38–46.

88. Vermeulen A. The hormonal activity of the postmenopausal ovary. *J Clin Endocrinol Metab.* 1976;42:247.

89. Waterman MR, Simpson ER. Regulation of adrenal cytochrome P-450 activity and gene expression. *Rev Toxicol.* 1987;98:259–287.

90. Wotiz HH, Davis JW, Lemon HM, Gut M. Studies in steroid metabolism. V. The conversion of testosterone-4-C14-to estrogens by human ovarian tissue. *J Biol Chem.* 1956;222:487.

91. Gambrell RD Jr. The menopause: benefits and risks of estrogen-progestogen replacement therapy. *Fertil Steril.* 1982;37(4):457–474.

92. Rabinovici J, Rothman P, Monroe SE, Nerenberg C, Jaffe RB. Endocrine effects and pharmacokinetic characteristics of a potent new gonadotropin-releasing hormone antagonist (Ganirelix) with minimal histamine-releasing properties: studies in postmenopausal women. *J Clin Endocrinol Metab.* 1992;75:1220.

93. Schiff M. The influence of estrogens on connective tissue. In: Asboe-Hansen G, ed. *Hormones and Connective Tissue.* Copenhagen: Munksgaard Press; 1967:282–341.

94. Applegarth LD. Emotional implications. *Reprod Endocrinol Surg Tech.* 1995;2:1953–1968.

95. Brodnitz F. Hormones and the human voice. *Bull NY Acad Med.* 1971;47:183–191.

96. Gramming P, Sundbert J, Ternstrom S, Leanderson R, Perkins W. Relationship between changes in voice pitch and loudness. *J Voice.* 1988;2:118–126.

97. Hammarback S, Damber JE, Backstrom T. Relationship between symptom severity and hormone changes in women with premenstrual syndrome. *J Clin Endocrinol Metab.* 1989;68:125.

98. Sunderberg J. *The Science of the Singing Voice.* Dekalb: Northern Illinois University Press; 1987.

99. Tarneaud J. *Traité Pratique de Phonologie et de Phoniatrie; La Voix, la Parole, le Chant.* Paris, France: Librairie Maloine; 1941.

100. Abitbol J. *Atlas of Laser Surgery.* San Diego, CA: Singular Publishing Group; 1995.

101. Abitbol J, Abitbol P. *Laser Voice Surgery* [movie 31 min]—21 Cases of Laser Voice Surgery. San Diego, CA: Singular Publishing Group; 1996.

102. Isshiki N. Mechanical and dynamic aspects of voice production as related to voice therapy and phonosurgery. *Otolaryngol Head Neck Surg.* 2000;122:782–793.

103. Abitbol J, Abitbol P. *The Feminine Voice and the Cycle of Life* [movie 22 min]. Bayacedez-Abitbol; 1998.

104. Abitbol J, Abitbol P. Sex hormones and the female voice. *J Voice.* 1999;13:444–446.

105. Lippe B. Turner's syndrome. *Endocrinol Metab Clin North Am.* 1991;20:121–152.

106. Ranke MB, Pfugler H, Rosendahl W, et al. Turner's syndrome: spontaneous growth in 150 cases and review of the literature. *Eur J Pediatr.* 1983;141:80–88.

107. Klinefelter HF. Klinefelter's syndrome: historical background and development. *South Med J.* 1986;79:1089–1094.

108. Bandmann HJ, Breite R, eds. *Klinefelter's Syndrome.* Berlin: Springer Verlag; 1984.

109. Sharland M, Burch M, McKenna WM, Paton MA. A clinical study of Noonan's syndrome. *Arch Dis Child.* 1992;67:178–183.

110. Del Castillo EB, Trabucco A, De la Balze FA. Syndrome produced by absence of the germinal epithelium without impairment of the Sertoli or Leydig cells. *J Clin Endocrinol Metab.* 1947;7:493–502.

111. Rebar RW, Erickson GF, Yen SSC. Idiopathic premature ovarian failure: clinical and endocrine characteristic, *Fertil Steril.* 1982;37:35–41.

112. Taylor AE, Schneyer A, Sluss P, Crowley WF Jr. Ovarian failure, resistance and activation. In: Adashi EY, Lung CK, eds. *The Ovary.* New York, NY: Raven Press; 1993.

113. Stein IF, Leventhal ML. Amenorrhea associated with bilateral polycystic ovaries. *Am J Obstet Gynecol.* 1935; 29:181–191.

114. Yen SSC. The polycystic ovary syndrome. *Clin Endocrinol.* 1980;12:177–208.

115. Tanner JM, Whitehouse RH. A note on the bone age at which patients with "isolated" growth hormone deficiency enter puberty. *J Clin Endocrinol Metab.* 1975;41: 788–790.

116. August GP, Lippe BM, Blethen SL, et al. Growth hormone treatment in the United States: demographic and diagnostic features of 2331 children. *J Pediatr.* 1990; 116:899–903.

117. Grunstein RR, Ho KY, Sullivan CE. Sleep apnea in acromegaly. *Ann Intern Med.* 1991;115:527–531.

118. Daughaday WH. Pituitary gigantism. *Endocrinol Metab Clin North Am.* 1992;21:633–637.

119. Pakarinen A, Hakkinen K, Alen M. Serum thyroid hormones, thyrotropin and thyroxine binding globulin in elite athletes during very intense strength training at one week. *J Sports Phys Fitness.* 1991;31:142–146.

120. Ziegler MG, Morrissey EC, Marshall LL. Catecholamine and thyroid hormones in traumatic injury. *Crit Care Med.* 1990;18:253–258.

121. Malinsky M, et al. Etude clinique et electrophysiologique des altérations de la voix au cours des thyrotoxicoses. *Ann Endocrinol (Paris).* 1977;38:171–172.

122. Watnakunakorn C, Hodges RH, Evans TC. Myxedema: a study of 400 cases. *Arch Intern Med.* 1965;116: 183–190.

123. Khaleeli AA, Griffith DG, Edwards RHT. The clinical presentation of hypothyroid myopathy and its relationship to abnormalities in structure and function of skeletal of muscle. *Clin Endocrinol.* 1983;19:365–376.

124. Siafakas NL, Salesiotou V, Filaditaki V, et al. Respiratory muscle strength in hypothyroidism. *Chest.* 1992; 102:189–194.

125. Klein DC. Photoneural regulation of the mammalian pineal gland. In: Evered D, Clark S, eds. *Photoperiodism, Melatonin and the Pineal. Ciba Foundation Symposium.* Vol. 117. London: Pitman; 1985:38–56.

126. Addison T. *On the Constitutional and Local Effect of Disease of the Supra Renal Capsules.* London: Highly; 1855.

127. Trousseau A. Bronze Addison's disease. *Arch Gen Med.* 1856;8:478–492.

128. Vita JA, Silverberg SJ, Goland RS, et al. Clinical clues to the cause of Addison's disease. *Am J Med.* 1985;78: 461–466.

129. Clements RS Jr. Diabetic neuropathy: New concepts of its etiology. *Diabetes.* 1979;28:608–611.

130. New MI, Gertner JM, Speiser PW, Del Balzo P. Growth and final height in classical and nonclassical 21-hydroxylase deficiency. *Acta Pediatr JPN.* 1988;30(suppl):79–88.

131. Ellenberg M. Diabetic neuropathy: clinical aspects. *Metabolism.* 1976;25:1627–1655.

132. Rontal M, Rontal E. Lesions of the vagus nerve: diagnosis, treatment and rehabilitation. *Laryngoscope.* 1977;87:72–86.

133. Cushing H. *The Pituitary Body and Its Disorders: Clinical States Produced by Disorders of the Hypophysis Cerebri.* Philadelphia, PA: JD Lippincott; 1912.

134. Ross J, Linch DC. Cushing's syndrome killing diseases: discriminatory value of signs and symptoms aiding early diagnosis. *Lancet.* 1982:646–649.

135. Urbanic RC, Georges JM. Cushing's disease: 18 years' experience. *Medicine.* 1981;60:14–24.

136. Abitbol J. *Les Coulisses de la Voix—Norma.* Bruxelles: Labor; 1994;42–65.

28

Laryngopharyngeal Reflux and Voice Disorders

Jamie A. Koufman, MD, FACS
S. Carter Wright, Jr., MD

It has been estimated that half of otolaryngology (ORL) patients with laryngeal and voice disorders have laryngopharyngeal reflux (LPR) as the primary cause or as a significant etiologic cofactor.[1] This appears to be true for patients with diverse clinical manifestations.[2-22] Many voice clinicians (including the authors) recommend that LPR be routinely assessed in patients with laryngeal and voice disorders; however, even among otolaryngologists who have a relatively high index of suspicion for LPR, it appears that this disorder is still often underdiagnosed and undertreated.[22] There appears to be a four-part explanation:

1. The symptoms, manifestations, patterns, and mechanisms of LPR and gastroesophageal reflux disease (GERD) are different.[2-4,22-35] Consequently, patients with LPR usually deny symptoms of heartburn and/or regurgitation.[2-4,26,28] Fewer than half of ORL patients with LPR documented by pH monitoring complain of heartburn or regurgitation, symptoms that clinicians have traditionally felt must be present to diagnose reflux disease.[2-4,26]

2. The findings of LPR on laryngeal examination vary considerably, and laryngeal edema, a hallmark of LPR, is often unappreciated as a positive finding.[36-38] Most otolaryngologists rely solely on the findings of erythema or of posterior laryngitis (red arytenoids and piled-up, hypertrophic, posterior commissure mucosa) as the diagnostic *sine qua non* of LPR. Unfortunately, those findings are not present in many LPR patients. In the authors' experience, edema (and not erythema) is the principal, and most common, finding of LPR. The edema may be diffuse, or it may create the illusion of sulcus vocalis, an appearance that is the result of subglottic edema in Reinke's space.[38] When the edema involves both the true and false vocal folds, it may cause the laryngeal ventricles to swell shut. This relatively common finding is termed *ventricular obliteration*.

3. Traditional diagnostic tests for gastroesophageal reflux disease (GERD) lack both sensitivity and specificity for LPR. Barium esophagography, radionuclide scanning, the Bernstein acid-perfusion test, and esophagoscopy with biopsy are all often negative in LPR patients.[3] This is probably because most LPR patients do not develop esophagitis, which is typically observed in gastroenterology patients with GERD.[2,3,26-28] In addition, LPR is frequently intermittent, and exacerba-

tions depend to some extent on ever-changing dietary and lifestyle factors.[3]

4. Therapeutic trials using traditional antireflux therapy [39-46] often fail in LPR patients, so that clinicians may falsely conclude that LPR is not present.[40,46] The traditional treatment for GERD, particularly in a patient with esophagitis, includes dietary and lifestyle modifications and use of antacids, H2-blockers, and/or single-daily-dose proton pump inhibitors (PPIs). Such treatment fails to control LPR in up to 50% of patients.[3,42-46] In many cases, the treatment dose is inadequate (as most LPR patients require b.i.d. PPI treatment); also, the duration of the therapeutic trial is often too "short."[22] Many clinicians believe that a therapeutic trial of antireflux therapy of few weeks duration is adequate, but that is not the case. Patients with long-standing LPR often require 6 months or more of optimal treatment (acid suppression) with PPIs to resolve their symptoms and findings. Also, PPI resistance in LPR patients is not uncommon, being about 10%.[22,42]

Within the last two decades, with the availability of new diagnostic methods and treatments, researchers have begun to elucidate the clinical patterns and mechanisms of LPR.[2-5,26-33] It now appears that patients with LPR are quite different from typical gastroenterology (GI) patients with heartburn and esophagitis (ie, GERD). How are LPR patients different than those with GERD? Why do ORL patients usually deny heartburn? What are the differences in the mechanisms of LPR and GERD?

Previously, the diagnosis of LPR was erroneously based on the gastroenterologist's esophagitis model of GERD. Improved diagnostic technology and effective treatments are beginning to yield important information about LPR and how it differs from GERD.

In a relative sense, ambulatory 24-hour double-probe (simultaneous esophageal and pharyngeal) pH monitoring (pH-metry) has become the diagnostic gold standard for LPR[2,3,24,25]; however, as a diagnostic, it is expensive and it is not widely available. Nevertheless, pH-metry effectively documents LPR with a high degree of specificity and sensitivity. The next tier of reflux-testing, impedance,[43] may prove to be even better for diagnosis in certain LPR subgroups, such as those with a chief complaint of chronic cough.

Transnasal esophagoscopy (TNE) is performed in the clinic setting without anesthesia or sedation (other than topical numbing of the nose).[26-28] TNE has allowed the otolaryngologist to screen the esophagus. In a large series, Postma et al[28] reported that 50% of the patients had positive findings on TNE, including, esophagitis 17%, hiatal hernia 8%, Barrett's metaplasia 5%, candida esophagitis 5%, and stricture 4%.

The treatment of LPR took a giant leap forward with the introduction of proton pump inhibitors (PPIs) into the United States in 1989. Compared to previous treatments, PPIs more effectively reduce gastric acid production.[22] In addition, antireflux surgery has been shown to be very effective for patients with recalcitrant or life-threatening LPR.[47]

HOW AND WHY ARE ORL PATIENTS WITH LPR DIFFERENT FROM GI PATIENTS WITH GERD?

Ossakow et al[4] compared the symptoms and findings of reflux disease in two discrete groups: ORL patients (n = 63) and GI patients (n = 36). They reported that hoarseness was present in 100% of the ORL patients and 0% of the GI patients and that heartburn was present in 89% of the GI patients, but in only 6% of the ORL patients. Other authors also have reported a low incidence of heartburn as a symptom in ORL patients with LPR.[2,3,26] Heartburn is a symptom of esophagitis, and most ORL patients do not have esophagitis. Wiener et al[2] studied 32 ORL patients with hoarseness and found that although pH-metry was abnormal in 78%, esophageal manometry was normal in 100%, and esophagoscopy with biopsy was normal in 72%. Koufman[3,26] found that fewer than 20% of ORL patients with LPR had findings of esophagitis by TNE or barium esophagogram. By comparison, esophagitis is found in most GI patients.

It may seem counterintuitive that LPR patients do not also have GERD, and this is an important reason why some clinicians remain skeptical of the diagnosis LPR. It is hard for some people to believe that one could have reflux-related disease without having heartburn or regurgitation. The explanation lies in examination of the pathophysiology of the two conditions; the mechanisms of LPR and GERD differ significantly. Both LPR and GERD are caused by mucosal injury from acid and pepsin exposure.[3] Esophageal epithelium, however, has protective mechanisms that make it more resistant to peptic injury than that of the laryngopharynx.[3,32,34,35] Furthermore, it is important to recognize that pepsin and not acid produces most reflux-related tissue injury or damage.[2,35]

Research is now exploring the cell biology of LPR, and it confirms that mucosal damage from pepsin is related to depletion of important cellular defense-proteins, such as carbonic anhydrase, E-cadherin (the material that makes up the "mortar" between squamous epithial cells, the tight junctions), COX-2, and the stress proteins.[34-35] In addition, it takes much less acid/pepsin exposure to cause tissue damage in the pharynx and larynx than in the esophagus.[35] Thus, even patients without enough esophageal reflux to develop esophagitis (and its principal symptom heartburn) still may develop symptomatic LPR.

The clinical manifestations and findings of reflux disease are different in GI and ORL patients, because the mechanisms of GERD and LPR are different. Usually, GI patients have esophageal dysmotility and lower esophageal sphincter (LES) dysfunction, whereas ORL patients generally have good esophageal motor function, but faulty upper esophageal sphincter (UES) function.[3,29,34]

GI patients with GERD experience abnormal nocturnal (supine) esophageal reflux, but only uncommonly experience daytime (upright) reflux; in contrast, LPR patients experience abnormal daytime upright reflux, but not supine nocturnal reflux.[1-3] Not surprisingly, esophageal motility is more frequently abnormal in GI patients than in ORL patients.[29] In addition, it has been shown experimentally that instilling acid in the distal esophagus of normal subjects and of patients with esophagitis usually results in a prompt increase in tone of the UES.[31] This physiologic response does not appear to be intact in ORL patients with LPR.

In summary, it appears that significant differences in esophageal (dys)function and reflux pattern may explain many of the clinical differences between LPR and GERD. Table 28–1 summarizes those differences.

CLINICAL MANIFESTATIONS OF LPR

In a large series of patients with LPR, dysphonia (hoarseness) was found to be the most common symptom (92%).[3] The pattern of dysphonia was either chronic or intermittent. Patients with intermittent dysphonia often complained that they suffered from "laryngitis" that lasted for days or weeks, several times a year.[3] Additional symptoms were experienced by the majority of the patients: chronic throat clearing (50%), chronic cough (44%), globus (33%), and dysphagia (27%). More than half the patients denied having any heartburn whatsoever; 13% had two or fewer episodes per week, and only 10% complained of more frequent or daily heartburn.[3]

Although most patients with LPR present with mild to moderate dysphonia as the primary symptom, some suffer from more serious, even life-threatening, conditions (Table 28–2). Other laryngeal manifestations of

Table 28–1. Typical Differences Between LPR and GERD

	GERD	LPR
Symptoms		
Heartburn and/or regurgitation	Yes	No
Hoarseness, cough, dysphagia, globus	No	Yes
Findings		
Esophagitis	Yes	No
Laryngeal inflammation	No	Yes
Test results		
Esophageal biopsy (esophagitis)	90%	20%
Abnormal esophageal manometry	Yes	Sometimes
Abnormal esophageal pH monitoring	Yes	Sometimes
Abnormal pharyngeal pH monitoring	No	Yes
Pattern of reflux		
Supine (nocturnal)	Yes	Sometimes
Upright (awake)	Sometimes	Yes
Response to treatment		
Dietary and lifestyle modifications	Sometimes	Sometimes
Success with H2-blockers	50%	50%
Success with proton pump inhibitors (PPIs)*	90%	90%

GERD = Gastroesophageal reflux disease

LPR = Laryngopharyngeal reflux

*Assuming adequate dosage and duration of therapy (i.e., b.i.d. PPIs for LPR).

Table data derived from Koufman.[2]

Table 28–2. LPR Symptoms and Associated Laryngeal Conditions

Symptoms

Chronic dysphonia

Intermittent dysphonia

Vocal fatigue

Vocal breaks

Chronic throat clearing

Excessive throat mucus

"Postnasal drip"

Chronic cough

Dysphagia

Globus

Conditions in Which LPR Is the Cause or a Causative Cofactor

Reflux laryngitis

Subglottic stenosis

Carcinoma of the larynx

Contact ulcers and granulomas

Posterior glottic stenosis

Arytenoid fixation

Paroxysmal laryngospasm

Vocal nodules

Polypoid degeneration

Laryngomalacia

Sudden infant death syndrome

Pachydermia laryngis

Recurrent leukoplakia

LPR include laryngospasm,[20-22] laryngeal stenosis, and carcinoma.[12,21] LPR is also associated with the development of polypoid degeneration (Reinke's edema), vocal nodules, and functional voice disorders.[1,13-19]

Reflux and Functional ("Nonorganic") Voice Disorders

The term functional voice disorder (FVD) applies to a variety of vocal abuse, misuse, or overuse syndromes. These conditions are also called muscle tension dysphonias (MTDs), because transnasal fiberoptic laryngoscopy (TFL) shows consistently abnormal patterns of laryngeal biomechanics. The most commonly observed pattern is supraglottic contraction, either anteroposterior contraction (foreshortening of

the vocal folds) and/or false vocal fold approximation/compression.[11]

The FVD group of conditions is often associated with the secondary development of histopathologic changes of vocal folds, which include hematomas, nodules, ulcers, cysts, pseudocysts, granulomas, and Reinke's edema. With the availability of pH-metry, data suggest that 70% of patients with these functional lesions have LPR in addition to abnormal laryngeal biomechanics.[1]

As part of the evaluation of each patient with an FVD, the clinician should elicit a reflux history. In addition, patients who have laryngeal erythema, edema, or thick mucus in the endolarynx should be suspected of having LPR. Although the treatment of LPR alone will not resolve most FVDs, some cases will resolve. Certainly, failure to treat LPR, when it is present, will delay or prevent resolution of the FVD.

It is important to note that the laryngeal findings of LPR may be subtle in the face of significant supraglottic contraction. The appearance of a (subglottic) groove giving each of the vocal folds the appearance of a sulcus (pseudosulcus)[38] should alert the clinician to the possibility of LPR. Likewise, the presence of thick endolaryngeal mucus is often a sign of LPR. This finding is probably the result of a local tissue inflammatory response to chronic irritation and not "postnasal drip."

Granulomas

The etiology of granulomas of the vocal process is multifactorial, but LPR is almost always a cofactor. Granulomas usually result from the combination of acute mucosal ulceration of the vocal process, LPR, and chronic vocal trauma caused by throat clearing and/or a hard glottal attack.[16,17] By itself, chronic vocal trauma can lead to vocal fold ulcers and granulomas; however, in the majority of cases, LPR is a cofactor. The clinician should, in each case, consider each of the possible contributing etiologic factors and correct each if therapy is to be effective. In the case of granulomas, effective antireflux therapy is sufficient to allow healing in the majority of patients within 8 months, as long as vocally abusive behaviors also are corrected.[16,17]

Paroxysmal Laryngospasm

Laryngospasm is an uncommon complaint, but patients who experience this frightening symptom are usually able to describe events in vivid detail.[3] If the clinician mimics severe inspiratory stridor, the patient will confirm that his or her breathing during an attack does indeed sound similar. Some patients are aware of a relationship between LPR and laryngospasm, others are not.[7]

In a canine model, Loughlin et al[8] showed that chemoreceptors ("taste buds") on the epiglottis responded to acid stimulation at pH of 2.5 (or lower) by triggering reflex laryngospasm. The afferent limb of this reflex is supplied by the superior laryngeal nerve, and nerve interruption abolished the laryngospasm reflex.[8]

In the authors' experience, the majority of patients with paroxysmal laryngospasm respond well to PPI therapy. Antireflux surgery (fundoplication) may be necessary in patients who fail medical treatment.[47] LPR-related laryngospasm may also be related to (or a cause of) the sudden infant death syndrome (SIDS).[6,9]

Polypoid Degeneration (Reinke's Edema)

Polypoid degeneration results from chronic laryngeal irritation over a period of many years. It is almost always bilateral and occurs most frequently in elderly female smokers. It is also seen in nonsmoking patients with LPR or hypothyroidism.

Polypoid degeneration may improve with antireflux therapy and cessation of smoking, but most patients with these lesions will require concomitant surgical treatment. Most patients with polypoid degeneration have abnormal pH-metry.[1] Consequently, LPR should be considered a key component in the pathogenesis of this condition, and patients undergoing surgical therapy should receive intense antireflux treatment for several months prior to surgery and during the perioperative period. This usually will help avoid surgical complications.[18]

Laryngeal Stenosis

Excluding trauma, LPR is the primary cause of subglottic and posterior laryngeal stenosis.[3,20] Chronic, intermittent, or chronic-intermittent LPR can cause, or indefinitely perpetuate, a laryngeal disorder. Using a canine model, it has been shown that intermittent (three times per week only) applications of acid and pepsin to the subglottic region following mucosal injury results in nonhealing ulceration of the cricoid, and even subglottic stenosis.[3,20] LPR documented by pH-metry has been found in 92% of stenosis cases.[3] In the authors' experience, intensive antireflux treatment (with PPIs or fundoplication) is highly successful in leading to decannulation in the majority of patients with stenosis.

The traditional dichotomy between mature and immature stenoses probably represents an oversimplification. Immature implies that massive edema and granulation tissue are present and that the inflammatory process is ongoing. Mature implies that acute inflammation has resolved, and that the stenosis is composed of mature fibrous tissue with thin (normal) overlying epithelium. Surgical attempts to correct immature stenosis usually fail unless the underlying inflammatory process is controlled. Conversely, mature stenoses are more often successfully corrected. In reality, many cases are neither mature nor immature, but somewhere in between. The same also may be true of many acquired laryngeal webs. In the authors' opinion, pH-metry and tight LPR control are indicated in all stenosis cases.

Carcinoma of the Larynx

The most important (identified) risk factors for the development of laryngeal carcinoma are tobacco and alcohol; however, LPR also appears to be an important cofactor, especially in nonsmokers.[3,12,21] The senior author reported 50 consecutive cases of laryngeal carcinoma in which LPR was documented in 84%, but only 58% were active smokers. The exact relationship between LPR and malignant degeneration remains to be proved, but the available pH-metry data suggest that most patients who develop laryngeal malignancy both smoke and have LPR. In addition, leukoplakia and other premalignant appearing lesions may resolve with antireflux therapy.

Tobacco and alcohol adversely influence almost all the body's antireflux mechanisms—they delay gastric emptying, decrease lower esophageal sphincter pressure and esophageal motility, decrease mucosal resistance, and increase gastric acid secretion[3]—and thus, strongly predispose one to reflux. pH-metry, followed by rigorous antireflux treatment, is recommended for all patients with laryngeal neoplasia, with or without other risk factors. Treatment for this group of patients probably should be lifelong.

DIAGNOSIS

When a patient presents with dysphonia, globus, dysphagia, chronic throat clearing and cough, or complains of "too much throat mucus," symptoms that suggest LPR, the clinician should perform a complete otolaryngologic examination, fiberoptic laryngoscopy, and consider pH-metry or impedance testing as well as a screening examination of the esophagus (ie, transnasal esophagoscopy).

The reflux symptom index (RSI)[23] and the reflux finding score (RFS)[36] are also useful in the assessment process, especially after initiation of therapy. Both indices have been shown to be good treatment outcome measures.[23,36,37]

At present, double-probe pH-metry and impedance testing have tremendous advantages over any other diagnostic method because they are both highly sensitive and specific.[3,24,25] Furthermore, they reveal the pattern of reflux, so that subsequent treatment can be customtailored for each patient.[3] For example, if the patient does not have supine nocturnal reflux, then elevation of the head of the bed need not be recommended.

pH-metry has been available for many years, and standards (normal values) have been established in many laboratories.[1,2,5,24,25] For the esophageal probe, the most important parameter is considered to be the percentage of time that the pH is less than 4, and this measurement is usually recorded for time in the upright position, time in the supine position, and the total time of the study.[2,24,25] For the upright period, the upper limit of normal is approximately 8.0% and for the supine, approximately 2.5%.[2,29,30] However, in many patients (especially professional voice users), lesser exposures may be associated with clinical symptoms.

The Pharyngeal Probe Is Essential in Diagnosing LPR

Pharyngeal (double-probe) pH monitoring, with the second (proximal) probe being placed just above the cricopharyngeus, when positive, is by definition diagnostic of LPR.[3,24] At our institutions, and at most others doing such testing, any pharyngeal acid exposure is considered to be abnormal.[3] Figure 28–1 shows an example of a portion of a double-probe pH study in which reflux is seen in both the esophageal and the pharyngeal probes.

Double-probe pH-metry is particularly important in ORL patients because the diagnosis of LPR can be missed in a patient with a "normal" esophageal study. It has been shown that the sensitivity of single-probe esophageal pH monitoring for LPR is only 62%, and its positive predictive value only 49%.[48] Were it not for the pharyngeal probe findings, many LPR patients would escape physical detection. Pharyngeal pH monitoring is necessary in ORL/LPR patients because it dramatically increases the diagnostic accuracy and is an effective method to assess therapeutic efficacy.

Screening Examinations of the Esophagus

Patients with significant LPR should have a screening examination of the esophagus. Although a barium esophagram is not a sensitive test for diagnosing LPR, it may be useful in patients with primary complaints of globus and/or dysphagia. Otherwise, unsedated, in-office, transnasal esophagoscopy (TNE) is recommended.[26-28] In a series of more than 700 patients undergoing such TNE, half had some esophageal abnormality, such as esophagitis, stricture, hiatal hernia, or Barrett's esophagus.[28]

Figure 28–2A shows the appearance of a peptic stricture that was an incidental finding. The patient presented with dysphonia, chronic throat clearing, cough, and dysphagia. He had grossly abnormal pH-metry (upright and supine). A biopsy of the esophagus was recommended, but the patient refused. He

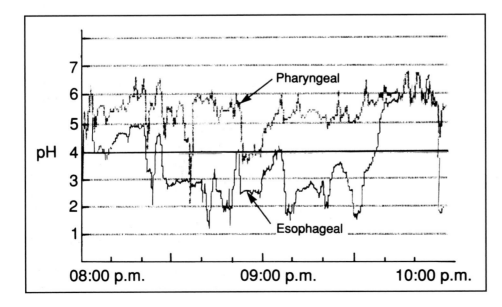

Figure 28–1. Example of a double-probe pH study. Pharyngeal reflux is shown. For a pharyngeal reflux event to be considered positive, a precipitous pH drop (below 4.0) in the pharyngeal probe must be immediately preceded by a similar pH drop in the esophageal probe.

bulatory pH monitoring. *Am J Gastroenterol.* 1989;84: 1503–1508.

3. Koufman JA. The otolaryngologic manifestations of gastroesophageal reflux disease (GERD): a clinical investigation of 225 patients using ambulatory 24- hour pH monitoring and an experimental investigation of the role of acid and pepsin in the development of laryngeal injury. *Laryngoscope.* 1991;101(suppl 53):1–78.

4. Ossakow SJ, Elta G, Colturi T, Bogdasarian R, Nostrant TT. Esophageal reflux and dysmotility as the basis for persistent cervical symptoms. *Ann Otol Rhinol Laryngol.* 1987;96:387–392.

5. Toohill RJ, Kuhn JC. Role of refluxed acid in pathogenesis of laryngeal disorders. *Am J Med.* 1997;103:100S–106S.

6. Wetmore RF. Effects of acid on the larynx of the maturing rabbit and their possible significance to the sudden infant death syndrome. *Laryngoscope.* 1993;103:1242–1254.

7. Loughlin CJ, Koufman JA. Paroxysmal laryngospasm secondary to gastroesophageal reflux. *Laryngoscope.* 1996;106:1502–1505.

8. Loughlin CJ, Koufman JA, Averill DB, et al. Acid-induced laryngospasm in a canine model. *Laryngoscope.* 1996;106:1506–1509.

9. Duke SG, Postma GN, McGuirt Jr. WF, Ririe D, Averill DB, Koufman JA. Laryngospasm and diaphragmatic arrest in the immature canine after laryngeal acid exposure: a possible model for sudden infant death syndrome (SIDS). *Ann Otol Rhinol Laryngol.* 2001;110:729–733.

10. Al Sabbagh G, Wo JM. Supraesophageal manifestations of gastroesophageal reflux disease. *Semin Gastrointest Dis.* 1999;10:113–119.

11. Koufman JA, Blalock PD. Functional voice disorders. *Otolaryngol Clin North Am.* 1991;24:1059–1073.

12. Koufman JA, Burke AJ. The etiology and pathogenesis of laryngeal carcinoma. *Otolaryngol Clin North Am.* 1997;30:1–19.

13. Rothstein SG. Reflux and vocal disorders in singers with bulimia. *J Voice.* 1998;12:89–90.

14. Kuhn J, Toohill RJ, Ulualp SO et al. Pharyngeal acid reflux events in patients with vocal cord nodules. *Laryngoscope.* 1998;108:1146–1149.

15. Ross JA, Noordzji JP, Woo P. Voice disorders in patients with suspected laryngopharyngeal reflux disease. *J Voice.* 1998;12:84–88.

16. Koufman JA. Contact ulcer and granuloma of the larynx. In: Gates G, ed. *Current Therapy in Otolaryngology-Head and Neck Surgery.* 5th ed. St. Louis, MO: Mosby Publishers; 1993:456–459.

17. Havas TE, Priestley J, Lowinger DS. A management strategy for vocal process granulomas. *Laryngoscope.* 1999;109:301–306.

18. Holland BW, Koufman JA, Postma GN, McGuirt Jr., WF. Laryngopharyngeal reflux and laryngeal web formation in patients with pediatric recurrent respiratory papillomas. *Laryngoscope.* 2002;112:1926–1929.

19. Koufman JA, Belafsky PC. Unilateral or localized Reinke's edema (pseudocyst) as a manifestation of vocal fold paresis: the paresis podule. *Laryngoscope.* 2001;111:576–580.

20. Little FB, Koufman JA, Kohut RI, Marshall RB. Effect of gastric acid on the pathogenesis of subglottic stenosis. *Ann Otol Rhinol Laryngol.* 1985;94:516–519.

21. Ward PH, Hanson DG. Reflux as an etiological factor of carcinoma of the laryngopharynx. *Laryngoscope.* 1988;98:1195–1199.

22. Koufman JA, Aviv JE, Casiano RR, Shaw GY. Position statement of the American Academy of Otolaryngology-Head and Neck Surgery on laryngopharyngeal reflux. *Otolaryngol Head Neck Surg.* 2002;127:32–35.

23. Belafsky PC, Postma GN, Koufman JA. Validity and reliability of the reflux symptom index (RSI). *J Voice.* 2002;16:274–277.

24. Postma GN. Ambulatory pH monitoring methodology. *Ann Otol Rhinol Laryngol.* 2000;184(suppl):10–14.

25. Grontved AM, West F. pH monitoring in patients with benign voice disorders. *Acta Otolaryngol Suppl.* 2000;543:229–231.

26. Koufman JA, Belafsky PC, Daniel E, Bach KK, Postma GN. Prevalence of esophagitis in patients with pH-documented laryngopharyngeal reflux. *Laryngoscope.* 2002;112:1606–1609.

27. Belafsky PC, Postma GN, Koufman JA. Transnasal esophagoscopy (TNE). *Otolaryngol Head Neck Surg.* 2001;125:588–589.

28. Postma GN, Cohen JT, Belafsky PC, et al. Transnasal esophagoscopy revisited (over 700 consecutive cases). *Laryngoscope.* 2005;115:321–323.

29. Postma GN, Tomek MS, Belafsky PC, Koufman JA. Esophageal motor function in laryngopharyngeal reflux is superior to that of classic gastroesophageal reflux disease. *Ann Otol Rhinol Laryngol.* 2001;110:1114–1116.

30. Halum SL, Postma GN, Johnston C, Belafsky PC, Koufman JA. Patients with isolated laryngopharyngeal reflux are not obese. *Laryngoscope.* 2005;115:1042–1045.

31. Gerhardt DC, Shuck TJ, Bordeaux RA, Winship DH. Human upper esophageal sphincter. Response to volume, osmotic and acid stimuli. *Gastroenterology.* 1978;75:268–274.

32. Helm JF, Dodds WJ, Riedel DR, Teeter BC, Hogan WJ, Arndorfer RC. Determinants of esophageal acid clearance in normal subjects. *Gastroenterology.* 1983;85:607–612.

33. Korsten MA, Rosman AS, Fishbein S, Shlein RD, Goldberg HE, Biener A. Chronic xerostomia increases esophageal acid exposure and is associated with esophageal injury. *Am J Med.* 1991;90:701–706.

34. Axford SE, Sharp N, Ross PE, et al. Cell biology of laryngeal epithelial defenses in health and disease: preliminary studies. *Ann Otol Rhinol Laryngol.* 2001;110:1099–1108.

35. Johnston N, Ross PE, Bulmer D, et al. Cell biology of laryngeal epithelial defenses in health and disease: further studies. *Ann Otol Rhinol Laryngol.* 2003;112:481–491.

36. Belafsky PC, Postma GN, Koufman JA. The validity and reliability of the reflux finding score (RFS). *Laryngoscope.* 2001;111:1313–1317.

37. Belafsky PC, Postma GN, Koufman KA. Laryngopharyngeal reflux symptoms improve before changes in physical findings. *Laryngoscope.* 2001;111:979–981.

38. Belafsky PC, Postma GN, Koufman JA. The association between laryngeal pseudosulcus and laryngopharyngeal reflux. *Otolaryngol Head Neck Surg.* 2002;126:649–652.

39. Jansen JB, Van Oene JC. Standard-dose lansoprazole is more effective than high-dose ranitidine in achieving endoscopic healing and symptom relief in patients with moderately severe reflux oesophagitis. The Dutch Lansoprazole Study Group. *Aliment Pharmacol Ther.* 1999;13:1611–1620.

40. Chiverton SG, Howden CW, Burget DW, Hunt RH. Omeprazole (20 mg) daily given in the morning or evening: a comparison of effects on gastric acidity, and plasma gastrin and omeprazole concentration. *Aliment Pharmacol Ther.* 1992;6:103–111.

41. Maton PN, Orlando R, Joelsson B. Efficacy of omeprazole versus ranitidine for symptomatic treatment of poorly responsive acid reflux disease—a prospective, controlled trial. *Aliment Pharmacol Ther.* 1999;13:819–826.

42. Amin MR, Postma GN, Johnson P, Digges N, Koufman JA. Proton pump inhibitor resistance in the treatment of laryngopharyngeal reflux. *Otolaryngol Head Neck Surg.* 2001;125:374–378.

43. Tambankar AP, Peters JH, Portale G, et al. Omeprazole does not reduce gastroesophageal reflux: new insights using multichannel impedance technology. *J Gastroenterol Surg.* 2004;8:888–895.

44. Leite LP, Johnston BT, Just RJ, Castell DO. Persistent acid secretion during omeprazole therapy: a study of gastric acid profiles in patients demonstrating failure of omeprazole therapy. *Am J Gastroenterol.* 1996;91:1527–1531.

45. Peghini PL, Katz PO, Bracy NA, Castell DO. Nocturnal recovery of gastric acid secretion with twice-daily dosing of proton pump inhibitors. *Am J Gastroenterol.* 1998;93:763–767.

46. Bough ID Jr, Sataloff RT, Castell DO, Hills JR, Gideon RM, Spiegel JR. Gastroesophageal reflux laryngitis resistant to omeprazole therapy. *J Voice.* 1995;9:205–211.

47. Westcott CJ, Hopkins MB, Bach KK, Postma, GN, Belafsky, PC, Koufman, JA. Fundoplication for laryngopharyngeal reflux. *J Am Coll Surg.* 2004;199:23–30.

48. Johnson PE, Koufman JA, Nowak LJ, Belafsky PC, Postma GN. Ambulatory 24-hour double-probe pH monitoring: the importance of manometry. *Laryngoscope.* 2001;111:1970–1975.

49. Johnston N, Knight J, Dettmar PW, Lively MO, Koufman JA. Pepsin and carbonic anhydrase as diagnostic markers for laryngopharyngeal reflux disease. *Laryngoscope.* 2004;114:2130–2134.

50. Knight J, Lively MO, Johnston N, Dettmar PW, Koufman JA. Sensitive pepsin immunoassay for detection of laryngopharyngeal reflux. *Laryngoscope.* 2005;115:1473–1478.

51. Tasker A, Dettmar PW, Panetti M, Koufman JA, Birchall JP, Pearson, JP. Reflux of gastric juice and glue ear in children. *Lancet.* 2002;359:493.

52. Little PJ, Matthews BL, Glock MS, et al. Extraesophageal pediatric reflux: 24-hour double-probe pH monitoring of 222 children. *Ann Otol Rhinol Laryngol Suppl.* 1997;169:1–16.

53. Faubion WA Jr, Zein NN. Gastroesophageal reflux in infants and children. *Mayo Clin Proc.* 1998;73:166–173.

29

Infectious and Inflammatory Disorders of the Larynx

Robert S. Lebovics, MD, FACS
H. Bryan Neel III, MD, PhD

LARYNGEAL PHYSIOLOGY AND IMMUNOLOGICAL RESPONSES

The larynx is a complex organ situated in the mid-neck that is involved in the functions of phonation and respiration as well as protection of the airway and aiding in deglutition. This organ consists of a network of cartilages and glandular elements, lined by either squamous or respiratory epithelium. The cricoarytenoid joint is a synovial joint, subject to systemic disorders that also affect joints elsewhere in the body. The larynx is innervated by an extensive neural network, subjecting it to disorders of impaired neural function. The lymphatic drainage and anatomic boundaries also have major therapeutic implications when dealing with malignancy. This chapter focuses on those disorders that alter normal laryngeal physiology by either an infectious organism or secondary to a systemic immune disorder mediated by a common inflammatory pathway.

Humans possess an efficient system of physical, cellular, and molecular host defenses. Usually the first level of protection is provided by a specialized epithelium and additional epidermal barriers. Local secretions from the sinonasal tract can contain such antimicrobial substances as lysozyme, or certain types of immunoglobulin G and A (IgG and IgA) antibodies that block microbial adherence and proliferation. The regular flow of fluids through the hollow tube of the pharynx and larynx, in addition to normal mucociliary flow, further prevents the internal spread of infectious organisms that might be colonizing the airway. Environmental trauma, systemic disorders, and large bacterial or viral burdens may, however, overwhelm the physical integrity of these natural barriers.

When external tissue surfaces are penetrated, additional immune mechanisms are recruited, and thus an inflammatory response is elicited. Inflammation can be regarded as the body's natural response to injury. Teleologically it serves to contain and/or eliminate the offending stimulus, and thereby allow for eventual tissue healing.

Although inflammation is a necessary protective response, it is clearly a double-edged sword. Severe, prolonged, or inappropriate inflammatory responses can occur in the larynx as in any organ system, and can result in the loss of normal function with consequent morbidity. Often, the challenge for the physician or surgeon is to provide supportive care for the patient until the inflammatory process subsides, or to modulate the inflammatory response through pharmacologic intervention.

Inflammation is a complex cascade of events, involving elements of both cellular and humoral immunity. Either antigen-specific or nonspecific responses may occur. However, the less specific ones have the advantage of being rapidly available during periods of acute infection and may permit the survival of the host until specific focused responses arrive via the immune system. The early or acute phase is characterized by vasodilation, increased vascular permeability, localized release of chemical mediators, and activation of reflex neuronal mechanisms. These lead to Virchow's classic signs of inflammation: pain, redness, heat, and swelling.

Polymorphonuclear leukocytes, lymphocytes, and macrophages are the host's primary acute-phase defense cells. They are highly mobile and short lived in blood cells, and yet they rapidly enter sites of infection to ingest and destroy bacteria. Chemotactic factors produced at the site of inflammation often direct the mobilized pool of polymorphonuclear cells to the site of injury. Several hours later, monocytes are recruited and transform into tissue macrophages. These cells are responsible for the presentation of antigen to T cells, and the production of interleukin-1 (IL-1), tumor necrosis factor (TNF), and interleukin-6 (IL-6) (Table 29–1).

The various stimulating factors, singly or in combination, may promote fever, stimulate hepatic acute-phase responses, and trigger catabolic responses. Lymphocytes and macrophages may respond with an elaborate array of colony-stimulating factors, which will further promote the production of leukocytes in the bone marrow. Depending on the nature of the infection or tissue insult, either a predominantly neutrophilic or a monocytic-lymphocytic infiltrate will predominate. This complex interplay of cascading and amplification continues either until the offending stimulus is eradicated and the tissue returns to normal, or until it is effectively walled off by a granulomatous inclusion. This allows a state of chronic inflammation to persist without a formal and complete resolution of the initial insult.

The larynx, because of its numerous structures and complex architecture, in addition to its critical life-sustaining functions, can frequently present symptoms in a rapid and forceful manner. Because it is the conduit of the body's airflow to and from the lungs, decreased ventilation or complete obstruction can result in either morbidity or mortality.[1] It is, therefore, of critical importance to all clinicians to recognize and diagnose inflammatory and infectious alterations of the larynx promptly, so that normal physiology can be restored and, in more extreme cases, life can be preserved.

COMMON INFECTIOUS DISORDERS OF THE LARYNX

Signs and Symptoms of Laryngeal Disease

A focused history includes information about changes in voice, breathing patterns, and swallowing, in addition to allergic, infectious, and systemic disorders. Persistent unexplained changes in the voice are pathognomonic of a laryngeal disorder. Other symptoms include cough, which can be dry or productive. Pain may be present or referred through branches of the vagus nerve to other regions of the head and neck, for ex-

Table 29–1. Cells of the Inflammatory Response

	Time	Products	Function
Mast cells	Immediate	Histamine, arachidonic acid metabolites	Central to initiation of allergic response
Neutrophils	0 to 6 hours	Proteolytic enzymes, oxygen radicals	Early phagocytosis control of extracellular pathogens
Monocytes	>6 hours	Pro-inflammatory cytokines: IL-1, IL-6, TNF-α Anti-inflammatory cytokines: IL-10	Initiation and modulation of cellular immunity antigen processing
Lymphocytes T cells B cells	Hours to days	T cells: lymphokines, IL-2, γ-interferon B cells: antibody	Antigen-specific responses to pathogens

ample, the ears. Dysphagia and odynophagia may be associated with neoplastic lesions of the larynx. Besides examination of the neck and throat, physical examination should include, when safe, an indirect mirror examination, flexible fiberoptic endoscopy, and/or rigid endoscopy preferably with a stroboscope. Vocal fold dysfunction, mucosal alterations, purulent infections of the larynx, mass lesions, structural abnormalities, and occasionally subglottic lesions will be evident on these examinations. Listening to the voice and to the sounds of breathing can also shed light on a pathologic process.

Acute Epiglottitis

Rapidly progressive cellulitis of the epiglottis and its surrounding tissues in the supraglottic airway can cause acute airway obstruction. In infants and children, the causative agent is almost always *Haemophilus influenzae* type B, and bacteremia is present invariably. In adolescents and adults with acute bacterial epiglottitis, the clinical presentation may be less fulminant, and other organisms may be causative. Frequently, the patient complains of dysphagia, odynophagia, and fever that progress over 1 to 2 days. Depending on the degree of respiratory obstruction, stridor may or may not be present. Like a child, an adult with epiglottitis prefers to lean forward, occasionally drooling secretions. Because the caliber of the airway is larger in the adult, intubation or tracheotomy may not be necessary, but the *possibility of imminent complete airway obstruction* mandates prompt management.[2] An edematous, cherry-red epiglottis and surrounding pharyngeal mucosa are the characteristic findings on examination, which *in adults* is best done with fiberoptic instrumentation to confirm the diagnosis. *In infants and children, fiberoptic examination is contraindicated.* A lateral x-ray of the neck may reveal an enlarged epiglottis or the so-called thumb sign. Most hospitals in the United States have protocols established in conjunction with departments of otolaryngology, pediatrics, and anesthesiology to both diagnose and manage the pediatric patient with epiglottitis. In children, an airway must always be secured.

Older patients can be managed by admission to an intensive care unit where adequate clinical monitoring is available until the possibility of airway obstruction has passed. Although fiberoptic examinations are recommended in adults, these procedures should be performed only after preparation has been made to secure an airway by either endotracheal intubation or tracheotomy. After blood cultures are obtained, appropriate antibiotic treatment should be initiated. This is usually a combination of ampicillin and chloramphenicol, although in many centers today a cephalosporin such as cefuroxime has been substituted. Oxygen is administered as dictated by oxygen saturation measurement, using pulse oximetry or arterial blood gas determination. Humidified air by face tent is advisable. If respiratory obstruction worsens, airway protection is required, preferably with endotracheal intubation. Glucocorticoids have been administered as part of the treatment, but are of unproven benefit. With an appropriate antibiotic, resolution of acute symptoms usually occurs within 48 hours. A child should not be extubated, nor an adult patient removed from an intensive care setting, unless the acute cellulitis of the epiglottis has resolved, as confirmed endoscopically.

Croup (Laryngotracheal Bronchitis)

Croup is a syndrome produced by acute infection of the lower air passages. It is seen most commonly in children below the age of 3 years. The most common pathogen is the parainfluenza virus, although a variety of respiratory viruses can also be found. *Mycoplasma pneumoniae* can produce laryngotracheal bronchitis and/or a crouplike syndrome. The pathophysiology is primarily one of circumferential mucosal inflammation in the subglottic larynx and trachea, and there are variable involvement and spasms of the vocal folds. The epiglottis is usually not involved. The clinical hallmarks include a barking cough with or without stridor and hoarseness. Croup can be distinguished clinically from epiglottitis by lateral x-rays of the neck. Management of severe croup requires hospitalization with close observation and possible intensive care observation. Humidification and oxygen supplementation are given, but rarely is endotracheal intubation required. Nebulized racemic epinephrine can be used and usually helps temporarily. The use of intravenous steroids still remains controversial.

OTHER BACTERIAL INFECTIONS OF THE LARYNX

Laryngeal Diphtheria

Diphtheria still occurs in certain areas of the United States and in other countries, and can infect children who are either immune-compromised or who have not received appropriate immunizations. Laryngeal diphtheria may be insidious because it can occur in a clinical setting in which the pharynx appears normal, that is, there is no silver-gray membrane on the pharynx. Usually, diphtheric laryngitis develops over several days with hoarseness that progresses to complete airway obstruction. Diagnosis is confirmed by a smear of the membranous exudate from either the pharynx or larynx, or if antimicrobial smears and cultures are positive for *Corynebacteria diphtheriae* organisms. In this clinical setting, antimicrobial treatment (frequently a penicillin) in addition to an antitoxin should be administered parenterally, concurrent to or after emergent securing of the airway. Paralysis of the palatal pharyngeal swallowing sequence may occur, and nasogastric tube feeding may be required to help minimize aspiration.[3] The incidence and severity of complications are usually related to the stage of disease at the time that diagnosis and treatment are initiated. Treatment with both antimicrobial agents and antitoxin should not be delayed until positive laboratory cultures are obtained, if there is reasonable clinical suspicion of the diagnosis. Laryngeal diphtheria now occurs almost exclusively in unimmunized individuals. In some patients, cardiomyopathy can occur secondary to the toxin.[3]

Perichondritis of the Larynx

Infection and/or inflammation, followed by necrosis of the laryngeal cartilage, can be associated with different types of acute and chronic diseases. The mucoperichondrium over the laryngeal cartilage is generally a tough resilient barrier to infectious organisms. However, once it is penetrated, its limited vascular supply predisposes to the formation of granulation tissue and/or necrosis and suppuration of the underlying larynx. Etiologic mechanisms are varied; they include iatrogenic causes such as trauma, including trauma from laryngeal surgery or tracheotomy. Inappropriately large endotracheal tubes and feeding tubes are also among the iatrogenic causes of cartilage destruction.[4-6] More commonly today in the United States, external beam irradiation to the larynx can predispose to perichondritis, particularly because of a diminished vascular supply to the tissues. In addition, the normal flora of the oropharynx, hypopharynx, and larynx can be altered by treatment with external beam irradiation. As such, gram-negative rods become part of the normal colonizing bacteria within this portion of the aerodigestive tract, and they may become causative pathogens in laryngeal perichondritis.

Signs and symptoms may vary, depending upon the extent of the problem and stage of inflammation. A patient may present with localized tenderness, dysphagia, odynophagia, fetor, or soft tissue swelling over the region of the larynx. Some early features of infection are severe pain, particularly radiating to the ear, in addition to hoarseness and odynophagia. Inflammation and edema of the arytenoid may result in im-

paired vocal fold mobility, in addition to audible voice changes. If inflammation extends into the cricoarytenoid joint, this may present clinically with fixation of one or both vocal folds. Inflammation of the cricoid cartilage may cause painful swelling, as well as edema over the posterior lamina of cricoid cartilage. This will result in absence of the normal laryngeal crepitus on physical examination. Major necrosis of the cricoid cartilage heralds complete collapse of the upper airway, necessitating emergency tracheotomy.

Initial treatment consists of identifying the cause of inflammation or infection. Any pockets of pus should be drained in the context of securing a stable airway. It must be emphasized, however, that at this stage, surgery is primarily for diagnosis, with only the airway requiring emergent intervention. A complete pathologic and microbiologic diagnosis is necessary to successful long-term management. In most circumstances, treating the underlying infectious or immune disorder will antedate definitive management of the laryngotracheal complex. Additional treatment during the diagnostic phase may include strict voice rest and analgesics. Because it is frequently easier to prevent severe perichondritis of the larynx than to treat the condition, the otolaryngologist should be involved promptly in the management of patients following both blunt and penetrating laryngeal trauma. Apparently adequate respirations and a seemingly normal voice in these cases may be misleading, and major complications can possibly be avoided with early diagnosis.

Tuberculous Laryngitis

The incidence of tuberculosis in the United States has been found to be increasing during the past several years. The majority of tuberculous infections of the larynx are secondary to pulmonary tuberculosis.[7-9] However, atypical forms of acid-fast bacteria can infect the larynx, particularly in patients with altered cellular immunities. Anatomically, the interarytenoid fold in the posterior portion of the larynx is the most common site of active acid-fast disease. The granulomatous, destructive process of the larynx is slow and insidious. Symptoms such as hoarseness, pain, and dysphagia may occur late in the disease process. It is highly advisable that all patients being treated for pulmonary tuberculosis have the larynx and the remainder of the upper aerodigestive tract examined by the otolaryngologist (Figure 29–1).

There are isolated cases of primary laryngeal tuberculosis, but these are uncommon. While the diagnosis of disease is generally established based on characteristic skin testing, chest radiographs, sputum examination, and early morning gastric lavage, the diagnosis of acid-fast involvement of the larynx requires histoly in the immunocompetent host, *C. albicans* is uncommon, although laryngeal thrush may be a sign of HIV infection. Oral fluconazole is the drug of choice for laryngeal infection.

IMMUNE DISEASES

Sarcoid of the Larynx

Sarcoid is a systemic granulomatous disease whose etiology is unclear. It primarily affects the lungs and mediastinal lymph nodes. However, multisystem involvement is common. Approximately 5% of patients with pulmonary sarcoid have laryngeal manifestations of their disease.[41] While the presentation of most laryngeal infections is similar, that is, progressive hoarseness and occasional pain, sarcoid needs to be distinguished both pathologically and immunologically from other diseases, particularly those involving *Mycobacterium tuberculosis.*

Pulmonary function tests may demonstrate characteristic tracings of extrathoracic pulmonary obstruction. There is a characteristic "honking" voice of sarcoid.[42] On examination, pink, edematous, and turbanlike enlargement of supraglottic structures may be considered pathognomonic for laryngeal sarcoid.[43] The incidence of malignancies for patients with sarcoid is greater than the expected incidences for thyroid cancer, laryngeal cancer, and leukemia. The increased cancer risk may be secondary to immunologic factors associated with sarcoid.

Histologically, sarcoid is characterized by noncaseating granulomas, as opposed to infectious organisms of the larynx. On presentation, laryngeal sarcoid usually involves the epiglottis, and contiguous structures such as the aryepiglottic folds and arytenoids often show diffuse, boggy, pale enlargements. Occasionally, the subglottic larynx becomes involved, producing significant airway symptoms. Pain is not a major complaint in most patients.

The diagnosis of sarcoid requires histologic confirmation. In addition, certain laboratory and radiographic findings support the diagnosis of sarcoid. Hypercalcemia and adenopathy of the chest or neck, in the presence of noncaseating granulomata of the lung or epiglottis, help to confirm the diagnosis. Although rarely used today, the Kveim skin test supports the diagnosis. As laryngeal swelling can cause airway obstruction, tracheotomy is required occasionally to support the airway.

Microscopic examination of the involved tissue reveals multiple hard tubercles that are often similar in size to those of acid-fast disease. The tubercle consists of a collection of epithelial cells surrounded by giant cells. In contrast to the findings in other granulomas, the surrounding zone of lymphocytes may be narrow or even absent.[44,45] This might explain why the sarcoid lesions do not undergo caseation necrosis.

Once a diagnosis of laryngeal sarcoid is made, the patient should be referred to an immunologist for systemic evaluation. While no definitive therapy exists, systemic steroids are frequently used in order to minimize symptoms. In cases of less severe obstruction, intralesional injections of steroids have been shown to be helpful, in addition to oral prednisone.[43,46]

AMYLOIDOSIS

Amyloidosis is a group of disorders characterized by deposition of acellular proteinaceous material in tissues.[47] Amyloid aggregates are composed of homogeneous subunits of different proteins which share several common features. All demonstrate a similar tertiary protein structure, the twisted β-pleated sheet. All amyloid deposits contain amyloid P protein, which is identical to serum amyloid P, and all of the primary protein structures are rich in aspartic acid and glutamic acid residues. The resulting structure has a highly polyanionic surface, which may predispose the formation of a β-pleated structure, and presumably contributes to the great stability of the protein aggregates. This characteristic, in turn, allows amyloid to accumulate as a nonreactive proteinaceous deposit that causes structural damage simply by pressure effects on adjacent tissues.[48]

Several subtypes of amyloidosis have been defined, based on the protein makeup of the amyloid deposits and the clinical characteristics of the patient. Primary amyloid (AL) is a product of an immunocyte (plasmacyte) dyscrasia. The proteins in AL amyloid are derived exclusively from immunoglobulin λ and κ chains. This type of amyloidosis occurs in patients with primary systemic amyloidosis, myeloma-associated amyloid, and in most cases of localized amyloidosis such as those involving the larynx.[47,49] There is significant evidence that suggests that the λ chains in AL are more amylogenic than the κ chains.[50] Whereas primary amyloidosis is characterized by the deposition of amyloid in mesenchymal tissues such as the tongue, heart, and gastrointestinal tract, secondary (AA) amyloidosis is associated with deposits mainly in reticuloendothelial organs such as the liver and spleen.[50] AA amyloidosis is associated with chronic destructive inflammatory and infectious diseases such as long-standing tuberculosis and rheumatoid arthritis, and inherited disorders such as familial Mediterranean fever. A third type of amyloid, AF, is a familial variant in which the amyloid subunits are derived from a genetic variant of prealbumin.[51] The protein deposits in AS, "senile" or age-related amyloidosis, are derived from the plasma protein transthyretin. Finally, other variants of amyloidosis include one associated with chronic dialysis in which β_2-microglobulin is the protein which forms the protein aggregates.[49]

Laryngeal involvement in amyloidosis is rare, accounting for <1% of all benign laryngeal tumors.[50] Only about 200 cases have been reported in the literature. Those laryngeal lesions that are reported typically are of primary amyloidosis, although a few cases exist of laryngeal involvement as a result of generalized secondary amyloidosis.[50] Prognostic significance has been attached to the appearance of laryngeal amyloidosis as a presenting symptom versus its appearance later in the course of systemic amyloidosis.

The typical patient who presents with laryngeal amyloidosis is in the 40 to 60 age range, and there is a male-to-female predominance of approximately 2:1.[50,52] Amyloidosis is a chronic, slowly progressive disease of insidious onset, characterized by hoarseness, dyspnea, cough, stridor, or odynophagia,[51] and rarely, hemoptysis.[48] The typical lesion of laryngeal amyloidosis is a firm, nonulcerated, orange-yellow to gray submucosal nodule. Less commonly it may present as one or multiple discrete pedunculated polypoid lesions which may involve any part of the larynx. Several series have noted that the location of amyloid deposits tends to be highest on the ventricles and false vocal folds, somewhat less common in the subglottis and on the aryepiglottic folds, and least common on the true vocal folds.[49,52] The most common clinical presentation is, however, for multiple sites of the larynx to be involved.[49] It is extremely rare for vocal fold fixation or cicatricial stenosis to occur in the context of laryngeal amyloidosis unless other predisposing factors are also present.[10] Various clinical descriptions of amyloidosis include that of a cystic lesion on the true vocal fold[53]; an infiltrating tumor of the true vocal folds and subglottis[51]; multinodular deposits in the subglottis, trachea, and mainstem bronchus[51]; a diffuse infiltrative subglottic narrowing[50]; and an ulcerative process of the anterior commissure with submucosal posterior commissure fullness extending into the subglottis.[50]

Four histologic patterns of amyloidosis have been described. These include amorphous random masses, deposits around blood vessel walls, deposits in continuity with the basement membrane of seromucinous glands, and deposits within adipose tissue.[50,54] Finally, in one series where the laryngeal deposits were carefully subtyped, the amyloidosis was found to be exclusively of the AL type, with more than 60% of the laryngeal deposits displaying a λ light chain staining pattern and 25% with a κ pattern.[49]

In the rare instances of laryngeal amyloidosis secondary to a chronic disease, management focuses upon control of the primary disease. In the much more common isolated laryngeal amyloidosis, the primary treatment is endoscopic surgical removal of nodules that interfere with laryngeal or airway function. In many series it has been demonstrated that if the lesion can be completely excised, there is little or no tendency for recurrence. Because the likelihood of recurrent or residual disease is significant, special care must be taken to avoid traumatization of adjacent normal laryngeal tissues.[53] Removal of amyloid lesions may be complicated by bleeding, because of the propensity of amyloid to infiltrate blood vessels. Advocates of CO_2 laser excision cite improved control of hemorrhage as one advantage of the laser. However, it is cautioned that laser use should be avoided in more extensive lesions because of the significant likelihood of extensive scarring postoperatively.[51,53] In large lesions it often becomes necessary to use external approaches. Although an early study indicated that "coring out" a subglottic lesion was a lasting and effective treatment,[52] more recent series employ laryngofissure for treatment of diffuse subglottic and tracheal amyloidosis. In such studies, excision and curettage of gross lesions has been used, and some have found that repeated curettage as necessary ultimately allows stabilization of the lesions and subsequent decannulation of tracheotomy-dependent patients.[50] Local or systemic steroids are ineffective in controlling or reversing the lesions of amyloidosis.[48,50,55]

In patients with significant subglottic amyloid deposits, bronchoscopy may be merited to determine the extent of the lesions. In addition, pulmonary function tests including flow-volume loops provide a helpful baseline of the patient's airway obstruction as well as differentiating between upper and lower airway obstruction.[48]

Overall, the prognosis for laryngeal amyloidosis is quite good. The need for a tracheotomy is rare,[10] although extensive subglottic lesions may require such measures until they can be controlled or resected.[50] Rarely, death has been reported secondary to amyloidosis; this occurs typically from diffuse tracheobronchial disease and pulmonary failure.[49]

WEGENER'S GRANULOMATOSIS

Wegener's granulomatosis is a multisystem inflammatory disease characterized by vasculitis, granulo-

16. Liu TC, Qiu JS. Pathological findings on peripheral nerves, lymph nodes, and visceral organs of leprosy. *Int J Lepr Other Mycobact Dis.* 1984;52:377–383.

17. Pillsbury HC, Sasaki CT. Granulomatous diseases of the larynx. *Otolaryngol Clin North Am.* 1982;15:539–551.

18. McNulty JS, Fassett RL. Syphilis: an otolaryngologic perspective. *Laryngoscope.* 1981;91:889–905.

19. Lacy PD, Alderson DJ, Parker AJ. Late congenital syphilis of the larynx and pharynx presenting at endotracheal intubation. *J Laryngol Otol.* 1994;108:688–689.

20. Andraca R, Edson RS, Kern EB. Rhinoscleroma: a growing concern in the United States? Mayo Clinic experience. *Mayo Clin Proc.* 1993;68:1151–1157.

21. Soni NK. Scleroma of the larynx. *J Laryngol Otol.* 1997;111:438–440.

22. Fajardo-Dolci G, Chavolla R, Lamadrid-Bautista E, et al. Laryngeal scleroma. *J Otolaryngol.* 1999;28:229–231.

23. Postma GN, Wawrose S, Tami TA. Isolated subglottic scleroma. *Ear Nose Throat J.* 1996;75:306–308.

24. Amoils CP, Shindo ML. Laryngotracheal manifestations of rhinoscleroma. *Ann Otol Rhinol Laryngol.* 1996;105:336–340.

25. Zitsch RP III, Bothwell M. Actinomycosis: a potential complication of head and neck surgery. *Am J Otolaryngol.* 1999;20:260–262.

26. Nelson EG, Tybor AG. Actinomycosis of the larynx. *Ear Nose Throat J.* 1992;71:356–358.

27. Tsuji DH, Fukuda H, Kawasaki Y, et al. Actinomycosis of the larynx. *Auris Nasus Larynx.* 1991;18:79–85.

28. Hughes RA, Paonessa DF, Conway WF. Actinomycosis of the larynx. *Ann Otol Rhinol Laryngol.* 1984;93:520–524.

29. Shaheen SO, Ellis FG. Actinomycosis of the larynx. *J R Soc Med.* 1983;76:226–228.

30. Dumich PS, Neel HB. Blastomycosis of the larynx. *Laryngoscope.* 1983;93:1266–1270.

31. Reder PA, Neel HB. Blastomycosis in otolaryngology: review of a large series. *Laryngoscope.* 1993;103:53–58.

32. Mikaelian AJ, Varkey B, Grossman TW, et al. Blastomycosis of the head and neck. *Otolaryngol Head Neck Surg.* 1989;101:489–495.

33. Suen JY, Wetmore SJ, Wetzel WJ, et al. Blastomycosis of the larynx. *Ann Otol Rhinol Laryngol.* 1980;89:563–566.

34. McCune MA, Rogers RS, Roberts GD. Laryngeal presentation of blastomycosis. *Int J Dermatol.* 1980;19:263–269.

35. Hajare S, Rakusan TA, Kalia A, et al. Laryngeal coccidioidomycosis causing airway obstruction. *Pediatr Infect Dis J.* 1989;8:54–56.

36. Boyle JO, Coulthard SW, Mandel RM. Laryngeal involvement in disseminated coccidioidomycosis. *Arch Otolaryngol Head Surg.* 1991;117:433–438.

37. Sataloff RT, Wilborn A, Prestipino A, et al. Histoplasmosis of the larynx. *Am J Otolaryngol.* 1993;14:199–205.

38. Gerber ME, Rosdeutscher JD, Seiden AM, et al. Histoplasmosis: the otolaryngologist's perspective. *Laryngoscope.* 1995;105:919–923.

39. Reibel JF, Jahrsdoerfer RA, Johns MM, et al. Histoplasmosis of the larynx. *Otolaryngol Head Neck Surg.* 1982;90:740–743.

40. Negroni R, Palmieri O, Koren F, et al. Oral treatment of paracoccidioidomycosis and histoplasmosis with itraconazole in humans. *Rev Infect Dis.* 1987;9(suppl 1):S47–S50.

41. Ellison DE, Canalis RF. Sarcoidosis of the head and neck. *Clin Dermatol.* 1986;4:136–142.

42. Gallivan GJ, Landis JN. Sarcoidosis of the larynx: preserving and restoring airway and professional voice. *J Voice.* 1993;7:81–94.

43. Neel HB III, McDonald TJ. Laryngeal sarcoidosis: report of 13 patients. *Ann Otol Rhinol Laryngol.* 1982;91:359–362.

44. Sakamoto M, Ishizawa M, Kitahara N. Polypoid type of laryngeal sarcoidosis—case report and review of the literature. *Eur Arch Otorhinolaryngol.* 2000;257:436–438.

45. Benjamin B, Dalton C, Croxson G. Laryngoscopic diagnosis of laryngeal sarcoid. *Ann Otol Rhinol Laryngol.* 1995;104:529–531.

46. Bower JS, Belen JE, Weg JG, et al. Manifestations and treatment of laryngeal sarcoidosis. *Am Rev Respir Dis.* 1980;122:325–332.

47. Raymond AK, Sneige N, Batsakis JG. Amyloidosis in the upper aerodigestive tracts. *Ann Otol Rhinol Laryngol.* 1992;101:794–796.

48. Finn DG, Farmer JC. Management of amyloidosis of the larynx and trachea. *Arch Otolaryngol.* 1982;108:54–56.

49. Lewis JE, Olsen KD, Kurtin PJ, et al. Laryngeal amyloidosis: a clinicopathologic and immunohistochemical review. *Otolaryngol Head Neck Surg.* 1992;106:372–377.

50. Fernandes CM, Pirle D, Pudifin DJ. Laryngeal amyloidosis. *J Laryngol Otol.* 1982;96:1165–1175.

51. Simpson GT II, Strong MS, Skinner M, et al. Localized amyloidosis of the head and neck and upper aerodigestive and lower respiratory tracts. *Ann Otol Rhinol Laryngol.* 1984;93:374–379.

52. Djalilian M, McDonald TI, Devine KD, et al. Nontraumatic, nonneoplastic subglottic stenosis. *Ann Otol.* 1975;84:757–763.

53. Talbot AR. Laryngeal amyloidosis. *J Laryngol Otol.* 1990;104:147–149.

54. Barnes EL, Zofar T. Laryngeal amyloidosis: clinicopathological study of seven years. *Ann Otol.* 1977;86:856–862.

55. Mitrani M, Biller HF. Laryngeal amyloidosis. *Laryngoscope.* 1985;95:1346–1347.

56. Hoare TJ, Jayne D, RhysEvans P, et al. Wegener's granulomatosis, subglottic stenosis, and antineutrophil cytoplasm antibodies. *J Laryngol Otol.* 1989;103:1187–1197.

57. Rasmussen N, Petersen J. Cellular immune responses and pathogenesis in C-ANCA positive vasculitides. *J Autoimmun.* 1993;6:227–236.

58. Case records of the Massachusetts General Hospital. Weekly clinicopathological exercises. Case 31-1986. A 39-year-old woman with stenosis of the subglottic area and pulmonary artery. *N Engl J Med.* 1986;7:378–387.

59. Lebovics RS, Hoffman GS, Leavitt RY, et al. The management of subglottic stenosis in patients with Wegener's granulomatosis. *Laryngoscope.* 1992;102:1341–1345.

60. Lu SY, Chen WJ, Eng HL. Lethal midline granuloma: report of three cases. *Changgeng Yi Xue Za Zhi.* 2000;23:99–106.

61. Barker TH, Hosni AA. Idiopathic midline destructive disease—does it exist? *J Laryngol Otol.* 1998;112:307–309.

62. Case records of the Massachusetts General Hospital. Weekly clinicopathological exercises. Case 19-1992. A 56-year-old man with Waldenstrom's macroglobulinemia and cutaneous and oral vesicles. *N Engl J Med.* 1992;326:1276–1284.

63. Nousari HC, Anhalt GJ. Pemphigus and bullous pemphigoid. *Lancet.* 1999;354:667–672.

64. Saunders MS, Gentile RD, Lobritz RW. Primary laryngeal and nasal septal lesions in pemphigus vulgaris. *J Am Osteopath Assoc.* 1992;92:933–937.

65. Estes SA. Relapsing polychondritis. A case report and literature review. *Cutis.* 1983;32:471–476.

66. Batsakis JG, Manning JT. Relapsing polychondritis. *Ann Otol Rhinol Laryngol.* 1989;98:83–84.

67. Gaffney RJ, Harrison M, Blayney AW. Nebulized racemic ephedrine in the treatment of acute exacerbations of laryngeal relapsing polychondritis. *J Laryngol Otol.* 1992;106:63–64.

30

Neurologic Disorders and the Voice

Marshall E. Smith, MD
Lorraine Olson Ramig, PhD

The laryngeal mechanism is subject to highly complex, extensive neural control; therefore, it is not surprising that disorders of the nervous system have effects on the voice. The phonatory function of the larynx, as well as its roles in respiration and swallowing, can be affected by a wide range of neurologic disorders. These span the entire spectrum of central to peripheral *etiologies* and include trauma, cerebral vascular accidents, tumors, and diseases of the nervous system. Except for the more common problem of laryngeal nerve paralysis and the unusual, but disabling, entity of spasmodic dysphonia, neurologically based voice disorders until recently have been a neglected topic for both basic and clinical research in the fields of otolaryngology, speech pathology, and neurology. It is now more apparent that laryngeal dysfunction is a component of many neurologic disorders and should be a critical consideration in patient assessment and management.[1]

While there have been advances in knowledge of neurologic control of vocalization,[2-5] it is readily apparent that there is little information on laryngeal pathophysiology of many neurologic disorders. The integration between the basic science and clinical realm in neurolaryngology is far from complete. Advances in clinical and research laryngology have begun to bridge this gap. Laryngeal imaging has greatly assisted our ability to visually examine and record laryngeal function.[6-8] In this way, the laryngeal examination has become more accessible as part of a neurologic assessment. Other voice examination techniques include acoustic analysis, glottography, and aerodynamic and electromyographic measures.[9-12] These also have emerging roles in documentation, diagnosis, and assessment of treatment efficacy for neurologic voice disorders.[13-17]

The causes of neurologic disorders of the voice range from common to obscure, depending on the disorder. The "immobile vocal fold" is a frequently encountered clinical problem in otolaryngology. Though speech problems are often associated with the common neurologic conditions of stroke and head injury, the association of *voice* disorders with these conditions has not been systematically described. Eighty-

447

nine percent of the 1.5 million patients with Parkinson's disease in the United States have voice disorders.[18] Essential tremor is the most common movement disorder; it affects the voice in 4 to 20% of cases.[19] Less often encountered are the voice disorders associated with neurologic diseases such as Huntington's disease and cerebellar ataxia. Koufman reviewed a series of 100 consecutive patients seen in a practice with voice complaints.[20] Sixteen had neurologic disorders of the voice, 8 with vocal fold paralysis, and 8 with a variety of other neurologic diseases, including Parkinson's disease, vocal tremor, and myasthenia gravis.

One *framework* for studying neurologic diseases and the voice has come from studies of speech disorders. Research by Darley et al[21,22] identified different clinically distinguishable types of dysarthrias that could be correlated with pathology in specific areas of the central and peripheral nervous systems. Because many of these neurologic disorders also involve dysphonias, a similar "site-of-lesion" approach was adopted as a tool for classification of neurologic voice disorders.[7,23,24] A general outline of this classic approach is given in Table 30–1.

Aronson has categorized neurologic voice disorders according to the nature of the voice production, whether constant or variable.[25] Five types were described: (1) Relatively constant neurologic voice disorders, including flaccid, spastic (pseudobulbar), mixed flaccid-spastic, and hypokinetic (parkinsonian) dysphonias; (2) Arrhythmically fluctuating neurologic voice disorders, including ataxic, choreic, and dystonic dysphonias; (3) Rhythmically fluctuating dysphonias, including dysphonias of essential voice tremor and palatopharyngolaryngeal myoclonus; (4) Paroxysmal neurologic voice disorder, the sudden abberant phonatory bursts of Gilles de la Tourette syndrome; and (5) Neurologic voice disorders associated with loss of volitional phonation, such as apraxia of speech and phonation associated with cerebrovascular accidents. A strength of this classification scheme is its focus on the resulting voice production. However, it does not give direction to the clinician regarding phonatory function to guide treatment interventions.

Recently, Ramig and Scherer[26] proposed a system for considering neurologic voice disorders with specific application to *treatment*. Rather than relating the neurologic disorder to the site of neural damage, this classification system focuses on the existing phonatory dysfunction and resulting voice characteristics. The following categories of neural-based phonatory dysfunction were proposed: *adduction* problems (hypoadduction and hyperadduction), *stability* problems (long-term, eg, tremor and short-term, eg, hoarseness), and *coordination* problems (phonatory incoordination, eg, dysprosody). These categories were used to organize approaches to treatment of neurologic

Table 30–1. Traditional Classification of Neurologic Voice Disorders Based on Cause

Classification	Examples
I. Flaccid paresis or paralysis (lower motor neuron)	
A. Muscle	Myopathies, muscular dystrophies
B. Neuromuscular junction	Myasthenia gravis
C. Peripheral nerve	
1. RLN	Trauma, tumor, idiopathic, iatrogenic (surgery, drugs, radiation),
2. SLN	collagen—vascular, Guillain-Barré
3. Upper vagus nerve	
D. Brainstem nucleus	Stroke (Wallenberg's syndrome), Arnold-Chiari malformation, syringobulbia, tumor, trauma
II. Spastic paresis (upper motor neuron)	Pseudobulbar palsy
III. Dyskinetic movement disorders (extrapyramidal system)	Parkinson's disease, essential tremor, dyskinesias, myoclonus, choreas, laryngeal dystonias
IV. Ataxias (cerebellar)	Degeneration, hemorrhage, infarction
V. Apraxias (cortical and subcortical)	Trauma, stroke, tumor, cerebral palsy
VI. Mixed disorders	Amyotrophic lateral sclerosis, multiple sclerosis, Shy-Drager syndrome

voice disorders, which focused on modification of laryngeal physical pathology with corresponding changes in perceptual characteristics of voice and *improved functional speech production*. This classification system, in a modified form (Table 30–2) is used to organize the description of neurologic voice disorders in this chapter on the dimensions of *adduction/abduction* and *stability*. It includes mixed disorders that combine features of these two dimensions. Miscellaneous disorders comprise the fourth and fifth types listed by Aronson.[25] Phonatory coordination problems (eg, dysprosody, voice-voiceless contrasts) have been reviewed elsewhere[26] and will not be repeated here as neurologic disorders affecting this dimension frequently overlap with the first two dimensions. It should be recognized that phonatory function in neurologic disorders can vary and show features of hypoadduction, hyperadduction, malabduction, instability, and/or incoordination at the same time, or that these features may vary during the course of an individual's disease. Nonetheless, the classification provides an outline for observing and interpreting the effects of neurologic disorders on voice that can then guide treatment interventions, be they behavioral, medical, and/or surgical. Treatment of neurologic voice disorders is reviewed briefly in this chapter but covered extensively elsewhere in this book.

DISORDERS OF ADDUCTION

Disorders of vocal fold adduction accompanying neurologic disorders can range from inadequate adduction (hypoadduction) to excessive adduction (hy-

Table 30–2. Classification of Neurologic Voice Disorders Based on Phonatory Dysfunction

Classification	Examples
I. Adduction or abduction problems	
A. Hypoadduction	All lower motor neuron laryngeal paresis or paralysis
	Myasthenia gravis
	Parkinson's disease
	Parkinsonism
	Shy-Drager syndrome
	Progressive supranuclear palsy
	Traumatic brain injury
B. Hyperadduction	Pseudobulbar palsy
	Huntington's disease
	Adductor laryngeal dystonia (spasmodic dysphonia)
C. Malabduction	Abductor laryngeal dystonia (spasmodic dysphonia)
II. Phonatory instability	
A. Short-term (cycle-to-cycle perturbation, aperiodicity, subharmonics)	Nearly all neurologically based voice disorders
B. Long-term (tremor)	Essential vocal tremor
	Parkinson's disease
	Dystonic tremor
	Cerebellar tremor
	Amyotrophic lateral sclerosis vocal "flutter"
	Palatopharyngolaryngeal myoclonus
	Other respiratory or vocal tract sources
III. Mixed disorders (adduction, abduction, instability)	Amyotrophic lateral sclerosis
	Multiple sclerosis
	Ataxic (cerebellar) dysphonia
	Mixed (abductor-adductor-tremor) spasmodic dysphonia
	Progressive supranuclear palsy
	Shy-Drager syndrome
IV. Miscellaneous disorders	Apraxic dysphonia of cortical dysfunction
	Involuntary phonation of Tourette syndrome

peradduction) to inappropriately timed abduction (malabduction).

Hypoadduction

Hypoadduction is observed in many forms and degrees in many neurologic disorders. Damage to any component of the motor unit (muscle, neuromuscular junction, nerve, or nucleus) may result in vocal fold hypoadduction. The most common example of this is vocal fold paralysis. It is also recognized that hypoadduction is found in neurologic diseases of central origin, including Parkinson's disease[27,28] and closed head injury.[29] A primary consequence of hypoadduction is reduced vocal loudness and breathiness.

Hypoadduction Associated with Disorders of the Muscle

Inflammatory myopathies, including polymyositis and dermatomyositis, are unusual conditions that may affect laryngeal function, particularly swallowing.[30] Muscular dystrophies are inherited diseases that yield progressive weakness that is variable in age of onset, distribution, and disability.[30,31] The main laryngeal symptomatology concerns swallowing, yielding oropharyngolaryngeal weakness. Ramig[32] reported increased acoustic aperiodicity and weak, hoarse, and nasal voices in patients with myotonic muscular dystrophy. Myotonic dystrophy is associated mainly with velopharyngeal incompetence.[33,34]

Hypoadduction Associated With Disorders of the Neuromuscular Junction

Interruption of transmission of nerve impulses at the neuromuscular junction may lead to flaccid paresis or paralysis of the vocal folds. Myasthenia gravis (MG) is a neuromuscular disease manifested by weakness and fatigability of voluntary muscles. The incidence of MG has been reported from 2 to 10 per 100,000.[35,36] Overall, it is seen twice as frequently in women as men, with an even higher ratio in the third and fourth decades. Men usually develop MG in their 50s or 60s.[80] Alhough neonatal and juvenile forms exist, voice and speech symptoms as initial or secondary symptoms occur primarily in the adult form. An association has been made with thymomas.

MG frequently presents with otolaryngologic symptoms. The most common presenting symptoms are ocular (ptosis and diplopia). It is important to recognize that other head and neck symptoms may be present as an initial manifestation of MG. Carpenter et al reviewed 175 patients with MG.[37] Thirty percent had primary symptoms of dysphagia, dysarthria, or dysphonia. Dhillon and Brookes reviewed 48 patients with MG.[38] Nine of their patients had only head and neck symptoms initially, 6 of these complained of dysphonia, usually in conjunction with dysphagia. Calcaterra et al had an even higher percentage of patients in their series present with voice complaints.[39] Of 50 patients with MG, 26 had initial speech complaint: 13 with dysarthria, 5 with hypernasality, 4 with stridor, and 4 with vocal weakness. Vocal fatigue is the major voice complaint in individuals with MG. It may be misdiagnosed as a superior laryngeal nerve paralysis or bilateral vocal fold paresis/paralysis.[40] These and other reports[41] make the neurolaryngologist and speech pathologist aware that voice and laryngeal involvement may occur as an initial or secondary symptom in MG.

Examination of the larynx in patients suspected of MG should involve observation of the velopharynx for inadequate closure, as well as glottal insufficiency—incomplete adduction or bowing of the vocal folds. The patient should be "stressed" with repetitive vocalizing tasks (reading or counting out loud for 5 minutes) to induce fatigability of involved structures. Phonating or singing a sustained high note for several minutes may induce fatigue with a noticeable drop in pitch of the voice.[42] Fatigability may also be assessed by testing for stapedial reflex decay.[43] Laryngoscopy may raise the suspicion of the examiner to suspect sluggish vocal fold mobility or asymmetry, suggestive of superior laryngeal nerve (SLN) paralysis. Laryngeal EMG of the cricothyroid muscles is helpful to differentiate SLN paralysis from MG.[40] A fluctuation in vocal fold mobility during repeated examinations is suggestive of MG.[80] The diagnosis is made by a *Tensilon* (edrophonium) test. Edrophonium, a short-acting anticholinesterase drug, administered intravenously results in prompt reversal of symptoms. Improvement in voice and resonance characteristics on spectrograms following edrophonium injection has been documented.[44] Because of the concern for progression to respiratory involvement that may occur in MG, prompt neurologic referral is warranted if MG is suspected.[45] Treatment of MG involves anticholinesterase drugs (eg, pyridostigmine). Steroids are used for severe cases. The effect of thymectomy in treatment of MG is controversial, but is generally recommended in younger patients.[46]

Hypoadduction Associated with Disorders of the Peripheral Nerve (Recurrent Laryngeal Nerve)

Vocal fold paralysis is a common problem resulting in vocal fold hypoadduction, probably the most common neurologic voice disorder seen by the otolaryngologist.[20] This section will generally concern *unilateral vocal fold paralysis* (UVP), as this commonly affects the voice and is much more frequently seen than bilateral vocal fold paralysis. It should be mentioned, however, that bilateral vocal fold weakness may also present with dysphonia and requires an extensive evaluation.[47] Many surveys have reported on the etiologies of vocal fold paralysis. The results of nine surveys involving 1,019 patients were compiled by Terris et al.[48] Thirty-six percent of cases were from neoplasm with 55% of these caused by lung cancer. Twenty-five percent were postsurgical, mainly from thyroidectomy. Other causes included idiopathic (14%), inflammatory or medical (13%), and central neurologic (6%). Medical etiologies should be sought in obscure cases, such as vincristine (a chemotherapeutic drug) induced laryngeal neuropathy,[49] or postpolio syndrome associated laryngeal paresis or paralysis.[50-53] The distinction between "idiopathic" and "inflammatory" causes of laryngeal paralysis may be blurred; in many cases "idiopathic" UVP is felt to be an isolated neuropathy caused by virus.[54-56]

Patient symptoms in UVP vary widely. Complaints of hoarse voice and breathy voice are frequent, although it is important to recognize that the voice may be fairly normal.[57] Problems with swallowing, choking, coughing, and aspiration can be found and may be of more immediate concern in considering intervention.

The voice in a patient with UVP is usually perceived as reduced in loudness, hoarse, and breathy. Diplophonia may be present. Acoustic findings that often accompany UVP include increased aperiodicity, reduced pitch range and variation, reduced vocal intensity, and decreased harmonics-to-noise ratio.[57] Variations in glottographic patterns may be seen.[58-60] Glottal aerodynamics often demonstrate high mean airflow rates, and an offset of airflow from baseline ("DC leak"), reflecting glottal insufficiency.[57,61]

Several factors influence glottal dynamics and resulting voice in UVP. These include: (1) individual variations in laryngeal framework anatomy[62] and peripheral innervation[63]; (2) the degree and extent of reinnervation[64]; (3) the degree of laryngeal muscle atrophy[65,66]; (4) the time variation of the second and third factors; and, very importantly, (5) individual vocalizing behaviors and laryngeal biomechanics that attempt to compensate for the glottal insufficiency.[67] The particular voice symptoms are created by the complex interaction of the above factors that influence laryngeal biomechanics, particularly in UVP relating to the geometry of the glottic (anterior and posterior) aperture, the three-dimensional position and orientation of the arytenoids, the vertical position of the folds relative to each other, muscle stiffness asymmetries and resulting body-cover relationships, and the interaction of these with glottal airflow and pressures.[7,68]

Laryngoscopy (flexible and rigid telescope) is of critical importance in the evaluation of UVP, as in other voice disorders. Laryngostroboscopy is also very helpful for viewing the effects of UVP on vocal fold position and movement, and glottal closure, mucosal wave asymmetries, and vocal process vertical position.[69] Tomography has also been used in UVP to demonstrate vocal folds on different vertical levels.[70]

The relationship between the location of peripheral laryngeal nerve lesion and the position of the affected vocal fold in UVP seen on laryngoscopy has been a source of controversy. A common notion, promulgated as the "Wagner-Grossman theory," related the position of the vocal fold in vocal fold paralyses to the activity of the cricothyroid muscle.[71] Clinical relevance has been ascribed to this theory by relating glottal configuration to the topognostic localization of site of laryngeal nerve injury.[55,72] In vivo studies have yielded conflicting results.[71,72] Several recent clinical studies have questioned this dogma, pointing to the wide variability in glottal position at various locations of injury.[73-75] A factor complicating this issue is that, in many cases, the exact site and degree of nerve injury are unknown.[7] Neuroanatomic studies have shed light on this controversy. Sanders et al described multiple and variable ipsilateral and crossed interconnections in the peripheral innervation of the human larynx between the superior and recurrent laryngeal nerves.[63] These variations may help explain the spectrum of glottal configurations seen in UVP.

The management of dysphonia secondary to UVP includes behavioral therapy[76] and a variety of surgical techniques. These are covered extensively in other chapters of this book.

Hypoadduction Associated with Disorders of the Peripheral Nerve (Superior Laryngeal Nerve)

Superior laryngeal nerve (SLN) paralysis is less common than recurrent laryngeal paralysis.[77] Causes include surgical trauma (eg, thyroidectomy, carotid endarterectomy), blunt neck trauma, and idiopathic cases. Its presentation may be subtle. Voice complaints may be only of a mild hoarseness, vocal fatigue, or difficulty with projection or singing despite normal speaking voice.[40,78] The laryngeal examination findings in unilateral SLN paralysis have been described as a rotation of the anterior commissure away from and posterior glottis toward the affected (paralyzed) side.[7,77] This maneuver may only be evident by having the patient attempt to phonate at high pitch.[79] Shortening of the vocal fold, unilateral bowing, or scissoring of the vocal folds may be observed.[80] The asymmetry of laryngeal vibration in SLN paralysis may be seen on laryngostroboscopy.[81] This asymmetry has been demonstrated in mathematical simulations[68,82] and animal phonation models of SLN paralysis.[83]

Hypoadduction Associated with Disorders of the Nucleus

Injury to the lower motor neurons of the tenth nerve nucleus results in flaccid laryngeal paralysis and hypoadduction.[23,24] The injury can occur via vascular brainstem infarction of the posterior inferior cerebellar artery. This vascular accident when associated with symptoms of dysphagia and dysarthria, ipsilateral Horner's syndrome, ipsilateral face, and contralateral body pain-temperature impairment, is known as Wallenberg's (lateral pontomedullary) syndrome. Other causes include Arnold-Chiari malformation, syringobulbia, tumor, and trauma.

Hypoadduction Associated with Parkinson's Disease

Hypoadduction is *commonly* associated with the extrapyramidal disorder of idiopathic Parkinson's disease (IPD), a nigrostriatal disorder characterized by dopamine deficiency.[84] Rigidity, tremor, and reduced range of motion are the primary physical pathologies associated with IPD. One in every 100 individuals over 60 and 1 in every 1,000 individuals under age 60 have IPD. While IPD is frequently considered a disease of the elderly, patients have been diagnosed as early as the third decade of life. Patients can live 10 to 20 years after diagnosis. At least 89% of the 1.5 million individuals with IPD in the United States have a voice disorder.[18]

The voice disorder in IPD is generally characterized by reduced loudness, monotone, hoarseness, and tremor. Reduced volume may be the first *or an early sign of IPD*.[25,85] These voice characteristics are frequently observed in the context of a generalized dysarthria which includes imprecise articulation. The patient with IPD may be unaware that his voice is soft; the reason for this self-perceptual impairment is unclear.[86] The perception of reduced loudness is supported by an acoustic study reporting statistically significantly (2-4 dB at 30 cm) reduced sound pressure level (SPL) in individuals (n = 29) with IPD across a variety of speech tasks when compared to an age-matched control group (n = 14).[87] Reduced SPL has been associated with glottal incompetence and/or

bowed vocal folds,[27,28] and with reduced subglottal air pressure.[88] Two recent electromyographic studies of laryngeal muscles in IPD report evidence of reduced activation of the TA when compared to a healthy aging group.[11] Decreases in the rate and increases in the variability of motor unit firing in the TA of both aged and IPD males were reported by Luschei et al.[12] These findings were interpreted to reflect reduced central drive to the laryngeal motoneuron pools. In contrast, one study[89] reported thyroarytenoid recordings of a single subject with IPD. Loss of reciprocal suppression of the TA during inspiration was found, indicative of parkinsonian rigidity. No neurogenic changes were seen to indicate a peripheral neuropathology. Although recordings of reciprocal muscles (posterior cricoarytenoid) were not made, it was thought that the hypokinetic laryngeal movement in IPD was related to deterioration in the reciprocal adjustment of the antagonistic muscles.

Although dopaminergic (levadopa) treatment has positive effects on the general function of IPD, voice and speech symptoms are not consistently alleviated by these pharmacologic treatments.[27,90] Neurosurgical interventions (eg, pallidotomy, adrenal and fetal cell transplants) have been conducted.[91] Findings following these procedures support improved limb function and reduction of medication, but changes in laryngeal and speech mechanism function are not clear.[92,93]

Speech therapy has historically been ineffective for IPD.[94,95] However, a recent approach by Ramig and associates,[96-98] the Lee Silverman Voice Treatment (LSVT), which focuses on *improved phonation and sensory awareness*, has generated short and long-term efficacy data.[15-17,99] Significant functional changes in vocal loudness with co-occurring changes in sound pressure level, subglottal air pressure,[88] and vocal fold adduction[28] have been reported following intensive voice treatment (16 sessions in one month). In addition, data support generalized effects of this treatment to articulation,[97] swallowing,[100] and facial expression (J. Spielman and L. Ramig, unpublished data). Recent PET scan findings support evidence of neural changes following treatment.[101] Details of this treatment are summarized elsewhere.[102]

Hypophonia Accompanying Closed Head Injury

Traumatic brain injury yields complex neurologic insults. They usually affect the cortical and subcortical structures as well as others. These injuries may result in voice and speech problems. Voice problems in these patients are described as having decreased loudness. One study found decreases in laryngeal airway resis-

laryngoscope allows examination of the larynx, pharynx, palate, and velopharyngeal sphincter at rest and during a variety of tasks, including connected speech, sustained phonation, coughing, singing, and swallowing. This capability is extremely helpful in the assessment of neurologic voice disorders. The rigid laryngeal telescope is also helpful, but not useful in every case. It provides superior image quality for view of the larynx at rest and during sustained vowel phonation, and for viewing the vocal fold mucosal waves under stroboscopic lighting.[10] Video documentation for review and patient education is also an important aspect of the laryngeal imaging examination.

The patient with a neurologic voice disorder may have other neurologic examination findings that aid the physician in diagnosis. These have been reviewed in an excellent summary by Rosenfield.[247] While this neurologic assessment may not replace a complete evaluation by a neurologist, it helps the laryngologist to understand the nature of the illness of which the voice may only be a part. It also facilitates communication with the neurologist about the patient's problem. Components include a cranial nerve examination, assessment of muscle strength and tone (motor and extrapyramidal), and coordination (cerebellar). Although cranial nerve testing is familiar to the otolaryngologist, other aspects of neurologic examination are not. However, these should be routinely performed in cases of suspected neurologic voice disorders. In the elderly patient, a screening examination for tone (resistance to passive movement) may be more revealing than an assessment of muscle strength.[105] Increased tone on passive movement of the limbs may be an upper motor neuron sign, and rigidity of wrist or elbow movement may be an early sign of Parkinson's disease. Coordination and cerebellar function are assessed by observation of gait and Romberg's sign. Following the Romberg test the coordination of the upper extremities is evaluated by finger-nose testing. Observation of the outstretched limbs allows evaluation of postural (cerebellar) tremor. Resting tremor that improves with movement is seen in Parkinson's disease. During the examination the patient is observed for adventitious (unintended or involuntary) movements (eg, tremor of head or limbs, circumoral twitches, blepharospasm, dyskinesias, or dystonias). Observation of the patient's handwriting may be helpful in identifying ataxia or tremor.

Special diagnostic tests are indicated in selected cases. Laryngeal electromyography has been found to be helpful in the diagnostic assessment of vocal fold paralysis, differentiating paralysis from fixation, and in determining prognosis for recovery.[74,250-253] It can provide helpful information in determining etiology

and treatment of a variety of neurolaryngologic disorders.[254] The workup of vocal fold paralysis, in the absence of identifiable etiology, involves imaging studies along the entire course of the nerve on the affected side.[48] Regarding spasmodic dysphonia, in the absence of secondary causes for dystonia,[104,255] Rosenfield et al[111] recommended additional medical evaluation with a thyroid-stimulating hormone level (TSH) to identify concomitant hypothyroidism, and Swenson et al[255] suggested a complete blood count and sedimentation rate to rule out systemic vasculitis. In the patient with suspected myasthenia gravis a *Tensilon* test should be performed. Those with presumed underlying central neurologic lesions are evaluated with MRI.

TREATMENT ISSUES RELATED TO NEUROLOGIC DISORDERS OF THE LARYNX

This chapter organized neurologic disorders of the larynx according to the phonatory dysfunctional dimensions of hypoadduction, hyperadduction, malabduction, and short- and long-term instabilities, and mixed abnormalities. This classification system lends itself to treatment planning that spans the various etiologic factors.

When planning treatment for neurologic disorders of the larynx, it is important to consider that patients often have disorders of multiple speech subsystems. Enhancing laryngeal function must be considered in relation to the impact of each subsystem on functional speech production. Recent findings support the key role of phonation in enhancing oral communication in neurologic disorders.[97] Treatment goals must also consider the role of language or cognitive disorders (aphasia, dementia) and the progressive nature of many neurologic diseases when planning treatment to maximize functional communication.

There are various forms of treatment that may affect neurologic disorders of the larynx. Some treatments (neuropharmacologic or neurosurgical) are designed to treat the neurologic disorder and may have co-occurring effects on laryngeal or speech function. Other treatments (behavioral, laryngeal-surgical) are designed to directly treat the phonatory dysfunction and improve the voice. These are ideally conducted by an interdisciplinary, collaborative group such as that formed by the speech pathologist, neurologist, and otolaryngologist to provide the patient who has a neurologic disorder of the larynx with optimal speech intelligibility.[26]

Acknowledgments This work was supported by NIH Grants K08-DC00132 and R01-DC01150 from the National Institute of Deafness and Communication Disorders.

REFERENCES

1. Blitzer A, Brin MF, Sasaki CT, et al, eds. *Neurologic Disorders of the Larynx*. New York, NY: Thieme Medical Publishers; 1992.
2. Barlow SM, Netsell R, Hunker CJ. Phonatory disorders associated with CNS lesions. In: Cummings CW, et al, eds. *Otolaryngology-Head and Neck Surgery*. 1st ed. St Louis, MO: CV Mosby; 1986;2087–2093.
3. Larson CR. Brain mechanisms involved in the control of vocalization. *J Voice*. 1998;2:301–311.
4. Gacek RR, Malmgren LT. Laryngeal motor innervation—central. In: Blitzer A, et al, eds. *Neurologic Disorders of the Larynx*. New York, NY: Thieme Medical Publishers; 1992;29–35.
5. Larson CR, Yoshida Y, Sessile BJ, Ludlow CR. Higher level motor and sensory integration. In: Titze IR, ed. *Vocal Fold Physiology: Frontiers in Basic Science*. San Diego, CA: Singular Publishing Group; 1993;227–275.
6. Ward PH, Berci G, Calcaterra TC. Advances in endoscopic examination of the respiratory system. *Ann Otol Rhinol Laryngol*. 1974;83:754–760.
7. Hanson DG. Neuromuscular disorders of the larynx. *Otolaryngol Clin North Am*. 1991;24:1035–1051.
8. Yanagisawa E. Physical examination of the larynx and videolaryngoscopy. In: Blitzer A, et al, eds. *Neurologic Disorders of the Larynx*. New York, NY: Thieme Medical Publishers; 1992;82–97.
9. Baken R, Orkikoff RF. *Clinical Measurement of Speech and Voice*. 2nd ed. San Diego, CA: Singular Publishing Group; 2000.
10. Bless DM. Measurement of vocal function. *Otolaryngol Clin North Am*. 1991;24:1023–1033.
11. Baker K, Ramig L, Luschei E, Smith M. Thyroarytenoid muscle activity associated with hypophonia in Parkinson disease and aging. *Neurology*. 1998;51(6):1592–1598.
12. Luschei E, Ramig L, Baker K, Smith M. Discharge characteristics of laryngeal single motor units during phonation in young and older adults and in persons with Parkinson disease. *J Neurophysiol*. 1999;81:2131–2139.
13. Ramig LO, Scherer RC, Klasner ER, et al. Acoustic analysis of voice in amyotrophic lateral sclerosis: a longitudinal case study. *J Speech Hear Disord*. 1990;55:2–14.
14. Countryman S, Ramig LA. Effects of intensive voice therapy on voice deficits associated with bilateral thalamotomy in Parkinson's disease: a case study. *J Med Speech-Lang Pathol*. 1993;1:233–249.
15. Ramig L, Sapir S, Fox C, Countryman S. Changes in vocal loudness following intensive voice treatment (LSVT) in individuals with Parkinson disease: a comparison with untreated patients and normal age-matched controls. *Mov Disord*. 2001;16:79–83
16. Ramig L, Countryman S, Thompson L, et al. Comparison of two forms of intensive speech treatment for Parkinson disease. *J Speech Lang Hear Res*. 1995;38:1232–1251.
17. Ramig L, Countryman S, O'Brien C, et al. Intensive speech treatment for patients with Parkinson disease: short and long-term comparison of two techniques. *Neurology*. 1996;47:1496–1504.
18. Logemann JA, Fisher HB, Boshes B, et al. Frequency and occurrence of vocal tract dysfunctions in the speech of a large sample of Parkinson's patients. *J Speech Hear Disord*. 1978;42:47–57.
19. Elble RJ, Koller WC. *Tremor*. Baltimore, MD: Johns Hopkins University Press; 1990.
20. Koufman JA, Isaacson G. The spectrum of vocal dysfunction. *Otolaryngol Clin North Am*. 1991;24:985–988.
21. Darley F, Aronson A, Brown J. Differential diagnostic patterns of dysarthria. *J Speech Hear Res*. 1969;12:246–269.
22. Darley F, Aronson A, Brown J. Clusters of deviant speech dimensions in the dysarthrias. *J Speech Hear Res*. 1969;12:462–496.
23. Ward PH, Hanson DG, Berci G. Photographic studies of the larynx in central laryngeal paresis and paralysis. *Acta Otolaryngol (Stockh)*. 1981;91:353–367.
24. Ward PH, Hanson DG, Berci G. Observations on central neurologic etiology for laryngeal dysfunction. *Ann Otol Rhinol Laryngol*. 1981;90:430–441.
25. Aronson AE. *Clinical Voice Disorders*. 3rd ed. New York, NY: Thieme; 1990.
26. Ramig LO, Scherer RC. Speech therapy for neurological disorders of the larynx. In: Blitzer A, et al, eds. *Neurologic Disorders of the Larynx*. New York, NY: Thieme Medical Publishers; 1992:163–181.
27. Hanson DG, Gerratt BR, Ward PH. Cinegraphic observations of vocal pathology in Parkinson's disease. *Laryngoscope*. 1984;92:348–353.
28. Smith ME, Ramig LO, Dromey C, et al. Intensive voice treatment in Parkinson's disease: laryngostroboscopic findings. *J Voice*. 1995;10:354–361.
29. McHenry MA, Wilson RL, Minton JT. Management of multiple physiologic system deficits following traumatic brain injury. *J Med Speech-Lang Pathol*. 1994;2:59–74.
30. Younger DS, Lange DJ, Lovelace RE, et al. Neuromuscular disorders of the larynx. In: Blitzer A, et al, eds. *Neurologic Disorders of the Larynx*. New York, NY: Thieme Medical Publishers; 1992;246.
31. Mastaglia FL. Genetic myopathies. In: Swash M, Oxbury J, eds. *Clinical Neurology*. New York, NY: Churchill Livingstone; 1991;1286.
32. Ramig LA, Scherer RC, Titze IR, et al. Acoustic analysis of voices of patients with neurological disease: rationale and preliminary data. *Ann Otol Rhinol Laryngol*. 1988;97:164–172.
33. Salomonson J, Kawamoto H, Wilson L. Velopharyngeal incompetence as the presenting symptom of myotonic dystrophy. *Cleft Palate J*. 1988;25:296–300.
34. Hillarp B, Ekberg O, Jacobsson S, Nylander G, Aberg M. Myotonic dystrophy revealed at videoradiography of deglutition and speech in adult patients with velopha-

ryngeal insufficiency: presentation of four cases. *Cleft Palate Craniofac J.* 1994;31:125–133.

35. Fenchiel GM. Clinical syndromes of myasthenia in infancy and childhood. *Arch Neurol.* 1978;35:97–103.

36. Scadding GK, Harvard CWH. Pathogenesis and treatment of myasthenia gravis. *Br Med J.* 1981;283:1008–1019.

37. Carpenter RJ, McDonald TJ, Howard FM. The otolaryngologic presentation of myasthenia gravis. *Laryngoscope.* 1979;89:922–928.

38. Dhillon RS, Brookes GB. Myasthenia gravis in otolaryngological practice. *Clin Otolaryngol.* 1984;9:27–34.

39. Calcaterra TC, Stern F, Herrmann C, et al. The otolaryngologist's role in myasthenia gravis. *Trans Am Acad Ophthalmol Otolaryngol.* 1972;76:308–312.

40. Dursun G, Sataloff RT, Spiegel JR, Mandel S, Heuer RJ, Rosen DC. Superior laryngeal nerve paresis and paralysis. *J Voice.* 1996;10:206–211.

41. Neiman RF, Mountjoy JR, Allen EL. Myasthenia gravis focal to the larynx: report of a case. *Arch Otolaryngol.* 1975;101:569–570.

42. Walker FO. Voice fatigue in myasthenia gravis: the sinking pitch sign. *Neurology.* 1997;48:1135–1136.

43. Warren WR, Gutmann L, Cody RC, et al. Stapedius reflex decay in myasthenia gravis. *Arch Neurol.* 1977;34:496–497.

44. Rontal M, Rontal E, Leuchter W, et al. Voice spectrography in the evaluation of myasthenia gravis of the larynx. *Ann Otol Rhinol Laryngol.* 1978;87:722–728.

45. Tyler HR. Neurology of the larynx. *Otolaryngol Clin North Am.* 1984;17:75–79.

46. Oosterhuis JHGH. Myasthenia gravis and other myasthenic syndromes. In: Swash M, Oxbury J, eds. *Clinical Neurology.* New York, NY: Churchill Livingstone; 1991;1368.

47. Dray TG, Robinson LR, Hillel AD. Idiopathic bilateral vocal fold weakness. *Laryngoscope.* 1999;109:995–1002.

48. Terris DJ, Arnstein DP, Nguyen HH. Contemporary evaluation of unilateral vocal cord paralysis. *Otolaryngol Head Neck Surg.* 1992;107:84–90.

49. Annino DJ, MacArthur CJ, Friedman EM. Vincristine-induced recurrent laryngeal nerve paralysis. *Laryngoscope.* 1992;102:1260–1262.

50. Cannon S, Ritter FN. Vocal cord paralysis in postpoliomyelitis syndrome. *Laryngoscope.* 1987;97:981–983.

51. Nugent KM. Vocal cord paresis and glottic stenosis: a late complication of poliomyelitis. *South Med J.* 1987;80:1594–1595.

52. Driscoll BP, Gracco C, Coelho C, et al. Laryngeal function in postpolio patients. *Laryngoscope.* 1995;105:35–41.

53. Robinson LR, Hillel AD, Waugh PF. New laryngeal muscle weakness in post-polio syndrome. *Laryngoscope.* 1998;108:732-734.

54. Blau JN, Kapadia R. Idiopathic palsy of the recurrent laryngeal nerve: a transient cranial mononeuropathy. *Br Med J.* 1972;4:259–261.

55. Ward PH, Berci G. Observations on so-called idiopathic vocal cord paralysis. *Ann Otol Rhinol Laryngol.* 1982;91:558–563.

56. Bachor E, Bonkowsky V, Hacki T. Herpes simplex virus type I reactivation as a cause of a unilateral temporary paralysis of the vagus nerve. *Eur Arch Otorhinolaryngol.* 1996;253(4-5):297–300.

57. Colton RH, Casper JK. *Understanding Voice Problems: A Physiological Perspective for Diagnosis and Treatment.* 2nd ed. Baltimore, MD: Williams & Wilkins; 1996.

58. Gerratt BR, Hanson DG, Berke GS. Glottographic measures of laryngeal function in individuals with abnormal motor control. In: Baer T, Sasaki C, Harris K, eds. *Laryngeal Function in Phonation and Respiration.* Boston, MA: Little, Brown, and Co; 1987;521–534.

59. Hanson DG, Gerratt BR, Karin R, et al. Glottographic measures of vocal fold vibration: laryngeal paralysis. *Laryngoscope.* 1988;98:348–353.

60. Jiang J, Lin E, Hanson DG. Glottographic phase difference in recurrent nerve paralysis. *Ann Otol Rhinol Laryngol.* 2000;109:287–293.

61. Woo P, Colton R, Shangold L. Phonatory airflow analysis in patients with laryngeal disease. *Ann Otol Rhinol Laryngol.* 1987;96:549–555.

62. Hirano M, Kurita S, Yukizane K, et al. Asymmetry of the laryngeal framework: a morphological study of cadaver larynges. *Ann Otol Rhinol Laryngol.* 1989;98:135–140.

63. Sanders I, Wu BL, Mu L, et al. The innervation of the human larynx. *Arch Otolaryngol Head Neck Surg.* 1993;119:934–939.

64. Crumley R, McCabe B. Regeneration of the recurrent laryngeal nerve. *Otolaryngol Head Neck Surg.* 1982;92:442–447.

65. Kirchner JA. Atrophy of laryngeal muscles in vagal paralysis. *Laryngoscope.* 1966;76:1753–1765.

66. Quiney RE, Michaels L. Histopathology of vocal cord palsy from recurrent laryngeal nerve damage. *J Otolaryngol.* 1990;19:237–241.

67. Pinho SM, Pontes PA, Gadelha ME, Biasi N. Vestibular vocal fold behavior during phonation in unilateral vocal fold paralysis. *J Voice.* 1999;13(1):36–42.

68. Smith ME, Berke GS, Gerratt BR, et al. Laryngeal paralyses: theoretical considerations and effects of laryngeal vibration. *J Speech Hear Res.* 1992;35:545–554.

69. Hirano M, Bless DM. *Videostroboscopic Examination of the Larynx.* San Diego, CA: Singular Publishing Group; 1993:167–169.

70. Isshiki N, Ishikawa T. Diagnostic value of tomography in unilateral vocal cord paralysis. *Laryngoscope.* 1976;86:1573–1578.

71. Dedo HH. The paralyzed larynx: an electromyographic study in dogs and humans. *Laryngoscope.* 1970;80:1455–1517.

72. Woodson GE. Configuration of the glottis in laryngeal paralysis. II: animal experiments. *Laryngoscope.* 1993;103:1235–1241.

73. Woodson GE. Configuration of the glottis in laryngeal paralysis. I: clinical study. *Laryngoscope.* 1993;103:1227–1234.

74. Hirano M, Nozoe I, Shin T, Maeyama T. Electromyography for laryngeal paralysis. In: Hirano, M, Kirchner JA, Bless DM, eds. *Neurolaryngology: Recent Advances.* Boston, MA: College-Hill; 1987:232–248.

75. Koufman JA, Walker FO, Joharji GM. The cricothyroid muscle does not influence vocal fold position in laryngeal paralysis. *Laryngoscope.* 1995;105:368–372.

76. Heuer RJ, Sataloff RT, Emerich K, et al. Unilateral recurrent laryngeal nerve paralysis: the importance of "pre-operative" voice therapy. *J Voice.* 1997;11(1):88–94.

77. Ward PH, Berci G, Calcaterra TC. Superior laryngeal nerve paralysis: an often overlooked entity. *Trans Am Acad Ophthalmol Otolaryngol.* 1977;84:78–89.

78. Adour KK, Schneider GD, Hilsinger RL. Acute superior laryngeal nerve palsy: analysis of 78 cases. *Otolaryngol Head Neck Surg.* 1980;88:418–424.

79. Tanaka S, Hirano M, Umeno H. Laryngeal behavior in unilateral superior laryngeal nerve paralysis. *Ann Otol Rhinol Laryngol.* 1994;103:93–97.

80. Sataloff RT, Mandel S, Rosen DC. Neurologic disorders affecting the voice in performance. In: Sataloff RT, ed. *Professional Voice: The Science and Art of Clinical Care.* 2nd ed. San Diego, CA: Singular Publishing Group; 1997;479–498.

81. Koufman JA. Approach to the patient with a voice disorder. *Otolaryngol Clin North Am.* 1991;24:989–998.

82. Isshiki N, Tanabe M, Ishizaka K, et al. Clinical significance of asymmetrical vocal cord tension. *Ann Otol Rhinol Laryngol.* 1977;86:58–66.

83. Berke G, Moore D, Hantke D, et al. Laryngeal modeling: theoretical, in-vitro, in-vivo. *Laryngoscope.* 1987;97:871–881.

84. Hornykiewicz O. Metabolism of brain dopamine in human parkinsonism: neurochemical and clinical aspects. In: Costa E, Cote L, Yahr M, eds. *Biochemistry and Pharmacology of the Basal Ganglia.* New York, NY: Raven Press; 1966.

85. Stewart C, Winfield L, Hunt A, et al. Speech dysfunction in early Parkinson's disease. *Mov Disord.* 1995;10:562–565.

86. Ho AK, Bradshaw JL, Iansek T. Volume perception in parkinsonian speech. *Mov Disord.* 2000;15:1125–1131.

87. Fox C, Ramig L. Speech and voice characteristics of men and women who are elderly and have idiopathic Parkinson disease. *Am J Speech Lang Pathol.* 1997;6, 85–94.

88. Ramig L. Dromey C. Aerodynamic mechanisms underlying treatment related changes in SPL in patients with Parkinson disease. *J Speech Hear Res.* 1996;39:798–807.

89. Hirose H, Joshita Y. Laryngeal behavior in patients with disorders of the central nervous system. In: Hirano M, Kirchner JA, Bless DM, eds. *Neurolaryngology: Recent Advances.* Boston, MA: Little, Brown, and Co; 1987;258–266.

90. Larson K, Ramig L, Scherer R. Preliminary speech and voice analysis during drug-related fluctuations in Parkinson's disease. *J Med Speech-Lang Pathol.* 1994;2:211–226.

91. Freed C, Breeze R, Rosenberg N, et al. Survival of implanted fetal dopamine cells and neurologic improvement 12 to 46 months after transplantation for Parkinson disease. *New Engl J Med.* 1993;327:1549–1555.

92. Schultz G, Peterson T, Sapienza C, et al. Voice and speech characteristics of persons with Parkinson's disease pre- and post-pallidotomy surgery: preliminary findings. *J Speech Lang Hear Res.* 1999;42:1176–1194.

93. Baker K, Ramig L, Johnson A, Freed C. Preliminary speech and voice analysis following fetal dopamine transplants in five individuals with Parkinson disease, *J Speech Lang Hear Res.* 1997;40:615–626.

94. Sarno MT. Speech impairment in Parkinson's disease. *Arch Phys Med Rehab.* 1968;49:269–275.

95. Weiner WJ, Singer C. Parkinson's disease and non-pharmacologic treatment programs. *J Am Geriatr Soc.* 1989;37:359–363.

96. Ramig LO, Bonitati C, Lemke J, et al. Voice treatment for patients with Parkinson disease: development of an approach and preliminary efficacy data. *J Med Speech-Lang Pathol.* 1994;2(3):191–210.

97. Dromey C, Ramig L, Johnson A. Phonatory and articulatory changes associated with increased vocal intensity in Parkinson disease: a case study. *J Speech Lang Hear Res.* 1995;38:751–764.

98. Ramig LO, Dromey C: Aerodynamic mechanisms underlying treatment related changes in SPL in patients with Parkinson disease. *J Speech Lang Hear Res.* 1996;39:798–807.

99. Ramig L, Sapir S, Countryman S, et al. Intensive voice treatment (LSVT) for individuals with Parkinson disease: a two-year follow-up. *J Neurol, Neurosurg Psychiatry.* 2001;71:493–498.

100. El Sharwaki A, Ramig L, Logemann J, et al. Swallowing and voice effects of Lee Silverman Voice Treatment (LSVT): a pilot study. *J Neurol, Neurosurg Psychiatry.* In review.

101. Liotti M, Vogel D, New P, et al. *A PET study of functional reorganization of premotor regions in Parkinson's disease following intensive speech and voice treatment (LSVT).* A paper presented to the Academy of Neurology. Toronto, Canada; November, 1998.

102. Ramig L, Pawlas A, Countryman S. *The Lee Silverman Voice Treatment: A Practical Guide for Treating the Voice and Speech Disorders in Parkinson Disease.* The National Center for Voice and Speech (NCVS) and The LSVT Foundation; Louisville, CO; 1995.

103. McHenry M. Acoustic characteristics of voice after severe traumatic brain injury. *Laryngoscope.* 2000;110(7):1157–1161.

104. Brin MF, Fahn S, Blitzer A, et al. Movement disorders of the larynx. In: Blitzer A, Brin MF, Sasaki CT, et al, eds. *Neurologic Disorders of the Larynx.* New York, NY: Thieme Medical Publishers; 1992;248–278.

105. Glick TH. *Neurologic Skills: Examination and Diagnosis.* Boston, MA: Blackwell Scientific Publications; 1993.

106. Duffy J. *Motor Speech Disorders.* St. Louis, MO: Mosby; 1995.

107. Duffy J, Folger W. *Dysarthria in unilateral central nervous system lesions.* Paper presented at the annual convention of the America Speech-Language Hearing Association. Detroit, MI; 1986.

108. Aring CD. Supranuclear (pseudobulbar) palsy. *Arch Int Med.* 1965;115;19.

109. Penney JB, Young AB, Shoulson I, et al. Huntington's disease in Venezuela: 7 years of follow-up on symptomatic and asymptomatic individuals. *Mov Disord.* 1990;5:93–99.

110. Ramig LA. Acoustic analyses of phonation in patients with Huntington's disease: preliminary report. *Ann Otol Rhinol Laryngol.* 1986;95:288–293.

111. Rosenfield DB, Donovan DT, Sulek M, et al. Neurologic aspects of spasmodic dysphonia. *J Otolaryngol.* 1990;19:231–236.

112. Izdebski K. Symptomatology of adductor spasmodic dysphonia: a physiologic model. *J Voice.* 1992;6:306–319.

113. Cannito M, Johnson H. Spastic dysphonia: a continuum disorder. *J Commun Disord.* 1981;14:215–223.

114. Blitzer A, Lovelace RE, Brin MF, et al. Electromyographic findings in focal laryngeal dystonia (spastic dysphonia). *Ann Otol Rhinol Laryngol.* 1985;94:591–594.

115. Blitzer A, Brin MF, Fahn S, et al. Clinical and laboratory characteristics of focal laryngeal dystonia: study of 110 cases. *Laryngoscope.* 1988;98:636–640.

116. Freeman FJ, Cannito M, Finitzo-Hieber T. Classification of spasmodic dysphonia by visual perceptual and acoustic means. In: Gates GA, ed. *Spastic Dysphonia: State of the Art.* New York, NY: The Voice Foundation; 1985:5–18.

117. Finitzo T, Freeman F. Spasmodic dysphonia: whether and where: results of seven years of research. *J Speech Hear Res.* 1989;32:541–555.

118. Blitzer A, Brin MF. The dystonic larynx. *J Voice.* 1992;6:294–297.

119. Hanson DG, Logemann JA, Hain T. Differential diagnosis of spasmodic dysphonia: a kinematic perspective. *J Voice.* 1992;6:325–337.

120. Cannito MP, Kondraske GV, Johns DF. Oral-facial sensorimotor function in spasmodic dysphonia. In: Moore CA, Yorkston KM, eds. *Dysarthria and Apraxia of Speech: Perspectives on Management.* Baltimore, MD: Paul H. Brookes Publishing Co; 1991;205–225.

121. Jacome DE, Yanez GF. Spastic dysphonia and Meigs disease [letter]. *Neurology.* 1980;30:349.

122. Robe E, Brumlik J, Moore P. A study of spastic dysphonia (neurologic and electroencephalic abnormalities). *Laryngoscope.* 1960;70:219–245.

123. Finitzo-Hieber T, Freeman FJ, Gerling IJ, et al. Auditory brainstem response abnormalities in adductor spasmodic dysphonia. *Am J Otolaryngol.* 1982;3:26–30.

124. Tolosa E, Montserrat L, Bayes A. Blink reflex studies in focal dystonias: enhanced excitability of brainstem interneurons in cranial dystonia and spasmodic torticollis. *Mov Disord.* 1988;3:61–69.

125. Cohen LG, Ludlow CL, Warden BS, et al. Blink reflex excitability recovery curves in patients with spasmodic dysphonia. *Neurology.* 1989;39:572–577.

126. Devous MD, Pool KD, Finitzo T, et al. Evidence for cortical dysfunction in spasmodic dysphonia: regional cerebral blood flow and quantitative electrophysiology. *Brain Lang.* 1990;39:331–344.

127. Schaefer SD, Freeman FJ, Finitzo T, et al. Magnetic resonance imaging findings and correlations in spasmodic dysphonia patients. *Ann Otol Rhinol Laryngol.* 1985;94:595–601.

128. Lee MS, Lee SB, Kim WC. Spasmodic dysphonia associated with a left ventrolateral putaminal lesion. *Neurology.* 1996; 47:827–828.

129. Pool KD, Freeman FJ, Finitzo T, et al. Heterogeneity in spasmodic dysphonia: neurologic and voice findings. *Arch Neurol.* 1991;48:305–309.

130. Davis PJ, Bartlett D, Luschei E, Berke GS. Coordination of the respiratory and laryngeal systems in breathing and vocalization. In: Titze IR, ed. *Vocal Fold Physiology: Frontiers in Basic Science.* San Diego, CA: Singular Publishing Group; 1993:189–226.

131. Ludlow CL, VanPelt F, Koda J. Characteristics of late responses to superior laryngeal nerve stimulation in humans. *Ann Otol Rhinol Laryngol.* 1992;101:127–134.

132. Ludlow CL, Schulz GM, Yamashita T, Deleyiannis FW. Abnormalities in long latency responses to superior laryngeal nerve stimulation in adductor spasmodic dysphonia. *Ann Otol Rhinol Laryngol.* 1995;104:928–935.

133. Bielamowicz S, Ludlow CL. Effects of botulinum toxin on pathophysiology in spasmodic dysphonia. *Ann Otol Rhinol Laryngol.* 2000;109:194–203.

134. Bloch CS, Hirano M, Gould WJ. Symptom improvement of spastic dysphonia in response to phonatory tasks. *Ann Otol Rhinol Laryngol.* 1985;94:51–54.

135. Ginsberg BI, Wallack JJ, Srain JJ, et al. Defining the psychiatric role in spastic dysphonia. *Gen Hosp Psychiatry.* 1988;10:132–137.

136. Murry T, Cannito MP, Woodson GE. Spasmodic dysphonia: emotional status and botulinum toxin treatment. *Arch Otolaryngol Head Neck Surg.* 1994;120:310–316.

137. Roy N, Bless DM, Heisey D. Personality and voice disorders: a superfactor trait analysis. *J Speech Lang Hear Res.* 2000;43:749–768.

138. Ludlow CL, Sedory SE, Fujita M. Neurophysiological control of vocal fold adduction and abduction for phonation onset and offset during speech. In: Gauffin J, Hammarberg B, eds. *Vocal Fold Physiology: Acoustic, Perceptual, and Physiological Aspects of Voice Mechanisms.* San Diego, CA: Singular Publishing Group; 1991:197–206.

139. Woodson GE, Zwirner P, Murry T, et al. Functional assessment of patients with spasmodic dysphonia. *J Voice.* 1992;6:338–343.

140. Woodson GE, Zwirner P, Murry T, et al. Use of flexible fiberoptic laryngoscopy to assess patient with spasmodic dysphonia. *J Voice.* 1991;5:85–91.

141. Koufman JA, Blalock PD. Classification of laryngeal dystonias. *The Visible Voice.* 1992;1(3):4–5,19–23.

142. Zwirner P, Murry T, Swenson M, et al. Effects of botulinum toxin therapy in patients with adductor spasmodic dysphonia: acoustic, aerodynamic, and videoendoscopic findings. *Laryngoscope* 1992;102:400–406.

143. Hartman DE, Aronson AE. Clinical investigations of intermittent breathy dysphonia. *J Speech Hear Disord.* 1981;46:428–432.

144. Merson RM, Ginsberg AP. Spasmodic dysphonia: abductor type. a clinical report of acoustic, aerodynamic, and perceptual characteristics. *Laryngoscope*. 1979;89:129–139.

145. Wolfe VI, Bacon M. Spectrographic comparison of two types of spastic dysphonia. *J Speech Hear Disord*. 1976;41:325–332.

146. Zwitman DH. Bilateral cord dysfunctions: abductor type spastic dysphonia. *J Speech Hear Disord*. 1979;44:373–378.

147. Koufman JA, Blalock PD. Diagnosis of spasmodic dysphonia by spectral analysis. *The Visible Voice*. 1992;1(3):6–7,15–18.

148. Watson BC, Schaefer SD, Freeman FJ, et al. Laryngeal electromyographic activity in adductor and abductor spasmodic dysphonia. *J Speech Hear Res*. 1991;34:473–482.

149. Van Pelt F, Ludlow CL, Smith PJ. Comparison of muscle activation patterns in adductor and abductor spasmodic dysphonia. *Ann Otol Rhinol Laryngol*. 1994;103:192–200.

150. Ludlow CL, Naunton RF, Terada S, et al. Successful treatment of selected cases of abductor spasmodic dysphonia using botulinum toxin. *Otolaryngol Head Neck Surg*. 1991;104:849–855.

151. Deleyiannis FW, Gillespie M, Bielamowicz S, Yamashita T, Ludlow CL. Laryngeal long latency response conditioning in abductor spasmodic dysphonia. *Ann Otol Rhinol Laryngol*. 1999;108:612–619.

152. Rontal M, Rontal E, Rolnick M, et al. A method for the treatment of abductor spasmodic dysphonia with botulinum toxin injections: a preliminary report. *Laryngoscope*. 1991;101:911–914.

153. Blitzer A, Brin MF, Stewart C, et al. Abductor laryngeal dystonia: a series treated with botulinum toxin. *Laryngoscope*. 1992;102:163–167.

154. Bidus KA, Thomas GR, Ludlow CL. Effects of adductor muscle stimulation on speech in abductor spasmodic dysphonia. *Laryngoscope*. 2000;110:1943–1949.

155. Titze IR. *Principles of Voice Production*. Upper Saddle River, NJ: Prentice Hall; 1994.

156. Titze IR. Measurements for the assessment of voice disorders. In: Cooper JA, ed. *Assessment of Speech and Voice Production: Research and Clinical Applications*. NIDCD Monograph. Vol 1. 1991;42–49.

157. Giovanni A, Ouaknine M, Guelfucci R, Yu T, Zanaret M, Triglia JM. Nonlinear behavior of vocal fold vibration: the role of coupling between the vocal folds. *J Voice*. 1999:13:465–476.

158. Larson C, Kempster G, Kistler M. Changes in voice fundamental frequency following discharge of single motor units in cricothyroid and thyroarytenoid muscles. *J Speech Hear Res*. 1987;30:552–558.

159. Titze IR. A model for neurologic sources of aperiodicity in vocal fold vibration. *J Speech Hear Res*. 1991;34:460–472.

160. Davies P, McGowan R, Shadel C, Scherer R. Practical flow duct acoustics applied to the vocal tract. In: Titze IR, ed. *Vocal Fold Physiology: Frontiers in Basic Science*. San Diego, CA: Singular Publishing Group; 1993:93–142.

161. Rothenberg M. Acoustic interaction between the glottal source and the vocal tract. In: Stevens KN, Hirano M, eds. *Vocal Fold Physiology*. Tokyo, Japan: University of Tokyo Press; 1979:305–328.

162. Orlikoff RF, Baken RJ. The effect of the heartbeat on fundamental frequency perturbation. *J Speech Hear Res*. 1989;32:576–583.

163. Orlikoff RF. Vowel amplitude variation associated with the heart cycle. *J Acoust Soc Am*. 1990;88:2091–2098.

164. Titze IR, Baken RJ, Herzel H. Evidence of chaos in vocal fold vibration. In: Titze IR, ed. *Vocal Fold Physiology: Frontiers in Basic Science*. San Diego, CA: Singular Publishing Group; 1993:143–188.

165. Scherer RC, Gould WJ, Titze IR, et al. Preliminary evaluation of selected acoustic and glottographic measures for clinical phonatory function analysis. *J Voice*. 1988;2:230–244.

166. Heiberger VL, Horii Y. Jitter and shimmer in sustained phonation. In: Lass NJ, ed. *Speech and Language: Advances in Basic Research and Practice*. Vol. 7. New York, NY: Academic Press; 1982:299–332.

167. Ramig LA, Ringel RL. The effects of physiological aging on selected acoustic characteristics of voice. *J Speech Hear Res*. 1983;26:22–30.

168. Linville SE. Intraspeaker variability in fundamental frequency stability: an age-related phenomenon? *J Acoust Soc Am*. 1988;83:741–745.

169. Wilcox K, Horii Y. Age and changes in vocal jitter. *J Gerontol*. 1980;35:194–198.

170. Horii Y. Jitter and shimmer differences among sustained vowel phonations. *J Speech Hear Res*. 1982;25:12–14.

171. Ramig LA, Scherer RC, Titze IR, et al. Acoustic analysis of voices of patients with neurologic disease: rationale and preliminary data. *Ann Otol Rhinol Laryngol*. 1988;97:164–172.

172. Ludlow C, Coulter D, Gentges F. The differential sensitivity of frequency perturbation to laryngeal neoplasms and neuropathologies. In: Bless DM, Abbs JH, eds. *Vocal Fold Physiology: Contemporary Research and Clinical Issues*. San Diego, CA: College-Hill Press; 1983:381–392.

173. Zwirner P, Murry T, Woodson GE. Phonatory function in neurologically impaired patients. *J Commun Disord*. 1991;24:287–300.

174. Baken RJ. Irregularity of vocal period and amplitude: a first approach to the fractal analysis of voice. *J Voice*. 1990;4:185–197.

175. Herzel H, Steinecke I, Mende W, et al. Chaos and bifurcations during voiced speech. In: Mosekilde E, ed. *Complexity, Chaos and Biological Evolution*. New York, NY: Plenum Press; 1991:41–50.

176. Gleick J. *Chaos: Making a New Science*. New York, NY: Viking Penguin; 1987.

177. Herzel H, Berry D, Titze IR, Saleh M. Analysis of vocal disorders with methods from nonlinear dynamics. *J Speech Hear Res*. 1994;37:1008–1019.

31

Vocal Fold Paralysis

Glendon M. Gardner, MD
Michael S. Benninger, MD

This chapter discusses the presentation, evaluation, and treatment of patients with unilateral or bilateral vocal fold immobility or hypomobility. Some of the surgical procedures will be described in detail; others are covered more completely in other chapters. The chapter begins with a discussion of vocal fold position and then addresses the clinical assessment and treatment of unilateral and then bilateral vocal fold paralysis.

POSITION OF THE VOCAL FOLDS FOLLOWING LARYNGEAL PARALYSIS

Vocal fold position following motor nerve paralysis has been a subject of some controversy. Classic teaching stated that the site of the neurologic injury can be determined based on the position of the vocal fold. The position of vocal folds as traditionally described with various neural injuries is shown in Figure 31–1. With the advent of laryngeal electromyography, recent studies have shown a poor correlation between specific injuries and vocal fold position.[1] Therefore, clinical determination of site of lesion based on vocal fold position alone is often difficult. The following section presents some of the arguments in this controversy.

Unilateral Superior Laryngeal Nerve Paralysis

The superior laryngeal nerve (SLN) provides supraglottic sensation via its internal branch and motor innervation to the cricothyroid (CT) muscle via its external branch.[2,3] Paralysis of the SLN affects vocal fold position by altering CT function. The CT is described traditionally as containing two bellies: the more medial pars recta, which originates on the anterior inferior cricoid cartilage and inserts on the inferior cornua of the thyroid cartilage, and the more lateral pars oblique, which runs obliquely to insert on the inferior border of the thyroid cartilage.[3,4] The action of the CT muscle in an intact larynx is to "tilt the cricoid lamina backward through the cricothyroid joint, thus lengthening, tensing, and adducting the vocal cords."[3] The effect of isolated SLN paralysis on vocal fold positioning has long been the subject of debate, owing in part to imprecise and confusing terminology. Recently, though, a consensus has been evolving in the literature regarding position of the vocal folds following SLN lesion. Canine and human electromyographic and videostroboscopic studies show that, following local anesthesia and/or sectioning of the SLN, the true vocal fold (TVF) on the affected side appears normal at rest. During phonation, due to the unopposed action

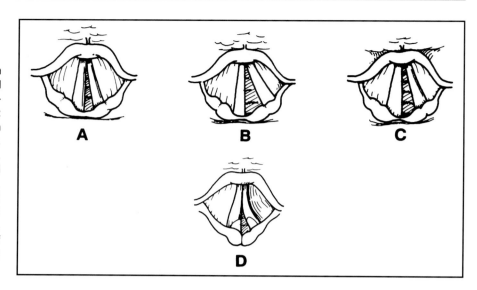

Figure 31–1. Vocal fold position following right sided laryngeal nerve injury as traditionally described. Position during phonation: **A.** Paramedian position. Seen with compensated unilateral RLN injury. **B.** Lateral (cadaveric) position. Seen with combined SLN and RLN injury. **C.** Intermediate position. Seen with poorly compensated RLN injury or well compensated combined SLN and RLN injury. **D.** Isolated SLN injury with shift of posterior commissure to the right and bowing of false vocal fold.

of the contralateral cricothyroid muscle, the anterior portion of the cricoid cartilage is pulled, upward and laterally, toward the intact side. This rocking motion results in deviation of the posterior portion of the larynx to the paralyzed side.[2] Other authors feel that, if the cricothyroid joints are intact, the thyroid cartilage can only move in its natural direction regardless of whether one CT muscle is paralyzed or not, and that no deviation of the thyroid cartilage relative to the cricoid cartilage is possible.[5] The proposed rocking motion is also thought to lengthen the aryepiglottic fold on the intact side and shorten the aryepiglottic fold on the paralyzed side. As a result of the loss of tension on the affected side, the ipsilateral vocal fold may appear wavy during phonation. It may also appear to be at a lower level during inspiration and at a higher level during expiration.[2,4,6,7] Ipsilateral bowing of the true vocal fold, prolapse of the false vocal fold, and altered waveform on videostroboscopy have been reported in a canine study (Elizabeth Ransom, personal communication, 1993) and is also seen in humans shortly after injury[8] (Figures 31–1 and 31–2). Videostroboscopic analysis after lidocaine injection of the SLN in humans reveals moderate traveling wave asymmetry, decreased velocity and excursion of the involved side, and decreased tension of the vocal fold on the involved side.[9]

Clinically, patients with unilateral SLN paralysis are said to be at higher risk of aspiration due to their sensory deficit. Patients with unilateral SLN injury have been reported to suffer from lower pitched, weak, monotonous and easily tired voice[6] (Elizabeth Ransom, personal communication, 1993)

Koufman reported on 26 patients with unilateral vocal fold paralysis and demonstrated with laryngeal

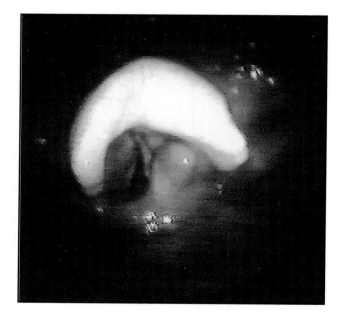

Figure 31–2. Isolated left superior laryngeal nerve paralysis. Note shift of posterior commissure to left and prominence of left false vocal fold.

EMG that the status of the cricothyroid muscle did not influence the vocal fold position.[10]

Bilateral Superior Laryngeal Nerve Paralysis

Not often described, this lesion is said to cause no change in vocal fold positioning due to the symmetric loss of movement with phonation. However, close scrutiny usually reveals a "floppy" epiglottis and vocal folds that are bowed and lower than usual in the membranous portion. An increased risk of aspiration has been suggested, presumably secondary to a loss of supraglottic sensory innervation.[2] Additionally, the patient experiences loss of high pitch.

Unilateral Recurrent Laryngeal Nerve Paralysis

The recurrent laryngeal nerve innervates the lateral cricoarytenoid, thyroarytenoid, vocalis, and aryepiglottic muscles via its anterior branch and the posterior cricoarytenoid and interarytenoid muscles via its posterior branch.[3] Innervation of the interarytenoid muscle is classically described as bilateral, being the only intrinsic laryngeal muscle to receive bilateral innervation. One study suggests that not only does the interarytenoid muscle receive bilateral innervation via the RLN, but that the SLN also contributes to interarytenoid innervation.[8] Unilateral paralysis of the RLN results in nonfunction of all intrinsic laryngeal muscles with the exception of the interarytenoid and cricothyroid muscles. The vocal fold has classically been described as assuming a paramedian position (Figures 31–1 and 31–3). On phonation, the true vocal fold may display apparent active adduction due to the unopposed action of the cricothyroid muscle or the interarytenoid muscle.[2] Vocal fold waveform is often seen on the involved side by videostroboscopic analysis but marked wave asymmetry, lower velocity, and later onset of vibration are seen on the paralyzed side.[9] Breathiness, rapid air escape, and diplophonia are characteristic vocal findings.[4,6,9]

Despite these well-described positions related to unilateral recurrent laryngeal nerve paralysis, clinical determination of site of lesion based on vocal fold position alone is often difficult. Electromyography may be necessary to isolate the site of lesion.

Bilateral Recurrent Laryngeal Nerve Paralysis

With bilateral RLN paralysis, which is occasionally encountered following thyroid surgery, both vocal folds assume the median to paramedian position. Here, too, apparent active adduction results from the unopposed action of the cricothyroid muscles. Symmetric movement is expected, and although incomplete closure may occur, no shifting of the posterior portion of the larynx is seen due to the action of bilateral cricothyroid muscles.

The position of the vocal folds in bilateral paralysis depends somewhat on the site of lesion. Because bilateral paralysis typically is secondary to injury to the two RLNs, the unopposed action of the cricothyroid muscles can result in good approximation and vibration with adduction resulting in good voice. Even if the vocal folds are in a paramedian position, the myoelastic and aerodynamic forces can result in good vocal fold waveform, which is usually symmetric as viewed by videostroboscopy. The lack of activity of both posterior cricoarytenoid muscles results in an inadequate glottic chink for respiration. The rare high vagal bilateral paralysis (usually central paralysis) results in poor closure and a poor airway (Figures 31–4 and

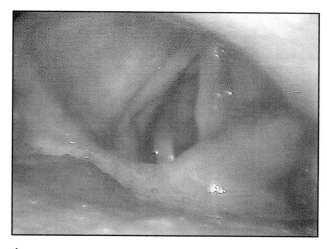

A

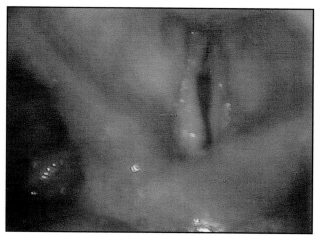

B

Figure 31–3. Right recurrent laryngeal nerve paralysis. **A.** Abduction. **B.** Adduction. Note vocal fold in paramedian position. Vocal fold excursion is greater on uninvolved (*left*) side.

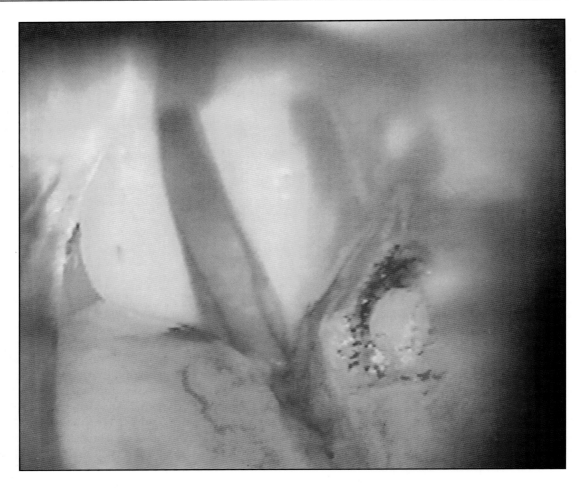

Figure 31–4. Patient with bilateral vocal fold paralysis due to diabetic neuropathy at beginning of right CO_2 laser arytenoidectomy showing initial incision.

31–5) Infants with Arnold-Chiari malformation will present with airway compromise.

Complete Vagal Section (Superior and Inferior Laryngeal Nerve Paralysis)

In instances of complete loss of vagal motor input, the vocal folds have been reported to assume an intermediate or "cadaveric" position.[11] The folds are more lateral than with isolated RLN injury due to the loss of adduction otherwise provided by the cricothyroid muscle when the SLN is intact.[2,9] (Elizabeth Ransom, personal communication, 1993) The authors' recent studies in dogs have shown that, immediately following sectioning of the SLN and RLN on the same side, the vocal fold assumes a paramedian position at rest. With adduction during phonation, the characteristic findings of a shift of the posterior portion of the larynx to the side of lesion and fullness of the false vocal fold

noted with a SLN injury are also seen (Elizabeth Ransom, personal communication, 1993). It is possible that the lateralized position that has been described is due to the long-term effects of a sustained paralysis unlike the more acute effects immediately following injury. When a SLN injury is induced on one side while a RLN injury occurs on the other, the individual effects of the two separate lesions are seen immediately following denervation: the vocal fold assumes a paramedian position on the side of the RLN paralysis and posterior shifting is noted toward the side of the SLN paralysis with attempts at phonation. Long term effects may, however, differ (Figures 31–6 and 31–7). Videostroboscopy may show the vocal folds vibrating at different levels with profound asymmetry of the traveling wave. Loss of vocal fold tension on the involved side with decreased traveling wave velocity and excursion is seen. The uninvolved vocal fold may be positioned higher than the paralyzed fold.[9]

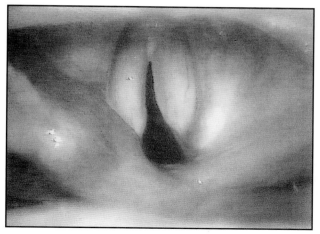

A

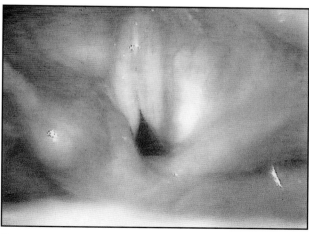

B

Figure 31–5. A different patient with bilateral vocal fold paralysis following thyroidectomy. Patient is status post right laser arytenoidectomy and temporary stitch lateraliza- tion. She had been tracheostomy-dependent due to airway insufficiency and is now decannulated. **A.** Quiet respiration. **B.** Phonation

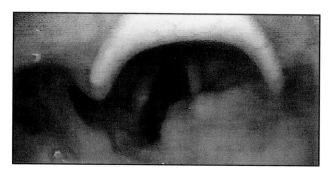

A

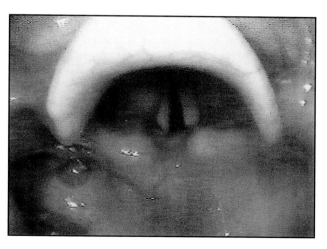

B

Figure 31–6. Poorly compensated right vocal fold paraly- sis 6 months following resection of vagus nerve during skull base surgery. Note lateralized position. **A.** Abduction. **B.** Adduction

EVALUATION OF VOCAL FOLD PARALYSIS

Evaluation of vocal fold paralysis is aimed at deter- mining the cause of the immobility and the severity of the symptoms in order to guide treatment. Often, the cause is obvious, such as a known transection of the nerve with trauma, or during surgery for a malignan- cy involving the recurrent laryngeal nerve. Frequent- ly, the etiology is not readily apparent as in the case of idiopathic paralysis. Furthermore, immobile vocal folds may not be paralyzed.

We will address the presentation for unilateral and bi- lateral vocal fold immobility in separate sections, focus- ing on the many different etiologies for these conditions.

Presentation of Unilateral Vocal Fold Immobility.

Dysphonia is by far the most common presenting complaint for patients with a unilateral immobile vo- cal fold, followed by aspiration and weak cough.[12] The

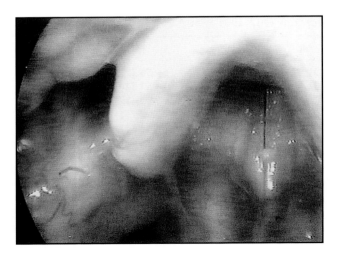

Figure 31–7. Well-compensated, left vocal fold paralysis 12 months following resection of vagus nerve during skull base surgery. Note prominence of left false vocal fold, which is also seen in isolated superior laryngeal nerve paralysis (adduction).

voice is usually characterized as weak and breathy, hoarse or rough. Onset can be noted immediately after extubation following iatrogenic injury to the recurrent laryngeal nerve or after external trauma. Patients with idiopathic vocal fold paralysis often report awakening with a dysphonic voice with a normal voice just the previous day. Other patients will report a slow (days to weeks) gradual onset. These patients are often found to have an enlarging neoplasm (usually malignant) impinging on the RLN or vagus nerve. Patients with SLN motor dysfunction (extrinsic branch) note difficulty with high pitch and aspiration if it is primarily a sensory problem (intrinsic branch).

If the etiology is obvious from the history (thyroidectomy) and the physical examination is consistent (not suggestive of arytenoid dislocation), then no further workup is necessary. A review of previously reported studies suggests that thyroid surgery was once the most common cause of unilateral and bilateral vocal fold paralysis.[13,14] Recently, extralaryngeal malignancies have been found to be the most common cause.[15,16] A review of 251 consecutive cases of vocal fold paralysis (159 unilateral and 92 bilateral) at Henry Ford Hospital has shown that nonlaryngeal malignancies, primarily pulmonary, are the cause of the majority of unilateral paralysis accounting for 25% and for a large percentage of bilateral paralyses[17] (Table 31–1). Treating these underlying causes will occasionally result in return of motion of the vocal fold.

Surgical Trauma

As noted in most early studies, surgery of the thyroid or parathyroid glands was the most common cause of

unilateral vocal fold paralysis. This was due to the intimate relationship of the thyroid vessels and the RLN and SLN. Today, some other surgical procedures that have become more common have also resulted in unilateral vocal fold paralysis. The anterior approach to the cervical spine is a very popular approach to the anterior vertebral bodies from C3 to T1 and results in unilateral vocal fold paralysis in 2% to 7% of cases.[18] Interestingly, the right RLN is injured more often during these cases than the left. This may be due to the shorter course of the right RLN and the resultant less slack in the nerve making it more prone to stretch-induced trauma from retraction.[18]

An increasingly aggressive surgical approach to pulmonary malignancies has made this an increasingly common cause of unilateral vocal fold paralysis. The left RLN is at higher risk due to its more intrathoracic course.

Non-neoplastic pulmonary processes, such as invasive aspergillosis have also been reported to cause unilateral vocal fold paralysis. While this is more common in immunocompromised patients, it can occur in otherwise healthy individuals.[19]

Other Anatomic Causes of Unilateral Vocal Fold Paralysis

Ortner's syndrome, also known as cardiovocal syndrome, consists of a left recurrent laryngeal nerve palsy secondary to cardiac disease such as a dilated left atrium in the case of mitral valve stenosis compressing the RLN against the aortic arch. Other causes include aneurysms of the large intrathoracic vessels.[20]

The high incidence of extralaryngeal malignancies, cardiomegaly, and mediastinal adenopathy as possible etiologies implies that, unless the cause is readily apparent, close vigilance to rule out these causes is necessary. We have found that a thorough history, office laryngoscopy, careful head and neck examination, chest x-ray (CXR), and CT scan or MRI scan from the skull base through the superior mediastinum is a sufficient workup to identify these tumors. MRI or CT of the chest has not revealed unsuspected neoplasms, nor is the routine cost of these procedures justified. Of the 251 patients discussed above, no pulmonary or mediastinal neoplasm that was not noted on CXR was identified, and all surviving patients have had at least 1 year of follow-up.[17] Conceivably, this is because a neoplasm would have to be large enough to be identified by CXR to cause enough external compression of the RLN to result in a paralysis. Some, however, do advocate routine chest CT and esophagram for all idiopathic vocal fold paralyses.[21]

As described earlier, immobility and paralysis are not necessarily synonymous. An immobile fold may

Table 31–1. Cases of Vocal Fold Immobility Seen at Henry Ford Hospital, 1987-1991

Etiology	Unilateral	Bilateral	Total
Nonlaryngeal malignancy	39 (25)*	17 (19)	56 (23)
Idiopathic	37 (23)	14 (15)	51 (20)
Thyroidectomy	16 (10)	16 (17)	32 (12)
Neurologic	14 (9)	12 (13)	26 (11)
Trauma	17 (10)	14 (16)	31 (13)
Iatrogenic (nonthyroidectomy)	19 (12)	5 (5)	24 (9)
Postintubation	6 (4)	11 (12)	17 (7)
Cardiomegaly/thoracic aneurysm	8 (5)	0 (0)	8 (3)
Mediastinal adenopathy/TB	3 (2)	0 (0)	3 (1)
Rheumatoid arthritis	0 (0)	3 (3)	3 (1)
TOTAL	159	92	251

*( ) = %

be secondary to paralysis or cricoarytenoid joint fixation, and at times a paralysis of the recurrent laryngeal nerve may not result in immobility of the vocal fold because of the actions of the uninvolved intrinsic and extrinsic laryngeal muscles. A mechanically immobile arytenoid should be suspected when the problem arises immediately after extubation when the surgery was not likely to injure the laryngeal nerves, after external trauma to the neck, or in the case of severe rheumatoid arthritis. Palpation of the joint in the office or under anesthesia may be necessary. If direct laryngoscopy is done, a dislocated arytenoid can be reduced at the time of endoscopy.[22] Endotracheal intubation can cause true vocal fold paralysis.[23] It is thought that the endotracheal tube cuff in the subglottis (rather than in the trachea) can compress the anterior branch of the recurrent laryngeal nerve where it enters the larynx between the cricoid and thyroid cartilages.[23] Following long-standing unilateral paralysis, some joint fixation may occur.

A unilateral immobile vocal fold due to central neurologic disease is unlikely to be an isolated finding. A complete history and physical examination should reveal other neurologic dysfunction.

The next issue to consider is whether the immobility is permanent or only a temporary paresis or paralysis? Fortunately, laryngeal electromyography (EMG) has been helpful in assessing the innervation of laryngeal muscles. The EMG can be conveniently used to assess the thyroarytenoid and posterior cricoarytenoid muscles innervated by the RLN and the cricothyroid muscle innervated by the SLN. Koufman has developed a workable scale for interpretation of laryngeal EMG in vocal fold paralysis[1] (Table 31–2). Laryngeal muscles do have some dissimilarities to splanchnic muscles, and experience is necessary to be able to make an appropriate evaluation. Furthermore, reinnervation potentials do not necessarily mean that normal vocal fold movement will occur, nor does denervation imply that reinnervation will not take place. However, our experience has shown that the absence of significant recruitment despite signs of reinnervation (polyphasic motor units) at 6 months invariably results in permanent immobility or severe hypomobility, probably due to synkinesis.

The quality of voice with unilateral vocal fold immobility should be assessed and can help in treatment planning. The most important parameter is the patient's perception of his or her own voice quality which can be assessed using the voice handicap index (VHI) questionnaire[24,25] (see chapter 21). The otolaryngologist's and the speech-language pathologist's perceptions are also critical and can be measured systematically for research purposes. Tape recording speech samples helps to assess changes in voice quality over time or with treatment. Objective evaluations that assess voice are numerous and are beyond the scope of this chapter. Nonetheless, certain basic determinations are valuable in the assessment of any voice disorder: perceptual assessment; determination of pitch, range, and perturbation; evaluation of vibration with videostroboscopy; and airflow rates.

Table 31–2. Interpretation of Laryngeal EMG in Vocal Fold Paralysis

Class	Spontaneous Activity	Individual Motor Recruitment	Unit Morphology	Interpretation
I	Absent	Normal	Normal	Normal
II	Absent	Reduced	Polyphasic units	Old injury
III	Present	Reduced	Polyphasic units	Equivocal*
IV	Present	Absent	Fibs, myokimea, etc	Denervation

*In this situation, the EMG may indicate either ongoing denervation or early recovery

The ability to examine the larynx directly with a laryngeal mirror is helpful for a global assessment of the larynx. Flexible fiberoptic nasopharyngolaryngoscopy allows for more specialized evaluation of laryngeal function, particularly during running speech. It allows for sniffing, which maximally stimulates the posterior cricoarytenoid muscles demonstrating the best airway in cases of bilateral vocal fold immobility. Videostroboscopy will help to determine whether normal vocal fold vibration is present; to assess the character, quality, symmetry and excursion of the traveling wave; and, most importantly, to assess closure. Closure is most affected by the various procedures that medialize the immobile vocal fold. In some cases, videostroboscopy can be useful to rule out other pathologies or to help assess for hyperfunctional voice behaviors, and it is critical in the evaluation of post-treatment results. Occasionally, patients with unilateral paralysis without treatment accommodate sufficiently to achieve complete closure and allow return of normal vocal fold vibration, as viewed by videostroboscopy (Figure 31–7). Airflow rates can be indirectly measured utilizing maximum phonation time (MPT), which can be performed in any office setting with a stopwatch or more directly assessed with the aid of spirometry or sophisticated airflow instruments such as the Nagashima Phonatory Function Analyzer. Increased airflow rates and shortened phonation times are expected with unilateral vocal fold paralysis whereas normal values may be seen with bilateral vocal fold paralysis. Fundamental frequency and pitch range decrease with unilateral vocal fold paralysis but may be within normal ranges in bilateral vocal fold paralysis. Caution must be exercised when using such tasks in that compensatory behaviors frequently develop as a result of the disorder, making objective tests difficult to interpret. Compensatory (often hyperfunctional) voice behaviors may persist after surgical intervention and interfere with accurate assessment of treatment results. Retesting following voice rehabilitation will give more accurate determinations of ultimate voice function. Despite these limitations, we feel

that the combination of practitioner and patient perceptual assessment (Voice Handicap Index, VHI), evaluation of pitch range, vocal fold vibratory characteristics (stroboscopy), and airflow rates are all valuable in evaluating a patient with vocal fold immobility and judging the results of therapy. Frequency and intensity perturbations are generally assessed, but may be difficult to interpret, although they have been found to be helpful in some patients.

A further difficulty is determining which patients will compensate for their paralysis even if the immobility is permanent. Despite electromyography showing denervation and in situations where reinnervation is not likely or possible, many patients will compensate satisfactorily for their occupational, social, or avocational needs. This is particularly true in young, otherwise healthy patients with good vocal fold bulk. In such patients, waiting to see if sufficient accommodation will take place under the care and instruction of a skilled speech-language pathologist is indicated. Usually, a 6- to 12-month interval is sufficient although we have seen return of function up to 18 months after injury. In patients with near-aphonia or those having difficulty with aspiration, early intervention is often indicated. Some now proceed with intervention at the time or shortly after major neurologic, base of skull, or pulmonary surgery where significant aspiration and subsequent sequelae are expected.[26] We now recommend such early intervention in selected cases, and some authors advocate voice therapy in virtually all cases of vocal fold paralysis or paresis.[27]

Idiopathic vocal fold immobility presents many difficulties in treatment planning. Is recovery likely to occur? Will return of function be normal or synkinetic, or will the patient accommodate sufficiently? Although the general sense is that idiopathic vocal fold paralyses tend to recover spontaneously, the literature suggests that this may not be the case.[17] In the Henry Ford Hospital series, only 13.5% of unilateral and 21% of bilateral idiopathic paralyses recovered spontaneously. It is likely that both the true rate of idiopathic paralysis and recovery from these insults is greater than would be gleaned from these reports. Havas reported a 75% recovery rate among patients with idiopathic palsies while Ramadan et al reported only a 19% recovery rate in the same population.[28,29] Many temporary idiopathic pareses result in either mild or quickly resolving dysphonias, and the patient does not seek general medical or otolaryngological care.

The real challenge in idiopathic vocal fold paralysis may be in early identification resulting in earlier intervention, which may prevent prolonged or permanent sequelae. It is well accepted that herpetic involvement in cranial nerve injury (such as occurs in herpes zoster oticus) is often polyneuropathic. In otologic/facial nerve herpes infection, systemic steroids and/or an antiherpetic medication may be offered. Such approaches may be applicable to idiopathic vocal fold paralysis if identified early. Anecdotal use of Acyclovir has been reported in the literature.[30] Large, multi-institutional studies may be needed to determine if any efficacy or indication exists.

Once the etiology is determined and recovery is not expected, decisions about potential intervention can be made. At the time of patient presentation, counseling and conservative treatment, such as voice therapy, should begin despite not knowing the etiology.

TREATMENT OF UNILATERAL VOCAL FOLD PARALYSIS

Treatment of unilateral vocal fold paralysis aims at improving voice quality and preventing aspiration. The site of injury (RLN or combined SLN plus RLN), the bulk of the vocal fold, the degree of compensation (see Figures 31–6 and 31–7), the general health and pulmonary status of the patient, and degree of proprioceptive integrity will all play a role in the quality of voice after unilateral vocal fold paralysis. The surgeon must evaluate carefully all these parameters and discuss potential options while weighing the benefits, simplicity, and risks of surgery with the patient and should consult with other members of the voice team prior to proceeding.

The Role of Voice Therapy

Voice therapy is very important in the general treatment of patients with a unilateral vocal fold paralysis. Assessment can help determine the degree or likelihood of accommodation and can assess whether any compensatory behaviors have developed that will inhibit rehabilitation. Many patients may develop hyperfunctional voice behaviors in an attempt to compensate. Such behaviors will be counterproductive to effective vocalization alone or after surgical treatment. Voice therapy alone may provide sufficient improvement in many patients. If surgical intervention is planned, preoperative voice therapy will facilitate postoperative rehabilitation.[27]

Surgical Treatment of Unilateral Vocal Fold Paralysis

Many different techniques are available for treatment of unilateral vocal fold paralysis. In an effort to standardize nomenclature for laryngoplastic procedures, a classification has been developed by the Speech, Voice, and Swallowing Disorders Committee of the American Academy of Otolaryngology-Head and Neck Surgery (AAO-HNS) and adopted by the Board of the AAO-HNS (Table 31–3).

The goal of all surgical approaches to unilateral vocal fold paralysis is to improve closure. We may think of these different procedures as being static, dynamic, permanent, or temporary. The static procedures put the immobile vocal fold in the midline so that the mobile vocal fold may approximate it, whereas the dynamic procedures attempt to restore the motion of the immobile vocal fold, hopefully restoring the glottis to as near-normal a situation as possible. The dynamic procedures all involve reinnervation or electrical pacing of the immobile vocal fold, and the static procedures consist of using some substance to better position the vocal fold. These substances include Teflon, Gelfoam, fat, fascia, Silastic, collagen, hydroxylapatite, Gore-Tex, tissue expanders, and others.

Injection Laryngoplasty (IL)

In the not too distant past, certainly the most commonly performed procedure for the treatment of a paralyzed unilateral vocal fold was Teflon injection into the immobile vocal fold. This may still be the most common procedure performed by general otolaryngologists. Teflon was introduced as a supposedly inert substance that can medialize the vocal fold and can be injected either transorally[31] or transcutaneously.[32] Proper placement is lateral to the vocal process of the arytenoid, deep in the thyroarytenoid muscle (as far lateral as possible, up against the thyroid cartilage) in the midportion (on the vertical axis). In experienced hands, Teflon is a quick and effective way of improving voice.[33,34] It has significant drawbacks, which may have prompted interest in other methods of medialization. These include improper amount (too much) or site of placement (too superficial, too inferior, too anterior), which can result in bolus shifting, and/or

Table 31–3. Laryngoplastic Phonosurgery Classification

A. Laryngeal Framework Surgery (LFS) with

      Arytenoid adduction   (AA)

      Medialization   (M)

      Lateralization   (L)

      Anterior Commissure

            Retrusion (relaxation)   (ACR)

            Protrusion (tensing)   (ACP)

      Cricothyroid Approximation (CTA)

      Medialization laryngoplasty can be qualified by method of medialization

          Medialization laryngoplasty with:

               s - Silastic

               c - cartilage

               e - expander

               o - other

B. Injection Laryngoplasty ((L)

    D - Direct

    I - Indirect

          Injection laryngoplasty with:

               t - Teflon

               g - Gelfoam

               col - collagen

               f - fat

               o - other

    Abbreviations may be used, ie:

      Laryngeal framework surgery with medialization—silastic (LFS-M-s)

      Laryngeal framework surgery with arytenoid adduction (LFS-AA)

      Injection laryngoplasty—direct—Teflon (IL-D-t)

granuloma formation. Even with proper injection, granulomas may occur as Teflon does promote a foreign body reaction.[35,36] The result is often a very stiff, nonvibrating vocal fold and a less than acceptable voice.[37] The surgical removal of Teflon is difficult due to its infiltration into the muscle fibers and is generally ungratifying.[38] Finally, although experienced laryngologists find the results to be predictable, many find that the results are suboptimal. Although other modalities of treatment have pre-empted the use of Teflon, for some it remains an important treatment option. Its ease of use and transoral approach provide effective medialization for patients with significant systemic disease, incurable neoplasms affecting the recurrent laryngeal nerve in individuals where aspiration is the primary problem, or those not requiring subtle voice changes.[12]

Gelfoam, a temporary injectable substance, has been used in patients with acute needs for medialization where vocal fold movement may return and a perma-

nent procedure is not necessarily indicated. It can also be used to help predict results from other permanent injected substances.

Autologous fat has been advocated as an alternative to Teflon.[39,40] The advantage is that it is abundant in supply and is a homograft. The unpredictability of the degree of resorption, concerns over the best methods to harvest and process the fat, and lack of long-term results have prevented more widespread acceptance. Studies in cats suggest that the fat does not last more than 12 months; other studies in dogs shows that it remains viable longer.[41-43] All authors recommend over-injection of the fat. The expected resorption is seen as a drawback for permanent correction of this problem, but may make fat an ideal substance for short-term (6-12 months) improvement when recovery is possible.[44-47]

Collagen is a bioimplant substance that is integrated into host tissues. It is used to provide bulk and soften scar.[48] It has been advocated as a method to medialize vocal fold paralysis, particularly in the face of

mised airway. Bilateral vocal fold paralyses, therefore, almost always require intervention although many patients will delay treatment until they get into trouble or succumb from their underlying disease. Patients frequently have a tracheotomy early in the course of their disease and most patients will have a tracheotomy at some time during their treatment, although some surgeons perform the definitive airway-expanding procedure without doing a tracheotomy. A suture lateralization can be done "early" and tracheotomy be avoided.[98] Most surgeons, however, prefer to first secure the airway with tracheotomy and then consider treatment options to improve breathing and allow for decannulation. One of the difficulties with treating bilateral vocal fold paralysis is that the better the airway, the worse the voice and the greater the risk for aspiration. Thorough preoperative counseling is advisable to prevent unrealistic expectations on the part of the patient. It may be necessary to perform conservative surgery initially so that overeager vocal fold lateralization does not result in significant dysphonia. The patient needs to be cautioned that more than one operation may be necessary to allow both decannulation and quality voice production.

Medical Treatment

Treatment of inflammatory conditions may or may not improve the mobility of the vocal folds.[79,80,99] Therapy will, however, create a more favorable environment for healing with less scarring after surgical repair has been performed. This treatment should be instituted before the surgery takes place.

Systemic steroids will reduce mucosal edema, which can improve the airway short-term, but are unlikely to provide a definitive solution unless the etiology is a connective tissue disorder. If that is the case, long-term steroids may be the treatment of choice and at least one month of steroids should be used. Start with one week of prednisone 1mg/kg/day and then taper. Reassess at the end of the month for a beneficial effect.

Indications for Surgical Intervention

The goal of surgery is to improve the posterior glottic airway. Surgical procedures can be categorized as dynamic, in which the normal mobility of the vocal folds is restored; static conservative, in which the airway is enlarged without irreversibly destroying tissue; and static destructive, in which normal tissue is removed to improve the airway in a static manner. Although the first two methods are preferable, the last category

yields the most consistently adequate airway results, but may adversely affect voice and swallowing. Tracheotomy bypasses the problem entirely.

Not all stenotic airways should be treated surgically. Some patients are only mildly symptomatic. Some are dyspneic only with strenuous exertion. Some are too ill to tolerate surgery or do not have the pulmonary reserve to tolerate any aspiration, which may occur postoperatively. The advantages and potential complications of each procedure must be discussed thoroughly with the patient preoperatively. With several surgical techniques the voice result is very unpredictable, as is the effect on swallowing. Although we consider the need for tracheotomy to be a failure in these situations, some patients would rather keep a tracheotomy than risk any change in voice or dysphagia. The patient must always be advised that keeping or undergoing a tracheotomy is a viable option.

History

Tracheotomy is the oldest surgical treatment of BVFI or PGS. In 1922, Chevalier Jackson removed the entire vocal fold and ventricle, which, although it provided an excellent airway, caused severely breathy dysphonia and aspiration.[100] The King procedure is an open operation in which a mobilized arytenoid is fixed laterally.[101] Kelly and Woodman provided further modifications of King's procedure.[102,103]

Thornell described the first endoscopic arytenoidectomy in 1948.[104] Whicker and Devine reported an initial success rate of 82% in a series of 147 patients treated with Thornell's technique, which improved to 92% when some of the failures underwent a contralateral procedure. They reported a 96% voice preservation rate,[105] although this does not imply a completely normal voice.

Endoscopic Surgery

There are various endoscopic techniques for enlarging the posterior glottic airway in a static manner. These procedures involve excision of tissue at or anterior to the arytenoid so as to gain as much cross-sectional area as possible without disturbing the majority of the membranous vocal folds, which are crucial for voice production.

Ossoff et al described the classic CO_2 laser arytenoidectomy and partial cordectomy in 1983.[106] This procedure involves vaporization of the mucosa overlying the arytenoid cartilage, the cartilage itself, and a portion of the posterior aspect of the membranous vocal fold (see Figures 31–4 and 31–5). The defect must be flush with the inner aspect of the cricoid cartilage. At least the anterior half of the membranous vocal fold remains intact to make contact with the unoperated side. At the end of the procedure, the defect is quite large. Initially, the voice is breathy and the patient may aspirate liquids. As the wound heals, however, the defect contracts considerably and voice and swallowing improve. The airway decreases in area, but in most cases remains adequate for decannulation or relief of symptoms. In 1990, Ossoff et al reported an 86% rate of decannulation in a series of 28 patients.[107]

There have been many modifications of the technique described above. Remacle et al preserve a shell of the posterior aspect of the arytenoid cartilage. They feel that this stabilizes the posterior aspect of the airway, preventing prolapse of the mucosa into the glottic gap. They report excellent airway results in 40 of 41 patients with only 1 posterior synechia and 2 granulomas, which resolved spontaneously. A good or normal voice resulted in 39 of the 41 patients.[75]

Others, including the author, have modified Ossoff's technique by preserving the mucosa along the medial aspect of the arytenoid cartilage.[108] (L. Arick Forrest, MD, personal communication, 1995). This may be sutured laterally after resection of the arytenoid cartilage and a portion of the posterior vocalis muscle and vocal ligament is complete. The final airway result also seems more predictable with this submucosal technique. Some investigators have resected varying portions of the arytenoid cartilage while preserving the mucosa and suturing it laterally.[109,110]

Dennis and Kashima utilize a more conservative procedure for enlarging the posterior airway. A C-shaped portion of the membranous vocal fold is removed with the CO_2 laser just anterior to the vocal process without exposing cartilage. This can be done unilaterally, bilaterally, or in a stepwise manner as need dictates.[111] Eckel et al compared Kashima's technique with Ossoff's and found that both procedures were equally effective in achieving an adequate airway and both affected voice to an unpredictable degree. Partial cordectomy was faster and easier to perform and arytenoidectomy was more likely to cause subclinical aspiration as seen on flexible endoscopic evaluation of swallow (FEES).[112]

Suture lateralization of one immobile vocal fold in BVFI was described by Ejnell as an alternative to tracheotomy in cases where the prognosis is favorable for recovery of activity of at least one vocal fold or as a long-term solution. He and other authors have reported results comparable to those described above.[98,113-116] The procedure is quite easy to perform. While one surgeon observes the larynx via direct laryngoscopy, a second surgeon passes a 16-gauge needle through the thyroid cartilage aiming for just superior to the vocal

process of the arytenoid cartilage and an 0 nylon suture is passed through the needle. The needle is then passed just inferior to the vocal process and the suture threaded by the endoscopist out the needle, taking care not to sever the suture on the needle. The suture is tied tightly enough to achieve the desired airway with the arytenoid rotated to a paramedian position. Voice is minimally affected if the vocal fold is not lateralized too far.[113-116] A lateral position results in a very breathy voice and reoperation with loosening of the suture may be required. No complications are reported. The procedure is reversible should the activity of either vocal fold return.

Suture lateralization has also been combined with standard arytenoidectomy and partial cordectomy procedures. Lichtenberger[117] designed an endo-extralaryngeal needle carrier to facilitate this procedure.

Variations on endoscopic approaches to BVFI are numerous. Linder and Lindholm create a groove along the lateral superior aspect of the true vocal fold including the vocal process with the CO_2 laser. Fibrin glue is injected into the groove to hold the medial aspect of the fold laterally. They report a success rate of 5/9 after one procedure and 8/9 after several. Patients who required bilateral procedures had "breathy but still intelligible voices."[118]

Rontal and Rontal describe a precise lysis of the interarytenoid and thyroarytenoid attachments to the arytenoid cartilage, as well as removal of the vocal process to allow the arytenoid cartilage to move laterally, thereby improving the airway in 8 patients with BVFI. They report 100% success regarding airway and excellent postoperative voices.[119]

Expansion of the posterior glottic airway can be achieved endoscopically by splitting the posterior cricoid lamina with a laser and placing a cartilage graft. Inglis et al report that the procedure is more likely to be successful if only posterior glottic stenosis (PGS) is present rather than both PGS and subglottic stenosis.[120]

Open Surgery

The posterior glottis may be approached via anterior laryngofissure. This provides excellent exposure from the inferior aspect of the cricoid ring to the superior aspect of the arytenoid cartilages. The anterior thyroid cartilage must be divided exactly in the midline at the anterior commissure to avoid disruption of the anterior vocal folds. The posterior cricoid lamina can be easily divided and a rib graft placed, as described above. This has been done successfully by the author for both pediatric and adult cases. Other areas of stenosis are easily addressed at the same time.

Arytenoidectomy may be done via an external approach, either anterior laryngofissure or a lateral approach, with resection of the posterior aspect of the thyroid cartilage and elevation of the piriform sinus mucosa to gain access to the arytenoid cartilage.

Reinnervation

For BVFI due to paralysis of both recurrent laryngeal or vagus nerves, reinnervation of one or both posterior cricoarytenoid (PCA) muscles would be the ideal solution to open the posterior glottis. This would restore laryngeal function with glottic opening on inspiration, without destroying intrinsic laryngeal structures. For the technique to be successful, at least one arytenoid must be passively mobile.

Reinnervation for BVFI was first described by Tucker in 1976 when he mobilized a branch of the ansa hypoglossi and a small block of muscle from the anterior belly of the omohyoid and sutured it to the PCA. His first series of 5 patients was initially 100% successful and in 1989 he reported a 74% success rate in 214 patients with BVFI with a minimum of 2-year follow-up.[121,122] Baldissera et al and Doyle et al reported success in the cat model when using phrenic nerve. Baldissera's group performed two anastamoses involving the phrenic nerve and RLNs to reinnervate both PCA muscles. Reinnervation with restoration of motion was successful in 6 of 6 cats unilaterally and 5 of 6 contralaterally.[123] Doyle et al transplanted the phrenic nerve directly into the PCA of cats and achieved inspiratory abduction of the paralyzed vocal fold in 9 of 12 subjects.[124] Crumley first transferred the phrenic nerve to the omohyoid muscle in 3 monkeys and then transferred the muscle to denervated PCA muscles achieving success in all 3 animals. This study demonstrated the possibility of replacing the PCA if necessary.[125]

Maniglia has investigated reinnervation of the posterior cricoarytenoid muscle with the motor branch of the superior laryngeal nerve and reported good results in an animal model.[126] These procedures are attractive because they do not prevent other treatments and may be reasonable first-line approaches in infants and small children.

Laryngeal Pacing

Laryngeal electrical pacing involves implanting a pacing device similar to a cardiac pacemaker with the electrode inserted in or laid on the PCA muscle. The device triggers with inspiration. One arytenoid must be passively mobile, as with laryngeal reinnervation procedures. The first report of electrical pacing in the human larynx was by Zealear et al in 1996.[127] This patient has also received injections of botulinum toxin A to the thyroarytenoid muscles to improve the airway and has been successful (Mark Courey, MD, personal communication, June, 1999).

Botulinum Toxin A

Cohen and Thompson injected botulinum toxin A (BOTOX) into the cricothyroid muscles of dogs in whom the recurrent laryngeal nerves had been sectioned.[128] They noted that the vocal folds lateralized after injection with an improved airway, and this effect lasted the expected time based on the different doses given.

CONCLUSIONS

Treatment of vocal fold paralysis relies on satisfactory history and voice evaluation, determination of etiology of paralysis, and assessment of compensation and expected recovery. Many patients with unilateral vocal fold paralysis will accommodate satisfactorily for their own voice needs either independently or more usually with the aid of an experienced voice pathologist. In patients where compensation is not sufficient, interventional treatment is necessary. Bilateral vocal fold paralysis presents different problems and requires different solutions.

The type of treatment should be based on the patient's needs, the experience of the physician, and the cost and ease of the procedure. Because this is a rapidly evolving area, the clinician should be aware of the advantages and disadvantages of new techniques as they develop. He or she should be experienced in more than one technique as different situations may require different approaches. Finally, the clinician should evaluate the pre- and postoperative voice and airway results of the procedures used so that he or she can modify approaches based on personal experience and developments in the field.

REFERENCES

1. Koufman JA. Laryngeal electromyography (EMG): clinical applications. *The Visible Voice.* 1993;2:49–53.
2. Levine H, Tucker H. *Surgical management of the paralyzed larynx.* Philadelphia, PA, Saunders 1975.
3. Hollingshead W. *Anatomy for surgeons.* 3rd ed. Philadelphia, PA: Harper and Row; 1982,
4. Bevan K, Griffiths M, Morgan M. Cricothyroid muscle paralysis: its recognition and diagnosis. *J Laryngol Otol.* 1989;103:191–195.
5. Woodson GE. Laryngeal neurophysiology and its clinical uses. [Review] [60 refs]. *Head Neck.* 1996;18:78–86.

6. Abelson T, Tucker H. Laryngeal findings in superior laryngeal nerve paralysis: a controversy. *Otolaryngol Head Neck Surg.* 1981;89:463–470.

7. Hirano M. Surgical anatomy and physiology of the vocal folds. In: Gould W, Sataloff R, Spiegel J, eds. *Voice surgery.* St. Louis, MO: CV Mosby; 1993:135–158.

8. Liancai M, Sanders I, Wu B, et al. The intramuscular innervation of the human interarytenoid muscle. *Laryngoscope.* 1994;104:33–38.

9. Sercarz J, Berke G, Gerratt B, et al. Videostroboscopy of human vocal fold paralysis. *Ann Otol Rhinol Laryngol.* 1992;101:567–576.

10. Koufman JA, Walker FO, Joharji GM. The cricothyroid muscle does not influence vocal fold position in laryngeal paralysis. *Laryngoscope.* 1995;105:368–372.

11. Pressman, Kellman (revised by Kirchner J). *Physiology of the larynx.* Washington, DC: AAO-HNS Foundation; 1986.

12. Gardner GM, Shaari CM, Parnes SM. Long-term morbidity and mortality in patients undergoing surgery for unilateral vocal cord paralysis. *Laryngoscope.* 1992;102:501–508.

13. Maisel R, Ogura J. Evaluation and treatment of vocal cord paralysis. *Laryngoscope.* 1974;84:302–316.

14. Tucker H. Vocal cord paralysis—1979: etiology and management. *Laryngoscope.* 1979;90:585–590.

15. Parnell F, Brandenburg J. Vocal cord paralysis. A review of 100 cases. *Laryngoscope.* 1970;80:1036–1045.

16. Barondess J, Pompei P, Schley W. A study of vocal cord palsy. *Trans Am Clin Climatol Assoc.* 1985;97:141–148.

17. Benninger MS, Gillen JB, Altman JS. Changing etiology of vocal fold immobility. [Review] [15 refs]. *Laryngoscope.* 1998;108:1346–1350.

18. Weisberg NK, Spengler DM, Netterville JL. Stretch-induced nerve injury as a cause of paralysis secondary to the anterior cervical approach. *Otolaryngol Head Neck Surg.* 1997;116:317–326.

19. Nakahira M, Saito H, Miyagi T. Left vocal cord paralysis as a primary manifestation of invasive pulmonary aspergillosis in a nonimmunocompromised host. [Review] [6 refs]. *Arch Otolaryngol Head Neck Surg.* 1999;125:691–693.

20. Thirlwall AS. Ortner's syndrome: a centenary review of unilateral recurrent laryngeal nerve palsy secondary to cardiothoracic disease. *J Laryngol Otol.* 1997;111:869–871.

21. Altman JS, Benninger MS. The evaluation of unilateral vocal fold immobility: is chest X-ray enough? *J Voice.* 1997;11:364–367.

22. Sataloff RT. Arytenoid dislocation: techniques of surgical rduction. *Op Tech Otolaryngol Head Neck Surg.* 1998;9:196–202.

23. Laursen RJ, Larsen KM, Molgaard J, Kolze V. Unilateral vocal cord paralysis following endotracheal intubation. *Acta Anaesthesiol Scand.* 1998;42:131–132.

24. Jacobson B, Johnson A, Grywalski C, et al. The Voice Handicap Index (VHI): development and validation. *J Speech Lang Pathol.* 1997;6:66–70.

25. Benninger MS, Ahuja AS, Gardner G, Grywalski C. Assessing outcomes for dysphonic patients. *J Voice.* 1998;12:540–550.

26. Netterville JL, Stone RE, Luken ES, Civantos FJ, Ossoff RH. Silastic medialization and arytenoid adduction: the Vanderbilt experience. A review of 116 phonosurgical procedures. *Ann Otol Rhinol Laryngol.* 1993;102:413–424.

27. Heuer R, Sataloff R, Emerich K, et al. Unilateral recurrent laryngeal nerve paralysis: the importance of "preoperative" voice therapy. *J Voice.* 1997;11:88–94.

28. Havas T, Lowinger D, Priestley J. Unilateral vocal fold paralysis: causes, options and outcomes. *Aust N Z J Surg.* 1999;69:509–513.

29. Ramadan HH, Wax MK, Avery S. Outcome and changing cause of unilateral vocal cord paralysis. *Otolaryngol Head Neck Surg.* 1998;118:199–202.

30. Benninger MS. Acyclovir for the treatment of idiopathic vocal cord paralysis. *Ear Nose Throat.* 1992;71:207–208.

31. Dedo H. Injection and removal of Teflon for unilateral vocal cord paralysis. *Ann Otol Rhinol Laryngol.* 1992;101:81–85.

32. Strasnick B, Berke G, Ward P. Transcutaneous Teflon injection for unilateral vocal cord paralysis. *Laryngoscope.* 1991;101:785–787.

33. Livesey JR, Carding PN. An analysis of vocal cord paralysis before and after Teflon injection using combined glottography. *Clin Otolaryngol Allied Sci.* 1995;20:423–427.

34. Harries ML, Morrison M. Management of unilateral vocal cord paralysis by injection medialization with teflon paste. Quantitative results. *Ann Otol Rhinol Laryngol.* 1998;107:332–336.

35. Dedo H, Carlsoo B. Histologic evaluation of Teflon granulomas of human vocal cords. *Acta Otolaryngol.* 1982;93:475–484.

36. Lewy R. Responses of laryngeal tissue to granular teflon in situ. *Arch Otolaryngol Head Neck Surg,* 1966;83:355–359.

37. Gardner GM, Parnes SM. Status of the mucosal wave post vocal cord injection versus thyroplasty. *J Voice.* 1991;5:64–73.

38. Netterville JL, Coleman JR, Jr, Chang S, Rainey CL, Reinisch L, Ossoff, RH. Lateral laryngotomy for the removal of Teflon granuloma. *Ann Otol Rhinol Laryngol.* 1998;107:735–744.

39. Mikaelian D, Lowry L, Sataloff R. Lipoinjection for unilateral vocal fold paralysis. *Laryngoscope.* 1991;101:465–468.

40. Brandenburg J, Kirkham W, Koshkee D. Vocal cord augmentation with autogenous fat. *Laryngoscope.* 1992;102:495–500.

41. Saccogna PW, Werning JW, Setrakian S, Strauss M. Lipoinjection in the paralyzed feline vocal fold: study of graft survival. *Otolaryngol Head Neck Surg.* 1997;117:465–470.

42. Wexler D, Gray S, Jiang J, et al. Phonosurgical studies: fat-graft reconstruction of injured canine vocal cords. *Ann Otol Rhinol Laryngol.* 1989;98:668–673.

43. Archer SM, Banks ER. *Intracordal injection of autologous fat for augmentation of the mucosally damaged canine vocal fold: a long-term histological study.* Paper presented at the Second World Congress on Laryngeal Cancer; 1994; Sydney, Australia.

44. Laccourreye O, Crevier-Buchman L, Pimpec-Barthes F, Garcia D, Riquet, M, Brasnu D. Recovery of function after intracordal autologous fat injection for unilateral recurrent laryngeal nerve paralysis. *J Laryngol Otol.* 1998; 112:1082–1084.

45. Burns JA, Kobler JB, Zeitels SM. Microstereo-laryngoscopic lipoinjection: practical considerations. [Review] [15 refs]. *Laryngoscope.* 2004;114(10):1864–1867.

46. Laccourreye O, Papon JF, Kania R, Crevier-Buchman L. Brasnu D. Hans S. Intracordal injection of autologous fat in patients with unilateral laryngeal nerve paralysis: long-term results from the patient's perspective. [Review] [23 refs]. *Laryngoscope.* 2003;113(3):541–545.

47. McCulloch TM, Andrews BT, Hoffman HT, Graham SM, Karnell MP, Minnick C. Long-term follow-up of fat injection laryngoplasty for unilateral vocal cord paralysis. *Laryngoscope.* 2002;112(7 pt 1):1235–1238.

48. Bless D, Ford C, Loftus J. Role of injectable collagen in the treatment of glottic insufficiency: a study of 199 patients. *Ann Otol Rhinol Laryngol.* 1992;101:237–246.

49. Rihkanen H, Reijonen P, Lehikoinen-Soderlund S, Lauri ER. Videostroboscopic assessment of unilateral vocal fold paralysis after augmentation with autologous fascia. *Eur Arch Oto-Rhino-Laryngol.* 2004;261(4):177–183.

50. Belafsky PC, Postma GN. Vocal fold augmentation with calcium hydroxylapatite. *Otolaryngol Head Neck Surg.* 2004;131(4):351–354.

51. Green D, Ward P. The management of the divided recurrent laryngeal nerve. *Laryngoscope.* 1977;100:779–794.

52. Chhetri DK, Gerratt BR, Kreiman J, Berke GS. Combined arytenoid adduction and laryngeal reinnervation in the treatment of vocal fold paralysis. *Laryngoscope.* 1999;109:1928–1936.

53. Tucker HM. Reinnervation of the unilaterally paralyzed larynx. *Ann Otol Rhinol Laryngol.* 1977;86:789–794.

54. Crumley R. Update: ansa cervicalis to recurrent laryngeal nerve anastomosis for unilateral laryngeal paralysis. *Laryngoscope.* 1991;101:384–387.

55. Sercarz JA, Nguyen L, Nasri S, Graves MC, Wenokur R, Berke GS. Physiologic motion after laryngeal nerve reinnervation: a new method. *Otolaryngol Head Neck Surg.* 1997;116:466–474.

56. Isshiki N, Morita H, Okamura H, et al. Thyroplasty as a new phonosurgical technique. *Acta Otolaryngol.* 1974;78: 451–456.

57. Isshiki N. Recent advances in phonosurgery. *Folia Phoniatr (Basel.)* 1980;32:119–124.

58. Koufman JA. Laryngoplasty for vocal cord medialization: an alternative to Teflon. *Laryngoscope.* 1986;96:726–731.

59. Slavitt D, Maragos N. Physiologic assessment of arytenoid adduction. *Ann Otol Rhinol Laryngol.* 1992;101:321–326.

60. Montgomery WW, Montgomery SK. Montgomery thyroplasty implant system. *Ann Otol Rhinol Laryngol.*1997;170(suppl):1–16.

61. Cummings C, Purcell L, Flint P. Hydroxylapatite laryngeal implants for medialization: preliminary report. *Laryngoscope.* 1993;102:843–851.

62. McCulloch TM, Hoffman HT. Medialization laryngoplasty with expanded polytetrafluoroethylene. Surgical technique and preliminary results. *Ann Otol Rhinol Laryngol.* 1998;107:427–432.

63. Cohen JT. Bates DD. Postma GN. Revision Gore-Tex medialization laryngoplasty. *Otolaryngol Head Neck Surg.* 2004;131(3):236–240.

64. Schneider B. Denk DM. Bigenzahn W. Acoustic assessment of the voice quality before and after medialization thyroplasty using the titanium vocal fold medialization implant (TVFMI). *Otolaryngol Head Neck Surg.* 2003;128(6): 815–822.

65. Kraus DH, Orlikoff RF, Rizk SS, Rosenberg DB. Arytenoid adduction as an adjunct to type I thyroplasty for unilateral vocal cord paralysis. *Head Neck.* 1999;21:52–59.

66. Zeitels SM, Hochman I, Hillman RE. Adduction arytenopexy: a new procedure for paralytic dysphonia with implications for implant medialization. [Review] [110 refs]. *Ann Otol Rhinol Laryngol.* 1998;173(suppl):2–24.

67. Gardner GM. Posterior glottic stenosis and bilateral vocal fold immobility. *Otolaryngol Clin North Am.* 2000;33:855–877.

68. Cavo J, Jr. True vocal cord paralysis following intubation. *Laryngoscope.* 1985;95:1352–1359.

69. Holley H, Gildea J. Vocal cord paralysis after tracheal intubation. *JAMA.* 1971;215:281–284.

70. Minuck M. Unilateral vocal cord paralysis following endotracheal intubation. *Anesthesiology.* 1976;45:448–449.

71. Nuutinen J, Karaja J. Bilateral vocal cord paralysis following general anaesthesia. *Laryngoscope.* 1981;91:83–86.

72. Talmi YP, Wolf M, Bar-Ziv J, Nusem-Horowitz S, Kronenberg J. Postintubation arytenoid subluxation. *Ann Otol Rhinol Laryngol.* 1996;105:384–390.

73. Chatterji S, Gupta N, Mishra T. Valvular glottic obstruction following extubation. *Anesthesia.* 1984;39:246–247.

74. Inomata S, Nishikawa T, Suga A, Yamashita S. Transient bilateral vocal cord paralysis after insertion of a laryngeal mask airway. *Anesthesiology.* 1995;82:787–788.

75. Remacle M, Lawson G, Mayne A, Jamart J. Subtotal carbon dioxide laser arytenoidectomy by endoscopic approach for treatment of bilateral cord immobility in adduction. *Ann Otol Rhinol Laryngol.* 1996;105:438–445.

76. Stack B, Ridley M. Arytenoid subluxation from blunt laryngeal trauma. *Am J Otolaryngol.* 1994;15:68–73.

77. Miller F, Wanamaker J, Hicks D, et al. Cricoarytenoid arthritis and ankylosing spondylitis. *Arch Otolaryngol Head Neck Surg.* 1994;120:214–216.

78. Hussain M. Relapsing polychondritis presenting with stridor from bilateral vocal cord palsy. *J Laryngol Otol.* 1991;105:961–964.

79. Saluja S, Singh RR, Misra AK, et al. Bilateral recurrent laryngeal nerve palsy in systemic lupus erythematosus. *Clin Exp Rheumatol.* 1989;7:81–83.

80. Teitel A, MacKenzie C, Stern R, et al. Laryngeal involvement in systemic lupus erythematosus. *Semin Arthritis Rheum.* 1992;22:203–214.

81. Zvaifler N. Neurologic manifestations. In: Schur P, ed. *The clinical management of systemic lupus erythematosus.* New York, NY: Grune & Stratton; 1983:167–188

82. Lewis J, Olsen K, Inwards C. Cartilaginous tumors of the larynx: clinicopathologic review of 47 cases. *Ann Otol Rhinol Laryngol.* 1997;106:94–100.

83. Chang CY. Martinu T. Witsell DL. Bilateral vocal cord paresis as a presenting sign of paraneoplastic syndrome: case report. *Otolaryngol Head Neck Surg.* 2004; 130(6):788–790.

84. Holinger L, Holinger P, Holinger P. Etiology of bilateral abductor vocal cord paralysis. *Ann Otol Rhinol Laryngol.* 1976;85:428–436.

85. Sommer D, Freeman J. Bilateral vocal cord paralysis associated with diabetes mellitus: case reports. *J Otolaryngol.* 1994;23:169–171.

86. Thompson JW, Stocks RM. Brief bilateral vocal cord paralysis after insecticide poisoning. A new variant of toxicity syndrome [see comments]. *Arch Otolaryngol Head Neck Surg.* 1997;123:93–96.

87. Newman DS, Gardner GM, Jacobson B. *Management of laryngospsam in amyotrophic lateral sclerosis.* Paper presented at the 9th Annual Symposium on ALS/MND; 1998.

88. Aronson A. Laryngeal-phonatory dysfunction in closed-head injury. *Brain Inj.* 1994;8:663–665.

89. Griffiths C, Bough D. Neurologic diseases and their effect on voice. *J Voice.* 1989;3:148–156.

90. Job A, Raman M, Gnanmuthu C. Laryngeal stridor in myasthenia gravis. *J Laryngol Otol.* 1992;106:633–634.

91. Tyler H. Neurologic disorders. In: Fried M, ed. *The larynx: a multidisciplinary approach.* Boston, MA: Little, Brown; 1988:173–178

92. Driscoll BP, Gracco C, Coelho C, Goldstein J, Oshima K, Tierney E, Sasaki CT. Laryngeal function in postpolio patients. *Laryngoscope.* 1995;105:35–41.

93. Fukuda H, Kitani M, Imaoka K. A case of hereditary motor and sensory neuropathy with vocal cords palsy and diaphragmatic weakness. *Rinsho Shinkeigaku.* 1993;33:175–181.

94. Lin YC, Lee WT, Wang PJ, Shen YZ. Vocal cord paralysis and hypoventilation in a patient with suspected Leigh disease. *Pediatr Neurol.* 1999;20:223–225.

95. Ahmadian JL, Heller SL, Nishida T, Altman KW. Myotonic dystrophy type 1 (DM1) presenting with laryngeal stridor and vocal fold paresis. *Muscle Nerve.* 2002;25(4):616–618.

96. Donaghy M, Kennett R. Varying occurrence of vocal cord paralysis in a family with autosomal dominant hereditary motor and sensory neuropathy. *J Neurol.* 1999;246:552–555.

97. Manaligod JM, Smith RJ. Familial laryngeal paralysis. *Am J Med Genet.* 1998;77:277–280.

98. Rovo L, Jori J, Ivan L, Brzozka M, Czigner J. "Early" vocal cord laterofixation for the treatment of bilateral vocal cord immobility. *Eur Arch Oto-Rhino-Laryngol.* 2001; 258(10):509–513.

99. Smith G, Ward P, Berci G. Laryngeal involvement by systemic lupus erythematosus. *Trans Am Acad Ophth Otol.* 1977;84:124–128.

100. Jackson C. Ventriculocordectomy: a new operation for the cure of goitrous glottic stenosis. *Arch Surg.* 1922; 4:257–274.

101. King B. A new and function restoring operation for bilateral abductor cord paralysis. *JAMA.* 1939;112:814–823.

102. Woodman D. A modification of the extralaryngeal approach to arytenoidectomy for bilateral abductor paralysis. *Arch Otolaryngol.* 1946;43:63–71.

103. Kelly J. Surgical treatment of bilateral paralysis of the abductor muscles. *Arch Otolaryngol Head Neck Surg.* 1941;33:293–304.

104. Thornell W. Intralaryngeal approach for arytenoidectomy in bilateral abductor vocal cord paralysis. *Arch Otolaryngol Head Neck Surg.* 1948;47:505–508.

105. Whicker J, Devine K. Long-term results of Thornell arytenoidectomy in bilateral vocal cord paralysis. *Laryngoscope.* 1972;82:1331–1336.

106. Ossoff RH, Karlan MS, Sisson GA. Endoscopic laser arytenoidectomy. *Lasers Surg Med.* 1983;2:293–299.

107. Ossoff RH, Duncavage JA, Shapshay SM, Krespi YP, Sisson GA, Sr. Endoscopic laser arytenoidectomy revisited. *Ann Otology Rhinol Laryngol.* 1990;99:764–771.

108. el Chazly M, Rifai M, el Ezz AA. Arytenoidectomy and posterior cordectomy for bilateral abductor paralysis. *J Laryngol Otol.* 1991;105:454–455.

109. Benninger M, Bhattacharya N, Fried M. Surgical management for bilateral vocal fold immobility. *Op Tech Otolaryngol Head Neck Surg.* 1998;9:1–8.

110. Rontal M, Rontal E. Endoscopic laryngeal surgery for bilateral midline vocal cord obstruction. *Ann Otol Rhinol Laryngol.* 1990;99:605–610.

111. Dennis DP, Kashima H. Carbon dioxide laser posterior cordectomy for treatment of bilateral vocal cord paralysis. *Ann Otol Rhinol Laryngol.* 1989;98:930–934.

112. Eckel HE, Thumfart M, Wassermann K, Vossing M, Thumfart WF. Cordectomy versus arytenoidectomy in the management of bilateral vocal cord paralysis [published erratum appears in *Ann Otol Rhinol Laryngol.* 1995 Feb;104(2):119]. *Ann Otology, Rhinol Laryngol.* 1994;103: 852–857.

113. Ejnell H, Tisell LE. Acute temporary laterofixation for treatment of bilateral vocal cord paralyses after surgery for advanced thyroid carcinoma. *World J Surg.* 1993;17: 277–281.

114. Geterud A, Ejnell H, Stenborg R, Bake B. Long-term results with a simple surgical treatment of bilateral vocal cord paralysis. *Laryngoscope.* 1990;100:1005–1008.

115. Hawthorne MR, Nunez DA. Bilateral vocal cord palsy: the alternative to tracheostomy. *J Otolaryngol.* 1992;21: 364–365.

116. Moustafa H, el Guindy A, el Sherief S, Targam A. The role of endoscopic laterofixation of the vocal cord in the treatment of bilateral abductor paralysis. *J Laryngol Otol.* 1992;106:31–34.

117. Lichtenberger G, Toohill RJ. Technique of endo-extralaryngeal suture lateralization for bilateral abductor vocal cord paralysis. *Laryngoscope.* 1997;107:1281–1283.

118. Linder A, Lindholm CE. Vocal fold lateralization using carbon dioxide laser and fibrin glue. *J Laryngol Otol.* 1992;106:226–230.

119. Rontal M, Rontal E. Use of laryngeal muscular tenotomy for bilateral midline vocal cord fixation. *Ann Otol Rhinol Laryngol.* 1994;103:583–589.

120. Inglis AF Jr., Perkins JA, Manning SC, Mouzakes J. Endoscopic posterior cricoid split and rib grafting in 10 children. *Laryngoscope.* 2003;113(11):2004–2009.

121. Tucker HM. Human laryngeal reinnervation: long-term experience with the nerve-muscle pedicle technique. *Laryngoscope.* 1978;88:598–604.

122. Tucker HM. Long-term results of nerve-muscle pedicle reinnervation for laryngeal paralysis. *Ann Otol Rhinol Laryngol.* 1989;98:674–676.

123. Baldissera F, Cantarella G, Marini G, et al. Recovery of inspiratory abduction of the paralyzed vocal cords after bilateral reinnervation of the cricoarytenoid muscles by one single branch of the phrenic nerve. *Laryngoscope.* 1989;99:1286–1292.

124. O'Grady KF, Irish JC, Doyle DJ, Gullane P, Butany J. Effects of medialization laryngoplasty on airway resistance: a pilot study. *Laryngoscope.* 1999;109:419–424.

125. Crumley R. Muscle transfer for laryngeal paralysis: restoration of inspiratory vocal cord abduction by phrenic-omohyoid transfer. *Arch Otolaryngol Head Neck Surg.* 1991;117:1113–1117.

126. Maniglia A, Dodds B, Sorenson K, et al. Newer techniques of laryngeal reinnervation: superior laryngeal nerve (motor branch) as a driver of the posterior cricoarytenoid muscle. *Ann Otol Rhinol Laryngol.* 1989;98:907–909.

127. Zealear DL, Rainey CL, Herzon GD, Netterville JL, Ossoff RH. Electrical pacing of the paralyzed human larynx. *Ann Otol Rhinol Laryngol.* 1996;105:689–693.

128. Cohen S, Thompson J. Use of botulinum toxin to lateralize true vocal cords: a biomedical method to relieve bilateral abductor vocal cord paralysis. *Ann Otol Rhinol Laryngol.* 1987;96:534–541.

32

Management of the Spasmodic Dysphonias

Pamela R. Kearney, MD
Eric A. Mann, MD, PhD
Christy L. Ludlow, PhD

CHARACTERISTICS OF FOCAL DYSTONIAS

The spasmodic dysphonias (SDs) are currently understood to be focal dystonias affecting the laryngeal muscles during speech.[1-3] A dystonia is a syndrome of abnormal muscle contractions resulting in abnormalities in voluntary movement. Other focal dystonias include torticollis, blepharospasm, oral mandibular dystonia, and writer's cramp. [4-9] Each is a chronic, adult-onset, motor control disorder with abnormal levels of muscle tone. Abnormal muscle contractions can occur any time the patient is awake (eg, torticollis[10]), can be exacerbated by other movements involving the cranial musculature (eg, speaking can increase blepharospasm,[7,11]) and may occur only during performance of a particular task (eg, writer's cramp[9]). In each form, certain muscle contractions are affected, which become triggered or exacerbated during volitional movement. In some

forms, long periods of hyperactivity can be observed in a muscle while the patient is at rest.[4,12]

The focal dystonias are often task-specific,[13] that is, muscle tone abnormalities occur only during certain task(s). In oromandibular dystonia, for example, a patient may have jaw opening dystonia during speech, but not during chewing.[14] Similarly, only speech is usually affected in the SDs while laughter and crying are unaffected.[15] These characteristics have contributed to considerable misunderstanding of these patients,[13,16] who were previously thought to have a psychiatric disorder. With progression of the disorder, usually within the first 2 years, additional muscles and/or tasks may become affected. The spasmodic dysphonias are no exception.

DIAGNOSIS OF SPASMODIC DYSPHONIA

The diagnosis of the spasmodic dyphonias is based on symptoms.[17] Patients often first notice their symptoms during a period of increased stress, following an upper respiratory infection, or during a speech performance. The onset may be sudden or gradual. When the onset is gradual, the symptoms often first occur only in certain situations, waxing and waning dependent on stress or speaking demands. The symptoms will generally stabilize within 2 years after onset. In other cases, the symptoms may remain chronic at the initial severity level. Diagnosis is based on the particular type of voice symptoms in speech and the exclusion of other neurologic movement disorders that could account for laryngeal movement control abnormalities. Specific voicing tasks can be used to elicit the characteristics of each type of spasmodic dysphonia. Table 32–1 summarizes the usual speech symptom traits in the spasmodic dysphonias, as well as those of several other closely grouped disorders.

Adductor Spasmodic Dysphonia

Adductor spasmodic dysphonia is the most common of the SDs, comprising approximately 85% of the diagnosed cases. In adductor spasmodic dysphonia, speech is characterized by intermittent voice breaks in the middle of vowels. It is effortful, with strain and sometimes hoarseness, although the essential symptom is voice breaks. These are heard most often in continually voiced sentences, particularly when glottal stops mark word boundaries, such as in "we_eat," or when two voiced sounds occur in sequence within a word, such as "ye_ar" or "d_og." In the sentences, "We eat eels every day," "We mow our lawn all year," and "A dog dug a new bone," the voice breaks are due to rapid hyperadductions of the folds that interrupt phonation. These can be seen on fiberoptic nasolaryngoscopy.[18] During a break, there is a rapid shortening and/or squeezing of the vocal folds resulting in a quick glottic closure, which interrupts airflow through the glottis.

Specialists in this field are in agreement that patients with hyperadduction voice breaks in vowels have adductor SD. However, there is disagreement on whether patients with constant strain and hoarseness without intermittent voice breaks also have SD. Individuals

Table 32–1. Speech Symptoms Characteristic of Each of the Spasmodic Dysphonias

Type of Spasmodic Dysphonia	Voice Symptoms	Speech Materials Used to Test
Adductor spasmodic dysphonia	Voice breaks in vowels More severe cases have can have strained effortful voice with harsh voice	All voiced sentences (eg, "We eat eels every day") Repeated vowels (eg, "ee-ee-ee-ee")
Abductor spasmodic dysphonia	Prolonged voiceless consonants More severe cases can have constantly breathy voice	Sentences or syllables containing voiceless consonants (eg, "The puppy bit the tape" "When he comes home, we'll feed him") Repetitions of the syllables (eg, "see", "key," "he," "tea," and "pea"
Other Types of Dysphonia Vocal tremor: adductor	Regular voice breaks Frequency and intensity modulation at around 5 Hz.	Prolonged vowel (eg. "ah" or "ee") using a speaking voice in the habitual pitch range
Vocal tremor: abductor	Regular breathy breaks resulting in loss of volume during vowels	Prolonged vowel (eg, "ah" or "ee") using a speaking voice in the habitual pitch range
-Hyperfunctional voice	Constantly tight, strained	All voicing tasks are effortful and affected
-Muscular tension dysphonia	Effortful voice with glottal fry or harsh voice	All voicing tasks are affected.
-Breathy dysphonia	Constantly breathy voice	All voicing tasks are affected.
-Psychogenic dysphonia	Increased airflow or elevated habitual pitch	Symptoms abate on distraction, such as counting backwards by sevens.

with voices characterized by constant strain but without discernible voice breaks may be diagnosed with muscular tension dysphonia.[19] During fiberoptic videolaryngoscopy, these patients have anterior-posterior squeezing of the laryngeal inlet and hyperconstriction of the ventricular (false) vocal folds resulting in a "pinhole" appearance during speech. Their constantly tight voice is extremely effortful. Both groups, however, complain of effortful voice production.

A diagnosis of muscular tension dysphonia implies that such patients do not have a neurologic motor control disorder, but rather a functional voice production disorder due to excessive laryngeal tension.[20] However, the neurologic functioning of these patients has not yet been carefully studied. A holistic treatment approach is often used, combining voice therapy and psychological counseling. To date, no studies have determined whether these patients have neurophysiologic abnormalities similar to patients with SD.

Some patients with constantly tight voices may benefit from botulinum toxin injections; others do not. Patients with hyperfunctional voice may have no discernible differences from patients with SD on reports of stress or psychosocial difficulties. Until some objective methods become available for identifying the patients with SDs, it is best to make decisions based on individual patient characteristics. In general, however, the presence of voice breaks in speech should be the diagnostic criterion for adductor SD and administering botulinum toxin injections.

Abductor Spasmodic Dysphonia

Abductor SD is rare, accounting for approximately 15% of patients with spasmodic dysphonia. As in adductor SD, diagnosis is based on speech symptoms. These patients have prolonged voiceless consonants due to difficulties with voice onset following such voiceless sounds as /h/, /s/, /f/, /p/, /t/, and /k/. Some, but not all, patients with abductor SD will also have a breathy voice quality. On fiberoptic laryngoscopy, these patients have excessive and prolonged abduction during voiceless consonants. Vocal fold abduction interferes with closure of the vowel sound that follows. Patients with abductor SD, however, rarely have difficulties with vocal fold adduction for voice onset at the beginning of speech, except when speech begins with a voiceless consonant. Sustained prolonged vowels are usually normal, except in very severe cases who may have a breathy voice quality. The laryngeal gesture of producing partial glottal opening for a voiceless consonant with airflow (such as for /h/), followed by rapid adduction for a vowel, is particularly difficult for these patients.

To examine for symptoms of abductor SD, the patient's speech should be compared during voiced sentences such as "We mow our lawn all year," which should contain few abnormalities, with sentences containing a high proportion of voiceless consonants such as "The puppy bit the tape" and "When he comes home we'll feed him." Syllable repetitions can also be used comparing repetitions of "ee-ee-ee-ee-ee" with the vowel separated by glottal stops, which is relatively unaffected in abductor SD, to repetitions the same syllable containing a voiceless consonant such as "pea,""tea," "key," or "see," which is likely to be affected. In more severe cases, patients with abductor SD may have a breathy voice quality along with voiceless consonant prolongations.

Difficulties and disagreements can occur, however, concerning patients with constant breathiness or whispering dysphonia. Some patients with whispering dysphonia actually have a psychogenic dysphonia and are most appropriately managed using voice therapy.[21-23] These patients whisper constantly and do not have any greater difficulty with sentences that contain a high proportion of voiceless consonants than with those containing all voiced segments. Referral to a social worker, psychologist, or psychiatrist to examine the patient for any emotional basis for the voice disorder can sometimes be helpful. Some individuals, however, also have emotional stresses that are unrelated to their disorder.

Another confounding factor may be neurologic diseases that affect vocal fold movement control. We have had patients who initially were diagnosed as having abductor spasmodic dysphonia who later developed additional neurologic problems and were subsequently diagnosed as having Parkinson's disease. It is difficult to know whether the voice symptoms were an early manifestation of Parkinson's disease or a separate disorder.

Mixed Adductor and Abductor Spasmodic Dysphonia

Although extremely rare, a few patients have symptoms of both adductor and abductor SD. Diagnosis is made similarly to the pure adductor and abductor SDs, except that these patients will have difficulty with both types of tasks. Correct diagnosis is important, however, as it has implications for predicting treatment response. Mixed patients are difficult to treat as botulinum toxin injections can produce side effects with no benefit. In our experience, thyroarytenoid injections produce breathiness that exacerbates the disorder and posterior cricoarytenoid injections may provide little benefit.

Spasmodic Dysphonia with Tremor

Patients with adductor SD often have an associated tremor producing regular voice offsets, cyclic reductions in voice amplitude, or fundamental frequency. Tremor often is most evident in the speaking range and may disappear at higher pitch ranges. Identification of adductor tremor when mixed with adductor SD is important for predicting treatment following botulinum toxin injection. Frequently, these treatments will reduce the adductor spasms but not control the tremor, which then becomes more evident.[24] This may be due to differences in pathophysiology underlying the two types of symptoms; that is, reducing muscle activation seems to have a role in the reduction of adductor spasms but may have less effect on adductor tremor.

Additional Dysphonias to Consider

Voice Tremor

Voice tremor can occur in isolation as well as in combination with adductor or abductor SD. Sometimes a patient with voice tremor is thought to have adductor SD because the tremor causes voice breaks in vowels during speech. However, when the patient is asked to produce a prolonged vowel, the regularity of the glottal stops or frequency and amplitude variations can be heard, usually around 5 Hz.[25] It can best be detected on prolonged vowels when regularly spaced voice breaks or modulations in frequency and intensity are heard. This disorder affects women more often than men and may be a familial form of benign essential tremor. It occasionally appears in younger women in their twenties and remains a chronic disorder throughout life without progression. Frequently, however, it first appears in late middle age. Like the dystonias, tremor can be focal, affecting the muscles only in the vocal folds, and task-specific, occurring only during voicing. Treatment with botulinum toxin injections into the thyroarytenoid muscles is most effective when the disorder is both focal and task-specific. In one series, 60% of patients received benefit.[26] When the patient also has head tremor, laryngeal injections have limited effect. When many regions of the vocal tract are affected, such as the ventricular folds, posterior pharynx, or soft palate, botulinum toxin injections may not noticeably benefit the voice; however, the patient may experience reduced effort when speaking. Beta blockers, such as propanolol, also can be used in these patients in conjunction with botulinum toxin injection but have little measurable voice effect. A trial of methazolamide was disappointing in patients with vocal tremor.[27] Thus far, no pharmacologic trials have reported benefits in a series of voice tremor patients.

Recent reports of deep brain stimulation in the thalamus have benefited a few patients with vocal tremor.[28-39] These are preliminary reports in patients with tremor affecting many body regions. It is encouraging, however, that some benefit was found for the voice. These reports may also provide some insight into the mechanisms involved in tremor pathophysiology, at least in some patients.

Although much more rare, abductor tremor produces periodic breathy breaks in phonation and can be easily detected in prolonged phonation. This can occur in association with abductor spasmodic dysphonia or in isolation. On fiberoptic nasolaryngoscopy during prolonged vowels, the vocal folds have regular abductions during phonation, producing either regular reductions in amplitude and/or increases in fundamental frequency. This disorder is probably the most difficult to manage; botulinum toxin injection into the posterior cricoarytenoid muscle is usually of limited benefit and recurrent nerve surgery is not appropriate. We have seen patients who have undergone bilateral thyroplasty with limited benefit.

Psychogenic Voice Disorders

Although our voice team involves a multidisciplinary group, in most instances the final consensus regarding diagnosis depends mainly on the voice symptoms. We have found that patients who report intermittent symptoms with intervals of normal voice often have psychogenic dysphonias. Although symptoms in the SDs usually vary in severity dependent upon stress and fatigue, the symptoms rarely disappear entirely without intervention.[31] Patients with psychogenic dysphonia may also exhibit pitch switching; that is, their voice may become high-pitched for several minutes or hours at a time and then return to normal.

A patient profile in psychogenic voice disorders may include: (1) indifference to voice symptoms; (2) referral to one's different voices as independent of one's self with statements like, "See, it came again"; (3) habitual dependence on someone else to speak for them; and (4) a history of abuse or emotional crises in childhood that they were unable to resolve. Voice therapy aimed at teaching the patient how to produce a normal voice in a supportive, nonthreatening manner can be effective.

However, none of these observations is without exceptions. Some patients with adductor or abductor SD report that, after they first experienced symptoms, they abated for a year or two, then returned, and progressed. Further, many patients with SD have family and life events as devastating as those of patients with psychogenic dysphonia. Some patients with SD develop anxiety as a result of having a voice disorder which then abates with treatment.[32] On the other hand, some patients may have an unrelated psychiatric disturbance that should be treated concurrently with management of their voice disorder.[33]

Compensatory Speech Patterns

Patients with SD sometimes use compensatory techniques to communicate with less effort. Patients with adductor SD, for example, may speak in a whisper to have greater control with less effort. When a patient presents with a whispering aphonia, therefore, it is important to ask them to attempt to speak with voice. The more typical symptoms of adductor or abductor SD may then emerge. Others speak on inhalation, which opens the glottis, to overcome the hyperadduction and produce voice more easily. During testing, such patients should be encouraged to speak on exhalation to allow symptom evaluation. The muscular tension symptoms that some patients with SD develop in all likelihood began with an attempt to control the intermittent hyperadductions. This is often seen in voice tremor as well. Some patients with adductor SD learn to initiate speech with an /h/ to avoid hyperadduction of the folds. Similarly, patients with abductor SD may initiate voice with a glottal stop or anterior-posterior squeeze of the ventricular folds to prevent breathy interruptions. During evaluation, patients with mixed adductor and abductor symptoms should be asked to describe which techniques they were taught in therapy or what strategies they have developed to manage their symptoms when they are in situations where intelligible speech is essential.

Compensatory techniques can also interfere with symptom management. Patients may continue to use their compensatory techniques after botulinum toxin injection, which may interfere with the treatment result. When a patient has been using it for many years, speaking on inhalation is a compensatory technique that often requires voice therapy to reverse.

PATHOPHYSIOLOGY

For many years, spasmodic dysphonia was considered a psychological disorder. This idea was reinforced by the absence of symptoms in many patients with SD while laughing, singing, or following sedation with barbiturates.[15,34] Furthermore, many pa-

tients with SD who underwent psychological evaluation were thought to have an underlying emotional conflict or psychological disorder as the cause of their symptoms.[35] In recent years, however, abnormalities in various neurologic reflex responses in patients with SD[36,37] and the association of SD with other focal dystonias have shown that SD is, in fact, a neurologic disorder.[1] Psychological disorders such as depression, anxiety, and somatization appear to be more common in patients with SD when compared to control subjects.[38] However, these disorders may be a response to the debilitating voice effects of SD on social interactions and job performance, because these often resolve following successful treatment for SD.[32,38]

The name of the spasmodic dysphonias was changed in the early 1980s from spastic dysphonia to spasmodic dysphonia when bursts were observed in the laryngeal muscles during interruptions in phonation in a patient with SD.[39] Systematic studies of patient groups with SD, however, did not show the expected pattern of muscle tone abnormalities of increased thyroarytenoid activity in adductor SD and increased posterior cricoarytenoid activity in abductor SD. Schaefer et al[40] found greater variation of muscle activity in patients with adductor SD than in control subjects but no clear pattern of activation abnormality. The results differed across speech tasks with the greatest variation in thyroarytenoid levels found in the patients on repeated word and sentence tasks. To further investigate physiological differences in laryngeal muscle activity in adductor and abductor SD, Watson et al[41] examined thyroarytenoid and posterior cricoarytenoid muscles during sustained /i/ and /s/ productions. Some patients with adductor SD had normal levels of thyroarytenoid (TA) activity whereas some patients with abductor SD had higher levels of thyroarytenoid activity than the patients with adductor SD or the controls. Another study examined untreated adductor and abductor SD patients[42] during repetition of syllables that were particularly difficult for patients with SD: "ee" repetition with glottal stops between vowels (for adductor SD) and the syllable "see" (for abductor SD). Intrinsic (thyroarytenoid, cricothyroid and posterior cricoarytenoid) and extrinsic (thyrohyoid and sternothyroid) laryngeal muscles were measured while the patients produced the syllables, albeit with considerable difficulty. None of the EMG measures differed from normal in either patient group. The results suggested that the patients were using a normal pattern of muscle activation for speech and that voice breaks were due to the *intrusion* of spasmodic bursts overlaid on a normal muscle activation pattern.

Adductor Spasmodic Dysphonia

Nash and Ludlow[43] compared laryngeal muscle activity during speech with and without voice breaks and found increased levels of thyroarytenoid activity only during breaks in adductor spasmodic dysphonia. A nonsignificant trend for an increase in the cricothyroid muscle during speech breaks was also found. Thus, the abnormality in SD was not an overall abnormal level of muscle tone but rather the intrusion of spasmodic muscle bursts on an otherwise normal pattern of muscle recruitment.

When laryngeal muscle activity was studied in patients with adductor SD before and after botulinum toxin injection,[44] the investigators counted the number of spasmodic bursts in unidentified electromyographic recordings from the thyroarytenoid and cricothyroid muscles in normal controls and patients with adductor SD before and after treatment. The number of bursts was greater in the thyroarytenoid muscles in the patients. After treatment, the number of bursts was reduced both in the treated and untreated muscles. Further, the initial numbers of bursts and the change in bursts correlated well with the frequency of voice breaks pretreatment and their reduction after treatment. The problem in SD, then, is the intrusion of involuntary muscle bursts that account for the numbers of voice breaks before and after injection of botulinum toxin.

Neurophysiologic studies have addressed which mechanisms could be involved in the generation of spasmodic muscle bursts. The laryngeal adductor reflex is elicited by electrical stimulation of the superior laryngeal nerve.[45] With this specific type of stimulation, two separate responses have been noted in the thyroarytenoid muscle: an ipsilateral R1 response is followed by a later bilateral response, the R2. This reflex can be elicited by a single stimulus, but when stimuli are presented in pairs with short intervals between them, responses to the second stimulus are reduced in amplitude. This is known as a conditioning effect and demonstrates the presence of normal inhibitory mechanisms responsible for the control of these reflex responses.[36] Normally, central suppression of adductor responses to repeated stimuli may allow speakers to produce voice without eliciting reflexive spasms that could disrupt speech. Studies of patients with adductor spasmodic dysphonia have demonstrated that these conditioning effects are absent or reduced in most patients with adductor SD.[36] In a later study of abductor SD, similar abnormalities were found for a group of patients with abductor SD, although the abnormality was not quite as consistent as in adductor SD.[37]

Abductor Spasmodic Dysphonia

Only a few studies have examined the pathophysiology of this rare type of SD. In a clinical study of 10 patients with abductor SD, spasmodic bursts were found in a variety of muscles associated with prolonged voice offsets. Six of the patients had spasmodic bursts in the cricothyroid muscle; only a few had spasms in the posterior cricoarytenoid muscle. Many had simultaneous spasms in several muscles; the thyroarytenoid, posterior cricoarytenoid, and cricothyroid. One patient did not have spasmodic bursts in any muscle but rather a lack of activity was noted during phonation in the thyroarytenoid muscle. In another study,[41] a patient with abductor SD had higher levels of thyroarytenoid activation than either the controls or the patients with adductor SD.

The results to date, therefore, have been much less clear-cut in abductor SD than in adductor SD. Difficulties have included the lack of a clear-cut diagnosis, rarity of patients, and difficulty accessing the posterior cricoarytenoid muscle. One study compared thyroarytenoid, cricothryoid, and posterior cricoarytenoid muscle activity in patients with abductor SD with controls during speech breaks and in similar speech without breaks.[47] Levels of thyroarytenoid muscle activity were increased on the right side only in the patients. These findings corresponded with reduced left-sided movement in the patients during speech. This finding suggests that the voice is unstable both for initiating and sustaining phonation because of tension differences between the two sides of the larynx.

Vocal Tremor

Only a few studies have examined laryngeal muscle activity in voice tremor. Tomoda et al[48] studied the thyroarytenoid muscle in two patients and found tremor bursts associated with exhalation and phonation. They proposed that the tremor was activated during the expiratory part of the respiratory cycle. Koda and Ludlow[25] examined laryngeal muscle tremor in both intrinsic and extrinsic laryngeal musculature during inspiration, expiration, phonation, and whisper. A variety of muscles were affected with tremor bursts in the patients studied. Tremor occurred most frequently during phonation and less during inspiration. Although tremor was correlated between muscles on the right and left sides of the larynx, the sides were often out of phase by as much as 20 ms. The mechanism responsible for tremor generation is unknown but the recent results with thalamic stimulation suggest that the thalamus may be one part of the circuit.[28,29]

RISK FACTORS FOR THE DEVELOPMENT OF SPASMODIC DYSPHONIA

SD is an idiopathic disorder, that is, the cause and risk factors for the development of the disorder are unknown. Genetic studies have identified a gene mutation involved in the development of idiopathic torsion dystonia,[49] which usually begins in childhood. Some of the family members have only SD,[50] indicating that SD may be related to idiopathic torsion dystonia. Cases of familial spasmodic dysphonia are rare, however, and no associated genetic locus for SD has been found at the present time, as is the case for other focal dystonias.[51] There has been a single case report of a patient with an action myoclonus of the hands and arms and spasmodic dysphonia who had an A to G transition at nucleotide 8344 in mitochondrial DNA.[52] Current thinking, however, is that the pathogenesis of some focal dystonias is the result of a weak genetic predisposition interacting with acquired factors later in life. Some of the acquired factors may include head injury, chronic drug exposure, or peripheral injuries,[53] as well as a viral infection or life stress. Schweinfurth, et al[54] found in a retrospective case series that 65% of the patients with SD previously had the mumps or measles compared with a national average of 15% in a similar age group. They also found that 30% of patients associated the onset of their SD with an upper respiratory tract infection and 21% with a major life stress. Some factors reported associated with the onset of other focal dystonias include overuse in hand cramps,[13] pain following injury,[55] or extensive dental work in oral mandibular dystonia.[56] Patients with spasmodic dysphonia often have a higher incidence of other movement disorders.[1,34] Schweinfurth, et al[54] reported that 26% of the patients with SD had a concurrent essential tremor compared with 4% of first degree relative controls, while 11% had writer's cramp compared with 4% of the relatives. We have seen some patients who report onset following laryngeal surgery although the presence of SD prior to surgery could not be eliminated.

MANAGEMENT OF SPASMODIC DYSPHONIA

Currently, treatments for spasmodic dysphonia are only aimed at symptom reduction and do not alter the underlying central nervous system disorder. Until more is known about the underlying neurologic disorder, treatments cannot be expected to reverse it. The symptoms can, however, be managed. Several different treatment strategies have been employed in an attempt to control or reduce the speech symptoms of these patients.

The available treatments include both medical and surgical options. Among the medical options is botulinum toxin injection, the most commonly used SD treatment and for those with adductor SD, the most successful. Voice therapy can be useful to assist patients in developing strategies to decrease the symptom effects on their lives. Unfortunately, neuropharmacologic agents have been less consistent in assisting large numbers of these patients. Surgical strategies would be ideal if they could provide permanent relief from symptoms without a concomitant disability. The most frequently described procedures are recurrent laryngeal nerve section and avulsion. Many surgically treated patients have an eventual recurrence of symptoms and thus have both SD and a vocal fold paralysis; as a result, several other experimental surgical procedures have been described.

Medical Management of Spasmodic Dysphonia

Botulinum Toxin Injection

Botulinum toxin is a protease that induces chemical denervation by preventing the release of acetylcholine at neuromuscular junctions, resulting in a flaccid paralysis of the muscles. There are eight known serotypes—A, B, C1, C2, and D through G, each with a unique antigenicity and site of action.[57] Only botulinum toxin serotypes A and B are commercially available. Serotype A is marketed as BOTOX in the United States and Dysport in Europe. Clinical studies in humans indicate that BOTOX is more potent than Dysport on a per unit basis. However, there is no consensus in the literature regarding the relative potencies of the two formulations, with reported BOTOX: Dysport conversion factors ranging from 1:5 to 1:2.41.[58] All further references to botulinum toxin dosages in this chapter refer to the BOTOX formulation. Less commonly used is botulinum toxin serotype B, marketed as Myobloc. Currently, the most common use of Myobloc is in patients who have developed an apparent resistance to serotype A.

The first therapeutic use of botulinum toxin was by Dr. Alan Scott, an ophthalmologist, who reported benefit following injection of the extraocular muscles for the treatment of strabismus.[59,60] It was found that abnormalities due to muscle imbalances could be corrected for up to 3 months. Because of subsequent reinnervation of end plates, the denervation is only temporary and the symptoms return when muscle function returns. In 1985, successful treatment of patients with blepharospasm[61] and torticollis[62] demonstrated the potential for use in treatment of focal dystonias. The first reports in spasmodic dysphonia were in 1987 by Miller et al[63] and by Blitzer et al.[64] Miller and his associates used large unilateral injections (35 mouse units) into the thyroarytenoid muscle; Blitzer et al used much smaller bilateral thyroarytenoid injections of between 2.5 and 3.5 mouse units.[64]

Although not specifically approved by the Food and Drug Administration (FDA) for use in SD, botulinum toxin has been recognized by the American Academy of Otolaryngology-Head and Neck Surgery as a primary therapy for patients with this disorder.[65] In fact, botulinum toxin injection has become the treatment of choice for adductor SD, mainly because it is transient and less costly than surgery.[66] Rather than surgical approaches that permanently alter the larynx and produce neural or structural injury, patients can select botulinum toxin treatment without risk of a permanent alteration to their larynx. Its temporary nature is also the primary disadvantage of this treatment. The patient will benefit during the denervation phase but will have symptoms return following reinnervation. Reinjection is usually required every 4 to 5 months making treatment costly in the long run.

Effects and Side Effects. Often patients report some reductions in voice breaks by 48 hours and sometimes a reduction in effort as early as 6 to 12 hours after injection. Usually, however, no overt changes are noted for 48 to 72 hours. The effects of the toxin can continue to increase up to 7 days after injection, probably because of diffusion of the toxin through the muscle. This may be why some patients with adductor SD report that their voice is best 3 days after an injection into the thyroarytenoid muscle, followed by the onset of breathiness and other side effects by 5 days.

Because of the resultant motor weakness in the injected vocal fold, the most common side effect for adductor SD patients is breathiness. It can last 1 to 2 weeks and may be more pronounced following bilateral injections, particularly in males with mild to moderate symptom severity. Difficulty swallowing liquids is also commonly seen; however, the dysphagia usually dissipates in 3 to 5 days. During the affected time period, patients should be advised to sip through a straw and to avoid attempting to swallow liquids quickly.

Fortunately, the side effects can often be minimized with lower dosing, but this may be a tradeoff as the duration of intended duration of effects may also be shortened. The dosage-side effect profile is very individual among patients, with women often tolerating a larger dosage than men. Larger dosages (15–20 Units unilaterally, 4 Units bilaterally) can sometimes be administered in more severely affected women without the risk of significant side effects such as swallowing difficulties for liquids and breathiness. However, caution is advised in treating men. Often dosages greater than 15 Units unilaterally or 2 or 2.5 Units bilaterally can result in significant side effects, aspiration of liquids and prolonged voice loss for several weeks in men. This may be because the larger cartilages in the male larynx have different biomechanical effects following muscle denervation.

Injection Techniques. Currently, most laryngologists use electromyographic (EMG) guidance. The patient is grounded and a hollow, Teflon-coated hypodermic needle with a bared tip and hub is used as a monopolar electrode with a surface reference electrode at the skin. The needle hub is connected to one pole of a physiologic amplifier and the reference electrode to the other. The hypodermic needle is connected to a syringe filled with a solution of botulinum toxin diluted 25 Units per 1 milliliter of saline. The physiologic amplifier is connected to an oscilloscope and an audio speaker for visual and auditory monitoring of electrode activity. Once the electrode is thought to be in muscle, the patient is asked to perform a verification gesture. For the thyroarytenoid muscle (TA), this is a repeated /i/. For the cricothyroid (CT) muscle, the patient is asked to do a glide, with the muscle becoming active in the higher registers. The posterior cricoarytenoid (PCA) is activated during a sniff gesture and will be suppressed with swallowing. If a noticeable increase in muscle activity is observed during the verification gesture, then it is assumed that the electrode is in the appropriate location for injection of botulinum toxin.

Different techniques are used to approach the laryngeal muscles commonly injected with botulinum toxin. The percutaneous approach is perhaps the most commonly used to inject the TA muscle. The needle is inserted through the cricothyroid membrane between the cartilages and angled superiorly and slightly laterally into the body of the fold following the procedures described by Hirano and Ohala for locating and verifying placement in the thyroarytenoid muscle.[67] A transcartilaginous approach estimates that the anterior commissure of the vocal folds is midway between the thyroid notch and the inferior edge of the thyroid cartilage. A 27-gauge needle is placed directly through the thyroid cartilage 5 mm inferior and 5 mm lateral to this point.[68] Ford, et al[69] used a specially designed curved pharyngeal injector placed perorally to indirectly inject botulinum toxin into the superior-lateral aspect of the vocal folds. This technique requires topi-

ficial,[120] but others have suggested that this may be because he is seeing patients with psychogenic overlay.[121] Voice therapy, however, might be beneficial to patients with SD in gaining greater insight into their voice production control difficulties. At present, we recommend a trial of voice therapy for the following types of patients with SD:

1. patients with mild intermittent symptoms of adductor SD;
2. patients with a psychogenic dysphonia, psychogenic overlay, or symptom exaggeration;
3. patients requesting assistance with increasing benefit duration following botulinum toxin injection; and
4. patients with abductor SD receiving limited benefit from botulinum toxin injections.

We currently do not recommend voice therapy for patients with voice tremor or previously untreated patients with moderate to severe adductor SD without compensatory overlay, as they are usually not able to benefit from voice therapy. Until they have had some symptom reduction by botulinum toxin injection, voice therapy is only frustrating and could produce a negative attitude toward therapy postinjection when they might be able to benefit.

One of the greatest difficulties with voice therapy for patients with SD is the difficulty with patient compliance. With treatment alternatives such as botulinum toxin injection that offer more immediate symptom control, voice therapy can be an unattractive alternative.

Neuropharmacologic Therapy

No controlled studies to date demonstrate effective symptom control in SD or vocal tremor using neuropharmacologic agents. However, clinicians often have individual patients who have reported or evidenced significant symptom relief in an unblinded trial. Propranolol (Inderal), a beta-blocker, has been used in treating voice tremor patients to "blunt" the tremor but not significantly reduce it. Trihexyphenidyl HCl (Artane), an anticholinergic, has some benefit when patients have a severe dystonia. Benztropine mesylate (Cogentin), also an anticholinergic, has provided some patient benefit but little symptom change. Baclofen (Liorsal), a muscle relaxant, has provided some relief in a few individuals but has not significantly eliminated symptoms in patients with SD. Many patients are prescribed diazepam (Valium), a CNS depressant with muscle relaxant effects, or alprazolam (Xanax), a benzodiazepine, to reduce stress resulting

from the effects the disorder has on their daily lives. Many of these agents, however, have significant side effects such as impairment of cognition or dry mouth.

In general, the role of neuropharmacologic agents in SD has been to provide some patient relief without any demonstrable symptom reduction. Often positive responses are idiosyncratic to a few patients, while most do not report any benefit. Perhaps some patient benefits are due to suggestion, the presence of psychogenic overlay, or symptom exaggeration. To date, no controlled neuropharmacologic studies have demonstrated significant symptom reduction in patients with SD. At present, the role of these medications in the management of SD is only an adjunct to other approaches.

Surgical Management

At this time, botulinum toxin injections remain the gold standard of treatment for spasmodic dysphonia in most institutions. Unfortunately, its temporary nature causes it to be an expensive management technique in the long run. The goal remains to find a treatment or procedure that would provide permanent relief from the voice symptoms without causing permanent damage to the nerves or other structures of the larynx. Unfortunately, no such procedure yet exists. Various surgical procedures have been performed over the years with mixed results.

Because many of these techniques permanently alter the laryngeal structure[122] or can injure the recurrent laryngeal nerve[123] accurate diagnosis and objective symptom assessment need to be employed when such procedures are used. Diagnosis is presently based on symptoms, thus the need to exclude patients with a psychogenic or functional dysphonia is of great importance. Some of these patients could undergo spontaneous recovery.[31] Structural or neural alterations as a result of surgical intervention could interfere with their ability to regain a normal voice.

The more commonly reported procedures, as well as several more experimental ones will be reviewed.

Recurrent Laryngeal Nerve Section

Dedo[124] first introduced recurrent laryngeal nerve section as a treatment for adductor SD in 1976. Noting improvement in voice symptoms following temporary unilateral RLN paralysis with lidocaine injection, he subsequently removed a 1-cm segment of the RLN below the inferior pole of the thyroid gland in 34 patients. All patients demonstrated a reduction or elimination in voice breaks and associated facial and neck grimaces or tics. Although all were pleased with their voice improvement, several patients developed the breathiness, pitch control problems, and hoarseness that are characteristic of unilateral vocal fold paralysis.

Early enthusiasm for the procedure[125-127] was quickly tempered by reports of recurrent voice symptoms in some patients.[107-109,128-130] Aronson and DeSanto[131] noted an alarming 64% recurrence rate in 33 patients at 3 years following surgery, and 48% of failed patients had a worse voice than before surgery. Interestingly, the authors observed a higher failure rate in females compared to males (77% vs 36%). They attributed the recurrent symptoms in these patients to intensified activity of the contralateral innervated vocal fold and/or other surrounding muscles because return of vocal fold movement was not observed on the operated side. However, other studies have demonstrated reinnervation of the vocal fold on the operated side in cases of recurrence using electromyography[86,128] and histology.[132,133] Further, patients with recurrent symptoms have responded to revision surgery[128,130,134] or botulinum toxin injections[86,87] of the previously operated side, suggesting that reinnervation is the most likely cause of postsurgical recurrences.

Dedo reported recurrent symptoms in approximately 10 to 15% of his patients[135,136] and has maintained that his results are better than those of others for two reasons. First, he resects a portion of the nerve, turns back each stump, and ligates each end. Second, prior to and immediately following surgery, Dedo and his colleagues provide voice training so that the patients gain more insight into preventing overpressure and making the best use of their voice postsurgery. He has also suggested that laser thinning of the body of the vocal fold, to achieve lateralization of the vocal fold edge, can be helpful in reducing the overpressure seen in patients with recurrent symptoms.[136]

One obvious advantage of the recurrent nerve section is that, even using the conservative estimate of Aronson,[131] a minimum of 30 to 40% of patients could have a long-term benefit and may not need additional treatment.

There are several disadvantages of this approach. The patients will have a longstanding paralysis even when there has been reinnervation. In addition to the obvious voice difficulties, this can produce respiratory difficulties and an increased risk of laryngospasm.[137,138] The patient also has a greater risk of developing a bilateral paralysis in the future if there is injury to the opposite nerve, because one side is already paralyzed. In addition, if the patient develops an excessively breathy voice, additional vocal fold medialization procedures may be required, which can result in symptom recurrence.[136] Finally, the timing of reinnervation is difficult to predict. Some patients

have undergone vocal fold medialization for treatment of excessive breathiness 1 year following nerve section, only to have SD symptoms return at 3 years following the nerve section. In addition, reports vary regarding the effectiveness of botulinum toxin after prior surgical intervention. Ludlow et al[86] found that patients who fail surgery can be treated using botulinum toxin injections with somewhat similar results to those obtained in patients without prior surgical intervention. Sulica et al[87] found that, although botulinum toxin is somewhat effective in surgical failures, the patients' perception of, and satisfaction with, their voices never reached that of patients who had not undergone recurrent nerve surgery. Hence, it adversely affects voice function and makes botulinum toxin injections less satisfactory.[87]

Overall, the inability to predict whether the patient will have a positive result before surgery, the difficulties with SD diagnosis, and the controversy over long-term success rates make the nerve section less preferred to botulinum toxin injection at the present time.

Recurrent Nerve Avulsion

Because of the reports of reinnervation following recurrent nerve section,[128,134] Netterville and his colleagues[132] developed a more radical approach to nerve resection, termed recurrent laryngeal nerve avulsion. This more extensive removal of the recurrent nerve is an effort to reduce the risk of reinnervation of the sectioned recurrent laryngeal nerve. After mobilization of the ipsilateral thyroid lobe, all branches of the RLN are identified, traced, and avulsed from their muscular insertions deep to the cricopharyngeus muscle. The proximal end of the nerve is then dissected for 3 to 4 cm beneath the clavicle where it is suture ligated and divided. The total length of RLN removed averages 9 cm, in contrast to an average of 2 cm reported in previous RLN section studies. Intermediate follow-up on 12 patients, averaging 1.5 years following the procedure, showed no recurrence of symptoms. The authors subsequently reported long-term follow-up of 3 to 7 years on 18 patients following recurrent laryngeal nerve avulsion.[133] Sixteen patients (89%) were free of SD symptoms at 3-year follow-up, although two of these patients later developed recurrent spasms following medialization laryngoplasty for treatment of weak voice. Thus, an overall recurrence rate of 22% (4/18) was reported for the series, which compares favorably to long-term recurrence rates for RLN section.[131,134] Of note, perceptual analysis of postoperative voices revealed some degree of abnormality (pitch, intensity, and/or quality) in all patients, consistent with the effects of unilateral vocal fold paralysis. Patients should be counseled regarding these potential effects preoperatively. Weed et al[137] recommend that nerve avulsion be reserved for patients who do not benefit from or do not tolerate botulinum toxin injections and for patients who have failed prior RLN section.

Experimental Surgical Approaches

Some experimental surgical approaches have been used in SD, usually by one investigator on a small number of patients.[122,139] Some of the more recent are selective laryngeal adductor denervation-reinnervation and thyroplasty. Nerve stimulation and myectomy techniques have also been mentioned.

Selective Laryngeal Adductor Denervation-Reinnervation. Berke et al[140] presented preliminary results with selective denervation of the laryngeal adductor muscles in an attempt to achieve a permanent bilateral adductor weakness that mimics the transient effects of Botox. Although unilateral selective denervation of laryngeal adductor muscles has been previously proposed[141] for the treatment of SD, the new procedure involves bilateral section of the adductor RLN branches to the thyroarytenoid and lateral cricoarytenoid muscles with intentional reinnervation of the proximal thyroarytenoid branches using branches of the ansa cervicalis nerve. The aim of this directed reinnervation is to prevent unwanted reinnervation by RLN efferents and to preserve adductor muscle tone.

This was a retrospective case series with 1- to 5-year follow-up on 21 patients with adductor SD who underwent the procedure. In general, symptoms and overall severity of SD improved from moderate to severe ratings preoperatively to mild to absent ratings postoperatively. All patients experienced severe vocal fold bowing and breathiness in the early postoperative period that improved after 3 to 6 months. Aspiration of greater than 2 weeks duration was noted in 2 patients, one of whom required hospitalization for aspiration pneumonia. Additional treatments (Botox, voice therapy, collagen injection, thyroarytenoid myotomy) were also performed in several patients to enhance the postoperative voice result.

More recently Allegretto et al[142] published a smaller series using the same technique as Berke and his colleagues. Of 6 patients with adductor SD, patient satisfaction was high and 5 of the 6 no longer required botulinum toxin injections. The follow-up ranged from 11 to 29 months with a mean of 20.3 months. One patient was rated to have a postoperative voice worse than the preoperative one by a majority of the judges.

As noted by the authors of both studies, long-term follow-up in a larger patient population will be required to define the role of this procedure in the treatment of adductor SD. In particular, the effects of bilateral denervation on airway protection and fine-motor control of the larynx for speech (pitch variability, loudness range, and voice onset timing) require further objective assessment. Because the procedure is technically difficult and produces permanent structural and functional changes in the larynx, if done, it should be reserved for patients with relatively severe disease.

Thyroplasty. Isshiki et al[143] first described the use of the midline lateralization thyroplasty (Type II) in the year 2000 in a female patient with presumed adductor spasmodic dysphonia. Within a year, the series had grown to 6 patients with 1 failure[144] and by 2004 Isshiki and his colleagues had performed 26 midline lateralization thyroplasties.[145] The procedure is performed under local anesthesia. The thyroid cartilage is divided in the midline and the thyroid alae are retracted laterally to a distance determined by the improvement in the patient's voice, an average of 3 to 4 mm. The thyroid alae are either anchored apart with silicone shims[143,144] or a specially made titanium bridge.[145] In the early procedures, they widened the anterior commissure with a midline perforation, which was closed with a composite graft. Later procedures omitted this step. Their initial results appeared encouraging. Twenty-two of 26 patients were reported to be free of vocal symptoms. Four had voices that were improved, but were slightly hoarse or pressed. One patient initially had no benefit, but is currently free from vocal symptoms after the surgery was repeated using their new titanium bridge. Unfortunately, their results have not yet been replicated by others. Chan, et al[146] recently reported a series of 13 patients who underwent midline lateralization thyroplasty who were followed 11 to 20 months. There were 4 early failures and thus they subsequently followed 9 patients over the long term. Five of the 9 were eventually classified as failures. Only 4 of the original patients maintained moderate improvement. The authors were unable to recommend the procedure based on their experience.

One possible advantage of this technique is that it allows a wide range of lateralization of the anterior vocal folds to relieve overpressure and voice spasms. Revision procedures, if required, would be theoretically possible by adjusting the size of the silicone shim or titanium bridge. Furthermore, the procedure damages neither muscle nor nerve, and its success is not jeopardized by reinnervation, as seen with other used procedures. If the laryngeal mucosa is violated, there could be contamination of the operative field increasing the possibility of wound infection, but this was not observed in the cases reported. As with all other surgical procedures proposed for SD, long-term objective assessment of voice symptoms will be key in evaluating the usefulness of midline lateralization thyroplasty for this indication.

Type III thyroplasty was reported by Tucker[122] in a series of 18 patients with SD. This procedure was first recommended by Isshiki,[147] who proposed that it should help patients with spasmodic dysphonia because it would reduce vocal fold tension. The procedure involved sectioning the thyroid cartilage by a superior-inferior cut on either side of the thyroid keel. The keel is then repositioned into the larynx, which shortens, thickens, and medializes the vocal folds. The result is a lower fundamental frequency[148] and some reduction in the airway. Because the vocal folds become more medialized, this procedure could increase hyperadduction. Tucker[122] reported short-term relief of spasms in 9 out of 16 patients. No long-term assessment of results was provided to determine whether there is any sustained benefit in this subset of patients. As mentioned previously, we have seen patients who have undergone the procedure who had significant symptoms and did not respond to botulinum toxin injection. The ability to reverse the surgery is limited because of the difficulty in protruding and anchoring the thyroid keel. Furthermore, the lowering of the fundamental frequency in female patients may add to their voice abnormalities. Finally, this procedure may exacerbate vocal fold hyperadduction in adductor SD patients. At present, Type III thyroplasty is not recommended for treatment of adductor SD.

Blitzer et al[71] reported using medialization thyroplasty (Type I) to increase medialization on one side in three patients with abductor SD. This was used as a last resort when botulinum toxin injections into the posterior cricoarytenoid and the cricothyroid were not effective. Long-term follow-up is needed to determine if the partial benefits were maintained over time. Medialization thryoplasty may also be helpful in reducing breathiness following RLN section or avulsion,[133] although medialization may increase the risk of SD symptom recurrence in these patients.

Nerve Stimulation. Friedman has reported using a recurrent nerve stimulator in patients with spasmodic dysphonia.[123,139] Initially, the stimulator was implanted unilaterally in one patient with abductor spasmodic dysphonia using a cuff electrode around the recurrent laryngeal nerve. Close postoperative monitoring showed no stimulation-induced alterations in respiratory or cardiac rate and no cardiac arrhythmias. When the stimulator was set at rates between 10 and 25 Hz, the vocal fold on the side of the stimulator moved toward the midline. Stimulation under these conditions was associated with improvement in voice quality as assessed by the patient and the investigators.

Subsequently, Friedman et al[123] reported follow-up on 5 SD patients implanted with the recurrent laryngeal nerve stimulator. Global assessment of voice quality by the patients and investigators generally ranged between minimal change and marked improvement in all cases, but none achieved a near-normal voice. The authors did not specify whether the patients had adductor or abductor and no voice symptom analyses were conducted. Although no effects of stimulation on cardiac or respiratory function were observed, one patient developed a permanent vocal fold paralysis from the procedure. In the same study, the authors reported additional safety experience in 113 patients they had implanted with a vagus nerve stimulator to control epilepsy. The system and implantation technique were similar to those described for the SD patients except that a spiral electrode was placed around the vagus nerve. The most common adverse events associated with stimulation were hoarseness, throat pain, and cough. An additional patient developed a vocal fold paralysis as result of sustained stimulation from a system malfunction. Based on the established safety profile and greater ease of electrode placement, the authors recommended future study of vagal rather than recurrent nerve stimulator implantation for treatment of SD.

The stimulator may act by blocking or overriding any neural impulses that usually produce spontaneous muscle bursts resulting in the voice breaks. Thus, the neural stimulation may replace abnormal uncontrolled muscle spasms with tonic contractions. However, nerve stimulators can often produce nerve injury, either because of compression reducing blood supply to the nerve or, if there is movement, producing twisting or pressure directly on the nerve. As noted by the authors, this approach is currently experimental, and further well-controlled studies are required to establish the long-term safety, effectiveness, and practicality of nerve stimulation in the treatment of SD.

Posterior Cricoarytenoid Myoplasty with Medialization Thyroplasty. Shaw et al[149] surgically weakened the posterior cricoarytenoid muscles, then performed a medialization thyroplasty in 3 female patients with abductor SD who had been repeatedly resistant to botulinum toxin injections. One patient developed stridor on postop day 3 and required a tracheotomy. She was decannulated in 3 months and, although not symptom-free, was improved 1 year out. Another patient, who did not require a tracheotomy had similarly improved voicing. Only 1 of the 3 patients had no symptoms at a year out. Clearly, this procedure is experimental and more studies will have to be done before it can be routinely recommended in abductor SD.

Preclinical Studies. Genack et al[150] described a myectomy in rabbits that might have application for spasmodic dysphonia patients. Partial unilateral thyroarytenoid myectomy was performed in the rabbit model through a thryoplasty cartilage window. Follow-up electromyography on the myectomy side 3 months postoperatively revealed reduced compound muscle action potentials compared to the control side. Histologic studies on the operated side demonstrated replacement of excised muscle fibers with loose areolar connective tissue without evidence of muscle regeneration. The obvious benefit of this procedure over RLN section or avulsion is that it is not dependent on denervation for its therapeutic effect. The lack of muscle regeneration following partial myectomy in this study holds promise for a sustained therapeutic effect in patients with SD. The authors note that this procedure could be performed bilaterally to maintain adductor balance between the thyroarytenoid muscles. Further preclinical studies in this area are warranted and should include longer follow-up for assessment of muscle regeneration and electromyographic findings.

CONCLUSION

At present, management techniques for spasmodic dysphonia are only aimed at peripheral control of the voice symptoms. Botulinum toxin and recurrent nerve section have been studied most frequently, and the results with botulinum toxin seem most predictable in adductor SD. However, this treatment is costly and usually requires continued reinjection as long as the patient has the disorder. Improved treatments are needed for vocal tremor and abductor SD. Improved understanding of the etiology and pathophysiology of these disorders is needed to develop long-term and effective treatment alternatives.

REFERENCES

1. Blitzer A., et al. Clinical and laboratory characteristics of focal laryngeal dystonia: study of 110 cases. *Laryngoscope.* 1988;98:636–640.
2. Blitzer A., et al. Electromyographic findings in focal laryngeal dystonia (spastic dysphonia). *Ann Otol Rhinol Laryngol.* 1985;94:591–594.
3. Blitzer A, Brin MF. Laryngeal dystonia: a series with botulinum toxin therapy. *Ann Otol Rhinol Laryngol.* 1991; 100:85–89.
4. Fahn S. Concept and classification of dystonia. In: Fahn S, ed. *Advances in Neurology: Dystonia 2.* New York, NY: Raven Press; 1988:1–8.
5. Golper LA, et al. Focal cranial dystonia. *J Speech Hear Disord.* 1983;48(2):128–134.
6. Jankovic J. Etiology and differential diagnosis of blepharospasm and oromandibular dystonia. In: Jankovic J, Tolosa E, eds. *Advances in Neurology: Facial Dyskinesias.* New York, NY: Raven Press; 1988:103–117.
7. Jankovic J, Nutt JG. Blepharospasm cranial-cervical dystonia (Meige's syndrome): familial occurrence. In: Jankovic J, Tolosa E, eds. *Advances in Neurology: Facial Dyskinesias.* New York, NY: Raven Press; 1988:117–123.
8. Lagueny A., et al. Jaw closing spasms-a form of focal dystonia? An electrophysiological study. *J Neurol Neurosurg Psychiatr.* 1989;52:652–655.
9. Sheehy MP, Rothwell JC, Marsden CD. Writer's cramp. In: Fahn S, ed. *Advances in Neurology: Dystonia.* New York, NY: Raven Press; 1988:457–472.
10. Chan J, Brin MF, Fahn S. Idiopathic cervical dystonia: clinical characteristics. *Movement Disord.* 1991;6:119–126.
11. Tolosa E, Marti MJ. Blepharospasm-oromandibular dystonia syndrome (Meige's syndrome): clinical aspects. In: Jankovic J, Tolosa E, eds. *Advances in Neurology: Facial Dyskinesias.* New York, NY: Raven Press; 1988:225–237.
12. Berardelli A. et al. The pathophysiology of cranial dystonia. In: Fahn S, ed. *Advances in Neurology: Dystonia 2.* New York, NY: Raven Press; 1988:525–535.
13. Rosenbaum F, Jankovic J. Task-specific focal tremor and dystonia: categorization of occupational movememnt disorders. *Neurology.* 1988;38:522–527.
14. Paulson GW, Barnes J. Oral facial dystonia triggered by speech. Psychosomatics. 1988;29:236–238.
15. Bloch CS, Hirano M, Gould WJ. Symptom improvement of spastic dysphonia in response to phonatory tasks. *Ann Otol Rhinol Laryngol.* 1985;94:51–54.
16. Golper LE, et al. Focal cranial dystonia. *J Speech Hear Disord.* 1983;48:128–134.
17. Gates G. Introduction. *J Voice.* 1992;6.
18. Parnes SM, Lavorato AS, Myers EN. Study of spastic dysphonia using videofiberoptic laryngoscopy. *Ann Otol.* 1978;87:322–326.
19. Morrison MD, Rammage LD. Muscle misuse voice disorders: description and classification. *Acta Otolaryngol (Stockh).* 1993;113:428–434.
20. Morrison MD, Nichol H, Rammage RA. Diagnostic criteria in functional dysphonia. *Laryngoscope.* 1986;96:1–8.
21. Aronson AE. Importance of the psychosocial interview in the diagnosis and treatment of "functional" voice disorders. *J Voice.* 1990;4:287–289.
22. Aronson AE, et al. Spastic dysphonia: II..Comparison with essential (voice) tremor and other neurologic and psychogenic dysphonias. *J Speech Hear Disord.* 1968;33: 219–231.

23. Aronson AE, Peterson HW, Litin EM. Psychiatric symptomatology in functional dysphonia and aphonia. *J Speech Hear Disord.*. 1966;31:115–127.

24. Izdebski K, Shipp T, Dedo HH. Predicting postoperative voice characteristics of spastic dysphonia patients. *Otolaryngol Head Neck Surg.*1979;87428–434.

25. Koda J,Ludlow CL. An evaluation of laryngeal muscle activation in patients with voice tremor. *Otolaryngol Head Neck Surg.* 1992;107:684–696.

26. Hertegard,S, Granqvist S, Lindestad PA. Botulinum toxin injections for essential voice tremor. *Ann Otol Rhinol Laryngol.* 2000;109(2):204–209.

27. Busenbark K, et al. Methazolamide for essential voice tremor. *Neurology.* 1996;47(5):1331–1332.

28. Yoon MS, et al. Vocal tremor reduction with deep brain stimulation. *Stereotact Funct Neurosurg,* 1999;72(2-4):241–244.

29. Carpenter MA, et al. Reduction in voice tremor under thalamic stimulation. *Neurology.* 1998;50(3):796–798.

30. Sataloff RT, et al. Vocal tremor reduction with deep brain stimulation: a preliminary report. *J Voice.*. 2002; 16(1):132–135.

31. Chevrie-Muller C, Arabia-Guidet C, Pfauwadel MC. Can one recover from spasmodic dysphonia? *Br J Disord Commun.* 1987;22(2):117–128.

32. Murry T, Cannito MP, Woodson GE. Spasmodic dysphonia. emotional status and botulinum toxin treatment. Arch *Otolaryngol Head Neck Surg.* 1994;120:310–316.

33. Morrison, M., et al., The Management of Voice Disorders. San Diego, CA: Singular Publishing Group; 1998..

34. Brodnitz FS. Spastic dysphonia. *Ann Otol Rhinol Laryngol.* 1976;85:210–214.

35. Barton R. The whispering syndrome of hysterical dysphonia. *Ann Otol Rhinol Laryngol.* 1960;69:156–165.

36. Ludlow CL, et al. Abnormalities in long latency responses to superior laryngeal nerve stimulation in adductor spasmodic dysphonia. *Ann Otol Rhinol.Laryngol.* 1995;104:928–935.

37. Deleyiannis FW, et al. Laryngeal long latency response conditioning in abductor spasmodic dysphonia. *Ann Otol Rhinol Laryngol.* 1999;108(6):612–619.

38. Liu CY, et al. Emotional symptoms are secondary to the voice disorder in patients with spasmodic dysphonia. *Gen Hosp Psychiatry.* 1998;20(4):255–259.

39. Shipp T, et al. Intrinsic laryngeal muscle activity in a spastic dysphonic patient. *J Speech Hear Disord.* 1985;50: 54–59.

40. Schaefer SD, et al. Multichannel electromyographic observations in spasmodic dysphonia patients and normal control subjects. *Ann Otol Rhinol Laryngol.* 1992;101:67–75.

41. Watson BC, et al. Laryngeal electromyographic activity in adductor and abductor spasmodic dysphonia. *J Speech Hear Res.* 1991;34:473–482.

42. Van Pelt F, Ludlow CL, Smith PJ. Comparison of muscle activation patterns in adductor and abductor spasmodic dysphonia. *Ann Otol Rhinol.Laryngol.* 1994;103:192–200.

43. Nash EA, Ludlow CL. Laryngeal muscle activity during speech breaks in adductor spasmodic dysphonia. *Laryngoscope.* 1996;106:484–489.

44. Bielamowicz S, Ludlow CL. Effects of botulinum toxin on pathophysiology in spasmodic dysphonia. *Ann Otol Rhinol Laryngol.* 2000;109:194–203.

45. Ludlow CL, VanPelt F, Koda J. Characteristics of late responses to superior laryngeal nerve stimulation in humans. *Ann Otol Rhinol Laryngol.* 1992;101:127–134.

46. Ludlow CL, et al. Successful treatment of selected cases of abductor spasmodic dysphonia using botulinum toxin injection. *Otolaryngol Head Neck Surg.* 1991;104:849–855.

47. Cyrus CB, et al. Adductor muscle activity abnormalities in abductor spasmodic dysphonia. *Otolaryngol Head Neck Surg.* 2001;124(1):23–30.

48. Tomoda H, et al. Voice tremor: dysregulation of voluntary expiratory muscles. *Neurology.* 1987;37:117–122.

49. Kramer PL, et al. The DYT1 gene on 9q34 is responsible for most cases of early limb-onset idiopathic torsion dystonia in non-Jews. *Am J Hum Genet.* 1994;55:468–475.

50. Brin MF, Blitzer A, Stewart C. Laryngeal dystonia (spasmodic dysphonia): observations of 901 patients and treatment with botulinum toxin. *Adv Neurol.* 1998;78: 237–252.

51. Bressman SB, et al. Exclusion of the DYT1 locus in familial torticollis. *Ann Neurol.* 1996;40:681–684.

52. Peng Y, Crumley R, Ringman JM. Spasmodic dysphonia in a patient with the A to G transition at nucleotide 8344 in mitochondrial DNA. *Mov Disord.* 2003;18(6):716–718.

53. Jankovic J. Post-traumatic movement disorders: central and peripheral mechanisms [see comments]. *Neurology.* 1994;44(11):2006–2014.

54. Schweinfurth J, Billante M, Courey M. Risk factors and demographics in patients with spasmodic dysponia. *Laryngoscope.* 2002;112:220–223.

55. Berry DA, et al. Interpretation of biomechanical simulations of normal and chaotic vocal fold oscillations with empirical eigenfunctions. *J Acoust Soc Am.* 1994;95:3595–3604.

56. Sankhla C, Lai EC, Jankovic J. Peripherally induced oromandibular dystonia. *J Neurol Neurosurg Psychiatry.* 1998;65(5):722–728.

57. Brin MF. Botulinum toxin: chemistry, pharmacology, toxicity, and immunology.*Muscle Nerve.* 1997;6:S146–S168.

58. Dressler D, Rothwell J, Marsden C. Comparing biological potencies of Botox and Dysport with a mouse diaphragm model may mislead. *J Neurol.* 1998;245:332.

59. Scott AB. Botulinum toxin injection into extraocular muscles as an alternative to strabismus surgery. *Ophthalmology.* 1980;87(10):1044–1049.

60. Scott AB. Botulinum toxin injection of eye muscles to correct strabismus. *Trans Am Ophthalmol Soc.* 1981;79: 734–770.

61. Scott AB, Kennedy RA, Stubbs HA. Botulinum A toxin injection as a treatment for blepharospasm. *Arch Ophthalmol.* 1985;103:347–350.

62. Tsui JK, et al. A pilot study on the use of botulinum toxin in spasmodic torticollis. *Can J Neurol Sci.* 1985;12:314–316.

63. Miller RH, Woodson GE, Jankovic J. Botulinum toxin injection of the vocal fold for spasmodic dysphonia. *Arch Otolaryngol Head Neck Surg.* 1987;113:603–605.

64. Blitzer A, et al. Localized injections of botulinum toxin for the treatment of focal laryngeal dystonia (spastic dysphonia). *Laryngoscope.* 1988;98:193–197.

65. AAO-HNS. *Policy Statement on Botulinum Toxin Treatment.* Adopted 7/20/90; Reviewed 9/20/95; Revised 4/9/97; Reaffirmed 3/1/98, 1998.

66. NIH Consensus Development Conference Statement: Clinical use of botulinum toxin. *Arch Neurol.* 1991;48: 1294–1298.

67. Hirano M, Ohala J. Use of hooked-wire electrodes for electromyography of the intrinsic laryngeal muscles. *J Speech Hear Res.* 1969;12:362–373.

68. Green DC, et al. Point-touch technique of botulinum toxin injection for the treatment of spasmodic dysphonia. *Ann Otol Rhinol Laryngol.* 1992;101:883–887.

69. Ford CN, Bless CM, Lowery JD. Indirect laryngoscopic approach for injection of botulinum toxin in spasmodic dysphonia. *Otolaryngol Head Neck Surg.* 1990;103:752–758.

70. Rhew K, Fiedler DA, Ludlow CL. Technique for injection of botulinum toxin through the flexible naso*laryngoscope. Otolaryngol Head Neck Surg.* 1994;111:787–794.

71. Blitzer A, et al. Abductor laryngeal dystonia: a series treated with botulinum toxin. *Laryngoscope.* 1992;102: 163–167.

72. Bielamowicz S, et al. Assessment of posterior cricoarytenoid botulinum toxin injections in patients with abductor spasmodic dysphonia. *Ann Otol Rhinol Laryngol,* 2001;110(5 pt 1):406–412.

73. Rontal M, et al. A method for the treatment of abductor spasmodic dysphonia with botulionum toxin injections: a preliminary report. *Laryngoscope.* 1991;101:911–914.

74. Bastian RW, Delsupehe KG. Indirect larynx and pharynx surgery: a replacement for direct laryngoscopy. *Laryngoscope.* 1996;106(10):1280–1286.

75. Ludlow CL, et al. A comparison of different injection techniques in the treatment of spasmodic dysphonia with botulinum toxin. *J Voice.* 1992;6:380–386.

76. Bielamowicz S, et al. Unilateral versus bilateral injections of botulinum toxin in patients with adductor spasmodic dysphonia. *J Voice.* 2002;16(1):117–123.

77. Maloney AP, Morrison MD. A comparison of the efficacy of unilateral versus bilateral botulinum toxin injections in the treatment of adductor spasmodic dysphonia. *J Otolaryngol,* 1994;23:160–164.

78. Adams SG, et al. Unilateral versus bilateral botulinum toxin injections in spasmodic dysphonia: acoustic and perceptual results. *J Otolaryngol.* 1993;22:171–175.

79. Castellanos PF, et al. Anatomic considerations in botulinum toxin type A therapy for spasmodic dysphonia. *Laryngoscope.* 1994;104:656–662.

80. Davidson B, Ludlow CL. Long term effects of botulinum toxin injections in spasmodic dysphonia. *Otolaryngol Head Neck Surg.* 1996;105:33–42.

81. Jankovic J, Schwartz K, Donovan DT. Botulinum toxin treatment of cranial-cervical dystonia, spasmodic dysphonia, other focal dystonias and hemifacial spasm. *J Neurol Neurosurg Psychiatry.* 1990;53:633–639.

82. Ludlow CL. Treatment of speech and voice disorders with botulinum toxin. *JAMA.* 1990;264:2671–2675.

83. Ludlow CL, et al. Effects of botulinum toxin injections on speech in adductor spasmodic dysphonia. *Neurology.* 1988;38:1220–1225.

84. Zwirner P, et al. Effects of botulinum toxin therapy in patients with adductor spasmodic dysphonia: acoustic,aerodynamic, and videoscopic findings. *Laryngoscope.* 1992;102:400–406.

85. Truong DD, et al. Double-blind controlled study of botulinum toxin in adductor spasmodic dysphonia. *Laryngoscope.* 1991;101:630–634.

86. Ludlow CL, et al. Spasmodic dysphonia: Botulinum toxin injection after recurrent nerve surgery. *Otolaryngol Head Neck Surg.* 1990;102:122–131.

87. Sulica L, et al. Botulinum toxin management of adductor spasmodic dysphonia after failed recurrent laryngeal nerve section. *Ann Otol Rhinol Laryngol.* 2003; 112(6):499–505.

88. Rontal M, et al. A method for the treatment of abductor spasmodic dysphonia with botulinum toxin injections: a preliminary report. *Laryngoscope.* 1991;101(8):911–914.

89. Rhew K, Fiedler DA, Ludlow CL. Technique for injection of botulinum toxin through the flexible naso*laryngoscope. Otolaryngol Head Neck Surg.* 1994;111(6):787–794.

90. Ludlow CL. Treating the spasmodic dysphonias with botulinum toxin: a comparison of results with adductor and abductor spasmodic dysphonia and vocal tremor. In: Tsui J, Calne D, eds. *The Dystonias.* New York, NY: Marcel Dekker, Inc; 1995:431–446.

91. Adler CH, et al. Botulinum toxin type A for treating voice tremor. *Arch Neurol.* 2004;61(9):1416–1420.

92. Warrick P, et al. The treatment of essential voice tremor with botulinum toxin A: a longitudinal case report. *J Voice.* 2000;14:410–421.

93. Warrick P, et al. Botulinum toxin for essential tremor of the voice with multiple anatomical sites of tremor: a crossover design study of unilateral versus bilateral injection. *Laryngoscope.* 2000;110(8):1366–1374.

94. Maronian NC, et al. Tremor laryngeal dystonia: treatment of the lateral cricoarytenoid muscle. *Ann Otol Rhinol Laryngol.* 2004;113(5):349–355.

95. Greene P, Fahn S, Diamond B. Development of resistance to botulinum toxin A in patients with torticollis. *Mov Disord.* 1994;9:213–217.

96. Ludlow CL, et al. Therapeutic use of type F botulinum toxin. *New Engl J Med.* 1992;326:349–350.

97. Smith ME, Ford CN. Resistance to botulinum toxin injections for spasmodic dysphonia. Arch *Otolaryngol Head Neck Surg.* 2000;126(4):533–535.

98. Chen R, Karp B, Hallett M. Botulinum toxin type F for treatment of dystonia: long-term experience. *Neurology.* 1998(51):1494–1496.

99. Siegel LS. Evaluation of neutralizing antibodies to type A, B, E, F botulinum toxins in sera from human recipients of botulinum pentavalent (ABCDE) toxoid. *J Clin Microbiol.* 1989;27:1906–1908.

100. Adler CH, et al. Safety and efficacy of botulinum toxin type B (Myobloc) in adductor spasmodic dysphonia. *Mov Disord.* 2004;19(9):1075–1079.

101. Troung DD, et al. Double-blind controlled study of botulinum toxin in adductor spasmodic dysphonia. *Laryngoscope.* 1991;101(6 pt 1):630–634.

102. Aronson AE, et al. Botulinum toxin injection for adductor spastic dysphonia: patients self-ratings of voice and phonatory effort after three successive injections. *Laryngoscope.* 1993;103:683–692.

103. Ludlow CL, et al. Limitations of laryngeal electromyography and magnetic stimulation for assessing laryngeal muscle control. *Ann Otol,Rhinol Laryngol.* 1994;103:16–27.

104. Holds JB, Fogg SG, Anderson RL. Botulinum A toxin injection: failures in clinical practice and a biomechanical system for the study of toxin-induced paralysis. *Ophthalmic Plast Reconstr Surg.* 1990;6:252–259.

105. Freuh BR, et al. Treatment of blepharospasm with botulinum toxin: a preliminary report. *Arch Ophthalmol.* 1984;102:1464–1468.

106. Holds JB, et al. Motor nerve sprouting in human orbicularis muscle after botulinum A injection. *Invest Opthalmol Vis Sci.* 1990;31:964–967.

107. Alderson K, Holds JB, Anderson RL. Botulinum-induced alteration of nerve-muscle interactions in the human orbicularis oculi following treatment for blepharospasm. *Neurology.* 1991;41:1800–1805.

108. Harris CP, et al. Histologic features of human orbicularis oculi treated with botulinum A toxin. *Arch Ophthalmol.* 1991;109:393–395.

109. Borodic GE, Ferrante R. Effects of repeated botulinum toxin injections on orbicularis oculi muscle. *J Clin Neuro-opthalmol.* 1992;12:121–127.

110. Jaffe DM, et al. Comparison of concentric needle versus hooked-wire electrodes in the canine larynx. *Otolaryngol Head Neck Surg.* 1998;118:655–662.

111. Roy N, Ford CN, Bless DM. Muscle tension dysphonia and spasmodic dysphonia: the role of manual laryngeal tension reduction in diagnosis and management. *Ann Otol Rhinol.Laryngol.* 1996;105:851–856.

112. Murry T, Woodson GE. Combined-modality treatment of adductor spasmodic dysphonia with botulinum toxin and voice therapy. *J Voice.* 1995;9:460–465.

113. Aronson AE. *Clinical Voice Disorders: An Interdisciplinary Approach.* 2nd ed. New York, NY: Thieme-Stratton; 1995.

114. Colton RH, Casper JK. *Understanding Voice Problems: A Physiological Perspective for Diagnosis and Treatment.* Baltimore, MD: Williams & Wilkins; 1995..

115. Berstein DA, Borkovec TD. *Progressive Relaxation Training: A Manual for the Helping Professions.* Champaign, IL: Research Press; 1973.

116. Boone DR. Respiratory training in voice therapy. *J Voice.* 1988;2:20–25.

117. Blood G. Efficacy of a computer-assisted voice treatment protocol. *Am.J.Speech Lang Pathol.* 1994;3:57–66.

118. Fujita M, et al. A new surface electrode for recording from the posterior cricoarytenoid muscle. *Laryngoscope.* 1989;99:316–320.

119. Kuna ST, Smickly JS, Insalaco G. Posterior cricoarytenoid muscle activity during wakefulness and sleep in normal adults. *J Appl Physiol.* 1990;68:1746–1754.

120. Cooper M. *Stop Committing Vocal Suicide.* 1996.

121. Fox S, Trace R. Role of voice therapy varies in SD treatment. *Advance SLP & Aud.* 1993;December 20:11–12.

122. Tucker HM. Laryngeal framework surgery in the management of spasmodic dysphonia: preliminary report. *Ann Otol Rhinol Laryngol.* 1989;98:52–54.

123. Friedman M, Wernicke JF, Caldarelli DD. Safety and tolerability of the implantable recurrent laryngeal nerve stimulator. *Ann Otol Rhinol Laryngol.* 1994;104:1240–1244.

124. Dedo HH. Recurrent laryngeal nerve section for spastic dysphonia. *Ann Otol Rhinol Laryngol.* 1976;85:451–459.

125. Levine HL, et al. Recurrent layngeal nerve section for spasmodic dysphonia. *Ann Otol Rhinol Laryngol.* 1979;88(4 pt 1):527–530.

126. Bocchino JV, Tucker HM. Recurrent laryngeal nerve pathology in spasmodic dysphonia. *Laryngoscope.* 1978;88(8 pt 1):1274–1278.

127. Barton RT. Treatment of spastic dysphonia by recurrent laryngeal nerve section. *Laryngoscope.* 1979;89(2 pt 1):244–249.

128. Fritzell B, et al. Experiences with recurrent laryngeal nerve section for spastic dysphonia. *Folia Phoniatr.* 1982;34:160–167.

129. Aronson AE, DeSanto LW. Adductor spastic dysphonia: 1½ years after recurrent laryngeal nerve resection. *Ann Otol Rhinol Laryngol.* 1981;90(1 pt 1): 2–6.

130. Wilson FB, Oldring JD, Mueller K. Recurrent laryngeal nerve dissection: a case report involving return of spastic dysphonia after initial surgery. *J Speech Hear Disord.* 1980;45(1):112–118.

131. Aronson AE, Desanto LW. Adductor spasmodic dysphonia: three years after recurrent nerve section. *Laryngoscope.* 1983;93:1–8.

132. Netterville JL, et al. Recurrent laryngeal nerve avulsion for treatment of spastic dysphonia. *Ann Otol Rhinol Laryngol.* 1991;100(1):10–14.

133. Banoub M, et al. Recurrent postoperative stridor requiring tracheostomy in a patient with spasmodic dysphonia. *Anesthesiology.* 2000;92(3):893–895.

134. Fritzell B, et al. Long-term results of recurrent laryngeal nerve resection for adductor spasmodic dysphonia. *J Voice.* 1993;7:172–178.

135. Dedo HH, Izdebski K. Intermediate results of 306 recurrent laryngeal nerve sections for spastic dysphonia. *Laryngoscope.* 1983;93:9–16.

136. Dedo HH, Izdebski K. Problems with surgical (RLN section) treatment of spasmodic dysphonia. *Laryngoscope.* 1983;93:268–271.

137. Weed DT, et al. Long-term follow-up of recurrent laryngeal nerve avulsion for the treatment of spastic dysphonia. *Ann Otol Rhinol Laryngol.* 1996;105(8):592–601.

138. Salassa JR, Desanto LW, Aronson AE. Respiratory distress after recurrent laryngeal nerve section for spastic dysphonia. *Laryngoscope.* 1982;92:240–245.

139. Friedman M, et al. Implantation of a recurrent laryngeal nerve stimulator for the treatment of spastic dysphonia. *Ann Otol Rhinol.Laryngol.* 1989;98:130–134.

140. Berke GS, et al. Selective laryngeal adductor denervation-reinnervation: a new surgical treatment for adductor spasmodic dysphonia. *Ann Otol Rhinol Laryngol.* 1999;108(3): 227–231.

141. Carpenter RJ, Henley-Cohn JL, Snyder GG. Spastic dysphonia: treatment by selective section of the recurrent laryngeal nerve. *Laryngoscope.* 1979;89(12):2000–2003.

142. Allegretto M, et al. Selective denervation: reinnervation for the control of adductor spasmodic dysphonia. *J Otolaryngol.* 2003;32(3):185–189.

143. Isshiki N, et al. Midline lateralization thyroplasty for adductor spasmodic dysphonia. *Ann Otol Rhinol Laryngol.* 2000;109(2):187–193.

144. Isshiki N, et al. Thyroplasty for adductor spasmodic dysphonia: further experiences. *Laryngoscope.* 2001; 111(4):615–621.

145. Isshiki N, Yamamoto I, Fukagai S. Type 2 thyroplasty for spasmodic dysphonia: fixation using a titanium bridge. *Acta Otolaryngol.* 2004;124(3):309–312.

146. Chan SW, et al. Long-term results of Type II thyroplasty for adductor spasmodic dysphonia. *Laryngoscope.* 2004;114(9):1604–1608.

147. Isshiki N. Recent advances in phonosurgery. *Folia Phoniatr.* 1980;32:119–154.

148. Slavit DH, Maragos NE, Lipton RJ. Physiologic assessment of Isshiki Type III thyroplasty. *Laryngoscope.* 1990;100:844–848.

149. Shaw GY, Sechtem PR, Rideout B. Posterior cricoarytenoid myoplasty with medialization thyroplasty in the management of refractory abductor spasmodic dysphonia. *Ann Otol Rhinol Laryngol.* 2003;112(4):303–306.

150. Genack, SH, et al. Partial thyroarytenoid myectomy: an animal study investigating a proposed new treatment for adductor spasmodic dysphonia. *Otolaryngol Head Neck Surg.* 1993;108(3):256–264.

33

Psychological Aspects of Voice Disorders

Deborah Caputo Rosen, RN, PhD
Reinhardt J. Heuer, PhD
Steven H. Levy, MD
Robert T. Sataloff, MD, DMA, FACS

The first task of the otolaryngologist treating any patient with a voice complaint is to establish an accurate diagnosis and its etiology. Only as a result of a thorough, comprehensive history and physical examination (including state-of-the-art technology) can the organic and psychologic components of the voice complaint be elucidated. All treatment planning and subsequent intervention depend on this process. However, even minor voice injuries or health problems can be very disturbing for many patients and devastating to some professional voice users. In some cases, they even trigger responses that delay return of normal voice. Such stress, and fear of the evaluation procedures themselves, often heighten the problem and may cloud diagnostic assessment. Moreover, some voice disorders may be entirely psychogenic, and professional psychologic assessment may be required to complete a thorough evaluation.

Although "voice," the newest subspecialty of otolaryngology, now provides a greatly improved standard of care for all patients with voice disorders, most of the advances in this field resulted from interest in and the study of voice professionals. Professional performers are not only demanding, but also remarkably self-analytic. Like athletes, performers have forced health care providers to change our definition of normalcy. Ordinarily, physicians, psychotherapists, and other professionals are granted great latitude in the definition of "normal." For example, if a microsurgeon injures his or her finger, and the hand surgeon restores 95% of function, the surgeon-patient is likely to be satisfied. If the same result occurs in a world-class violinist, that last 5% (or 1%) may mean the difference between renown and obscurity. Traditionally, we have not been trained to recognize, let alone quantify and restore, these degrees of physical perfection. Arts-medicine practitioners have learned to do so, including those in the field of voice. The process has required advances in scientific knowledge, clinical management, technology for voice assessment, voice therapy, and surgical technique. The drive to expand our knowledge has also led to unprecedented teamwork and interdisciplinary collaboration. As a result, voice care professionals have come to recognize important psychologic problems commonly found in patients with voice disorders. Such problems were ignored in past years. Now they are looked for diligently throughout evaluation and treatment. When identified, they often require intervention by a psychologic professional with special knowledge about voice disorders, as well as by a speech-language pathologist (SLP) and other voice team members.

Arts medicine psychologists specializing in the management of performance anxiety are becoming more common, but there are still very few psychological professionals with extensive experience in diagnosing and treating other psychologic concomitants of voice disorders. It is important for the physician and all other members of the voice care team to recognize the importance of psychologic factors in patients with voice disorders and to be familiar with mental health professionals in various disciplines in order to build a multidisciplinary team, generate appropriate referrals, and coordinate optimal patient care.

Psychiatrists are licensed physicians who have completed medical training, residency in psychiatry, and often additional training. They are qualified not only to establish medical and psychiatric diagnoses and provide therapy, but also to prescribe medications. Psychologists make mental health diagnoses, administer psychologic tests, and provide therapy. They do not prescribe medications, but often work closely with a physician (usually a psychiatrist) who may prescribe and help manage psychotropic medications during the course of psychotherapy. Clinical psychologists have a Masters or Doctoral degree in psychology and may have subspecialty training. Other clinical disciplines (ie, social work, nursing, counseling) license graduate-level practitioners to provide psychotherapy. Laryngologists, phoniatrists, and speech-language pathologists are not formally mental health professionals, although all have at least limited training in psychologic diagnosis. Specialty definitions vary from country to country. In the United States, laryngologists are responsible for medical diagnosis and treatment, and voice surgery. They also prescribe any medications needed to treat organic voice problems and occasionally take responsibility for prescribing psychoactive medications. Speech-language pathologists are responsible for behavioral therapy for speech, language, and swallowing disor-

ders. In many other countries, phoniatrists perform behavioral therapy in addition to making diagnoses. Phoniatrists are physicians. Traditionally, in some countries they have been members of an independent specialty that does not include laryngeal surgery. In other countries, they have been subspecialists of otolaryngology. The European Union has recently determined that in the future, in member countries, phoniatry will be a subspecialty of otolaryngology. Both speech-language pathologists and phoniatrists include at least some psychologic assessment and support in their therapeutic paradigms. However, they are not fully trained mental health professionals and must be constantly vigilant to recognize significant psychopathology and recommend appropriate referral for treatment by a psychologist or psychiatrist. Finding a mental health professional familiar with the special needs and problems of voice patients, especially singers and actors, is not easy. Arts medicine psychology is a relatively new field, as was voice care in the early 1980s. Nevertheless, it is usually possible to find a psychological professional who is either knowledgeable or at least interested enough to become knowledgeable. Resources are available in the literature to assist the interested mental health professional,[1] and incorporating such a colleague into the voice care team is extremely beneficial.

PSYCHOLOGY AND VOICE DISORDERS: AN OVERVIEW

Patients seeking medical care for voice disorders come from the general population. Consequently, a normal distribution of comorbid psychopathology can be expected in a laryngology practice. Psychologic factors can be causally related to a voice disorder and/or consequences of vocal dysfunction. In practice, they are usually interwoven.

The essential role of the voice in communication of the "self" creates special potential for psychologic impact. Severe psychologic consequences of voice dysfunction are especially common in individuals in whom the voice is pathologically perceived to be the self, such as professional voice users. However, the sensitive clinician will recognize varying degrees of similar reaction among most voice patients who are confronted with voice change or loss.

Our work with professional voice users has provided insight into the special intensification of psychologic distress they experience in association with lapses in vocal health. This has proved helpful in treating all patients with voice disorders, and has permitted recognition of psychologic problems that may delay recovery following vocal injury or surgery.

Self-esteem comprises not only who we believe we are, but also what we have chosen to do as our life's work. A psychologic double-exposure exists for performers who experience difficulty separating the two elements. The voice is in, is therefore of, indeed, is the self. Aronson's extensive review of the literature supports the maxim that the "voice is the mirror of the personality"—both normal and abnormal. Parameters such as voice quality, pitch, loudness, stress pattern, rate, pauses, articulation, vocabulary, syntax, and content are described as they reflect life stressors, psychopathology, and discrete emotions.[2] Sundberg describes Fonagy's research on the effects of various states of emotion on phonation. These studies revealed specific alterations in articulatory and laryngeal structures and in respiratory muscular activity patterns related to ten different emotional states.[3] Vogel and Carter include descriptive summaries of the features, symptoms, and signs of communication impairment in their text on neurologic and psychiatric disorders.[4] The mind and body are inextricably linked. Thoughts and feelings generate neurochemical transmissions that affect all organ systems. Therefore, not only can disturbances of physical function have profound emotional effects, disturbances of emotion can have profound bodily and artistic effects.

PROFESSIONAL VOICE USERS: SPECIAL CASE

It is useful to understand in greater depth the problems experienced by professional voice users who suffer vocal injuries. Most of our observations in this population occur among singers and actors. However, it must be remembered that, although they are the most obvious and demanding professional voice users, many other professionals are classified as professional voice users. These include: politicians, attorneys, clergy, teachers, salespeople, broadcasters, shop foremen (who speak over noise), football quarterbacks, secretaries, telephone operators, and others. Although we are likely to expect profound emotional reactions to voice problems among singers and actors, many other patients may also demonstrate similar reactions. If we do not recognize these reactions as such, they may be misinterpreted as anger, malingering, or other difficult patient behavior. Some patients are unconsciously afraid that their voices are lost forever and are psychologically unable to make a full effort at vocal recovery after injury or surgery. This blocking of the frightening possibilities by rationalization ("I haven't

made a maximum attempt so I don't know yet if my voice will be satisfactory") can result in prolonged or incomplete recovery after technically flawless surgery. It is incumbent upon the laryngologist and other members of the voice team to understand the psychologic consequences of voice disturbance and to recognize them not only in extreme cases, but even in their more subtle manifestations.[1]

Typically, successful professional voice users (especially actors, singers, and politicians) may fall into a personality subtype that is ambitious, driven, perfectionistic, and tightly controlled. Externally, they present themselves as confident, competitive, and self-assured. Internally, self-esteem, the product of personality development, is often far more fragile. Children and adolescents do the best they can to survive and integrate their life experiences, utilizing psychologic defense strategies that develop early in childhood. All psychologic defense mechanisms are means to that end. Most of these defenses are not under conscious control. They are an habitual element of the fabric of one's response to life, especially in stressful or psychologically threatening situations.

All psychologic adjustment expresses itself through the personality of the patient, and it is essential to focus on the personality style of every performer who seeks psychologic help. This can best be done during psychologic assessment and evaluation by exploring daily activities, especially those pertaining to the performer's involvement with his or her art, the patient's growth and personality development as an artist, and relationships with people both within and outside his or her performing environment. Each developmental phase carries inherent coping tasks and responsibilities, which can play an important part in the patient's emotional response to vocal dysfunction. Learning about, valuing highly, and managing our unique, individual psychologic vulnerabilities are critical to adaptive psychologic function throughout life.

Research into body image theory provides a theoretical basis for understanding the special impact of stress or injuries to the voice in vocal performers. The body is essential to perception, learning, and memory and the body serves as a sensory register and processor of sensory information.[5] Body experience is deeply personal and constitutes a private world typically shared with others only under conditions of closest intimacy. Moreover, the body is an expressive instrument, the medium through which individuality is communicated verbally and nonverbally.[5] It is therefore possible to anticipate direct correspondence between certain physical illness or injury and body and self-image. Among these are psychosomatic conditions and/or body states with high levels of involvement of personality factors. In these cases, body illness or injury may reactivate psychopathologic processes that began in early childhood or induce an emotional disorder such as denial or inappropriately prolonged depression.[5] Psychologic reactions to a physical injury are not uniformly disturbing or distressing and do not necessarily result in maladjustment. However, Shontz[5] notes that reactions to body injury are more a function of how much anxiety is generated by the experience than by the actual location, severity, or type of injury itself.

Human beings are remarkably adaptive and capable of living with most types of difficulties, injuries, or disabilities if they feel there is a good reason for doing so. If one's life has broad meaning and purpose, any given disorder takes on less significance. When a physical disability or any given body part becomes the main focus of concern or has been the main source of self-esteem in a person's life, that life becomes narrowed and constricted. Patients adapt satisfactorily to a personal medical condition when the problems of living related to the injury cease to be the dominant element in their total psychologic life.

A unique closeness exists between one's body and one's identity; this body-self is a central part of self-concept. The interdependence of body image and self-esteem means that distortion of one will affect the other. The cognitive-behavioral model for understanding body image includes the perceptual and affective components, as well as attitudinal ones. From the cognitive perspective, any body image producing dysphonia results from irrational thoughts, unrealistic expectations, and faulty explanations.[6] Body-image constructs and their affective and cognitive outcomes relate to personality types and cognitive styles. For example, depressive personality types chronically interpret events in terms of deficiencies and are trapped by habitual self-defeating thoughts. Anxious personality types chronically overestimate risks and become hypervigilant. These types of cognitive errors generate automatic thoughts which intensify body-image-related psychopathology.[1]

It is the task of personality theorists to explain the process of the genesis of the self. There are numerous coherent personality theories, all substantially interrelated. The framework of Karen Horney (1885-1952) is particularly useful in attempting to understand the creative personality and its vulnerabilities. In simplification, she formulated a "holistic notion of the personality as an individual unit functioning within a social framework and continually interacting with its environment."[7] In Horney's model, there are three selves. The actual self is the sum total of the individual's experience; the real self is responsible for harmonious integration; and the idealized self sets up unrealistically high expectations which, in the face of disappointment, result in self-hatred and self-alienation. We have chosen Horney's theory as a working model in evolving therapeutic approaches to the special patient population of professional voice users. They are the laryngologist's most demanding consumers of voice care and cling to their physician's explanations with dependency.[1,8]

It may be useful, for theoretical clarity, to divide the experience of vocal injury into several phases. In practice, however, these often overlap or recur and the emotional responses are not entirely linear.

- The phase of problem recognition. The patient feels that something is wrong, but may not be able to clearly define the problem, especially if the onset has been gradual or masked by a coexisting illness. Usually, personal "first aid" measures will be tried, and when they fail, the performer will manifest some level of panic. This is often followed by feelings of guilt when the distress is turned inward against the self, or rage or blame when externalized.

- The phase of diagnosis. This may be a protracted period if an injured performer does not have immediate access to a laryngologist experienced in the assessment of vocal injury. He or she may have already consulted with voice teachers, family physicians, allergists, nutritionists, peers, or otolaryngologists and speech-language pathologists without specialized training in caring for professional voice users. There may have been several, possibly contradictory, diagnoses and treatment protocols. The vocal dysfunction persists, and the patient grows more fearful and discouraged. If attempts to perform are continued, they may exacerbate the injury and/or produce embarrassing performances. The fear is of the unknown, but it is intuitively perceived as significant.

- The phase of treatment: acute/rehabilitative. Now, fear of the unknown becomes fear of the known, and of its outcome. The performer, now in the sick role, initially feels overwhelmed and powerless. There is frequently a strong component of blame that may be turned inward. "Why me, why now?" is the operant, recurrent thought. Vocal rehabilitation is an exquisitely slow, carefully monitored, frustrating process, and many patients become fearful and impatient. Some will meet the criteria for major depression, which is discussed in additional detail, as is the impact of vocal fold surgery.

- The phase of acceptance. When the acute and rehabilitative treatment protocol is complete, the final prognosis is clearer. When there are significant lasting changes in the voice, the patient will experience mourning. Even when there is full return of vocal function, a sense of vulnerability lingers. These individuals are likely to adhere strictly, even ritualistically, to preventive vocal hygiene habits and may be anxious enough to become hypochondriacal.[1,8,9]

The psychologic professional providing care to this special population must be well versed in developmental psychology, be experienced in the world of the performer, and retain an unshakable empathy for the patient who has experienced the psychologically disorganizing impact of vocal injury. It is critical to harken back to one of the earliest lessons taught to all psychotherapists in training. That is, the therapist must, through accurate empathy, earn the right to make interpretations and interventions. When this type of insightful and accurate support is available to the professional voice user, the psychotherapist may well be the patient's rudder in the rough seas of diagnosis, treatment, and rehabilitation.

PSYCHOGENIC VOICE DISORDERS

Voice disorders are divided into organic and nonorganic etiologies. Various terms have been used interchangeably (but imprecisely) to label observable vocal dysfunction in the presence of emotional factors which cause or perpetuate the symptoms. Aronson argues convincingly for the term *psychogenic*, which is "broadly synonymous with functional, but has the advantage of stating positively, based on an exploration of its causes, that the voice disorder is a manifestation of one or more types of psychological disequilibrium, such as anxiety, depression, conversion reaction, or personality disorder, that interfere with normal volitional control over phonation."[2]

Psychogenic disorders include a variety of discrete presentations. There is disagreement over classification among speech-language pathologists, with some excluding musculoskeletal tension disorders from this heading. Aronson and Butcher et al conclude that the hypercontraction of extrinsic and intrinsic laryngeal muscles, in response to emotional stress, is the "common denominator" behind the dysphonia or aphonia in these disorders.[2,10] In addition, the extent of pathology visible on laryngeal examination is inconsistent with the severity of the abnormal voice. They cite four categories:

1. *Musculoskeletal tension disorders*: including vocal abuse, vocal nodules, contact ulcers, and ventricular phonation;

2. *Conversion voice disorders*: including conversion muteness and aphonia, conversion dysphonia, and psychogenic adductor spastic dysphonia;
3. *Mutational falsetto* (puberphonia);
4. *Childlike speech in adults.*

Psychogenic dysphonia often presents as total inability to speak, whispered speech, extremely strained or strangled speech, interrupted speech rhythm, or speech in an abnormal register (such as falsetto in a male). Usually, involuntary vocalizations during laughing and coughing are normal. The vocal folds are often difficult to examine because of supraglottic hyperfunction. There may be apparent bowing of both vocal folds consistent with severe muscular tension dysphonia, creating anterior-posterior "squeeze" during phonation. Long-standing attempts to produce voice in the presence of this pattern may even result in traumatic lesions associated with vocal abuse patterns, such as vocal fold nodules. Normal abduction and adduction of the vocal folds may be visualized during flexible fiberoptic laryngoscopy by instructing the patient to perform maneuvers that decrease supraglottic load, such as whistling or sniffing. In addition, the singing voice is often more easily produced than the speaking voice in these patients. Tongue protrusion and stabilization during the rigid telescopic portion of the examination will often result in clear voice. The severe muscular tension dysphonia associated with psychogenic dysphonia can often be eliminated by behavioral interventions by the speech-language pathologist, sometimes in one session. In many instances moments of successful voice have been restored during stroboscopic examination.

Electromyography may be helpful in confirming the diagnosis by revealing simultaneous firing of abductors and adductors. Psychogenic dysphonia has been frequently misdiagnosed as spasmodic dysphonia, partially explaining the excellent spasmodic dysphonia cure rates in some series.

Psychogenic voice disorders are not merely the absence of observable neurolaryngeal abnormalities. This psychiatric diagnosis cannot be made with accuracy without the presence of a psychodynamic formulation based on understanding of the personality, motivations, conflicts, and primary as well as secondary gain associated with the symptoms.[1,11,12]

Conversion disorders are a special classification of psychogenic symptomatology and reflect loss of voluntary control over striated muscle or the sensory systems as a reflection of stress or psychologic conflict. They may occur in any organ system, but the target organ is often symbolically related to the specifics of the unconsciously perceived threat. The term was first used by Freud to describe a defense mechanism that rendered an intolerable wish or drive innocuous by translating its energy into a physical symptom. The presence of an ego-syntonic physical illness offers primary gain: relief from the anxiety, depression, or rage by maintaining the emotional conflict in the unconscious. Secondary gain often occurs by virtue of the sick role.

Classic descriptions of findings in these patients include indifference to the symptoms, chronic stress, suppressed anger, immaturity and dependency, moderate depression, and poor sex role identification.[12,13] Conversion voice disorders also reflect a breakdown in communication with some of the emotional significance in the patient's life; wanting but blocking the verbal expression of anger, fear, or remorse, and significant feelings of shame.[1,2]

Confirmed neurologic disease and psychogenic voice disorders do coexist and are known as somatic compliance.[14,15] Of course, potential organic causes of psychiatric disorders must always be thoroughly ruled out. Insidious onset of depression, personality changes, anxiety, or presumed conversion symptoms may be the first presentation of central nervous system (CNS) disease.[16]

THE SPEECH-LANGUAGE PATHOLOGIST'S ROLE IN TREATING PSYCHOLOGIC DISTURBANCES IN PATIENTS WITH VOICE DISORDERS

Speech-language pathology is a relatively new profession in the United States. Its roots are in psychology. The original members of the field came primarily from a psychology background. Early interest in the psychologic aspects of voicing are evidenced in texts such as *The Voice of Neurosis*.[17] Luchsinger and Arnold present an excellent review of the early literature in their text, *Voice-Speech-Language*.[18] At the present time, speech-language pathologists need to be familiar with models of treatment from the psychologic tradition, the medical tradition, and the educational tradition. When discussing the speech-language pathologist's role in managing functional voice problems, it must be made clear at the outset that the speech-language pathologist does not work in isolation but as part of a team, including, at a minimum, a laryngologist and speech-language pathologist. Singing instructors, acting instructors, stress specialists, psychologists, neurologists, and psychiatrists must be readily available and cognizant of the special needs of voice patients.

Psychology is defined as the study of human behavior, and the speech-language pathologist's role in treating voice-disordered patients is normalizing the patient's speaking and communication behavior. In this sense, all the activities of speech-language pathologists with voice-disordered patients are psychologic. The purpose of this chapter is not to present a full description of the role of the speech-language pathologist but to describe those areas in which the speech-language pathologist must deal with issues not directly related to the physical vocal mechanism. However, a brief overview of the activities engaged in by the speech-language pathologist and the voice patient help set the groundwork for a discussion of psychologic issues. A more detailed description has been published elsewhere.[19]

Preparation for Treatment

The speech-language pathologist must be aware of, and able to, interpret the findings of the laryngologist, including strobovideolaryngoscopy. Particular attention should be paid to findings demonstrating muscle tension or lack of glottic closure not associated with organic or physical changes. The perceptions of the laryngologist regarding organic and functional aspects of the patient need to be known.

A case history is taken, reviewing and amplifying the case history reported by the laryngologist. The case history should include but not be limited to the topics summarized in Table 33–1.

Subjective and objective measures of the patient's vocal mechanism and communication skills need to be obtained, including, but not limited to, the parameters listed in Table 33–2.

The speech-language pathologist should be able to develop a plan of behavioral changes. The case history provides an adequate sample of the patient's voice use in an interview situation. It is important to note how the patient's voice changes when talking about certain topics and to note evidence of improvement or fatigue as the interview proceeds. It provides data on what speaking activities are most important to the patient and which may need to be addressed initially in therapy. It provides information of the patient's willingness to talk about stressful issues or needs beyond direct focus on voicing and speech skills, which may be important regarding referral to other specialists dealing with stress and emotional or physical health. It establishes an initial rapport, or lack of it, with the clinician that may predict success, or failure, in therapeutic intervention. It also provides the speech-language pathologist with a sample of the patient's communication style and verbosity.

Table 33–1. The History

1. Circumstances surrounding the onset, development, and progress of the voice disorder, including:
   - illnesses of the patient
   - recent changes in employment
   - speaking responsibilities associated with the patient's employment
   - effects of the voice disorder on employment
   - employment environment
   - speaking activities outside of employment
   - environment in which social speaking activities occur
   - effects of the voice disorder on social exchange and social activities
   - activities the patient has had to give up because of voice disorder
   - illness or difficulty among family members or friends
   - stress factors at work and at home
   - methods of dealing with stress

2. Exploration of the social structure of the patient and environment, including:
   - family and living arrangements
   - friends and social gathering places
   - relationships with coworkers and superiors

3. The patient's response to the voice disorder needs to be explored as follows:
   - what bothers the patient most about the voice disorder?
   - what has the patient done to change voicing and how effective have these attempts been?
   - estimates of the speaking times at work and socially, now and before the voice disorder.
   - how does the patient feel about speaking at the present time—stressed, indifferent, depressed, challenged?

4. General health issues should be addressed:
   - chronic illness, including asthma, allergies, diabetes, thyroid dysfunction, chronic fatigue
   - head and neck trauma, including whiplash, concussion, spinal degeneration, temporomandibular joint disease, facial injury
   - surgery
   - high fevers
   - nonvocal symptoms, including swallowing difficulty, pain on speaking or swallowing, numbness, neck stiffness or reduced range of motion, voice quality, speaking rate, movement limitations of the articulators, nasal regurgitation, tremor or shakiness

5. Medications
   - prescription medications
   - over-the-counter drugs, including nonsteroidal anti-inflammatory drugs (NSAIDs), cough drops, decongestants, antihistamines, mouthwash, vitamins, alcohol, tobacco and caffeine products, and water intake.

The physical assessment provides the speech-language clinician with objective support for what the clinician has heard and information about how the patient is producing the voice. As behavioral change instituted during the therapy is based on eradication of symptoms of maladaptive voice or communication, listing and evaluating confirmed symptoms at this stage lead to the developing of an overall therapeutic plan. Focus should be initially on identification of the underlying behavior or behaviors responsible for maintaining the current voice. Early attention to these underlying behaviors reduces the length of therapy and should predict improvement of voicing.

Therapeutic Stage

Information giving is essential at the beginning and throughout the course of therapy. Patients need to know the reason(s) for the activities in which they are engaging and why these activities are important in changing their current voice problem. Without a thorough un-

Table 33–2. Vocal Function Assessment

1. Average fundamental frequency and loudness of the patient's conversational voice.

2. Average fundamental frequency, loudness, and speaking rate during a selected reading passage, both in normal reading and in the professional voice (if a professional speaker).

3. Acoustic and aerodynamic measures of sustained vowels, including:
   * measures of perturbation
   * measures of breathiness and noise
   * measures of vocal breaks and quality change
   * measures of airflow
   * measures of glottic pressure

4. Preferred breathing patterns for speech:
   * shallow, deep, appropriate for phrase length
   * clavicular, thoracic, abdominal, or mixed
   * coordination with voicing—exhalation initiated before voicing, glottic closure prior to initiation of exhalation
   * coordinated breath/voicing

5. Neck and laryngeal use:
   * positioning of the larynx during speech—high, low, inflexible
   * tension in the extralaryngeal muscles, particularly the omohyoid
   * laryngeal/hyoid space—present, reduced
   * position of the hyoid—tipped, tense, discomfort on palpation of the cornu

6. Use of the articulators:
   * Oral examination, including lip movements and symmetry, tongue movements and symmetry, palatal sufficiency in nonspeech contexts, diadochokinetic rates
   * ability to separate jaw and anterior tongue activity during the production of /l/, /t/, /d/, /n/
   * tongue tension during speech
   * jaw tension and jaw jutting during speech
   * looseness of temporomandibular joint during speech movements

derstanding of the reasons for changing behavior the probabilities of behavioral change are reduced.

The patient needs to know that a voice disorder is not usually caused by a single agent, but is rather a combination of physical changes, such as communication demands on the voice, the patient's skills in producing speech, and the patient's attempts to compensate for vocal changes. The initial goal in therapy is to manage communicative demands and improve the patient's ability to produce more normal voice. Reassessment of the need for medical/surgical interventions for physical changes is planned with the patient. Reassurance is provided that the goal of therapy is not to change personality or limit communication opportunities, but to return these at least to the level of communication enjoyed prior to the onset of the voice problem.

Patients need to be educated regarding their current breathing pattern. It may be insufficient for the demands placed on the patient's voice or a contributor to increased tension in the vocal mechanism. Abdominal breathing is the natural and preferred method of breathing by the body. Abdominal breathing is not a new skill. Patients engage in abdominal breathing when they are relaxed and when they are sleeping.

Patients need to be informed that predominately clavicular or thoracic breathing is usually the product of stress, a societal preference toward tight clothing, and/or demands by parents, teachers, and society in maintaining a tight tucked-in stomach. All these factors lead to a reduction of abdominal release during inhalation that leads to restriction in diaphragmatic downward motion and maximal inflation of the lungs. Suggested techniques for teaching effective, relaxed breathing may be found in Appendix 33–1.

Instruction in behavior is provided so that the patient understands that the vocal folds are opened by the flow of air from the lungs and closed because of their own elasticity and Bernoulli's principle. The vocal folds are vibrating much too rapidly to be manipulated by laryngeal effort, and patients need to comprehend that the emotional system and the conscious speech system share control of voicing, which varies with emotional context. The patient needs to know that laryngeal control is primarily automatic and that efforts to produce voice are counterproductive. The quality of the patient's voice during physiologic sound-making, such as laughter, and a gentle cough, can predict the quality of sound when extra effort is removed. Humming and sighing are also effective means of demonstrating the effect of reduced effort. Modeling by the clinician of easy, well-supported, well-resonated voice during these conversations can be a highly effective means of modifying the patient's vocal production in the therapy setting. Suggested techniques for teaching these aspects of efficient, relaxed voice production are included in Appendix 33–1.

A pattern of frequent tension checks needs to be established with the cooperation of the client. These need not be elaborate warm-up exercises or cool-down practice. The patient may decide to practice abdominal breathing in the shower, blowing the water away from his or her face, or humming with a relaxed jaw while inhaling the warm steamy air. The patient may be able to stroke the face, jaw, or neck at each stop light while driving to or from work or take an easy belly breath followed by a relaxed sigh. The patient may check his or her jaw tension before picking up the telephone to say "hello." A brief reminding note can be taped to the inside of the telephone receiver.

Abdominal breathing can be practiced leaning over the desk while reading memos or correcting examination papers. A sip of water between tasks can help the patient focus on relaxation of the jaw or throat and can be preceded by a deep abdominal inhalation. The patient can be very creative and very helpful in identifying times when correct vocal behavior can be practiced. Multiple reminders during the busy day can be more effective than a half-hour practice in the isolation of the patient's home and more likely to be done.

All these exercises are helpful in aiding the patient to become aware of the subtle nature of tension in the speaking mechanism, but may be overwhelmed by overriding tension not associated directly with speaking behavior in the face and neck. A decision must be made as to whether the speech-language pathologist has the skill to develop a more stringent relaxation regimen or if the patient needs, and is amenable to, a referral to an expert in stress management.

A discussion of relevant and irrelevant talking is necessary if the patient talks excessively. The patient needs to know that total vocal rest, if extended past a week, can lead to muscle atrophy and additional voice problems. The concept of vocal naps during the day and the possibility of reducing talking, or more positively, becoming a better listener in noisy environments, should

be introduced. The patient is more knowledgeable than the therapist as to when and how long these quiet times can be inserted into the daily schedule.

Patients under stress will bring their "job-voice" home with them. The patient will often complain that family members nag about the use of too loud a voice, of being too demanding, or of using too many directions. A vocal nap during the ride home with an added cool-down protocol can be helpful in providing a positive transition. The patient should be reminded that singing in the car over the noise of traffic and radio and engine noises can be abusive.

The patient needs to know that most people utilize visual cues (lip read) in noisy environments. If the patient has been successful in developing open oral resonance and articulation patterns, the ability of the patient's listeners to understand in noisy situations is enhanced. A slower rate of talking is also helpful in improving comprehension. The patient should be instructed in the effective use of light to highlight his or her face during such conversations.

Voice patients under stress often violate the rules of conversation, including rules of relevance, brevity, and turn-taking. A discussion of these rules may lead to an awareness of inappropriate communication patterns or the revelation of an underlying personality difficulty that may lead to a referral to a psychologic professional. Often persons with difficulty in personal relationships and/or coping with their circumstances can admit to a voice disorder, but not the underlying personal difficulties. The experience of voice therapy, especially supportive rather than prescriptive voice therapy, may lead to the acceptance of a referral to a professional trained in dealing with these underlying difficulties that might have been rejected at initial interview. The combination of an inability to relax following focal voice exercises, an inability to modify communication behaviors, a tendency for the patient to revert to discussions of personal problems rather than focus on the process on communication, all assist the therapist in reinforcing the idea that the patient's problem lies outside the realm of traditional voice therapy. A statement by the therapist such as, "You have very real problems, but I am not trained to deal with them. I know someone who can help you," can be the beginning of a successful referral.

Finally, the patient needs to know that voice therapy is short-term and finite. The goal of therapy is to identify underlying behavioral, emotional, and physical factors, modify current vocal behaviors, and develop better communication skills. The therapist must be aware that the stressed patient can develop inappropriate dependence upon the therapist. If therapy sessions begin to focus more on the patient's day-to-day personal problems than on voice, the time for psychologic referral is long past. Patients need to know that voice therapy usually is successful in only a few sessions, unless there are other problems that maintain the maladaptive vocal behavior. The therapeutic goal in these cases is to identify the underlying problems and make the appropriate referrals. This is a difficult concept for some patients, particularly singers, who are used to taking singing lessons most of their life.

Patients often respond to a voice change by struggling to continue to use their voices in their daily jobs. Teachers will continue to teach, preachers will continue to preach, and sales personnel will continue to sell. The fear of losing their livelihood drives them to modify their speaking techniques, usually applying extra effort, which results in fatigue, pain, and progressive voice loss. They will stop doing enjoyable leisure activities that involve talking and begin to feel impoverished both personally and socially. Feelings of self-worth are also diminished. They feel as though they are not doing their job as well as possible and often consider job changes that do not suit their training or skills.

The speech-language pathologist (SLP) can be very helpful in reducing these feelings by focusing on a plan to return the patient to comfortable functioning in his or her current occupation. If the patient is successful in modifying the effortful and compromised voice using the techniques described above, these reactions subside. The SLP should develop a therapeutic program that will provide the most rapid return of better voicing. The patient needs to be evaluated for the key elements producing vocal fatigue and vocal quality changes. A program of vocal hygiene that can alleviate environmental and behavioral stresses in the workplace, a program of reasonable vocal rest during the workday, and the initiation of a program which will reinstate the balance between respiratory, voicing, and resonance effort in vocal technique are very important. A timetable of when the patient can resume specific activities or when the treatment program will be reviewed to assess alternative treatment options gives the patient something to work toward. Selected practical aspects of voice therapy are reviewed in Appendix 33–1.

EXAMPLES OF PSYCHOLOGIC ASPECTS OF VOICE DISORDERS

Case 1

Case 1 had been a fifth-grade schoolteacher for 20 years. She denied having any previous voice problems, other than vocal fatigue by the end of the week at the end of the school year. She also assisted her husband, a pediatrician, as his receptionist during evening office hours. However, she now presented with progressive hoarseness. She was diagnosed with vocal fold swelling, gastroesophageal reflux laryngitis, and pinpoint vocal nodules by a laryngologist. She was seen by a speech-language pathologist one month prior to the end of the school year.

Case history revealed important life differences. The previous summer the regular receptionist at her husband's office had taken a maternity leave, and she had volunteered her services over the summer months. It was a busy office, and she spent many hours on the telephone and talking with patients. Her voice did not feel rested at the beginning of the school year.

Because of her excellent teaching record she had been assigned a student teacher who required a great deal of counseling, typically after school hours. She found herself rushing from school to her husband's office without time to eat. She began eating after office hours, experiencing heartburn and disrupted sleep. Her voice was worse in the morning and even more fatigued after the school day. She was physically tired before the day began. She had been given a prescription for ranitidine (Zantac), but did not believe it was helping her.

She noted that her students, her husband, and the patients at her husband's office complained that she was "yelling at them." She was very worried about her ability to continue teaching with "no voice." She was worried about the status of her marriage. She was seriously considering quitting teaching but was ambivalent because she really enjoyed teaching and felt she had a great deal to give both to her students and student teachers. She felt that engaging in voice therapy would only complicate her already busy schedule. She stated: "The harder I try, the worse things seem to get." She then cried.

Evaluation of her voice revealed a shallow thoracic breathing pattern. She had developed a pattern of taking a quick breath and holding it prior to initiation of voicing, resulting in glottal attack rates of 54% (normal 15%). Her voice was loud, low-pitched, and rough. She was using a tense jaw, jutting forward during speech. These characteristics were even worse when demonstrating her current teaching voice. She felt her voice was very different in the classroom now than before her voice problems began.

The following therapeutic plan was developed. Direct voice therapy was deferred until July following the end of school and a brief vacation. In the meantime she was urged to continue using the ranitidine and to institute a more rigorous program to control her reflux. The matter of paperwork was discussed. She decided not to take a new student teacher in the fall, but to try to teach.

Therapy in July focused on reducing vocal effort, re-establishing abdominal breathing, reducing glottal stopping, jaw relaxation, and open oral resonance for loudness. Classroom teaching materials were used for exercises. She was able to modify her vocal behaviors easily, although she continued to voice concern about her ability to use them in the classroom. A probable set of voice rests during the school day was discussed and cool-down procedures to implement on the trip to the office were planned. At the end of the therapy, review by the laryngologist demonstrated a reduction in the size of the vocal nodules, resolution of vocal swelling, and reduced reflux findings. She decided to try teaching but was still worried. A plan was developed to see her for therapeutic review two weeks into the school year, then, as needed, mid-fall, at winter break, at spring break, and at the end of the school year. If she felt she did not need to come in, she would call and report how her voice was progressing.

At the meeting two weeks into the school year, she reported that she was "surviving." She was still concerned about whether she was using her voice correctly. Through discussion, she decided she would enlist her students as monitors, particularly for loudness. During the fall, she called to say she was doing well. Her voice was strong and she was much less tired. She reported that her class had taken their role in monitoring her voice very enthusiastically and seriously. Her admission of voice problems and need for help had become an advantage for noise control in her classroom and in student/teacher interactions. She was planning to develop a vocal hygiene section in her curriculum.

At winter break, she reported her voice was not as fatigued and she was eagerly looking forward to return to teaching after the break.

At spring break, she no longer experienced vocal fatigue. Glottal attack remained under 10%. She was sleeping all night. Her reflux appeared to be under control. She was dismissed from therapy but reminded to contact the therapist if she experienced any problems.

Some patients appear to react to life stresses by overuse of their voices and excessive tension focused in the speaking mechanism. They may consider themselves talkative and congenial persons but actually talk constantly, rapidly, or in an excessively loud voice. They appear to be afraid of silence or afraid that if they give up their turn to talk they will not be able to talk again. They often complain of pain and tension in the neck and jaw or of a feeling of breathlessness. They may seek treatment when their inappropriate speaking patterns lead to benign lesions of the larynx or when some other organic change in the vocal mechanism causes their voice to break down. Modeling slower, softer voicing and turn-taking during thera-peutic sessions can be very helpful in reducing these vocal faults and providing a more reasonable speaking pattern. The development of relaxation programs for the face and neck to be used frequently during the day is useful. Discussions of the rules of discourse (how to behave and interact during discussions) may be helpful.

Some patients bring with them a severe overall body reaction to the stresses of their life. They complain of fatigue, sleeplessness, tension, and pain. They are unable to turn off their "work voice" at home. They complain of lack of time to complete all the activities with which they are engaged. Standard therapeutic procedures often are ineffective because they are unable to distinguish the subtle changes in support, voicing, or resonation caused by the overriding levels of general tension. They appear to be out of harmony with their body. Focal relaxation of the vocal mechanism is unsuccessful. They usually deny having emotional problems and have difficulty dealing with daily stress, but continue to return to nonvocal issues during the course of therapy. The SLP can be helpful in allowing these patients to experience a supportive one-on-one relationship as a prelude to referral to a psychologic professional. Often after several sessions with the SLP protesting that, "We are talking about issues I am not able to help you with, but Dr. X can," the patient is receptive to referral. Often referral to a stress manager or professional trained in Feldenkreis or Alexander technique or some other relaxation/body awareness method can be useful. The patient may return to the SLP following resolution of some of these issues. The SLP needs to be careful not to continue the therapeutic relationship so long as the patient becomes dependent on an ineffectual but sympathetic ear.

Case 2

Case 2 presented with a large hemorrhagic cyst on one vocal fold and a reactive lesion directly opposite the cyst on the other vocal fold. She was married and had an adopted son. She was a grade-school teacher. She had been forced to take a sabbatical because her voice had deteriorated. On evaluation she presented with a loud, hoarse voice with frequent glottal attacks and frequent aphonic breaks. She was extremely verbal with frequent run-on sentences and sentence revisions. She demonstrated a pattern of taking a rapid, large chest breath followed by holding the breath with her larynx at the end of inhalation. She demonstrated excessive tension in the speech musculature. Her conversational style was repetitious. Interestingly, her teacher's voice was better controlled. She admitted that yelling at a sporting event probably caused the cyst. She was seen prior to surgery. Therapy consisted in promoting a softer, more breathy voice. The combination of being relieved from teaching duties and modifying voicing behaviors was successful in eliminating the reactive lesion. Surgery for the hemorrhagic cyst was planned and carried out successfully. She was able to complete a week of voice rest following the surgery. The following weeks of gradual increased voice use were difficult for her. Therapy focused on reducing glottal attacks, improving breath support, and monitoring loudness. Materials included readings and repeated sentences and phrases. Materials from her classroom texts were used in preparation for her return to the classroom. She made excellent progress. However, when therapy moved to monitoring her new skills in general conversation, it became clear that she was unable to recognize her loudness level, control her excessive talking, or identify hard glottal attack.

She returned to school and was seen on a limited schedule similar to that used with the previously described patient. She complained of continued vocal fatigue and hoarseness. She developed a pattern of bringing small gifts. She had limited success in developing self-monitoring skills outside of controlled materials or classroom activities. She successfully completed the school year with no return of vocal fold masses. However, her monitoring skills and general levels of tension remained unchanged. The termination of therapy was discussed. She was very anxious about the termination, citing the continued fatigue and difficulties in monitoring her speech outside the classroom. It was suggested that emotional factors might play a role in her lack of success in changing these behaviors and that she might wish to begin seeing the psychologist associated with the practice. At this point, she admitted to a long history of both physical and verbal abuse, first from her father and then from her husband. It became clear that her failures in therapy led to criticism by the therapist that satisfied her unconscious need for abuse.

PATIENTS WITH APHONIA

As illustrated in the following cases, there appear to be four categories of patients who have little voicing capability in the absence of structural or neurologic etiology. These include: whispered voice; tense aphonia with intermittent squeaky, high-pitched syllables or words (often misdiagnosed as spasmodic dysphonia); low-pitched, rough, strangled voice quality; and voluntary muteness.

Cases 3 and 4 describe patients with whispered voice without vocal paralysis, vocal injury, or other

pathology. Usually the vocal folds of such patients appear to be normal. Initial case history may or may not reveal psychologic trauma associated with the onset of the aphonia. Nonspeech sounds such as cough, laugh, cry, and throat clearing are present and normal. These sounds can often be extended gradually into speech with the help of a therapist. If the patient is ready to give up the aphonic behavior, therapy is relatively brief, often obtaining normal voice within one session.

Case 3

Case 3 presented with a loud, strained, whispered voice. The laryngologist had found no laryngeal pathology. Case history revealed no changes in lifestyle, or environment, at the time of onset. However, the voice problem began about one year after her husband's retirement as owner and manager of a large grocery store. The family lived in a small town some distance from any cultural area. She felt the voice loss was related to a bad cold and allergy she had experienced at the time of onset. Normal voice was observed during throat clearing, coughing, and laughter. When asked "what bothered her about her voice loss," she answered, "I can't talk to my friends!"

Therapy consisted of extending the throat clear to "ah" to "hum" to longer and longer "hum-m-m-m" sounds. She was then able to produce the "hum" which was extended into single "m" words. At this point, she reverted to a whisper. The process was repeated with additional focus on relaxed production. This time she was able to extend to days of the week, counting, short phrases, sentences and, finally, conversation. It is not unusual to have to start at the beginning several times with these patients. She was very relieved and thankful to be able to talk again. During the ensuing conversation, she said: "Now, maybe he will let me rejoin my bridge club." When requestioned about changes in her lifestyle, she admitted that since her husband's retirement her life had changed extensively. She had thought, however, that it was only part of what to expect when one's spouse retired. He had begun to criticize her housekeeping in the same managerial style he used with his employees at the store. He had always done this, but now that he was retired and home it became almost constant. She was resentful because he did not volunteer to help. After about a year, he became more and more concerned with expenses and living on a fixed income. He complained about her extravagance in entertaining her bridge club every other month, even though he continued to golf regularly and attend his bowling team matches. He finally forbade her to entertain her bridge club and essentially took away her only source of pleasure and enjoyment. It was at this point that her voice deteriorated.

The mechanism of conversion reaction was then discussed in terms of the conflict between anger, resentment, and frustration versus maintenance of a loving relationship that might suffer irreparable damage if feelings were verbalized. She agreed that this was what had happened. These matters were discussed with her husband and the couple consented to marriage counseling on their return to their local community.

Some patients achieve secondary gain from a voice disorder, as illustrated in case 4. Often these patients come to the voice pathologist at the insistence of others. There frequently is a lack of affect surrounding the patient's feeling about his or her voice problem.

Case 4

Case 4 was a very wealthy widowed woman. She was brought to the voice center at the insistence of her unmarried sister who had come to live with her after the death of her husband. The onset of her voice problem had been gradual, beginning with speech within the home. The laryngologist reported normal vocal folds with no evidence of structural or neurologic pathology. The patient demonstrated little concern about her voice problem other than an inconvenience. When asked how her voice interfered with her life, she stated, with a little smile: "Well, when I am at parties, everyone has to come up to me to converse, and of course, I cannot reprimand or manage the servants, and I can't do the grocery shopping, my sister has to do that." Although physiologic sounds were present in involuntary voice such as coughing and "fuller" sounds like "uh-huh," she was unable to extend them into any semblance of speech voicing. The effect was a modified form of a whisper. She took umbrage at the suggestion of counseling or any emotional etiology for her voice problem and terminated contact. She refused to have her case discussed with her sister. It appeared to be clear that her voice problem would not improve until her sister and friends stopped reinforcing the positive impact of her voice problem.

Cases 5 and 6 exemplify a second group of aphonic patients who present with tense aphonic speech with intermittent squeaky, high-pitched syllables or words. They are often misdiagnosed with spasmodic dysphonia, currently thought to be a neurologic disorder. Careful differential diagnosis is important. However, initial evaluation and treatment are similar regardless of the diagnosis.

These patients may present with a history of emotional disorder or severe stress, reflux, asthma, and/or chemical sensitivity resulting in laryngospasm.

Strobovideolaryngoscopy usually reveals severe muscle tension with anterior-posterior constriction, elevated laryngeal position, reduced abduction and adduction and, in many cases, evidence of reflux laryngitis. Evaluation of the vocal mechanism finds the larynx held high in the neck. There is tension in the jaw, tongue, and extralaryngeal muscles. Breathing is high in the chest with excessive inspiratory effort. Therapy includes Aronson's digital manipulation,[2] yawn-sigh, swallow, and gargling activities to lower and relax the larynx. Tongue and jaw must be relaxed, using techniques described previously. Good abdominal breathing must be developed. Therapy needs to be intensive, on a daily basis. Appointments on a weekly basis allow too much time for the tension reactions to re-establish themselves, reducing the effectiveness of therapeutic intervention. Referral to a stress manager or psychologist is sometimes necessary. If voice therapy is successful in establishing normally pitched voice with little evidence of tension, but spasmodic aphonic breaks persist, the patient should be re-evaluated for the presence of spasmodic dysphonia.

Case 5

Case 5 presented with a high-pitched squeaky voice with frequent aphonic breaks. He felt his voice problem was directly related to his work situation. He was a middle manager in a utility company. He felt his company was in the process of downsizing, but instead of firing employees, the company designated some employees as eligible for upgrade training. The training consisted of EST-like sessions with no bathroom or food breaks and constant berating of the employee. Several of his fellow employees quit. He vowed to fight the system. However, at this point he lost his voice. He was transferred within the company from sales to a computer-intensive position. His voice returned to the presenting squeaky quality. He felt the stress of his treatment at work and resulting stress at home were directly related to his problem. Evaluation revealed high, tense laryngeal position, pain on palpation of the hyoid bone supporting the tongue, and "chest heave" breathing pattern. He was seen for a period of three days. Initially he was unable to maintain a relaxed lowered laryngeal position. He was able to monitor his larynx position digitally and was aware of the mechanism. When his larynx was lowered he produced normally pitched but breathy voice. Cues to make his voice louder improved voice quality but tended to introduce laryngeal tension and lifting of the larynx. Continued therapy, to relax the tongue and jaw and to develop abdominal breathing, were effective in producing normal voice. He refused suggestions for referral to the voice team psychologist. He contacts the therapist on occasion and continues to be symptom-free.

Case 6

Case 6 was a teacher's assistant in a preschool program. She came to school early one day and found the janitor cleaning the floors with a strong disinfectant liquid cleaner. Excessive cleaning fluid had spilled from the container and had spread across the floor. She was unable to breathe and was sent to the hospital emergency room where she received muscle relaxants and oxygen to restore breathing. Her breathing improved but her voice became high-pitched and squeaky. She experienced two other incidents of breathing difficulties associated with the smells in a new store and when buying carpet. She was unable to use commercial cleaning products in her home without experiencing shortness of breath. She was diagnosed with laryngospasm. Strobovideolaryngoscopy revealed severe muscle tension and elevated larynx, but normal laryngeal function. Voice evaluation revealed high laryngeal positioning, extreme tension in the neck and extralaryngeal muscles, and a rapid, shallow, thoracic breathing pattern. The patient was convinced that her voice problem was related to "damage while hospitalized" and was considering suing the hospital. Gentle digital massage and head and neck relaxation exercises restored her voice to normal. Therapy then focused on reducing fears of breathing and voicing. She was given strategies, including slow, deep, abdominal breathing and jaw and throat relaxation patterns to counteract the return of the laryngeal spasms. She consented to referral to a stress management/psychology professional. Therapy with the psychologist focused on deep relaxation and hypnotic suggestion to reduce fears and anxiety. She was able to return to work. She still avoided areas with strong smells but was able to utilize her compensation techniques. She has not required hospitalization for breathing difficulties since.

A third group of aphonic patients present with aphonia accompanied with a low-pitched, rough, strangled voice quality, such as case 7. Strobovideolaryngoscopy reveals extreme supralaryngeal tension with both anterior/posterior and medial compression of supralaryngeal structures. Often laryngeal examination is discontinued and voice therapy pursued because of the difficulty in viewing the vocal folds beneath the extreme supralaryngeal closure. Emotional trauma is usually present in these cases. Again, these patients are often misdiagnosed as having spasmodic dysphonia. Frequently, the same techniques utilized with whispering patients are helpful in modifying the vocal be-

havior toward normal. In addition, inhalation speech can be helpful in breaking the supraglottic tension.

Case 7

Case 7 lost her voice following the death of her grandson. Her voice was low, rough, strangled, and intermittently aphonic. Voice evaluation demonstrated generalized reduction of movement in the respiratory and articulatory systems with excessive tension in the extralaryngeal musculature. During the history, she described the death of her grandson. Her daughter and son-in-law went out to dinner, leaving their son with her and her husband. During the evening, the child suffered a severe asthma attack and died in her arms despite CPR. During the telling of the story her voice became more and more strangled. The therapist commented that she sounded like she wanted to cry and offered a tissue. At this, she burst into tears and great sobbing. She began to cry in a normal voice: "I am so angry." The therapist asked if she was angry because of the death of her grandson. She replied: "No, I am angry because I have not had a chance to grieve." Continuing in a normal voice, she related that her husband, daughter, and son-in-law were devastated by the death, which left her to make all arrangements for the autopsy, funeral, and burial. Her anger was especially directed toward her husband, who did not help, nor give her any expression of sympathy or sensitivity to the depth of her feelings and about the death and its aftermath. At the end of this revelation, the therapist gently brought her attention to the fact that her voice had become quite normal. She said: "Yes, but that's not the problem." She agreed to and was immediately referred to the voice team psychologist. She was followed periodically by speech therapy. Her voice remained stable. The psychologist reported that her problems with her family were much more extensive than those she had related to the speech-language pathologist.

Case 8

Case 8 was referred from his local speech-language pathologist to be evaluated for possible spasmodic dysphonia. He had been unable to obtain any normal speech after several months of therapy. His therapy had focused on relaxation techniques and breathing.

The patient presented with severe muscle tension dysphonia and low-pitched rough voice with a predominating whisper. Laryngoscopy could not be completed because of the severe supraglottic constriction. He denied any emotional trauma associated with the onset of his voice problem. His wife, however, felt it might be related to the death of his mother, followed within a month by the death of his father. He was also in the process of beginning retirement. All direct attempts at relaxing his voice, including inhalation speech, were ineffective or caused his voice to become worse. During instruction episodes and general conversation, he produced an occasional normal word or phrase. The therapist decided that direct therapy was not effective and began modeling normal easy voicing in conversation. Normal words and phrases were pointed out, and he was asked to reproduce the same vocal feeling and style in further conversation. Conversation focused on positive experiences and pleasurable activities. Over the course of four sessions, the frequency of normal voice continued to increase. His wife reported episodes of normal voice at home. By the fifth session, his voice was consistently normal except for a reduction in vocal loudness. There was no evidence of spasm. At this point, strobovideolaryngoscopy was completed and was within normal limits. At the next session, the subject of his parent's deaths was broached. He denied that this was a problem "that a good man should not let it bother him. A man should be strong enough to deal with such an inevitable occurrence." He felt it had been inappropriate for his previous female therapist to focus on that problem and found it difficult to cooperate with her in relaxation and breathing tasks. He was not ready to discuss his reaction. At the next session, he maintained his voicing. He also was able to begin to modify his breathing pattern to increase support and loudness. At the next session, he announced that he felt his voice had returned to normal and terminated therapy. He was seen six months follow-up with the laryngologist and continued to maintain relatively normal voice.

Case 9 describes a fourth form of aphonia, voluntary muteness. Voluntary muteness in the absence of severe laryngeal pathology, developmental language delay, or severe hearing loss is very rare. In over 35 years of experience with voice patients, we have seen only one such case.

Case 9

Case 9 was a 12-year-old boy. His mother, a loquacious and verbal woman, brought him to the voice center. She was concerned about his preparation for bar mitzvah. She was planning a large ceremony and big party, which she thought he would enjoy. However, he would not talk to her about the event or talk to the cantor or rabbi during training lessons. She had taken him to a psychologist, but he would not talk to her either. He was doing well in school although she did not know how much talking he did there. She reported that his father was a soft-spoken man of few words. She

felt that voice therapy might be helpful in increasing his loudness and ability to perform at his bar mitzvah.

Strobovideolaryngoscopy demonstrated a normal larynx. However, the laryngologist was unable to get him to vocalize with any strength. The therapist agreed to attempt short-term therapy, but felt that the boy had found a powerful tool to control his mother.

He reluctantly participated in breathing exercises and better oral resonance. He would practice portions of the readings required at the bar mitzvah service, but only in exchange for a turn at a computer game.

He arrived at the third session more animated than he had ever been before. His teacher had given the class a book report assignment. Each student was to read a book and then report orally to the class about the story from the point of view of one of the characters in the book. The report could only be five minutes long. He had chosen *Tom Sawyer* and wanted to report in the guise of that character. He discussed in detail his plans for a costume and asked for help in presenting an already prepared presentation. We worked on appropriate breath support and phrasing, projection and open oral resonance, and editing for length. He asked for an additional session to give us more time prior to his presentation. It was hoped that a breakthrough had occurred. He was working as hard as any aspiring actor, reporting that he received an A+ on his presentation. However, when the work resumed on his bar mitzvah readings, the old reluctance returned. He was able to demonstrate his skills if rewarded, but continued to be silent at home. His mother reported that he would at least mumble to the cantor. Plans for a large bar mitzvah were canceled. His mother was reluctant to re-engage in psychotherapy, and the patient discontinued voice therapy.

VOICE PROBLEMS ASSOCIATED WITH PSYCHOSIS

Rarely does the voice of the psychotic patient present as the most prevalent symptom. Several studies have been published characterizing the speech of the schizophrenic. These characteristics are considered to be the byproduct of affect, aura, and relational disturbances. Speech therapy for those voice characteristics is rarely considered. However, occasionally such a patient will be encountered in a voice center, as illustrated by case 10.

Case 10

Case 10 had a successful career in a medical subspecialty. However, she aspired to a career in opera. She had taken many lessons, but had been discouraged by her family and teachers to pursue this professionally. She had been highly unsuccessful while auditioning for roles. She came to the voice center to have her singing/speaking voice evaluated. Strobovideolaryngoscopy revealed normal laryngeal structures. She revealed, during history-taking, that her voice was fine at work, because of the lead shielding at the hospital. However, at home, her voice was disrupted and changed in quality, particularly when she was practicing singing and acting and at auditions. When asked why, she reported that "they" were shooting laser beams at her and shocking her, which disrupted her voice and made her voicing very tense. When asked, "Who they were" she replied, "Certain others who are jealous of my talents and want to thwart my career in singing." She also reported that the beams "they" were using burned her and produced changes in her skin color around her neck and shoulders.

When reading a passage, she winced, dodged, and several times cried out in pain. When this behavior was questioned, she reported calmly that "they" had followed her to the center and were shooting laser beams and using electric shock on her. She was reluctant to work on her speaking voice because the problems of tension that she had were caused by an external force and not by her.

Her evaluation by our singing specialist was similar. She was urged by the entire team to submit to evaluation by a psychiatrist, but would not do so.

VOICE PROBLEMS ASSOCIATED WITH ADOLESCENCE

Mutational falsetto is high-falsetto voicing, often with frequent pitch breaks. The voice is thin and high-pitched. Falsetto voice requires a different shaping of the glottis and different breath support than typical voicing. The larynx must ride high in the neck to produce falsetto. It is a normal phenomenon; most males can produce it. It is used frequently in singing by rock and roll singers and developed extensively by classical countertenors, but is not a preferred means of speech communication. It occurs in some young men following the onset of laryngeal growth associated with adolescence. The techniques described above for use with patients with squeaky voices are useful in this group. Usually, normal voicing is easily achieved during the evaluation and trial therapy sessions. Often the patient has both falsetto and normal voice, but prefers the falsetto for various personal reasons. Most of these patients are nonmuscular young men with little self-confidence. It has often been misdiagnosed as spasmodic dysphonia because of the pitch breaks.

Case 11

Case 11 was a 23-year-old auto body repairman. He was concerned about laryngeal cancer. His girlfriend and parents accompanied him to the voice clinic. Strobovideolaryngoscopy revealed normal larynx and the presence of falsetto voicing. During the voice evaluation, he was asked if he had any other voices. In a normal deep baritone he answered "Yes." He used the deep voice around his colleagues at the auto body shop. He used the falsetto voice with his girlfriend, his family, and his high school friends. His life was organized around the premise that the two groups of people were never present at the same time. When asked why he needed the dichotomy of voice, he answered that he was afraid his girlfriend and family would not like this other voice. He was asked if he would be willing to try. His girlfriend was brought into the room and he used his deep voice. She, of course, was thrilled. He was relieved, and his voice problem was solved.

Case 12

Case 12 was a 19-year-old college student. He had just completed his freshman year at a religious college. He had attended a choir school during his primary school years and had sung many soprano solos. His best singing occurred just prior to adolescent voice change. He continued to sing soprano although his voice became thin and he had difficulty keeping his voice from cracking following vocal mutation. His speaking voice continued to be high, breathy, and characterized by pitch breaks.

When he arrived at college, he enrolled in the religious music department, hoping to continue a career in choral singing. His singing teacher, instead of being impressed by his high voice, referred him to a local speech-language pathologist. He was diagnosed with spasmodic dysphonia, presumably because of the numerous pitch breaks. He was referred for neurologic workup and Botox injections. His singing teacher was not convinced of this diagnosis and referred him to our voice center.

Strobovideolaryngoscopy revealed a normal larynx with falsetto voice patterning. He was convinced that "spasmodic dysphonia had destroyed his singing voice." He was counseled on the effects of adolescent voice change. We explored the large size and angular shape of his larynx, comparing it to the much smaller, rounded larynx of a child. The symptoms of spasmodic dysphonia were described and tapes of spasmodic dysphonic voices were played for him.

Attempts at producing low-pitched normal voice extending from cough and throat-clearing sounds were successful but transition into speech sounds was difficult. He was asked to put his finger across his "Adam's apple" and tuck his chin down toward his chest. This maneuver made falsetto voicing impossible. Normal low-pitched voicing was achieved and transferred to syllables, words, phrases, question/answers, and monologue. The positioning cues were gradually replaced by gentle downward-tactile cues. He was engaged in conversation using the "new" voice for at least 30 minutes. He was asked to use his new voice with other personnel, his family (who had accompanied him to the center), and on the telephone to his singing teacher. His family was relieved that Botox injections were not necessary. Breath support was practiced in context of his speech. By the end of the evaluation and trial therapy session, he was convinced that he was a baritone and could continue singing in that role. He no longer felt he had spasmodic dysphonia. The singing specialist at the voice center saw him and it was reported that he was able to maintain his speaking voice and begin some singing exercises focusing on lower range extension and breath support. He was asked to call the center the following day to report on continued use of the "new" voice. During that call, the patient reported that he had retained his lower voice. He was looking forward to returning to college and working with his singing teacher on developing his baritone voice.

Occasionally, males with mutational falsetto demonstrate personal conflicts with their fathers, attachment problems with their mothers, or gender confusion. These patients tend to produce normal voice reluctantly and fail to maintain it, often complaining that such a voice is not appropriate for them. Counseling and referral to a psychologic professional to focus on these difficulties is necessary.

Young women do not present with mutational falsetto. Rarely, a young postpubescent girl will present with immature voice. This is characterized by high pitch and melody, inflection, articulation, and word choice more reminiscent of a preschool child than a postpubertal young adult. Usually, strong dependent behaviors are described in the history.

Case 13

Case 13 was a 17-year-old high school student who aspired to a career in musical theater. She had been highly successful in obtaining roles as a child in productions of *Annie*. She had been thwarted lately in winning any role because of her voice. She was close to tears and appeared to be very depressed. Laryngologic examination demonstrated normal structures but muscle tension associated with high pitch. Her

voice was very high pitched and immature with a mild lisp and "r" sound distortions. She was seen in therapy and made progress in controlled contexts. However, she was unable to transfer her more mature voice to home and school environments. She was very unhappy about this and felt that something was blocking her ability to use her more mature voice outside the office. She readily accepted referral to psychologic services. However, because of travel distance she was seen by someone closer to her home.

SUMMARY

In summary, speech-language pathologists provide many services in the context of a team approach to functional voice disorders. The speech-language pathologist's task is to modify disordered voices into serviceable voices with sufficient stamina to endure the demands of lifestyle and environment. The speech-language pathologist provides a caring and supportive environment that allows patients to explore possible underlying causes. Speech-language pathologists assist in the differential diagnosis of functional from organic disorders. He or she must be able to discern the difference between functional voice patterns and those that require medical/surgical treatment, and to share such insights with the laryngologist responsible for making medical diagnoses. Sensitivity to the fact that the voice is the mirror of emotions is essential. Each speech-language pathologist must be aware of his or her own limitations and be prepared to provide prudent and appropriate referral to other professionals trained in dealing with the psychologic and emotional issues as necessary. Above all, each speech-language pathologist must develop strong and cooperative relationships with other professionals who care for patients with voice disorders.

THE MENTAL HEALTH PROFESSIONAL'S ROLE IN TREATING PSYCHOLOGIC DISTURBANCES IN PATIENTS WITH VOICE DISORDERS

Role of the Psychologic Professional

Both psychologists and psychiatrists specialize in attending to emotional needs and problems. Psychiatrists, as physicians, focus on the neurologic and biologic causes and treatment of psychopathology. Psychologists have advanced graduate training in psychologic function and therapy. They concern themselves with cognitive processes such as thinking, behavior, and memory; the experiencing and expression of emotions; significant inner conflict, characteristic modes of defense in coping with stress; and personality style and perception of self and others, including their expression in interpersonal behavior. Other mental health professionals also provide psychotherapy to performers. In the author's (RTS) practice, clinical psychologists and a psychiatrist serve as members of the voice team, along with SLPs, singing voice specialists, and others. They work directly with some patients and offer consultation to the physician and other professionals.

Assessment of patients is done throughout the physician's history-taking and physical examinations, as well as in a formal psychiatric interview when appropriate in our center. Personality assessment, screening for or evaluating known psychopathology, and assessing potential surgical candidates is performed. Occasionally, psychometric instruments are added to the diagnostic interview. Confidentiality of content is extended to the treatment team to maximize interdisciplinary care. Because of their special interest in voicing parameters, the voice team psychologists are especially attuned to the therapeutic use of their own voices for intensifying rapport and pacing or leading the patient's emotional state during interventions.[20-22]

Psychotherapeutic treatment is offered on a short-term, diagnosis-related basis. Treatment is designed to identify and alleviate emotional distress and to increase the individual's resources for adaptive functioning. Individual psychotherapeutic approaches include brief insight-oriented therapies, cognitive/behavioral techniques, gestalt interventions, stress management, skill building, and clinical hypnosis.

After any indicated acute intervention is provided, and in patients whose coping repertoire is clearly adequate to the stressors, a psychoeducational model is used. The therapy session focuses on a prospective discussion of personal, inherent life stressors, and predictable illnesses. Stress management skills are taught and audiotapes are provided. These offer portable skills and supplemental sessions may be scheduled by mutual decision during appointments at the center for medical examinations and speech or singing voice therapy. A group therapy model, facilitated by the psychologist, has also been used to provide a forum for discussion of patient responses during the various phases of treatment. Participants benefit from the perspective and progress of other patients, the opportunity to decrease their experience of isolation, and the sharing of resources.

Long-term psychodynamic psychotherapy, chronic psychiatric conditions, and patients requiring psychopharmacologic management are referred to other consultant mental health professionals with special interest and insight in voice-related psychologic problems, or to the psychiatrist on our team. The voice team's psychologists also serve in a liaison role when patients already in treatment come to our center for voice care. In addition, the psychologist participates in professional education activities in the medical practice. These include writing, lecturing, and serving as a preceptor for visiting professionals. Specially trained psychologists have proven to be an invaluable addition to the voice team, and close collaboration with team members has proven to be valuable and stimulating for psychologists interested in the care of professional voice users.

General Psychopathologic Presentations

Otolaryngologists and all other health care providers involved with patients with voice disorders should recognize significant comorbid psychopathology and should be prepared to consult an appropriate mental health professional. Psychologists and psychiatrists are responsible for psychologic diagnosis and treatment, but it is important to select mental health professionals with advanced understanding of the special problems associated with voice disorders (especially, but not exclusively, in professional voice users). Patterns of voice use may provide clues to the presence of psychopathology, although voice disturbance is certainly not the principal feature of major psychiatric illness. Nevertheless, failure to recognize serious psychopathology in voice patients may result not only in errors in voice diagnosis and failures of therapy, but, more importantly, in serious injury to the patient, sometimes even death.

Although a full depressive syndrome, including melancholia, can occur as a result of loss, it fulfills the criteria for a major depressive episode only when the individual becomes preoccupied with feelings of worthlessness and guilt, demonstrates marked psychomotor retardation and other biologic markers, and becomes impaired in both social and occupational functioning.[23] Careful listening during the taking of a history will reveal a flat affect, including slowed rate of speech, decreased length of utterance, lengthy pauses, decreased pitch variability, monoloudness, and frequent use of vocal fry.[1] Author William Styron described his speech during his depressive illness as "slowed to the vocal equivalent of a shuffle."[24]

Major depression may be part of the patient's past medical history, may be a comorbid illness, or may be a result of the presenting problem. The essential feature is a prominent, persistent despondent mood characterized by a loss of pleasure in nearly all activities. Appetite and sleep are disturbed and there may be marked weight gain or loss, hypersomnia, or one of three insomnia patterns. Psychomotor agitation or retardation may be present. Patients may be distracted easily and demonstrate memory disturbances and difficulty concentrating. Feelings of worthlessness, helplessness, and hopelessness are a classic triad. Suicidal ideation, with or without plan, and/or concomitant psychotic features, may necessitate emergency intervention.

Major affective disorders are classified as unipolar or bipolar. In bipolar disorder, the patient will also experience periods of mania, which is a recurrent elated state first occurring in young adulthood. First manic episodes in patients over 50 should alert the clinician to medical or CNS illness, or to the effects of drugs. The presentation of the illness includes the following major characteristics on a continuum of severity: elevated mood, irritability/hostility, distractibility, inflated self-concept, grandiosity, physical and sexual overactivity, flight of ideas, decreased need for sleep, social intrusiveness, buying sprees, and inappropriate collections of possessions. Manic patients demonstrate impaired social and familial behavior patterns. They are manipulative, alienate family members, and tend to have a very high divorce rate.[10,25] Vocal presentation will manifest flight of ideas (content), rapid-paced, pressured speech, and often increased pitch and volume. There may be disfluency related to the rate of speech, breathlessness, and difficulty in interrupting the language stream. Three major theories, based on neuroanatomy, neuroendocrinology, and neuropharmacology, are the most currently promulgated explanations for these disease states, but they are beyond the scope of this chapter.[20,25-33]

Treatment of affective disorders includes psychotherapy. Diagnosis and short-term treatment of reactive depressive states may be performed by the psychologist on the voice team, utilizing individual or group therapy modalities. Longer-term treatment necessitates a referral to a community-based psychotherapist, ideally one whose skills, training, and understanding of the medical and artistic components of the illness are well-known to the referring laryngologist. The use of psychopharmacologic agents is a risk/benefit decision. When the patient's symptom severity meets the criteria for major affective disorder, the physiologic effects of the disease, as well as the potential for self-destructive behavior, must be carefully considered.

Anxiety is an expected response in reaction to any medical diagnosis and the required treatment. However, anxiety disorders are seen with increasing incidence. Vocal presentations of anxiety vary with the continuum of psychiatric symptoms, ranging from depression to agitation and including impairment of concentration. Psychotherapy, including desensitization, cognitive/behavioral techniques, stress management, hypnosis, and insight-oriented approaches are helpful. Patients must learn to tolerate their distress and identify factors that precipitate or intensify their symptoms. Medication may be used to treat the neurotransmitter disturbances and decrease the frequency of episodes. However, it may leave the underlying conflict unresolved and negatively affect artistic quality.[1,8,27] Some medical conditions are commonly associated with a presenting symptom of anxiety. These include CNS disease, Cushing's syndrome, hyperthyroidism, hypoglycemia, the consequences of minor head trauma, premenstrual syndrome, and cardiac disease such as mitral valve prolapse and various arrhythmias. Medications prescribed for other conditions may have anxiety as a side effect. These include such drugs as amphetamines, corticosteroids, caffeine, decongestants, cocaine, and the asthma armamentarium.[4]

Although psychotic behavior may be observed with major affective disorders, organic CNS disease, or drug toxicity, schizophrenia occurs in only 1 to 2% of the general population.[32] Its onset is most prominent in mid to late adolescence through the late 20s. Incidence is approximately equal for males and females and schizophrenia has been described in all cultures and socioeconomic classes. This is a group of mental disorders in which massive disruptions in cognition or perception, such as delusions, hallucinations, or thought disorders, are present. The fundamental causes of schizophrenia are unknown but the disease involves excessive amounts of neurotransmitters, chiefly dopamine. There is a genetic predisposition. Somatic delusions may present as voice complaints. However, flattening or inappropriateness of affect, a diagnostic characteristic of schizophrenia, will produce voice changes similar to those described for depression and mania. Where hallucinatory material creates fear, characteristics of anxiety and agitation will be audible. Perseveration, repetition, and neologisms may be present. The signs and symptoms also include clear indications of deterioration in social or occupational functioning, personal hygiene, changes in behavior and movement, an altered sense of self, and the presence of blunted or inappropriate affect.[4,23,32] The disease is chronic and control requires consistent use of antipsychotic medications for symptoms management. Social support in regulating activities of daily living is crucial in maintaining emotional control. Family counseling and support groups offer the opportunity to share experiences and resources in the care of individuals with this difficult disease.

Psychoactive Medications

All psychoactive agents have effects that can interfere with vocal tract physiology. Treatment requires frequent, open collaboration between the laryngologist and the psychiatrist. The patient and physician need to carefully weigh the benefits and side effects of available medications. Patients must be informed of the relative probability of experiencing any known side effect. This is especially critical to the professional voice user and plays an important role in developing a treatment plan when there is no imminent serious psychiatric risk. An overview of psychoactive medications is provided in Appendix 33–2.

Ongoing psychiatric treatment of patients with voice disorders mandates a careful evaluation of current and prior psychoactive drug therapy. In addition, numerous psychoactive substances are used in the medical management of neurologic conditions such as Tourette's syndrome (haloperidol), chronic pain syndromes (carbamazepine), and vertigo (diazepam, clonazepam).

The laryngologist must thus identify symptoms that may be causally related to drug side effects and avoid drug interactions. It is appropriate (with the patient's consent) to consult with the prescribing physician directly to advocate the use of the psychoactive drug least likely to produce adverse effects on the voice while adequately controlling the psychiatric illness. Patients with major psychiatric disorders should be under the care of a psychiatrist. The voice team should be guided by his or her recommendations. The psychiatric disease is most likely to be the highest priority in terms of risk to the patient.[28]

Eating Disorders and Substance Abuse

The rapport of the laryngologist and voice team may also allow patients to reveal other self-defeating disorders. Among the most common in arts medicine are body dysmorphic (eating) disorders and substance abuse problems. Comprehensive discussion of these subjects is beyond the scope of this chapter but it is important for the laryngologist to recognize such conditions, not only because of their effects on the voice, but also because of their potentially serious general medical and psychiatric implications. In addition to posterior laryngitis and pharyngitis, laryngeal findings associated with bulimia include subepithelial vocal fold hemorrhages, superficial telangiectasia of the vocal fold mucosa, and vocal fold scarring.[27]

Bulimia is a disorder associated with self-induced vomiting following episodes of binge eating. It may occur sporadically, or it may be a chronic problem. Vomiting produces signs and symptoms similar to se-vere chronic reflux as well as thinning of tooth enamel. Bulimia nervosa can be a serious disorder and may be associated with anorexia nervosa. Bulimia may be more prevalent than is commonly realized. It has been estimated to occur in as many as 2 to 4% of female adolescents and female young adults, and this number is rising. Laryngologists must be attentive to the potential for anorexia and exercise addiction in the maintenance of a desirable body appearance in performers.

Appetite Suppressants

There is enormous popular interest in the use of appetite suppressants in weight management. Many myths persist about proper weight management approaches in singers and the value and/or risk of weight loss. The availability and popularity of appetite suppressant drugs, and marketing approaches which included making them available in franchised weight loss centers, led many Americans to explore the use of "Fen-Phen" (phentermine [Ionamine and others] and fenfluramine [Pondomin]). Another drug that gained popularity is dexfenfluramine hydrochloride (Redux). These medications have limited efficacy in changing metabolism and limiting cravings. Many patients took these drugs in combinations that were never approved for concomitant use. Laryngologists and psychologic professionals caring for singers and other performers should be certain to investigate the potential use of these medications, which were voluntarily withdrawn from the market by their manufacturer in 1997 because of a significant correlation with cardiac valve damage and with pulmonary hypertension. The laryngologist should question patients about the use of over-the-counter and "herbal" products such as ephedra and "Metabolife." These too are potentially harmful because of sympathomimetic effects.

Alcohol, benzodiazepines, stimulants, cocaine, and narcotics are notoriously readily available in the performing community and on the streets. Patients who demonstrate signs and symptoms, or who admit that these areas of their lives are out of control, have taken the first step to regaining control, and this should be acknowledged while efficiently arranging treatment for them. The window of opportunity is often remarkably narrow. The physician should establish close ties to excellent treatment facilities where specialized clinicians can offer confidential outpatient management, with inpatient care available when required for safety.[1]

Neurogenic Dysphonia

Patients with neurologic disease are likely to experience psychiatric symptoms, especially depression and anxiety. These disorders cause physiologic changes that may exacerbate or mask the underlying neurologic presentation. Metcalfe and colleagues cite the incidence of severe depression and/or anxiety in neurologic patients at one-third.[34] Site of lesion affects the incidence, with lesions of the left cerebral hemisphere, basal ganglia, limbic system, thalamus, and anterior frontal lobe more likely to produce depression and anxiety.[35] These same structures are important in voice, speech, and language production, so depression and anxiety logically coexist with voice and language disorders resulting from CNS pathology.[35,36] Dystonias and stuttering are also associated with both neurologic and psychogenic etiologies, and must be carefully distinguished by the laryngologist before instituting interdisciplinary treatment.[37]

Stress Management

Stress pervades virtually all professions in today's fast-moving society. A singer preparing for a series of concerts, a teacher preparing for presentation of lectures, a lawyer anticipating a major trial, a businessperson negotiating an important contract, or a member of any other goal-oriented profession, each must deal with a myriad of demands on his or her time and talents. In 1971, Brodnitz reported on 2,286 cases of all forms of voice disorders and classified 80% of the disorders as attributable to voice abuse or psychogenic factors resulting in vocal dysfunction.[38] However, regardless of the incidence, it is clear that stress-related problems are important and common in professional voice users. Stress may be physical or psychologic and it often involves a combination of both. Either may interfere with performance. Stress represents a special problem for singers, because its physiologic manifestations may interfere with the delicate mechanisms of voice production.[1]

Stress is recognized as a factor in illness and disease and is probably implicated in almost every type of human problem. It is estimated that 50 to 70% of all physicians' visits involve complaints of stress-related illness.[39] Stress is a psychologic experience that has physiologic consequences. A brief review of some terminology may be useful. *Stress* is a term that is used broadly. Our working definition is emotional, cognitive, and physiologic reactions to psychologic demands and challenges. The term *stress level* reflects the degree of stress experienced. Stress is not an all-or-none phenomenon. The psychologic effects of stress range from mild to severely incapacitating. The term *stress response* refers to the physiologic reaction of an organism to stress. A stressor is an external stimulus or internal thought, perception, image, or emotion that creates stress.[40] Two other concepts are important in a contemporary discussion of stress: coping and adaptation. Lazarus has defined coping as "the process of managing demands (external and internal) that are appraised as taxing or exceeding the resources of the person."[41] In the early 1930s, Hans Selye, an endocrinologist, discovered a generalized response to stressors in research animals. He described their responses using the term *general adaptation syndrome*. Selye (cited in Green and Snellenberger[40]) postulated that the physiology of the research animals was trying to adapt to the challenges of noxious stimuli. The process of adaptation to chronic and severe stressors was harmful over time. There were three phases to the observed response: alarm, adaptation, and exhaustion. These phases were named for physiologic responses during a sequence of events. The alarm phase is the characteristic fight or flight response. If the stressor continued, the animal appeared to adapt. In the adaptation phase, the physiologic responses were less extreme but the animal eventually became more exhausted. In the exhaustion phase, the animal's adaptation energy was spent, physical symptoms occurred, and some animals died.[40]

Stress responses occur in part through the autonomic nervous system. A stressor triggers particular brain centers, which in turn affect target organs through nerve connections. The brain has two primary pathways for the stress response, neuronal and hormonal, and these pathways overlap. The body initiates a stress response through one of three pathways: through sympathetic nervous system efferents which terminate on target organs such as the heart and blood vessels; via the release of epinephrine and norepinephrine from the adrenal medulla; and through the release of various other catecholamines.[40] A full description of the various processes involved is beyond the scope of this chapter. However, stress has numerous physical consequences. Through the autonomic nervous system, it may alter oral and vocal fold secretions, heart rate, and gastric acid production. Under acute, anxiety-producing circumstances, such changes are to be expected. When frightened, a normal person's palms become cold and sweaty, the mouth becomes dry, heart rate increases, his or her pupils change size, and stomach acid secretions may increase. These phenomena are objective signs that may be observed by a physician and their symptoms may be recognized by the performer as dry mouth and voice fatigue, heart palpitations, and "heartburn." More severe, prolonged stress is also commonly associated with increased muscle tension throughout the body (but particularly in the head and neck), headaches, decreased ability to concentrate, and insomnia. Chronic fatigue is also a common symptom. These physiologic alterations may lead not only to altered vocal quality, but also to physical pathology. Increased gastric acid secretion is associated with ulcers, as well as reflux laryngitis and arytenoid irritation. Other gastrointestinal manifestations, such as colitis, irritable bowel syndrome, and dysphagia are also described. Chronic stress and tension may cause numerous pain syndromes although headaches, particularly migraines in vulnerable individuals, are most common. Stress is also associated with more serious physical problems such as myocardial infarction, asthma, and depression of the immune system.[27,40] Thus, the constant pressure under which many performers live may be more than an inconvenience. Stress factors should be recognized, and appropriate modifications should be made to ameliorate them.

Stressors may be physical or psychologic and often involve a combination of both. Either may interfere with performance. There are several situations in which physical stress is common and important. Generalized fatigue is seen frequently in hard-working singers, especially in the frantic few weeks preceding major performances. In order to maintain normal mucosal secretions, a strong immune system to fight infection, and the ability of muscles to recover from heavy use, rest, proper nutrition, and hydration are required. When the body is stressed through deprivation of these essentials, illness such as upper respiratory infection, voice fatigue, hoarseness, and other vocal dysfunctions may supervene.

Lack of physical conditioning undermines the power source of the voice. A person who becomes short of breath while climbing a flight of stairs hardly has the abdominal and respiratory endurance needed to sustain him or her optimally through the rigors of performance. The stress of attempting to perform under such circumstances often results in voice dysfunction.

Oversinging is another common physical stress. As with running, swimming, or any other athletic activity that depends upon sustained, coordinated muscle activity, singing requires conditioning to build up strength and endurance. Rest periods are also essential for muscle recovery. Singers who are accustomed to singing for one or two hours a day stress their physical voice-producing mechanism severely when they suddenly begin rehearsing for 14 hours daily immediately prior to performance.

Medical treatment of stress depends upon the specific circumstances. When the diagnosis is appropriate but poorly controlled anxiety, the singer can usually be helped by assurance that his or her voice complaint is related to anxiety and not to any physical problem. Under ordinary circumstances, once the singer's mind is put to rest regarding the questions of nodules, vocal fold injury, or other serious problems, his or her training usually allows compensation for vocal manifestations of anxiety, especially when the vocal complaint is minor. Slight alterations in quality or increased vocal fatigue are seen most frequently. These are often associated with lack of sleep, oversinging, and dehydration associated with the stress-producing commitment. The singer or actor should be advised to modify these and to consult his or her voice teacher. The voice teacher should ensure that good vocal technique is being used under performance and rehearsal circumstances. Frequently, young singers are not trained sufficiently in how and when to "mark." For example, many singers whistle to rest their voices, not realizing that active vocalization and potentially fatiguing vocal fold contact occur when whistling. Technical proficiency and a plan for voice conservation during rehearsals and performances are essentials under these circumstances. A manageable stressful situation may become unmanageable if real physical vocal problems develop.

Several additional modalities may be helpful in selected circumstances. Relative voice rest (using the voice only when necessary) may be important not only to voice conservation but also to psychologic relaxation. Under stressful circumstances, a singer needs as much peace and quiet as possible, not hectic socializing, parties with heavy voice use in noisy environments, and press appearances. The importance of adequate sleep and fluid intake cannot be overemphasized. Local therapy such as steam inhalation and neck muscle massage may be helpful in some people and certainly do no harm. The doctor may be very helpful in alleviating the singer's exogenous stress by conveying "doctor's orders" directly to theater management. This will save the singer the discomfort of having to personally confront an authority and violate his or her "show must go on" ethic. A short telephone call by the physician can be highly therapeutic.

When stress is chronic and incapacitating, more comprehensive measures are required. If psychologic stress manifestations become so severe as to impair performance or necessitate the use of drugs to allow performance, psychotherapy is indicated. The goals of psychotherapeutic approaches to stress management include:

- changing external and internal stressors;
- changing affective and cognitive reactions to stressors;
- changing physiologic reactions to stress; and
- changing stress behaviors.

A psychoeducational model is customarily used. Initially, the psychotherapist will assist the patient in identifying and evaluating stressor characteristics. A variety of assessment tools are available for this purpose. Interventions designed to increase a sense of efficacy and personal control are designed. Perceived control over the stressor directly affects stress level and it changes one's experience of the stressor. Laboratory and human research has determined a sense of control to be one of the most potent elements in the modulation of stress responses. Concrete exercises that impose time management are taught and practiced. Patients are urged to identify and expand their network of support as well. Psychologic intervention requires evaluation of the patient's cognitive model. Cognitive restructuring exercises as well as classical behavioral conditioning responses are useful, practical tools that patients easily learn and utilize effectively with practice. Cognitive skills include the use of monitored perception, thought, and internal dialogue to regulate emotional and physiologic responses. A variety of relaxation techniques are available and are ordinarily taught in the course of stress-management treatment. These include progressive relaxation, hypnosis, autogenic training and imagery, and biofeedback training. Underlying all these approaches is the premise that making conscious normally unconscious processes leads to control and self-efficacy.[1]

As with all medical conditions, the best treatment for stress in singers is prevention. Awareness of the conditions that lead to stress and its potential adverse effect on voice production often allows the singer to anticipate and avoid these problems. Stress is inevitable in performance and in life. Performers must learn to recognize it, compensate for it when necessary, and incorporate it into their singing as emotion and excitement—the "edge." Stress should be controlled, not pharmacologically eliminated. Used well, stress should be just one more tool of the singer's trade.

Performance Anxiety

Psychologic stress is intrinsic to vocal performance. For most people, sharing emotions is stressful even in the privacy of home, let alone under spotlights in front of a room full of people. Under ordinary circumstances, during training, a singer or actor learns to recognize his or her customary anxiety about performing, to accept it as part of his or her instrument, and to compensate for it. When psychologic pressures become severe enough to impair or prohibit performance, careful treatment is required. Such occurrences usually are temporary and happen because of a particular situation such as short notice for a critically important performance, a recent family death, and so forth. Chronic disabling psychologic stress in the face of performance is a more serious problem. In its most extreme forms, performance anxiety actually disrupts the skills of performers; in its milder form it lessens the enjoyment of appearing in public.[1]

Virtually all performers have experienced at least some symptoms of hyperarousal during their performance history and all fear their re-emergence. Some fortunate people seem to bypass this type of trauma, exhibiting only mild symptoms of nervousness ahead of performance, which disappear the moment they walk on stage.[42] In these individuals, personal physiology works consistently for instead of against them.[1] The human nervous system functions exquisitely for the great majority of our needs, but in performance anxiety it begins to work against the performer in those very circumstances when he or she wants most to do well. Human autonomic arousal continues to be under the sway of primal survival mechanisms, which are the basic lines of defense against physical danger: they prepare the individual to fight or flee in response to the perception of threat.[1] They are essential to our survival in situations of physical danger. The dangers that threaten performers are not physical in nature, but the human nervous system cannot differentiate between physical and psychologic dangers, producing physiologic responses that are the same. When the physical symptoms associated with extreme arousal are enumerated, it is easy to understand why they can be major impediments to skilled performance and may even be disabling. They include rapid heart rate, dry mouth, sweating palms, palpitations, tremor, high blood pressure, restricted breathing, frequency of urination, and impaired memory.[1]

This process is cognitive, and Beck and Emery[42] describe the development of cognitive sets using an analogy to photography. The individual scans the relevant environment and then determines which aspect, if any, on which to focus. Cognitive processing reduces the number of dimensions in a situation, sacrifices a great deal of information, and induces distortion into the "picture." Certain aspects of the situation are highlighted at the expense of others, the relative magnitudes and prominence of various features are distorted, and there is loss of perspective. In addition, they describe blurring and loss of important detail. These are the decisive influences upon what the individual sees. They describe how the cognitive set influences the picture that is perceived. The existing cognitive sets determine which aspects of the scene will be highlighted, which glossed over, and which excluded. The individual's first impressions of an event provide information that either reinforces or modifies the pre-existing cognitive set. The initial impression is critical because it determines whether the situation directly affects the patient's vital interest. It also sets the course of subsequent steps in conceptualization and the total response to a situation.[42] According to the cognitive model, at the same time the individual is evaluating the nature of the threat, he or she is also assessing the availability and effectiveness of internal resources for dealing with it and deflecting potential damage. The balance between potential danger and available coping responses determines the nature and intensity of the patient's stress response. Two major behavioral systems are activated, either separately or together, in response to the threat: those mediated by the sympathetic branch of the autonomic nervous system, "the fight or flight response," and those related to the parasympathetic branch, "the freeze or faint response."

A major feature of performance anxiety is that the actual fear prior to entering the situation appears plausible. A complex web of factors in this situation may aggravate the patient's fears. These may include the relative status of the performer and of the evaluator, the performer's skill, his or her confidence in the ability to perform adequately in a given "threatening situation," and the appraisal of the degree of threat (including the severity of potential damage to one's career and self-esteem). The individual's threshold of automatic defenses that undermine performance and the rigidity of the rules relevant to the performance in question are also factored into the intensity of the response. Unfortunately, the experience also increases the likelihood of the undesirable consequences. A vicious cycle is created in which the anticipation of an absolute, extreme, irreversible outcome makes the performer more fearful of the effects and inhibited when entering the situation.[42] Negative evaluation by judges or audiences is the common psychic threat. The individual suffering from performance anxiety believes that he or she is being scrutinized and judged. Components under observation include fluency, artistry, self-assurance, and technique.

Although most fears tend to decline with continued exposure and expertise, Caine notes that even highly skilled performers do not always experience lessening of performance anxiety over time.[43] Indeed, she describes a dilemma for the expert performer in which a potentially humiliating and frightening mistake is less and less tolerable. A behavioral feedback loop becomes established. The act of performance becomes the stimulus perceived as a threat. In situations of danger, the individual's physiology primes him or her to become more alert and sensitive to all potential threats in the surrounding environment. Anticipating mistakes increases arousal, which further enhances access to memories of mistakes and feelings of humiliation, which activates more fears and more arousal. This

process is linked by catastrophic thoughts, physiologic manifestations of anxiety, and imagery. Unfortunately, this process is often initiated very early in a young performer's training.[1] This process can also be seen in other highly driven and perfectionistic groups of individuals, for example, many surgeons.

A variety of psychotherapeutic treatment approaches to performance anxiety have been described in the literature. The most effective of these are cognitive and behavioral strategies, which assist performers in modulating levels of arousal to more optimal levels. Cognitive therapy addresses the essential mechanism sustaining performance anxiety: the cognitive set a performer brings to the performance situation. The autonomic nervous system is merely responding to the threat as it is perceived, and the intensity of the response correlates to the degree of threat generated by the sufferer's catastrophic expectations and negative self-talk. Cognitive restructuring techniques are extremely effective in producing the necessary adjustments. Monitoring internal self-dialogue comprises the first step in recognizing the dimension of the problem. These excessively self-critical attitudes enhance the probability of mistakes. Homework exercises designed to monitor critical thoughts are assigned. In the second step of cognitive treatment, adaptive, realistic self-statements are substituted. Behaviorally based treatment approaches such as thought-stopping, paired relaxation responses and "prescribing the symptom" are also utilized. Hypnosis is efficacious, providing relaxation techniques and introducing positive, satisfying, and joyful imagery.[1]

Brief psychotherapeutic approaches produce effective outcomes, but some proponents of the psychodynamic approach argue that the underlying conflicts will resurface in some form of symptom substitution. This author's (DCR) clinical approach includes an exploration for secondary gain offered by disabling performance anxiety. The performer's unconscious fear must be addressed for these treatments to remain effective and to avoid eventual symptom substitution. Patients are asked: "What does this symptom accomplish for you?" The question may sound unsympathetic, and the patient may need to search deeply for the answer. This search requires significant courage. If the patient makes effective use of the treatment strategies, what might be expected of him or her? Where might success lead? Is he or she ready to go on to the next phase in a performance career, or does it remain safer to be immobilized? Which problem is honestly more terrifying: the symptom of performance anxiety or the possibility of success? What would be the consequences of resolving the immobilizing performance anxiety? The patient is asked to imagine life in which the problem is no longer present. This exploration is often conducted using the relaxation and enhanced perception available in hypnosis.[1] Most of these questions are painful ones to answer. For some performers, success beckons with one hand and signals caution with the other. Eloise Ristad describes this with extraordinarily pragmatic wisdom.[44]

The part of us that holds back knows that change involves challenges-losses as well as gains. Change always means dying a little; leaving behind something old and tattered and no longer useful to us even though comfortably familiar.

A successful psychotherapeutic response to disabling performance anxiety requires a thorough explanation of the personal meaning of the symptom to the patient as well as an extensive and exciting repertoire of strategies for effecting personal change.

Reactive Responses

Reaction to illness is a major source of psychiatric disturbance in patients with significant voice dysfunction. Loss of communicative function is an experience of alienation that threatens human self-definition and independence. Catastrophic fears of loss of productivity, economic and social status and, in professional voice users, creative artistry, contribute to rising anxiety. Anxiety is known to worsen existing communication disorders, and the disturbances in memory, concentration, and synaptic transmission secondary to depression may intensify other voice symptoms and interfere with rehabilitation.

The self-concept is an essential construct of Carl Rodgers' theories of counseling. Rodgers described self-concept as composed of perceptions of the characteristics of the self and the relationships of the self to various aspects of life, as well as the values attached to the perceptions. Rodgers suggested that equilibrium requires that patients' self-concepts be congruent with their life experiences. It follows, then, that it is not the disability per se, that psychologically influences the person, but rather the subjective meaning and feelings attached to the disability. According to Rodgers, the two major psychologic defenses which operate to maintain consistent self-concept are denial and distortion.[45]

Families of patients are affected as well. They are often confused about the diagnosis and poorly prepared to support the patient's coping responses. The resulting stress may negatively influence family dynamics and intensify the patient's depressive illness.[46] As the voice-injured patient experiences the process of grieving, the psychologist may assume a more prominent role in his or her care. Essentially, the voice-injured patient goes through a grieving process similar to pa-

tients who mourn other losses such as the death of a loved one. In some cases, especially among voice professionals, the patients actually mourn the loss of their self as they perceive it.

The psychologist is responsible for facilitating the tasks of mourning and monitoring the individual's formal mental status for clinically significant changes.[1,8,9] There are a number of models for tracking this process. The most easily understood is that of Worden,[47] as adapted by the author (DCR). Initially, the task is to accept the reality of the loss. The need for and distress of accepting this is vestigial during the phase of diagnosis, and is held consciously in abeyance during the acute and rehabilitative phases of treatment, but it is reinforced with accumulating data measuring the patient's vocal function. As the reality becomes undeniable, the mourner must be helped to express the full range of grieving affect. The rate of accomplishing this is variable and individual. Generally, it will occur in the style with which the person usually copes with crisis and may be florid or tightly constricted. All responses must be invited and normalized. The psychologist facilitates the process and stays particularly attuned to unacceptable, divergent responses or to the failure to move through any particular response.

As attempts to deny the loss take place and fail, the mourner gradually encounters the next task: beginning to live and cope in a world in which the lost object is absent. This is the psychoanalytic process of decathexis; it requires the withdrawal of life energies from the lost object and the reinvesting of them in the self. For some professional voice users, this may be a temporary state as they make adjustments required by their rehabilitation demands. In other cases, the need for change will be lasting: change in fach, change in repertoire, need for amplification, altered performance schedule or, occasionally, change in career.[1,8,9]

As the patient so injured seeks to heal his or her life, another task looms. Known as recathexis, it involves reinvesting life energies in other relationships, interests, talents, and life goals. The individual is assisted in redefining and revaluing the self as apart from the voice. The voice is then seen as the product of the self, rather than as the equivalent of the self. For many performers this is painfully difficult.[1,8,9,47] Rosen and Sataloff have described in detail research applying the various theoretical models of grief resolution to the perception of vocal injury in professional voice users.[8]

The Surgical Experience

When vocal fold surgery is indicated, many individuals will demonstrate hospital-related phobias or self-destructive responses to pain. Adamson et al describe the importance of understanding how the patient's occupational identity will be affected by surgical intervention.[48] Vocal fold surgery has an impact on the major mode of communication that all human beings utilize; the impact is extraordinarily anxiety-producing in professional voice users. Even temporary periods of absolute voice restriction may induce feelings of insecurity, helplessness, and dissociation from the verbal world. Carpenter details the value of an early therapy session to focus on the fears, fantasies, misconceptions, and regression that frequently accompany a decision to undergo surgery.[49]

Surgical discussion usually highlights vocal fold surgery as elective for benign disease. The patient chooses surgery as the best or only remaining means to regaining the previously "normal" voice, or a different but desirable voice. The standard of care includes a thorough preoperative discussion of the limits and complications of surgery, with recognition by the surgeon that anxiety affects both understanding and retention of information about undesirable outcomes. Personality psychopathology or unrealistic expectations of the impact of surgery on their lives are factors for which surgical candidates can be screened.[5,50,51] Recognizing such problems preoperatively allows preoperative counseling and obviates many postoperative difficulties.

Although a thorough discussion is outside the scope of this chapter, surgically treated voice patients include those undergoing laryngectomy, with or without a voice prosthesis. The laryngectomized individual must make major psychologic and social adjustments. These include not only those adjustments related to a diagnosis of cancer, but also to a sudden disability: loss of voice. With the improvement in prognosis, research has begun to focus on the individual's quality of life after the laryngectomy. There is wide variability in the quality of preoperative and postoperative psychologic support reported by patients during each phase of care. Special psychologic issues in professional voice users diagnosed with laryngeal cancer are discussed in detail in other works.[1] Providing this support is a crucial role for the voice team's psychologist.[21,24,52]

CONCLUSION

Psychophysiologic research informs our treatment and maximizes the benefits of medical interactions in every specialty. This is the rightful role of the arts medicine psychologist: to possess mastery of the knowledge bases of psychology and medicine and also an experiential understanding of the performing arts so that he or she may stand in alliance with the injured performer on the journey to explore, understand, and modify the psychologic impact of performance-related injuries. The speech-language pathologist must understand the psychologic factors that may cause, or be caused by, voice disorders. The speech-language pathologist must also recognize his or her limits as a psychologic counselor and know when to refer to and collaborate with a mental health professional while maintaining responsibility for voice modification and some degree of psychologic support. The laryngologist must recognize the need for therapy in individual patients, accurately diagnose the presence of organic and or or functional disorders, select and coordinate the therapy team, and retain overall responsibility for the therapeutic process and the patient's outcome. Those who are privileged to care for that uniquely human capability—the voice—quickly come to understand the essential role of psychologic awareness in our treatment failures and successes.

REFERENCES

1. Rosen DC, Sataloff RT. *Psychology of Voice Disorders.* San Diego, CA: Singular Publishing Group; 1997.
2. Aronson A. *Clinical Voice Disorders.* 3rd ed. New York, NY: Thieme Medical Publishers; 1990:117–145, 314–315.
3. Sundberg J. *The Science of the Singing Voice.* DeKalb, IL: Northern Illinois University Press; 1985:146–156.
4. Vogel D, Carter J. *The Effects of Drugs on Communication Disorders.* San Diego, CA: Singular Publishing Group; 1995: 31–143.
5. Shontz F. Body image and physical disability. In: Cash T, Pruzinsky T, eds. *Body Images: Development, Deviance and Change.* New York, NY: Guilford Press; 1990:149–169.
6. Freedman R. Cognitive behavioral perspectives on body image change. In: Cash TF, Pruzinsky T, eds. *Body Images: Development, Deviance and Change.* New York, NY: Guilford Press; 1990:273–295.
7. Horney K. Cited by: Meissner W. Theories of personality. In: Nicholi A, ed. *The New Harvard Guide to Psychiatry.* Cambridge, MA: Harvard University Press; 1988:177–199.
8. Rosen DC, Sataloff RT. Psychological aspects of voice disorders. In: Rubin JS, Sataloff RT, Korovin G, Gould WJ, eds. *Diagnosis and Treatment of Voice Disorders.* New York, NY: Igaku-Shoin Medical Publishers; 1995:491–501.
9. Rosen DC, Sataloff RT, Evans H, Hawkshaw M. Self-esteem in singers: singing healthy, singing hurt. *NATS J.* 1993; 49:32–35.
10. Butcher P, Elias A, Raven R. *Psychogenic Voice Disorders and Cognitive-Behavior Therapy.* San Diego, CA: Singular Publishing Group; 1993;3–22.
11. Ostwald P, Avery M, Ostwald LD. Psychiatric problems of performing artists. In: Sataloff RT, Brandfonbrenner A, Lederman R, eds. *Performing Arts Medicine.* San Diego, CA: Singular Publishing Group; 1997:337–348.

12. Nemiah J. Psychoneurotic disorders. In: Nicholi A, ed. *The New Harvard Guide to Psychiatry*. Cambridge, MA: Harvard University Press; 1988:234–258.

13. Ziegler FS, Imboden JB. Contemporary conversion reactions: II. conceptual model. *Arch Gen Psychiatry*. 1962;6: 279–287.

14. Hartman DE, Daily WW, Morin KN. A case of superior laryngeal nerve paresis and psychogenic dysphonia. *J Speech Hear Disord*. 1989;54:526–529.

15. Sapir S, Aronson AE. Coexisting psychogenic and neurogenic dysphonia: a source of diagnostic confusion. *Br J Disord Commun*. 1987;22:73–80.

16. Cummings JL, Benson DF, Houlihan JP, Gosenfield LF. Mutism: loss of neocortical and limbic vocalization. *J Nerv Ment Dis*. 1983;171:255–259.

17. Moses PJ. *The Voice of Neurosis*. New York, NY: Grune and Stratton; 1954.

18. Luchsinger R, Arnold E. *Voice-Speech-Language—Clinical Communicology: Its Physiology and Pathology*. Belmont, CA: Wadsworth; 1965.

19. Rulnick RK, Heuer RJ, Perez KS, Emerich KA, Sataloff RT. Voice therapy. In: Sataloff RT. *Professional Voice: Science and Art of Clinical Care*. 2nd ed. San Diego, CA: Singular Publishing Group; 1997:699–720.

20. Weissman MM. The psychological treatment of depression. Evidence for the efficacy of psychotherapy alone, in comparison with, and in combination with pharmacotherapy. *Arch Gen Psychiatry*. 1979;38:1261–1269.

21. Gardner WH. Adjustment problems of laryngectomized women. *Arch Otolaryngol*. 1966;83:31–42.

22. Lankton S. *Practical Magic: A Translation of Neuro-Linguistic Programming into Clinical Psychotherapy*. Cupertino, CA: Meta Publications; 1980:174.

23. American Psychiatric Association. *Diagnostic and Statistical Manual of Mental Disorders III*. Washington, DC: American Psychiatric Association; 1987:206–210.

24. Styron W. *Darkness Visible: A Memoir of Madness*. New York, NY: Random House; 1990:27.

25. Klerman G. Depression and related disorders of mood. In: Nicholi A, ed. *The New Harvard Guide to Psychiatry*. Cambridge, MA: Harvard University Press; 1988:309–336.

26. Ross E. Rush A. Diagnosis and neuroanatomical correlates of depression in brain-damaged patients: implications for a neurology of depression. *Arch Gen Psychiatry*. 1981;38:1344–1354.

27. Sataloff RT. Stress, anxiety and psychogenic dysphonia. In: Sataloff RT. *Professional Voice: The Science and Art of Clinical Care*. 2nd ed. San Diego, CA: Singular Publishing Group; 1997:195–200.

28. Sataloff RT, Lawrence VL, Hawkshaw M, Rosen DC. Medications and their effects on the voice. In: Benninger MS, Jacobson BH, Johnson AF, eds. *Vocal Arts Medicine: The Care and Prevention of Professional Voice Disorders*. New York, NY: Thieme Medical Publishers; 1994:216–225.

29. Schatzberg A, Cole J. *Manual of Clinical Psychopharmacology*. 2nd ed. Washington, DC: American Psychiatric Press; 1991:40, 50, 55, 58, 66, 68, 69, 72–77, 110–125, 158–165, 169–177, 185–227, 343–348.

30. Stam H, Koopmans J, Mathieson C. The psychological impact of a laryngectomy: comprehensive assessment. *J Psychosoc Oncol*. 1991;9:37–58.

31. Stroudmire A. *Psychological Factors Affecting Medication Conditions*. Washington, DC: American Psychiatric Press; 1995:187–192.

32. Tsuang M, Faraone S, Day M. Schizophrenic disorders. In: Nicholi A, ed. *The New Harvard Guide to Psychiatry*. Cambridge, MA: Harvard University Press; 1988:259–295.

33. Watkins J. *Hypnotherapeutic Techniques*. New York, NY: Irvington Publishers; 1987:114.

34. Metcalfe R, Firth D, Pollock S. Creed F. Psychiatric morbidity and illness behaviour in female neurological in-patients. *J Neurol Neurosurg Psychiatry*. 1988;51:1387–1390.

35. Gianotti G. Emotional behavior and hemispheric side of lesion. *Cortex*. 1972;8:41–55.

36. Alexander MP, LoVerne SR Jr. Aphasia after left hemispheric intracerebral hemorrhage. *Neurology*. 1980;30: 1193–1202.

37. Mahr G, Leith W. Psychogenic stuttering of adult onset. *J Speech Hear Res*. 1992;35:283–286.

38. Brodnitz FS. Hormones and the human voice. *Bull NY Acad Med*. 1971;47:183–191.

39. Everly GS. *A Clinical Guide to the Treatment of Human Stress Response*. New York, NY: Plenum Press; 1989:40–43.

40. Green J, Snellenberger R. *The Dynamics of Health and Wellness. A Biopsychosocial Approach*. Fort Worth, TX: Holt, Reinhardt and Winston; 1991:61–64, 92, 98, 101–136.

41. Lazarus RS, Folkman S. *Stress Appraisal and Coping*. New York, NY: Springer-Verlag; 1984;283.

42. Beck A, Emery G. *Anxiety Disorders and Phobias: A Cognitive Perspective*. New York, NY: Basic Books; 1985:38–50,151.

43. Caine JB. Understanding and treating performance anxiety from a cognitive-behavior therapy perspective. *NATS J*. 1991;47:27–51.

44. Ristad E. *A Soprano on Her Head: Right Side Up Reflections on Life and Other Performances*. Moab, UT: Real People Press; 1982:154–155.

45. Rodgers CA. A theory of personality and interpersonal relationships as developed in a client centered framework. In: Koch S, ed. *Psychology: A Study of a Science*. New York, NY: McGraw-Hill, 1959:184–256.

46. Zraick RJ, Boone DR. Spouse attitudes toward the person with aphasia. *J Speech Hear Res*. 1991;34:123–128.

47. Worden W. *Grief Counseling and Grief Therapy*. New York, NY: Springer-Verlag; 1982:7–18.

48. Adamson JD, Hersuberg D, Shane I. The psychic significance of parts of the body in surgery. In: Howells JG, ed. *Modern Perspectives in the Psychiatric Aspects of Surgery*. New York, NY: Brunner Mazel; 1976:20–45.

49. Carpenter B. Psychological aspects of vocal fold surgery. In: Gould WJ, Sataloff RT, Spiegel JR, eds. *Voice Surgery*. St Louis, MO: Mosby; 1993:339–343.

50. Macgregor FC. Patient dissatisfaction with results of technically satisfactory surgery. *Aesthetic Plast Surg*. 1981; 5:27–32.

51. Ray CJ, Fitzgibbon G. The socially mediated reduction of stress in surgical patients. In: Obourne DJ, Grunberg M, Eisner JR, eds. *Research and Psychology in Medicine*. Vol 2. Oxford, England: Pergamon Press; 1979:521–527.

52. Berkowitz JF, Lucente FF. Counseling before laryngectomy. *Laryngoscope*. 1985;95:1332–1336.

53. Cole JO, Bodkin JA. Antidepressant drug side-effects. *J Clin Psychiatry*. 1990;51:521–526.

54. *Physician's Desk Reference*. Oradell, NJ: Medical Economics Data; 1994:2000–2003, 2267–2270.

55. *Physician's Desk Reference*. Oradell, NJ: Medical Economics Data; 1996:B20.

56. *Physician's Desk Reference*. Oradell, NJ: Medical Economics Data. 2000:562, 1073, 1649, 2209, 3070, 3237.

57. *Physician's Desk Reference*. Oradell, NJ: Medical Economics Data. 1997:1615, 1878, 2239.

58. Janitec P, Davis J, Prescorn F, Ab S. *Principles and Practice of Psychopharmacology*. Baltimore, MD: Williams and Wilkins; 1998:164–184, 230–289, 433–439.

APPENDIX 33–1: SUGGESTED VOICE THERAPY TECHNIQUES

Breathing

Patients are taught that taking a deep, high-chest breath increases air pressure in the lungs greatly, triggering a Valsalva response with closure of the glottis and laryngeal and chest muscle tension. The kind of breath the patient takes may influence tension in other parts of the vocal mechanism. High-chest breathing can contribute to a feeling of breathiness and tightness in the chest. Abdominal breathing produces lesser increases of lung air pressure and removes the tension from the neck and larynx. The patient needs to know what he or she is about to say before he or she inhales the breath to say it, and this concept is discussed and practiced. This simple construct eliminates respiratory/laryngeal incoordination, reduces revisions and struggle during speaking, and allows the patient to focus on how he or she is saying something rather than on the content of what is being said. Speech should be a continuous breath event, beginning with inhalation of the appropriate amount of air, through easy transition to exhalation and voicing, to the end of the utterance. Instruction and discussion of these matters prior to the initiation of a program of breath-support exercises increases the patient's willingness to change and turns the reluctant patient into an active participant in the process of change. Specific breathing exercises to incorporate abdominal breathing are available in many other publications.

Similarly, the patient needs to know that modification of articulation postures and open, relaxed jaw positioning improve loudness and acuity in noisy environments and can be invaluable in improving communication without effort and fatigue in most speaking circumstances. Tongue tension or pulling the tongue back in the mouth leads to tension in the hyoid and larynx region. These effects can easily be demonstrated and discussed by having the patient tense the tongue or retract the tongue while digitally monitoring tension under the chin and at the sides of the larynx. The same effects can be demonstrated during talking activities. Patients need to learn to explore the feelings associated with tension and extra speaking effort.

Relax Jaw Movement and Articulation

Closed, tense jaw articulation and substitution of jaw movement for tongue and lip movements increase ten-
sion and fatigue in the face and increase the amount of pulling on the temporomandibular joint capsule. These same methods of speaking reduce lip reading and loudness in noisy speaking situations. Patients learn that in American English only six sounds, /s/, /z/, /ʃ/, /ʒ/, /tʃ/, and /dʒ/ require closure of the jaw. All other consonants and all vowels can be produced by modifying the position of the lips and tongue with no, or minor, jaw adjustment. Most of speech can be produced with the jaw in a relaxed, partially open neutral position. This can be demonstrated by monitoring tension in the masseter muscle, placing the fingers of both hands in front of the ears and alternately clenching and opening the jaw. The patient will be able to feel the bulking of the masseter during clenching and the stretching of the masseter muscle fibers when the jaw is wide open. The neutral speaking position is identifiable by the absence of muscle bulk or stretched fibers. The patient needs to experience the feeling of relaxation associated with this speaking position. The patient can then be instructed in producing the syllable /la/ by simply lifting the tongue and touching the roof of the mouth behind the upper front teeth and then dropping the tongue to a relaxed position behind, but touching, the lower front teeth. This is extended to other consonants (/ta/, /da/, /na/, /ka/, and /ga/). When the patient is proficient in eliminating jaw tension in these contexts, the effect of lip movement in addition to relaxed jaw and tongue by producing words such as, too, due, coo, load, coat, and so forth, is practical. Lip consonants without tensing the jaw are then added. The sounds /f/, /v/, /th/, /o/, and voiced th (/ð/) need to be monitored for jaw jutting. Open relaxed jaw with improved oral resonance and relaxed tongue can then be practiced in words and phrases. Then the patient can practice in sentences. Practice should initially be done monitoring jaw position and movement with fingers between the posterior molars and with a mirror. As the patient begins to feel comfortable with a relaxed jaw, the tactile monitoring and then the visual monitoring can be eliminated. At this point, the patient should identify phrases and sentences he or she uses frequently, such as; "Hello"; "Put them away"; "I don't like that behavior," and so forth, which can be used as frequent daily reminders in their normal speech of more normal oral resonance and speech production. This assists in carryover. Practice continues with sentences including jaw closure

sounds and open vowels, such as: "He is going"; "Let me have a piece of pie"; "I chose two friends to go with me," and so forth. The open relaxed jaw can then be extended into question and answer activities, monologue, and dialogue.

APPENDIX 33–2: PSYCHOACTIVE MEDICATIONS

Antidepressants

Antidepressant medications include compounds from several different classes. Tri- and tetracyclic antidepressants (TCAs) block the reuptake of norepinephrine and serotonin and have secondary effects on pre- and postsynaptic receptors.[29] An H1-H2-receptor blockade has also been demonstrated.

Schatzberg and Cole summarize the side effects of TCAs as:

- anticholinergic (dry mouth and nasal mucosa, constipation, urinary hesitancy, gastro-esophageal reflux),
- autonomic (orthostatic hypotension, palpitations, increased cardiac conduction intervals, diaphoresis, hypertension, tremor),
- allergic (skin rashes),
- CNS (stimulation, sedation, delirium, twitching, nausea, speech delay, seizures, extrapyramidal symptoms), and
- other (weight gain, impotence).[29]

These may be dose related and agent specific.

Monoamine oxidase inhibitors (MAOIs) are useful in depression that is refractory to tricyclics. The mode of action involves inhibiting monoamine oxidase (MAO), which allows a buildup of norepinephrine. The full restoration of enzyme activity may take two weeks after the drug is discontinued.

The side effects of MAOIs may be extremely serious and troublesome. The one most commonly reported is dizziness secondary to orthostatic hypotension. When MAOIs are taken, hypertensive crisis with violent headache and potential cerebrovascular accident, or hyperpyrexic crisis with monoclonus and coma, may be produced by ingesting foods rich in tyramine, or by many medications, including meperidine (Demerol), epinephrine, local anesthetics containing sympathomimetics, decongestants, selective serotonin reuptake inhibitors (SSRIs), venlafaxine HCl, and surgical anesthetics. Other side effects include sexual dysfunction, sedation, insomnia, overstimulation, myositislike reactions, myoclonic twitches, and a small incidence of dry mouth, constipation, and urinary hesitancy.[29]

A few antidepressants have been developed with different chemical structures and side effect profiles. Trazodone (Desyrel) is pharmacologically complex. It blocks serotonin reuptake, has antihistamine properties, has alpha-1 and serotonin-2 antagonism. It is helpful in depression associated with insomnia. Three side effects are particularly noteworthy: sedation, acute dizziness with fainting (especially when taken on an empty stomach), and priapism.[1,53-55] Effexor (venlafaxine HCl) is a potent reuptake inhibitor of serotonin and norepinephrine and a weak reuptake inhibitor of dopamine. It is useful in both major depression and generalized anxiety disorder.[56]

Nefazodone hydrochloride (Serzone) is another antidepressant. Its chemical structure is different from the SSRIs, tri/tetracyclics, and MAOIs. It appears to inhibit neuronal reuptake of serotonin and has serotonin-2 antagonism. It has been advertised as useful in depressions characterized by anxiety. Side effects include significant orthostasis, potential activation of mania, and a questionable potential for priapism. Decreased cognitive and motor performance, dry mouth, nausea, and dizziness, are also noted as well as other frequently recurring side effects. This drug has notable medication interactions with Halcion, Xanax, and Propulsid. It is not recommended for patients with unstable heart disease.[57]

Bupropion (Wellbutrin) was released in 1989. It blocks the reuptake of norepinephrine and dopamine. It is not anticholinergic. The most commonly reported complaint is nausea. However, a potential risk of seizures exists, and the drug is not recommended in patients with a history of seizures, head trauma, or anorexia or bulimia.[29,53]

A group of antidepressant drugs that selectively inhibit the reuptake of serotonin are most likely to be selected as first pharmacologic agents. These include fluoxetine (Prozac), sertraline (Zoloft), paroxetine (Paxil), and citalopram (Celexa). They appear to be effective in typical episodic depression and for some chronic refractory presentations.[29,53] Major side effects are significant degrees of nausea, sweating, headache, mouth dryness, tremor, nervousness, dizziness, insomnia, somnolence, constipation, and sexual dysfunction. There are drug interactions with the concomitant administration of tryptophan, MAOIs, warfarin, cimetidine, phenobarbital, and phenytoin. Clearance of citalopram may be reduced by concomittant administration of omeprazole, metoprolol, or macrolide antibiotics.[53,56,57]

Mood Stabilizing

Mood-stabilizing drugs are those that are effective in manic episodes and prevent manic and depressive recurrences in patients with bipolar disorder. These include lithium salts and several anticonvulsants. Lithium is available in multiple formulations, and prescribing is guided by both symptom index and blood levels. Lithium side effects are apparent in diverse organ systems. The most commonly noted is fine tremor, especially noticeable in the fingers. With toxic lithium levels, gross tremulousness, ataxia, dysarthria, and confusion or delirium may develop. Some patients describe slowed mentation, measurable memory deficit, and impaired creativity. Chronic nausea and diarrhea are usually related to gastrointestinal tract mucosal irritation, but may be signs of toxicity. Some patients gain weight progressively and may demonstrate edema or increased appetite. Lithium therapy affects thyroid function. In some cases it is transitory, but there may be goiter with normal T3 and T4 but elevated TSH levels.[29]

Polyuria and secondary polydipsia are complications of lithium and may progress to diabetes insipidus. In most cases, discontinuing the medication reverses the renal effects. Prescribed thiazide diuretics can double the lithium level and lead to sudden lithium toxicity. Non steroidal anti-inflammatory drugs (NSAIDs) decrease lithium excretion. Cardiovascular effects include the rare induction of sick sinus syndrome. The aggravation of psoriasis, allergic skin rashes, and reversible alopecia are associated with lithium therapy, as are teratogenic effects.[29]

Anticonvulsant

Three anticonvulsant compounds appear to act preferentially on the temporal lobe and the limbic system. Carbamazepine (Tegretol) carries a risk of agranulocytosis or aplastic anemia, and is monitored by complete blood counts and symptoms of bone marrow depression. Care must be taken to avoid the numerous drug interactions that accelerate the metabolism of some drugs or raise carbamazepine levels.[29]

Valproic acid (Depakote, Depakene) is especially useful when there is a rapid-cycling pattern. The major side effect is hepatocellular toxicity and pancreatitis. Thrombocytopenia and platelet dysfunction have been reported. Sedation is common, and tremor, ataxia, weight gain, alopecia, and fetal neural tube defects are all side effects that patients must comprehend.[29,58] Newer anticonvulsants (Topamax) as well as gabapentin (Neurontin) are also used as mood-stabilizing agents.[58]

Anxiolytics

Anxiolytics are the psychotropic drugs most commonly prescribed, usually by nonpsychiatric specialists, for somatic disorders. It behooves the laryngologist to probe for a history of past or current drug therapy in markedly anxious or somatically focused patients with

vocal complaints. Benzodiazepines produce effective relief of anxiety but have a high addictive potential that includes physical symptoms of withdrawal, including potential seizures, if the drug is stopped abruptly. It is important to remember that this class of drugs is commonly available on the streets and from colleagues. The most common benzodiazepine side effect is dose-related sedation, followed by dizziness, weakness, ataxia, decreased motor performance, and mild hypotension. Clonazepam (Klonopin) is a benzodiazepine and may produce sedation, ataxia, and malcoordination, as well as (rarely) disinhibition, agitation, or asituational anger.[29] Alterations of sensory input, either by CNS stimulants (cocaine, amphetamines, and over-the-counter vasoconstrictors) or depressants, are potentially dangerous in a voice professional. The patient who is unaware of these effects should be apprised of them promptly by the laryngologist.[1,28]

Phenobarbital and meprobamate are no longer commonly used as anxiolytics in the United States. Clomipramine (Anafranil) and fluvoxamine (Luvox) are useful in the anxiety evident in an obsessive-compulsive disorder. The side effects are similar to those of the tricyclic antidepressants: dry mouth, hypotension, constipation, tachycardia, sweating, tremor, and anorgasmia.[29] Fluoxetine (Prozac) has also proved effective for some patients with obsessive-compulsive disorder, and appears better tolerated.[29]

Hydroxyzine, an antihistamine, is occasionally prescribed for mild anxiety and/or pruritus. It does not produce physical dependence but does potentiate the CNS effects of alcohol, narcotics, CNS depressants, and tricyclic antidepressants. Side effects include notable mucous membrane dryness and drowsiness.[29]

Buspirone (BuSpar) is not sedating at its usual dosage levels, and it has little addictive potential. Side effects include mild degrees of headache, nausea, and dizziness. However, it is poorly tolerated in patients accustomed to the more immediate relief of benzodiazepines.[29]

Beta-blockers are used by some clinicians to mask physiologic symptoms of sympathetic arousal in performance anxiety. Their side effects are serious and may include bradycardia, hypotension, weakness, fatigue, clouded sensorium, impotence, and bronchospasm. There is controversy regarding their potential to induce depression.[29] Although the problem of upper respiratory tract secretion dryness was diminished and other symptoms of performance anxiety were lessened in two studies,[27] the drugs are potentially dangerous. Moreover, they leave the underlying conflict unresolved and negatively affect artistic quality.[27] Some authors still prefer them, especially in those patients who may be at risk for drug dependency.

Antacids

The principal ingredients of antacids fall into three categories:

1. aluminum and magnesium-containing compounds;
2. sodium bicarbonate and calcium carbonate;
3. alginate-containing preparations.

The first two groups directly neutralize acid; the third provides a glutinous raft that floats on the surface of stomach contents and, to some extent, corks the gastroesophageal sphincter and coats irritated esophageal mucosa. There are numerous proprietary, non-prescription compounds containing combinations and variations of these substances available over-the-counter from pharmacies.

Antacids do have a drying effect on the vocal tract and in some individuals may cause constipation, diarrhea, or bloating.[5] There have been some concerns expressed in the popular press over long-term usage of aluminum-containing compounds although the authors have not, to date, identified any objective evidence supporting these contentions. There may also be some concerns regarding long-term usage of compounds with significant quantities of bismuth.

Histamine H2-Receptor Antagonists

For symptoms of GER not satisfactorily managed by the above measures, especially for performers in whom abdominal support for voicing produces brisk upright reflux, medical management may require the use of a histamine H2-receptor antagonist (eg, cimetidine, famotidine, nizatidine, ranitidine). This group of antihistamines selectively blocks histamine-mediated production of gastric acid and is almost entirely free of the hypnotic side effects of their nonspecific cousins. Dryness of the vocal tract has been reported as have liver function alteration, gastrointestinal disturbance, headache, dizziness, rashes, confusion, and very occasional hypersensitivity reactions.

Proton Pump Inhibitors

The most recent group of drugs used to reduce gastric acid secretion is the proton pump inhibitors (eg, omeprazole, lansoprazole, pantoprazole, rabeprazole). These highly effective medications now appear to be the treatment of choice in the acute medical management of GER, especially where there is evidence of esophagitis. No other medication is as effective in hydrogen ion transfer blockade. It is also the drug of choice in the maintenance management of LPR-relat-ed conditions such as posterior laryngitis and arytenoid granuloma. Although biochemically different, the range of side effects is not dissimilar to those of the H2-receptor antagonists, for example, GI disturbance, headache, hypersensitivity reactions, liver enzyme, and hematologic changes.

Prokinetic Agents

As adjunctive treatment to acid-reducing medications, a prokinetic agent (eg, metoclopramide) may be considered in order to improve gastroesophageal sphincter function, and to speed gastric emptying. Until recently another drug in this category, cisapride, was proving very effective; however, it has recently been withdrawn on both sides of the Atlantic because of potentially hazardous cardiac side effects. As a result, at the time of writing, there are a significant number of patients with symptoms previously controlled by this drug who now require a careful reappraisal of their antireflux maintenance.

Caveat: Medications that modify symptoms of gastritis, GER, and LPR may also mask the early signs of malignant gastroesophageal disease. It is not uncommon clinical practice at the time of writing for a laryngologist to institute short-term treatment with one of the agents described above. It is recommended that the treating physician consider, in patients in whom long-term management is being suggested, a referral to a gastrointestinal physician.

HORMONES

The larynx has been shown to have a significant number of receptors for estrogens and androgens.[23-25] Timonen found 15.6% of women treated for voice disturbances to have endocrinologic causation.[26] Hormone medications may affect voice quality by alterations in fluid content or structural changes, the latter being particularly seen following administration of androgens.[27]

Sex Hormones

Androgen-containing agents have been used or recommended for such conditions as endometriosis, fibrocystic breast disease, postmenopausal sexual dysfunction, and as part of some chemotherapeutic regimens for cancer. Such medicines can have as side effects hirsutism, alopecia, and permanent lowering of the fundamental frequency of the voice. They should only be used when absolutely indicated and following a frank discussion of risk benefits.[5,28-30]

Similarly, estrogen-containing compounds have been used in males as part of some chemotherapeutic regimens for cancer of the prostate or during transsexual procedures. There is less information available regarding the long-term effects of such medications on the voice.

Birth control pills with relatively high progesterone content may produce androgenlike changes in the voice.[5,31] Most oral contraceptives currently prescribed in the Western world have a better estrogen-progesterone balance, and voice changes are uncommon (less than 5%) and tend to abate following discontinuation.[5]

At menopause there is a 10 to 20 fold drop in estradiol levels but the ovaries continue to secrete androgens.[32] As such the voice tends to lower in fundamental frequency.[33]

In recent years, hormone replacement therapy has become widespread throughout the western world. There are many reasons for giving a patient long-term replacement, and the cardiologic, skeletal, and emotional consequences of this are now becoming comprehensively documented. The million women study published in the Lancet in 2003[34] has dramatically changed prescribing of HRT and, in general, the approach of general practitioners to its use. The study demonstrated that HRT use increases the risk of breast cancer and quantified the risk of increased occurrence. In the post-million women study era, women and their doctors need to carefully review the risk-benefit of use of such agents. What are much less widely covered are the vocal consequences of hormone replacement therapy (HRT). Work relating to the measurable effects of HRT on postmenopausal women, for example, that of Lindholm et al[35] is scarce in the literature. Notwithstanding this gap in the evidence base, HRT is not infrequently prescribed in the hope of delaying age-related vocal changes, frequently with little prior knowledge of the estrogenic/progestegenic/androgenic capacity of the medication prescribed. Unforeseen problems, such as difficulty in pitch matching, register breaks and other symptoms, may occur. Empirically there is little doubt that HRT, if used appropriately, can help an aging voice. However caution is advised, and it is the authors' feeling that this is best done in conjunction with a gynecologic opinion.

Thyroid

Thyroid axis abnormalities can have an impact upon the larynx, frequently producing significant changes in vocal quality. Hypothyroidism causes accumulation of mucopolysaccharides throughout the body. It can cause the vocal folds to thicken. It is associated with loss of range, efficiency, and a "muffling" of the voice.[36] Medical correction of the hypothyroid state with thyroxine will frequently improve voicing parameters. Hyperthyroidism can also affect vocal quality.

BETA-BLOCKERS

Beta-blockers are a class of antihypertensive medication that lower heart rate and blood pressure. These agents have also been noted to reduce anxiety during performance and have been used by snooker players, musicians, singers, and others.[37,38] They also produce an increase in salivation.[37] They are potentially dangerous in individuals with underlying pulmonary problems and may induce asthma attacks. Gates[39] has concluded that in doses sufficient to reduce stage fright, beta-blockers may also cause a lackluster performance. Most laryngologists recommend against their use in performers. Individuals with crescendoing preperformance anxiety may be better advised to seek counseling (see chapter 33, Psychologic Aspects of Voice Disorders.)

MEDICATIONS WITH POTENTIAL ADVERSE EFFECTS

Many medications, when administered systemically, can have a deleterious impact on vocal performance either directly, through their effects on the vocal tract, or indirectly, through CNS or other manifestations. Psychotropic agents represent a typical example. The numbers of drugs available are legion and cannot possibly be discussed in full. A table is addended discussing certain side effects of many of these classes of drugs (Table 34–1). It is by nature incomplete but may prove helpful to the prescribing physician or the patient.

CONCLUSION

Caring for professional voice users is rewarding but, at the same time, can be quite demanding. It is incumbent upon the physician or caregiver to understand the potential effects of medications that they may prescribe on the patient's vocal tract. As noted, the most notable effects of medications on the vocal tract occur through the autonomic nervous system, an understanding of which is important. A thorough history of medications being taken, both prescription and nonprescription, is essential, as is monitoring while treatment is in progress.

Table 34–1. Partial List of Medications with Potential Adverse Effects on the Vocal Tract (*continues*)

General	More Specific	Potential Adverse Symptoms and Comments
Analgesics/Anti-Inflammatants	Aspirin	• Platelet dysfunction • Increased likelihood of submucosal hemorrhage • GI upset • Be wary of aspirin in other over-the-counter compounds
	Narcotic-containing	• CNS depression
	Nonsteroidal Anti-Inflammatants	• GI side effects • Some minor clotting abnormalities
	Paracetamol	• Potential for liver irritation at high dosages
Antibiotics		• GI disturbance • Increased likelihood of candida • Possibility of superinfection
Anticholinergics		• Dry vocal tract • Blurred vision
Antihistamines (H1-receptor blockers)		• Sedation • Dryness • Be wary of combinations with sympathomimetics
Antihypertensives		• Many with parasympathomimetic effects
	Diuretics	• Dry mucous membrane • Thickened secretions
	Reserpine and methyldopa	• Dryness
	Alpha-adrenergic agonists	• Dryness • Reduced secretions
	ACE inhibitors	• Cough
Anti-Parkinson's Agents		• Many with anticholinergic side effects
	L-dopa	• GI disturbance • Oral dryness • Blurred vision • CNS changes
	Amantadine	• Anticholinergic side effects
	Dopamine receptor agonists	• GI disturbance • CNS changes
	Monoamine Oxidase Inhibitors	See Psychotropic section
Antitussive Medications		• Be wary of combination agents and vehicle (eg, H1-receptor antagonists, sympathomimetics, alcohol)
	Opiate-containing	• Sedation • Constipation • Dryness

Table 34–1. Partial List of Medications with Potential Adverse Effects on the Vocal Tract (*continues*)

General	More Specific	Potential Adverse Symptoms and Comments
Antiviral Medications		• Agitation • Tachycardia • Xerostomia • Xerophonia
Corticosteroids		• Suppress immune system (increased risk of infection) • Suppress endogenous steroid production • GI disturbance • CNS irritability • Muscle wasting • Fluid redistribution • Increased glucose
GI Medications		
	Antacids	• Dryness of vocal tract • Constipation
	H2-receptor blockers	• Occasional dryness of vocal tract
	Proton Pump Inhibitors	• Bloating, • Abdominal pain • Nausea
Psychotropic Agents		• All have effects that can interfere with vocal tract physiology

	Tricyclic and Tetracyclic Antidepressants	• Anticholinergic side effects:
		  Dry vocal tract
		  GER
		• Autonomic side effects:
		  Palpitations
		  Sweating
		• Allergic:
		  Skin rashes
		• CNS:
		  Stimulation or sedation
		  Nausea
		  Seizures

	Monoamine Oxidase Inhibitors	• Dizziness • Hypertension from certain foods and medications • Sedation • Insomnia • Small incidence of dry mouth • Small incidence of constipation
	Serotonin Reuptake Inhibitors	• Weakly cholinergic but do cause some mucosal drying • Sedation • GI disturbance • Blurred vision

Table 34–1. Partial List of Medications with Potential Adverse Effects on the Vocal Tract (*continued*)

General	More Specific	Potential Adverse Symptoms and Comments
	Phenothiazines	• Strong H1-receptor antagonists • Dryness of vocal tract always seen
	Benzodiazepines	• High addictive potential • No anticholinergic effects • May affect speech production by action on CNS
	Lithium	• Nausea • Diarrhea • May affect mentation • May alter thyroid function
Sprays/Inhalants (laryngeal)		
	Anesthetic (Lidocaine)	• Not recommended • Increased likelihood of vocal fold injury/hemorrhage
	Vasoconstrictor	• Generally not recommended • Use only under emergent extreme circumstances
	Diphenhydramine	• Has anesthetic effect and may increase likelihood of vocal fold injury
	Oxymetazoline	• No anesthetic effect
	Corticosteroids	• Dryness • Affects mucosal blanket • Questionable atrophy • Increased candida
Sympathomimetics		• Increased dryness of vocal tract • Thickened secretions • Xanthines reduce lower esophageal sphincter pressure and may increase reflux

REFERENCES

1. Lawrence VL. Common medications with laryngeal effects. *Ear Nose Throat J.* 1987;66: 23–28.
2. Martin FG. Drugs and vocal function. *J Voice.* 1988; 2:338–344.
3. Harris TM. The pharmacological treatment of voice disorders. *Folia Phoniatr (Basel).* 1992;44:3–4;143–154.
4. Thompson AR. Pharmacological agents with effects on voice. *Am J Otol.* 1995;16:12–18.
5. Sataloff RT, Hawkshaw M, Rosen DC. Medications: Effects and side effects in professional voice users. In: Sataloff RT. *Professional Voice: Science and Art of Clinical Care.* 2nd ed. San Diego, CA: Singular Publishing Group; 1997:457–469.
6. Sooy CD, Boles R. Neuroanatomy for the otolaryngology head and neck surgeon. In: Paparella MM, Shumrick DA, Gluckman JL, Meyerhoff WL, eds. *Otolaryngology.* 3rd ed. Philadelphia, PA: WB Saunders Co; 1991:107–142.
7. Davies J, Duckert L. Embryology and anatomy of the head, neck, face, palate, nose and paranasal sinuses. In: Paparella MM, Shumrick DA, Gluckman JL, Meyerhoff WL, eds. *Otolaryngology.* 3rd ed. Philadelphia, PA: WB Saunders Co; 1991:59–106.
8. Goodman U, Rall T, Nies AS, et al. *Goodman and Gilman's The Pharmacologic Basis of Therapeutics.* New York, NY: Pergamon Press; 1990:658.
9. The safety of inhaled nasal corticosteroids. *Curr Prob Pharmacol Care.* 1999;24:8.
10. Findlay CA, MacDonald JF, Wallace AM, Geddes N, et al. Lesson of the week: childhood Cushing's syndrome induced by betamethasone oral drops and repeat prescriptions. *Br Med J.* 1998;317(7160):739–740.

11. Homer JJ, Gazis TG. Cushing's syndrome induced by betamethasone nose drops (12). *Br Med J.* 1999;318(7194):1355–1356.
12. Scadding G. Effects of intranasal steroids on childhood growth. *ENT News.* November/December, 1999;8(pt 5):27–28.
13. Schenkel EJ, Skoner DP, Bronsky EA. *One Year of Treatment With Mometasone Furoate Aqueous Nasal Spray (MFNS) Does Not Suppress Growth in Children.* Poster 31B, EAACI; Brussels, Belgium; July 1999.
14. Moren F. Drug deposition of pressurised inhalation aerosols. I. Influence of actuator tube design. *Int J Pharmacol.* 1978;1:205–212.
15. Dolovich M, Ruffin R, Newhouse MT. Clinical evaluation of a simple demand inhalation device: MDI aerosol delivery device. *Chest.* 1983;84:36–41.
16. Newman SP, Pavia D, Garland N. Effects of various inhalation modes on the deposition of radioactive pressurised aerosols. *Eur J Respir Dis.* 1982;119(suppl):57–65.
17. Berkowitz R, Rachelefsky G, Harris AG, Chen R. A comparison of triamcinolone acetonide MDI with a built-in tube extender and beclomethasone dipropionate MDI in adult asthmatics. *Chest.* 1998;114:757–765.
18. Lavy JA, Wood G, Rubin JS, Harries M. Dysphonia associated with inhaled steroids. *J Voice.* 2000;14:581–588.
19. *British National Formulary.* British Medical Association and the Royal Pharmaceutical Society of Great Britain.
20. Koufman JA. Infectious and inflammatory diseases of the larynx. In: Ballenger JJ, Snow JB, eds. *Otorhinolaryngology.* 15th ed. Philadelphia, PA: Williams and Wilkins (Lea & Febiger); 1996:535–555.
21. Koufman JA, Cummins M. The prevalence and spectrum of reflux in laryngology: a prospective study of 132 consecutive patients with laryngeal and voice disorders. Available at: wfubmc.edu/voice/reflux_prev_study.html; 2002.
22. Sataloff RT, Castell DO, Katz PO, Sataloff DM. *Reflux Laryngitis and Related Disorders.* San Diego, CA: Singular Publishing Group; 1999.
23. Abramson AL, Steinberg BM, Gould WJ, et al. Estrogen receptors in the human larynx. Clinical study of the singing voice. *Transcripts of the 13th Symposium on Care of the Professional Voice.* 1984;2:409–413.
24. Virolainen E, Tuohiman P, Aitasato A, et al. Steroid hormone receptors in laryngeal carcinoma. *Otolaryngol Head Neck Surg.* 1986;4:512–517.
25. Newman S-R, Butler J, Hammond EH, Gray SD. Preliminary report on hormone receptors in the human vocal fold. *J Voice.* 2000;14:72–81.
26. Timonen S, Sonninen A, Wichmann K. Endocrinological laryngopathy. In: Follio KE, Vara P, eds. *Annales Chirurgiae et Gynaecologiae Fenniae.* 1962;51:3–29.
27. Damste PH. Virilization of the voice due to anabolic steroids. *Folia Phoniatr.* 1968;16:10–18.
28. Baker J. A report on alterations to the speaking voices of four women following hormonal therapy with virilising agents. *J Voice.* 1999;13:496–507.
29. Pattie MA, Murdoch B, Theodoros D, Forbes K. Voice changes in women treated for endometriosis and related conditions: the need for comprehensive vocal assessment. *J Voice.* 1998;12:366–371.
30. Gerritsma EJ, Brocaar MP, Hakkesteegt MM, Birkenhager JC. Virilization of the voice in post-menopausal women due to the androgenic steroid nandrolone decanoate (Decadurabolin). The effects of medication for one year. *Clin Otolaryngol.* 1994;19:79–84.
31. Krahulec I, Urbanova O, Simko S. Voice changes during hormonal contraception. *Cesk Otolaryngol.* 1977;26:234–237.
32. Khaw K. The menopause and hormone replacement therapy. *Post-grad Med J.* 1992;68:615–623.
33. Boulet MJ, Oddens BJ. Female voice change around and after the menopause: an initial investigation. *Maturitas.* 1996;23:15–21.
34. Beral V, Million Women Study Collaborators. Breast cancer and hormone-replacement therapy in the million women study. *Lancet,* 2003;362:419–437.
35. Lindholm P, Vilkman E, Raudaskoski T, Suvanto-Lukkonen E, Kauppila A. The effect of postmenopause and postmenopausal HRT on measured voice values and vocal symptoms. *Maturitas.* 1997;28:47–53.
36. Sataloff RT, Spiegel JR, Rosen DC. The effects of age on the voice. In: Sataloff, RT. *Professional Voice: Science and Art of Clinical Care.* 2nd ed. San Diego, CA: Singular Publishing Group; 1997:259–267.
37. James IM. The effects of oxprenolol on stage fright in musicians. *Lancet.* 1977;2:952–954.
38. Brantigan CD. The effect of beta blockage and beta stimulation on stage fright. *Am J Med.* 1982;72:88–94.
39. Gates GA, Saegert J, Wilson N, et al. Effects of beta-blockade on singing performance. *Ann Otol Rhinol Laryngol.* 1985;94:570–574.

35

Corticosteroid Use in Otolaryngology

Andrew Spector, MD
Marc Rosen, MD

Steroid use in otolaryngology is ubiquitous. Physicians used them to treat nearly every ailment that we encounter either as the primary therapy, as an adjunct to treatment, or as anecdotal and unsupported, unsubstantiated force of habit. Many of our uses of corticosteroids are supported in the literature but others do not have very good, if any, evidence-based double-blinded, placebo-controlled basis for their use. Also, an overwhelming stigmata has surrounded the use of steroids. Initial zeal for administration after their early clinical use in the 1950s by Hench gave way to hesitancy and repugnance as side effects and complications were perceived to outweigh any perceived benefit. In modern therapeutics, after decades of use and research, corticosteroids have found their place in treatment as appropriate dosing, duration, indications, and complication prevention have been identified. A stigma is still attached to steroid use because of all the potential negative outcomes associated with high-dose, long-term use. Knowledge of the origins, actions, side effects, benefits, and uses of corticos-

teroids is essential for the appropriateuse of these powerful medications.

Most practicing otolaryngologist will have had patients who have wondered if steroids are bad for them, what the risks involved are, if they will gain weight, and if by taking these agents their body habitus will change; for example if they will become muscular, masculinized, feminized, and so on or even if use of such agents is legal. This is quite pertinent given recent media coverage of the occasional use and abuse of "steroids" by professional athletes, and the prohibition to steroids by several athletic organizations..

This chapter first covers endogenous steroids, their production in the adrenal glands, and the regulation of their production in the human body. Next follows a brief discussion on the various effects of corticosteroids on different body systems. Side effects and potential adverse events from endogenous and exogenous excess is described therein. Information will then be provided regarding the pharmacodynamics and pharmacokinetics of synthetic, exogenously given

561

corticosteroids including varying biologic activity and management strategies to optimize therapy while minimizing undesired outcomes. Finally, pertinent literature-based evidence will be provided for specific uses of steroids in otolaryngology. There are a significant number of systemic disorders with manifestations in the head and neck where corticosteroid therapy is indispensable. Diseases in which systemic treatment is important include, among others, systemic lupus erythematosis, Wegener's granulomatosis, relapsing polychondritis, sarcoidosis, and temporal arteritis, The rheumatologic literature contains in-depth discussions of certain of the systemic problems and is beyond the scope of this text. Of important note for this chapter, however, is the paucity of published studies relating to the use of steroids in disorders involving the larynx. It is certain that, in this rapidly evolving field, literature reflecting the use of corticosteroids will expand.

ENDOGENOUS STEROIDS

The adrenal cortex is responsible for the production of three types of hormones: sex steroids, mostly androgens; mineralocorticoids like aldosterone; and glucocorticoids including cortisol. Glucocorticoids act ubiquitously in the body to help regulate metabolism and support the individual during stress. For our purposes, the glucocorticoids, as well as the progestagens, are C21 derivatives with an 11-hydroxyl group needed for biologic effect. All the steroid hormones have the cyclopentanoperhydrophenanthrene structure with three cyclohexane rings and one cyclopentane ring as the primary building block.[1]

Within the adrenal cortex, cortisol is synthesized within the zona fasciculata at a rate of about 10 to 20 milligrams per day and is regulated by adrenal corticotropic hormone (ACTH) secretion. The mineralcorticoids like aldosterone are manufactured at rates of up to 100 to 150 µg per day in the zona glomerulosa under the control of angiotensin II levels. These decrease sodium excretion and increase that of potassium in the kidneys. Meanwhile, the adrenal androgens or sex steroids are produced at a rate of more than 20 milligrams daily in the zona reticularis.[1]

Cholesterol is the precursor of all adrenal steroids and is largely obtained from low-density lipoproteins (LDL). Once the LDL is taken into the adrenal cortex, it is hydrolyzed to yield free cholesterol. To a much lesser extent, cholesterol can be synthesized de novo within the cortex. Once the cholesterol enters the mitochondrion, it is cleaved by the P450 side-chain cleav-

age enzyme to form pregnenolone then progesterone within the cytoplasm. Next, as a precursor to glucocorticoid formation, the progesterone is 17-alpha hydroxylated. This hydroxylase is not found in the zona glomerulosa, the location of aldosterone synthesis. After 11-deoxycortisol is formed, it is converted to cortisol in the mitochondria.[1]

Mineralocorticoid production in the adrenal zona glomerulosa is under the regulation of angiotensin II, serum potassium levels, and somewhat by circulating ACTH. Although aldosterone is the principal mineralocorticoid, cortisol also helps in fluid homeostasis, sodium retention, and plasma volume.

Adrenal production of androgens is responsible for more than half of circulating sex hormones in the premenopausal female. This is smaller in males where testicular production is dominant.[1]

The production of adrenal cortisol is controlled in part by its participation in the feedback loop with hypothalamic corticotropin-releasing hormone (CRH) and adrenal corticotropic hormone (ACTH) secretion from the anterior pituitary gland. An understanding of this feedback system is important, because it assists in understanding why suppression of the hypothalamic-pituitary-adrenal (HPA) axis can be a severe complication of long-term, high-dose steroid administration. The HPA axis coordinates both basal and stress-induced cortisol secretion. Proper functioning of this system is important as the adrenal gland stores only insignificant amounts of cortisol. Prolonged steroid therapy can cause adrenal atrophy from constant negative feedback.[1]

ACTH is the primary regulator of glucocorticoid synthesis. It is the 39 amino acid peptide hormone from the 241 amino acid precursor pro-opiomelanocortin (POMC).[1] POMC secretion is controlled primarily by CRH from the paraventricular nucleus of the hypothalamus as well as arginine vasopressin, stress, circadian rhythm, and direct feedback inhibition from cortisol.[1]

In response to stress, cytokines like IL-1, IL-6, and tumor necrosis factor-alpha (TNF-α) can stimulate ACTH release. Accordingly, cortisol release can be prompted by surgery, fever, cold, burns, hypotension, exercise, and hypoglycemia.[1]

The positive stimulators are countered by the negative regulatory feedback from glucocorticoids themselves. Both adrenal and exogenously administered corticosteroids inhibit production of POMC, CRH, and arginine vasopressin thus inhibiting further production of adrenal glucocorticoids. The amount of negative feedback inhibition is directly dependent on the dose, potency, half-life, and duration of elevated endogenous or exogenous steroid exposure. Pharma-

as long as 6 weeks.[10] It does not, however, allow for immediate cessation of therapy in the event of untoward corticosteroid effects. A different strategy is often employed to treat severe complications of rheumatologic conditions. High-dosed pulse corticosteroids utilize doses of prednisone approaching 1000 mg daily for 3 days without HPA axis suppression or significant side effects.[4]

Alternative day therapy using a drug of intermediate duration results in minimal HPA axis suppression and limited side effects. This can be started after the disease state is controlled initially with daily therapy. Long-duration drugs defeat the purpose of every other day dosing, whereas short-acting steroids do not maintain sufficient levels of medication to treat illness.[23]

Surgery is one of the more potent stimulators of the HPA axis. ACTH levels rise at the time of incision, and peak during reversal of general anesthesia, extubation, and immediate recovery period. Daily secretion of cortisol increases from 15 to 20 mg/day to 75 to 150 mg/day. This elevation promotes survival via increased cardiac contractility and mobilization of energy stores.[21] Otolaryngologists occasionally operate on patients who chronically take steroids for other illnesses. It is important to remember that these patients will require supplemental stress doses of steroids because their adrenal glands will not respond normally to the stress of surgery. This should be considered in anyone receiving more than 20 mg of prednisone daily for 3 weeks within the past year.[21] A dose of 75 to 150 mg equivalents of hydrocortisone is required at the time of surgery to approximate what the body would secrete in response to surgical stress. This dose will need to be repeated every 6 to 8 hours for 48 to 72 hours.[4] Patients undergoing minor procedures may receive 100 mg of hydrocortisone at induction and return to their normal dose on the second postoperative day.[21]

USE OF STEROIDS IN OTOLARYNGOLOGY

There are very few instances in otolaryngology where glucocorticoid steroid therapy does not have a role. In general terms, it is used to limit neural injury and reduce inflammation. Each physician must carefully weigh potential risks with therapeutic benefit for individual patients. The only absolute contraindication to therapy is anaphylaxis to steroid (which may be due to a diluent or preservatives in IV preparations although skin testing has shown actual steroid allergy).[23,24] Anaphylaxis is felt to be a heterogeneous entity without recurring underlying cause.[19]

With acute spinal cord injury, very high megadoses of glucocorticoids are given to prevent lipid peroxidation by oxygen-free radicals and thus avoid neural degeneration.[25] Studied doses have included 30 mg/kg of methylprednisolone, a more effective inhibitor of peroxidation than dexamethasone, IV followed by a 5.4 mg/kg/hr infusion or the equivalent of more than 2600 mg of prednisone.[26] Otolaryngologists treat neural injury on a smaller scale but use comparatively miniscule doses of steroid. The action of these medications may not be the product of the glucocorticoids receptor activity because decadron is actually a more potent glucocorticoid. This information might have implications for our choice and quantity of drug in the treatment of facial nerve, vestibular nerve, cochlear nerve, and recurrent laryngeal nerve insults.

Bell's palsy, or idiopathic facial nerve paralysis, is a diagnosis of exclusion once other causes of facial nerve weakness have been eliminated. The common denominator of this disease is inflammation of or around the VIIth cranial nerve. Without treatment, 71% recover completely and 84% achieve near-normal function.[27] Multiple studies have either supported or argued against the use of glucocorticoids for the treatment of this disorder.

Austin et al from UCLA in 1993 determined in a randomized, double-blinded placebo-controlled study that the time difference to recovery was not affected by steroid administration, although the degree of residual paresis was. Their conclusion was that patients with higher grades of denervation would receive more benefit than those with a House-Brackman grade II through IV, for example.[28]

De Diego's 1998 results reflected the natural history of the disease in a group not treated with corticosteroids. His 93.6% recovery rate in the prednisone-treated group demonstrated statistical significance compared to the recovery rate in an acyclovir-treated group. The 77.7% rate of recovery in the latter group is similar to the previously discussed rates of spontaneous improvement.[29]

The Quality Standards Subcommittee of the American Academy of Neurology reviewed 230 articles on Bell's palsy treatment to determine if steroids improve facial nerve outcome. Nine articles were prospective and randomized comparing steroids to placebo. The most commonly reported regimen was 1 mg/kg prednisone daily for 6 days followed by a 4-day taper. They found that the 2 class I studies and 1 class II study showed no significantly improved outcomes in the treated patients. One class II and 1 class III study showed that treated patients were 1.2 times more likely to obtain good function. None showed improved time to recovery. None of the studies had good power, so they combined the class I and class II studies and demonstrated a significant association between steroid use and good outcomes. They concluded that, in addition to the 80% achieving good outcome with no treatment, an additional 14% will benefit from corticosteroids and that they are safe and probably effective in improving facial function.[30]

A meta-analysis from Ramsey presented in *Laryngoscope* in 2000 determined there was clinically and statistically significant improvement in recovery after administering steroids.[31] The authors looked at two subsets of patients—one group with paresis who have a good prognosis and the other group with complete paralysis, associated with poor recovery. The rates of spontaneous recovery quoted previously did not distinguish between the two groups, so improvement rates in paresis are actually better than those rates. This analysis found that corticosteroids improved the overall incidence of complete recovery by 17%, especially when more than 400 mg were used and started within 7 days of onset, although, preferably sooner. That is to say, for every 100 patients treated with complete paralysis, 40 recover regardless of therapy and 17 of the remaining 60 will recover with steroid use.[31]

Those who support using steroids generally agree that therapy should begin as soon as possible. If the patient presents after 3 weeks from onset, steroids are useless. The dose utilized varies among authors but high-dose administration, usually 60 to 80 mg prednisone equivalent daily with a subsequent taper, is usually supported.

Other studies have examined whether perioperative glucocorticoid administration affects the incidence and severity of facial nerve dysfunction after surgery. Lee looked at 49 patients receiving placebo, high- or low-dose steroids both before and 2 doses after parotid surgery. She concluded that there was no evidence to suggest that decadron was beneficial for short- or long-term function.[32] This result reflected the findings of Welling's study from Ohio State with one day of preoperative steroid administration in acoustic neuroma surgery. He found no statistical significance in facial nerve function when controlling for tumor size.[33] There have been some studies, however, that suggest improved nerve function and recovery after the topical application of steroid to crushed sciatic nerve in an animal model.[34] This particular study by Galloway was prompted by the author's experience that topical application of steroids in skull base surgery seems to decrease postoperative motor nerve dysfunction. Perhaps, an interesting area of research regarding cranial nerve injury would study corticosteroid doses approaching those used for spinal cord injury to determine if outcomes are improved.

Of potential interest to the laryngologist and relating to the previous section on facial nerve outcomes, there have been no double-blinded placebo-controlled studies designed to determine the outcome of prophylactic corticosteroid administration for thyroidectomy. This procedure frequently causes edema or trauma to the laryngeal nerve innervation despite meticulous surgical technique and can lead to temporary or permanent vocal fold dysfunction. This is particularly pertinent as both the superior and recurrent laryngeal nerves are at risk.

Sinonasal disease is another area where corticosteroids have a well-suited niche for controlling allergy and inflammation. An entire chapter could be devoted to both the topical application and oral administration of corticosteroids in both acute and chronic rhinosinusitis and allergic rhinitis where they act to block late-phase reactions. Needless to say, they are indispensable adjuncts to therapy in addition to antibiotic therapy, appropriately indicated surgery, decongestants, antihistamines, irrigation, immunotherapy, and antileukotrienes. There are countless studies on the efficacy, safety, systemic absorption, and subsequent adverse reactions of intranasal steroids. In sinus disease, steroids block the production of inflammatory mediators, decrease vascular permeability, suppress eosinophils, and can lead to the rapid regression of sinonasal polyposis.[10] Indeed, in vitro studies of corticosteroids have demonstrated inflammatory cell apoptosis. The same study, however, did not find a similar effect with topical application in vivo.[35] While decreasing polyp size, they also increase nasal airway conductance. Ten- to fourteen-day courses of an oral preparation can render the sinonasal cavity more amenable to topical treatment. They can also make the surgical field more accessible when given for several days preoperatively and can limit the amount of mucosal edema and rhinorrhea around the time of surgery.[10,36] This has been confirmed in MRI studies, which showed a more than 30% reduction of polypoid rhinosinusitis and an 80% reduction in related symptoms after a course of oral and topical steroids.[37]

Allergic fungal sinusitis is another area where corticosteroid use is a mainstay of therapy. As in its pulmonary counterpart, allergic bronchopulmonary aspergillosis, systemic steroids are employed for disease remission and flares when coupled appropriately with surgery, topical corticosteroids, and immunotherapy.[38]

Sudden sensorineural hearing loss may be defined as a 20 dB drop in hearing over 3 frequencies in less than 3 days.[39] Among the potential causes of sudden hearing loss are autoimmune disease, viral-induced inflammation, and vascular phenomena. It is intuitive that glucocorticoids have a role in therapy if inflam-

29. De Diego JI, Prim MP, De Sarria MJ, Madero R, Gavila J. Idiopathic facial paralysis: a randomized, prospective and controlled study using single-dose prednisone versus acyclovir three times daily. *Laryngoscope.* 1998; 108(4):573–575.

30. Grogan PM, Gronseth GS. Practice parameter: steroids, acyclovir, and surgery for Bell's palsy (an evidence-based review): Report of the Quality Standars Subcommitee of the American Academy of *Neurology. Neurology.* 2001;56(7):830–836.

31. Ramsey MJ, DerSimonian R, Holtel MR, Burgess L. Corticosteroid treatment for idiopathic facial nerve paralysis: a meta-analysis. *Laryngoscope.* 2000;110(3):335–341.

32. Lee KJ, Fee WE, Terris DJ. The efficacy of corticosteroids in postparotidectomy facial nerve paresis. *Laryngoscope.* 2002;112(11):1958–1963.

33. Welling DB, Thomas R, Slater P, Daniels RL, Goodman JH. Preoperative antibiotics and steroids in vestibular schwannoma excision. *Laryngoscope.* 1999;109(7):1081–1083.

34. Galloway EB, Jensen RL, Dailey AT, et al. Role of topical steroids in reducing dysfunction after nerve injury. *Laryngoscope.* 2000;110(11):1907–1910.

35. Saunders MW, Wheatley AH, George SJ, Lai T, Birchall MA. Do corticosteroids induce apoptosis in nasal polyp inflammatory cells? In vivo and in vitro studies. *Laryngoscope.* 1999;109:785–790.

36. Mabry R. Corticosteroids in rhinology. In: Goldman JL, ed. *The Principles and Practice of Rhinology.* New York, NY: John Wiley; 1987.

37. Damm M, Jungehulsing M, Eckel HE, Schmidt M, Theissen P. Effects of systemic steroid treatment in chronic polypoid rhinosinusitis evaluated with magnetic resonance imaging. *Otolaryngol Head Neck Surg.* 1999;120(4): 633–638.

38. DeShazo RD, Chapin K, Swain RE. Current concepts: fungal sinusitis. *N Engl J Med.* 1997;337(4):254–259.

39. Gianoli GJ, Li JC. Transtympanic steroids for treatment of seen hearing loss. *Otolaryngol Head Neck Surg.* 2001; 125(3):142–146.

40. Byl FM. Sudden hearing loss: eight years experience and suggested prognostic table. *Laryngoscope.* 1984;94:647–661.

41. Mattox DE, Simmons FB. Natural history of sudden sensorineural hearing loss. *Ann Otol Rhinol Laryngol.* 1977; 86:463–480.

42. Uri N, Doweck I, Cohen-Kerem R, Greenberg E. Acyclovir in the treatment of idiopathic sudden sensorineural hearing loss. *Otolaryngol Head Neck Surg.* 2003;128: 544–549.

43. Wilson WR, Byl FM, Laird N. Efficacy of steroids in the treatment of idiopathic sudden hearing loss: a double-blind clinical study. *Arch Otolaryngol.* 1980;106:772–776.

44. Moskowitz D, Lee KJ, Smith HW. Steroid use in idiopathic sudden sensorineural hearing loss. *Laryngoscope.* 1984;94:664–666.

45. Chen CY, Halpin C, Rauch SD. Oral steroid treatment of sudden sensorineural hearing loss: a ten-year retrospective analysis. *Otol Neurotol.* 2003;24:728–733.

46. Silverstein H, Choo D, Rosenberg SI, Kuhn J, Seidman M, Stein I. Intratympanic steroid treatment of inner ear disease and tinnitus. *Ear Nose Throat J.* 1996;75:476–478.

47. Chandrasekhar SS, Rubinstein RY, Kwartler JA, et al. Dexamethasone pharmacokinetics in the inner ear: comparison of route of administration and use of facilitating agents. *Otolaryngol Head Neck Surg.* 2000;122:521–528.

48. Guan-Min H, Hung-Ching L, Min-Tsan S, et al. Effectiveness of intratympanic dexamethason injection in sudden-deafness patients as salvage treatment. *Laryngoscope.* 2004;114(7):1184–1189.

49. Brooks GB. Circulating immune complexes in Meniere's disease. *Arch Otolaryngol Head Neck Surg.* 1986;112:536–540.

50. Shea JJ, Ge X. Dexamethasone perfusion of the labyrinth plus intravenous dexamethasone for Meniere's disease. *Otolaryngol Clin North Am.* 1996;29:353–358.

51. Hillman TM, Arriaga MA, Chen DA. Intratympanic steroids: do they acutely improve hearing in cases of cochlear hydrops? *Laryngoscope.* 2003;113(11):1903–1907.

52. Arriaga MA, Goldman S. Hearing results of intratympanic steroid treatment of endolymphatic hydrops. *Laryngoscope.* 1998;108:1682–1685.

53. Silverstein H, Isaacson JE, Olds MJ, Rowan PT, Rosenberg S. Dexamethasone inner ear perfusion for the treatment of Meniere's disease: a prospective, randomized, double-blinded crossover trial. *Am J Otol.* 1998;19:196–201.

54. Barrs DM, Keyser JS, Stallworth C, McElveen JT. Intratympanic steroid injections for intractable Meniere's disease. *Laryngoscope.* 2001;111(12):2100–2104.

55. Strupp M, Zingler VC, Arbusow V, et al. Methylprednisolone, valacyclovir, or the combination for vestibular neuritis. *N Engl J Med.* 2004;351(4):354–361.

56. Ohbayashi S, Oda M, Yamamoto M, et al. Recovery of the vestibular function after vestibular neuronitis. *Acta Otolaryngol Suppl.* 1993;503:31–34.

57. Catlin FI, Grimes WJ. The effect of steroid therapy on recovery from tonsillectomy in children. *Arch Otolaryngol Head Neck Surg.* 1991;117(6):649–652.

58. Tom LW, Templeton JJ, Thompson ME, Marsh RR. Dexamethasone in adenotonsillectomy. *Int J Pediatr Otorhinolaryngol.* 1996;37:115–120.

59. April MM, Callan ND, Nowak DM, Hausdorff MA, The effect of intravenous dexamethasone in pediatric adenotonsillectomy. *Arch Otolaryngol Head Neck Surg.* 1996;122: 117–120.

60. Goldman AC, Govindaraj S, Rosenfeld RM. A meta-analysis of dexamethason use with tonsillectomy. *Otolaryngol Head Neck Surg.* 2000;123:682–686.

61. Volk MS, Martin P, Brodsky L, Stanievich JF, Ballou M. The effects of preoperative steroids on tonsillectomy patients. *Otolaryngol Head Neck Surg.* 1993;109:726–730.

62. Ohlms LA, Wilder RT, Weston B. Use of intraoperative corticosteroids in pediatric tonsillectomy. *Arch Otolaryngol Head Neck Surg.* 1995;121(7):737–742.

63. Palme CE, Tomasevic P, Pohl DV. Evaluating the effects of oral prednisolone on recovery after tonsillectomy: a prospective, double-blind, randomized trial. *Laryngoscope.* 2000;110(2):2000–2004.

64. Williams PM, Strome M, Eliachar I, et al. Impact of steroids on recovery after uvulopalatopharyngoplasty. *Laryngoscope.* 1999;109(12):1941–1946.

65. Al-Ghamdi, SA, Manoukian JJ, Morielli A, et al. Do systemic corticosteroids effectively treat obstructive sleep apnea secondary to adenotonsillar hypertrophy? *Laryngoscope* 1997; 107:1382–1387.

66. Wei JL, Kasperbauer JL, Weaver AL, Bogust AJ. Efficacy of single-dose dexamethasone as adjuvant therapy for acute pharyngitis. *Laryngoscope.* 2002;112:87–93.

67. Johnson RF, Stewart MG, Wright CC. An evidence-based review of the treatment of peritonsillar abscess. *Otolaryngol Head Neck Surg.* 2003;128:332–343.

68. O'Brien JF, Meade JL, Falk JL. Dexamethasone as adjuvant therapy for severe acute pharyngitis. *Ann Emerg Med.* 1993;22:212–215.

69. Tateya I, Omori K, Kijima H, et al. Steroid injection for Reinke's edema using fiberoptic laryngeal surgery. *Acta Otolaryngol.* 2003;123:417–420.

70. Tateya I, Omori K, Kijima H, et al. Steroid injection to vocal nodules using fiberoptic laryngeal surgery under topical anesthesia. *Eur Arch Otorhinolaryngol.* 2004;261:489–492.

71. Nielsen VM, Hojslet PE. Topical treatment of Reinke's oedema with Beclomethasone Dipropionate inhalation aerosol. *J Laryngol Otol.* 1987;101:921–924.

72. Jackson C. Contact ulcer of the larynx. *Ann Otol Rhinol Laryngol.* 1928;37:227–238.

73. Hoffman HT, Overhold E, Karnell M, McCulloch TM. Vocal process granuloma. *Head Neck.* 2001;23:1061–1074.

74. Jaroma M, Pakareinen L, Nuuteinen J. Treatment of vocal cord granuloma. *Acta Otolaryngol.* 1989;107:296–299.

75. Roh HJ, Goh EK, Chon KM, Wang SG. Topical inhalant steroid (Budesonide, Pulmicort Nasal) therapy in intubation granuloma. *J Laryngol Otol.* 1999;113:427–432.

76. Watts CR, Clark R, Early S. Acoustic measures of phonatory improvement secondary to treatment by oral corticosteroids in a professional singer: a case report. *J Voice.* 2001;15:115–121.

77. Stannard W, O'Callaghan C. Management of croup. *Paediatr Drugs.* 2002;4:231–240.

78. Wright RB, Pomerantz WJ, Luria JW. New approaches to respiratory infections in children. Bronchiolitis and croup. *Emerg Med Clin North Am.* 2002;20:93–114.

79. Rittichier KK. The role of corticosteroids in the treatment of croup. *Treat Respir Med.* 2004;3:139–145.

80. Ho LI, Harn HJ, Lien TC, Hu PY, Wang JH. Postextubation laryngeal edema in adults: risk factor evaluation and prevention by hydrocortisone. *Intensive Care Med.* 1996;22:933–936.

81. Meade MO, Guyatt GH, Cook DJ, Sinuff T, Butler R. Trials of corticosteroids to prevent postextubation airway complications. *Chest.* 2001;120(suppl):464–468.

82. Tellez DW, Galvis AG, Storgion SA, et al. Dexamethasone in the prevention of postextubation stridor in children. *J Pediatr.* 1991;118:289–294.

83. Anene O, Meert KL, Uy H, Simpson P, Sarnaik AP. Dexamethasone for the prevention of postextubation airway obstruction: a prospective, randomized, double-blind, placebo-controlled trial. *Crit Care Med.* 1996;24:1666–1669.

36

The Role of the Speech-Language Pathologist in the Treatment of Voice Disorders

Thomas Murry, PhD
Clark A. Rosen, MD, FACS

Treatment of voice disorders by speech-language pathologists (SLPs) has steadily advanced over the past 25 years. The vast expansion of research in vocal fold physiology and voice disorders has increased the understanding of techniques and methods for behavioral management of voice disorders. More importantly, these advances have resulted in increased use of voice therapy to avoid surgery, prepare patients for voice surgery, and maximize vocal rehabilitation following surgery. Laryngology and speech-language pathology have melded a treatment rationale that combines the expertise of these two disciplines to maximize voice rehabilitation.

The modern SLP brings essential vocal mechanics, voice physiology information, and behavior management skills to the evaluation and treatment process.

The SLP uses behavioral techniques to reduce traumatic voice use, increase vocal efficiency, and produce a clearer tone. The SLP develops and applies perceptual cues to help the patient to identify and monitor changes in phonation. Voice therapy methods also include the application of cognitive strategies to complement acquisition of new motor skills. The therapeutic process requires SLPs to have a keen sense of observational and interventional treatment methods.

Successful voice therapy is grounded in an understanding of laryngeal anatomy; physiology of the respiratory, laryngeal, and articulatory systems; knowledge of physiological phonetics; and excellent auditory discrimination. Listening to a variety of voice samples and identifying their characteristics is an integral part of this training. These skills develop as the speech-language pathologist works in a voice care setting. In addition to the treatment skills, a thorough understanding of the voice problem from the patient's perspective is integral in counseling the patient as to his or her vocal needs. Continuously challenging one's listening acuity, coupled with knowledge of voice disorders and a keen understanding of the needs of the patient contributes to the successful treatment of voice disorders by the speech-language pathologist.

The professional singer presents with a specific set of needs that SLPs must take into consideration. Vocal difficulty in any individual is significant; however, for singers and other vocal performers such as actors, newscasters, and voice-over professionals, voice loss may mean career changes, loss of income, or other significant changes in life. Thus, SLPs must establish appropriate goals for vocal performers that account for a return to full voice use if appropriate. They must have the knowledge necessary to achieve the highest and best voice use for the patient.

The role of the SLP in the treatment of voice disorders complements the role of the laryngologist. The SLP is an essential member of the voice care team, and his or her role in the treatment of voice disorders extends from the time of the first visit until the patient has achieved the highest and best use of the voice. This chapter reviews the key aspects of treatment and focuses on the role of the speech-language pathologist in caring for those with a voice disorder.

THE VOICE EVALUATION

Ultimately, the goals of the voice evaluation are to establish a set of parameters that describe voice quality and voice usage and to relate these parameters to a well-designed treatment program. Figure 36–1 presents a typical algorithm for the voice evaluation process from evaluation to treatment. The model is a combined approach by the laryngologist and speech-language pathologist.

The role of the SLP in the evaluation process is significant because treatment is related not only to the pathology of the disorder, but also to the associated pathophysiology (often compensatory). The SLP should understand the medical and surgical options available for the patient's voice problem and treatment. Patients often ask questions regarding pending or future voice surgery. These discussions should be kept to a minimum, and the SLP should refer questions related to the type of surgery and the risks and benefits involved back to the surgeon. The SLP should know the surgical alternatives but focus on behavioral issues during the diagnostic process.

The voice evaluation consists of a detailed patient history relating previous voice use and training to current voice limitations. There has been a strong recent interest in better understanding the patient's concern about his or her problem. The Voice Handicap Index (VHI) developed by Jacobson et al was the first validated instrument to assess the patient's degree of voice handicap.[1] Since then, several other measures have been developed, all with the goal of assessing the degree to which the patient feels handicapped by his or her voice problem. More recently, the VHI-10, a validated modification of the VHI, was developed to reduce the time needed to assess the patient's perception of his or her handicap.[2]

Following a review of the VHI or similar tool, a thorough case history should precede testing or treatment. This may be done using a case history questionnaire[3] or simply through a narrative discussion of the patient's voice changes since their inception. Regardless of whether or not a questionnaire is used, the evaluation process focuses on voice use, both past and present, medical history, and changes in both speaking and singing. There are several key aspects to the patient history: (1) the chief complaint, (2) length of time of the problem, (3) circumstances surrounding the onset of the problem, (4) previous voice problems and treatments, (5) how the voice problem affects the patient's current and future work and social status, and (6) the patient's expectations.

General Observations and Perceptual Assessment

A perceptual assessment of the voice quality should also be done. This includes a perceptual rating of the appropriateness of pitch and loudness, voice qualities, and rate of speech. This may be done with a scale such as the GRBAS developed by Hirano[4] or the more recent CAPE-V scale proposed by the American Speech-Language and Hearing Consensus Conference and discussed by Behrman.[5] The CAPE-V uses an analog scale on which the rating parameters are scored, resulting in a continuous scale rather than a four-point scale of the original GRBAS. The perceptual assessment may also include singing range and the effects of vocal fatigue. If the patient has completed surgery prior to his or her first visit to the SLP, then the history should include a detailed description of the preoperative voice and the patient's comparisons of the pre- and postoperative voice. All diagnostic sessions should include perceptual judgments by the SLP regarding voice quality, loudness, and pitch range. Informal ratings may be done using sustained phonation or standardized voice tasks (sustained and connected speech). Previous investiga-

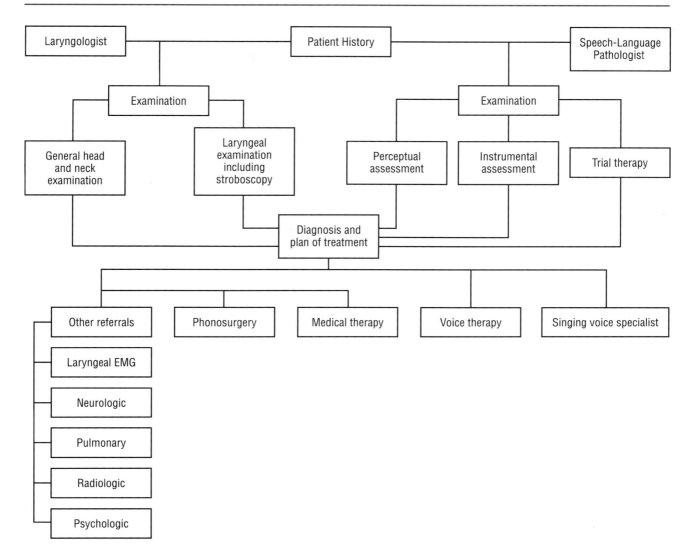

Figure 36–1. Voice Evaluation and Treatment Algorithm.

tions indicate that both are reliable when the patient is asked to produce the samples at his or her comfortable effort level.[6,7] The current approach to the assessment of the voice disorder involves instrumental assessment; however, both informal and formal perceptual assessments made by the clinician provide significant information on how the voice is used by the patient and a preliminary insight into the nature and severity of the voice disorder.

Additional aspects of the voice evaluation include the patient's posture and alignment during his or her normal speaking activities. The importance of a well-supported speaking voice cannot be underestimated. This begins with posture and how the individual uses the body to deliver the voice. The correct erect posture is standing upright with the feet slightly apart and the

knees unlocked. The shoulders should be loose, and the head should be over the shoulders and not extended out from the shoulders. Thus, in evaluating a university professor, it would be appropriate to observe and listen to a short segment of one of his or her lectures. For those who sit much of the time at their job, posture should be an erect back with shoulders relaxed and the feet flat on the floor. Thus, it is appropriate to ask secretaries or others who sit at their job most of the day to demonstrate their posture and alignment at a desk and observe their speech in this simulated setting. In some cases, it may be particularly helpful for the therapist to visit the patient's work environment and observe conditions and behaviors first hand.

Special attention should be given to patients in special situations such as stage performances, the coach's bench voice, courtroom voice use, or the elementary teacher who often is bending over children's desks. All of these postures may contribute to poor alignment and, therefore, poor support of the vocal mechanism.

Instrumental Assessment

The use of instrumental assessment procedures for voice care is now common. Acoustic analysis provides an objective measure of the patient's voice under controlled conditions. Common measures include frequency range, intensity range, and mean speaking fundamental frequency. These measures are done quite simply when the voice is not severely dysphonic. However, as dysphonia increases, the reliability of acoustic measures decreases.[8] Use of the voice range profile provides a dynamic assessment of the range of voice capable in the patient. The voice range profile is a valuable measure not only for singers but also for all patients with voice disorders undergoing treatment.[9] It should be mentioned, however, that if there is a suspicion of a lesion, the therapist must be sure that performing a voice range profile would not cause additional damage to the vocal folds. The Kay Computerized Speech Laboratory (CSL) and the multidimensional voice profile acoustic analyses systems (Kay Elemetrics, Englewood, NJ) are well-known systems for acoustic measurements. However, other systems are also available.

A physiological analysis of the interaction between pulmonary function and laryngeal function should also be done during the diagnostic process. Instrumentation is available to obtain mean airflow rate, estimates of subglottic air pressure, and the resultant laryngeal airway resistance value during voice production. These measures provide an objective assessment of the interaction of respiratory and phonatory components (ie, laryngeal valving efficiency).

Compliance

A third aspect of the voice evaluation is to determine through observation, as well as assessment, the patient's compliance or possible compliance with treatment programs. Whether the patient is to undergo surgery and voice therapy or voice therapy only, the issue of compliance is extremely important. One often gets a feel for the level of compliance as a result of questions regarding the importance of voice use by the patient. A trial of voice therapy is also part of the initial evaluation. It provides another way of evaluating the patient's voice and acts as a measure of assessing overall compliance with the treatment program. This is sometimes referred to as "unloading" and includes therapeutic procedures to determine the patient's ability to modify vocal function. It is at this point that communication among the SLP, the surgeon, and the patient is particularly important. Without an understanding of the need for compliance and the issues related to compliance, treatment is not likely to be successful. Communication between the SLP and the surgeon will help to formulate the treatment plan. For example, a patient with Reinke's edema is not likely to show much long-term improvement with surgery or voice therapy if she or he continues to smoke cigarettes and maintains the forceful, low-pitched voice usually seen in these patients. A behavioral management program of voice use, along with modification of personal habits related to smoking, should be integrated into an intensive treatment of these patients.[10]

Review of Results: Establishing the Diagnosis

When the medical diagnosis and speech-language pathology evaluations have been completed, the voice care team establishes a treatment plan with the patient's diagnostic information and the patient's needs in mind. Once the patient knows the diagnosis, a reasonable explanation as to how the vocal injury or voice disorder occurred is important. This often comes about as a result of an in-depth review of the case history by the speech-language pathologist. An explanation of relevant issues in each individual's case is often necessary so that the patient understands that it was not his or her singing teacher or something mysterious that caused the problem. If the patient understands the behavioral implications and their relationship to the voice disorder, he or she will be more likely to accept the voice therapy component of treatment. Moreover, he or she will be less likely to want a "magic pill" to correct the condition. Thorough understanding of how a vocal injury occurred is the first step toward prevention of another injury in the future.

The goals of treatment should address behavioral concerns; medication, if necessary; and the role and timing of phonosurgery (if needed). An appropriate model for patients with benign vocal fold lesions is one in which the laryngologist supports the need for behavioral modification and the speech-language pathologist supports the possible need for phonomicrosurgery. *Both of these treatment modalities should be presented to the patient (when indicated) at the same time so that the patient understands that the comprehensive management of his or her disorder is the most successful approach to recovery.*

TREATMENT

Once the diagnosis and plan of treatment are determined, the major role of the SLP is to provide voice therapy. Table 36–1 lists the most common voice disorders

TABLE 36–1. Common Voice Disorders for Which Voice Therapy Is the Initial Treatment of Choice

Vocal Fold Nodules
Vocal Fold Cyst
Vocal Fold Polyp
Reinke's Edema*
Muscle Tension Dysphonia, primary
Paradoxical Vocal Fold Motion Disorder
Vocal Fold Paresis
Vocal Fold Paralysis**
Neurogenic Voice Disorders
Functional Dysphonia
Vocal Fold Granuloma

*Unless significant airway restriction is present.

**Unless the patient is at high risk for aspiration or the vocal fold is in a lateral position

for which voice therapy is usually the initial treatment modality. Therapy may be provided in conjunction with surgical procedures that precede or (preferably) follow the therapy, or it may be the sole treatment modality. In some cases, voice therapy is also done in conjunction with psychotherapy to maximize the control of behavioral issues that coexist with the voice disorder.

Although voice therapy is a prominent treatment modality for treating many kinds of voice disorders, there is little agreement among SLPs regarding the specific techniques to be used. Moreover, in the past, "voice experts" advanced ideas that worked for them but were never tested for efficacy or outcomes. Nonetheless, even to this day, contributions by the so-called "experts" appear to be the primary basis for treatment. That is not to say that these treatments do not work. Rather, it is to say that the treatment of voice disorders remains ripe for studies of efficacy and outcome.

The medical referral process and the service delivery systems now in force in the United States govern voice therapy in the United States of America. Treatment often relies on third-party payers who limit the number of treatment sessions. Thus, modern-day SLPs must use existing information about the disorder, its pathophysiology, function, and objective measurements to guide the therapy within the number of sessions allowed. In the current health delivery system, there is little or no room for extraneous sessions to work for long periods of time on unitary aspects of voice production. The length of time of treatment varies from country to country and even within countries among individual SLPs.

The voice therapist incorporates breathing techniques with postural adjustments, muscle relaxation, and specific phonatory exercises targeted at the underlying cause of the dysphonia. The patient should be given a series of breathing and relaxation exercises to practice at home. It is important for the patient to begin an active daily treatment program from the first therapy visit. The importance of home practice of therapy skills cannot be overemphasized. Although some patients may show significant improvement in the time allotted to therapy by insurance plans, behavioral changes may require more time than originally allowed.

The physician and the therapist should take a proactive stand and provide information to the insurer documenting patient improvement and the rationale for further voice therapy. Follow-up instrumental assessments, laryngostroboscopic examination (with photos), or other indications such as reduced or lost work time should be used to justify additional treatment coverage. It is important for the speech pathologist and laryngologist to provide documentation and objective measures to demonstrate the efficacy of voice therapy as a viable treatment for voice disorders.

General Treatment Guidelines

Recently, Casper and Murry provided guidelines or general concepts essential to the success of any voice therapy program.[11] These concepts provide the framework for all treatment programs, regardless of the specific therapeutic techniques employed.

Patient education is the first step in all voice therapy. A thorough understanding of normal voice production will help to educate the patient about the dysphonic voice. Diagrams may be useful. Second, a review of the videolaryngoscopic examination may be helpful to point out lesions, movement disorders, or other aspects of the examination that are related to the dysphonia. Third, the patient should have an understanding of the voice therapy process. Fourth, the patient should understand what is meant by vocal hygiene. Finally, the patient must understand the goals of treatment. Treatment is not a long and extended process but rather a behavior-oriented approach to targeting specific behaviors that contribute to the dysphonia.

Once the patient understands the goals of voice therapy and the methods to achieve the goals, specific exercises and behavioral modifications are designed to reach the goals. The patient should understand that, in most cases, voice therapy does not eliminate such things as vocal fold paralysis, a vocal fold cyst, or a vocal fold polyp. Voice therapy, rather, provides the most efficient use of the voice, given the conditions of the voice, and leads to improvement in voice quality. For vocal nodules, however, it is expected that proper voice therapy with adequate compliance will reduce or eliminate the nodules in more than 95% of cases, unless the diagnosis is incorrect. This is similar to taking proper care of a callus, which disappears following the reduction of trauma to the callused area. Once the patient understands the process, basic vocal fold anatomy and physiology, and the goals of treatment, the therapy process may begin with both the therapist and the patient well aware of the goals of therapy and the methods needed to reach them.

Vocal Hygiene

Vocal hygiene is an essential component of treatment. In some cases, vocal hygiene may be the only form of treatment. Vocal hygiene encompasses three major areas:

1. The knowledge of what is traumatic or stressful to the vocal folds;
2. Techniques to improve or expedite recovery such as the use of steam or other hydration, the reduction of inhaled medications (if possible); and
3. The reduction or elimination of throat clearing.

The awareness of noxious stimuli, such as cigarette smoke, strong chemicals, or alcohol, must also be pointed out and monitored during the therapy program. For the singer or actor, specific reference must be made to the importance of voice rest before and after a performance and the avoidance of excessive speaking (especially before a performance such as for interviews, telephone calls or visits from well-wishers). Other aspects of vocal hygiene include understanding the effects of loud laughing, excessive coughing, or crying. All of these behaviors can lead to further vocal damage, and a program to monitor this behavior must be implemented at the start of therapy. Patients with voice disorders that involve lack of or poor vocal fold closure must also be taught to eliminate attempts to produce long phrases in loud or noisy conditions. This, in itself, will help to regulate the use of breathing more appropriately.

Vocal hygiene focuses on healthy use of the vocal organs. The importance of increased hydration, elimination of throat clearing, and other parts of a good vocal hygiene program, as noted in Table 36–2, must be spelled out in detail to the patient. A clear understanding of how the vocal mechanism works, and the many ways in which it can be injured, is also part of the vocal hygiene program. It should be pointed out that an effective vocal hygiene program for children, even as young as 4 or 5 years old will provide an effective deterrent to severe voice disorders.

TABLE 36–2. Critical Aspects of a Vocal Fold Hygiene Program

Eliminate smoking
Avoid singing when sick
Control gastroesophageal reflux
Reduce or eliminate throat clearing
Maintain adequate hydration
Eat a balanced diet
Use warm-up and cool-down period before and, after singing
Exercise to maintain good overall body condition
Know the effects of medications, over-the-counter preparations, alternative medicines, and prescription medicines on the voice
Avoid loud talking in the presence of background noise
Avoid inhaling of secondhand smoke and other irritants
Avoid extensive strained whispering
Exercise regularly to maintain body tone

A proper vocal hygiene program coupled with voice therapy can change behavior so that the vocal folds are not damaged further and a reactive lesion, if present, will be reduced. The patient must use his auditory and kinesthetic awareness to detect easier voice usage, improved voice quality, and less voice effort as part of the vocal hygiene program.

Voice Therapy (Direct)

For many voice disorders, voice therapy is the treatment of choice. It is a treatment based on behavioral methods that allows the patient to correct faulty vocal habits, develop awareness for good and bad voice quality, and understand the nature of healthy voice use for both the speaking and singing. A comprehensive program of voice care may include: (1) initial treatment and, if necessary, preparation for surgery; (2) an acute postoperative period and/or; (3) postoperative rehabilitation.

In some cases, preoperative treatment will be sufficient; and the patient may not require surgical treatment for the disorder.

The ultimate goals of voice therapy are:

1. To return the voice to optimal use;
2. To establish a vocal hygiene program that will be useful not only immediately but also following

surgery. It should also be one that is capable of being applied over long periods of time to establish a healthy vocal lifestyle.

3. To improve voice quality and increase vocal efficiency with minimal vocal effort;

Vocal rehabilitation must be planned and executed properly to ensure that the goals are met. The specific means to achieve the goals of therapy must be structured to the patient's needs. If surgery is involved, the timing of surgery must be selected based on voice requirements, performance requirements, or other job-related speaking and singing demands. Once the surgery date is scheduled, the voice therapist assists with establishing a preoperative voice use schedule, a postoperative voice rest schedule, and a coordinated follow-up treatment schedule to take advantage of the postoperative laryngeal examination and interaction with the laryngologist. Although voice care and rehabilitation are primarily done by the voice therapist, other disciplines such as psychiatry, gastroenterology, physical therapy, singing instruction, and pediatrics may be asked to play a role in the pre- and postoperative care of the patient on an as needed basis.

The Treatment Period

Voice therapy may be extensive if vocal habits are poor and the goal is to establish healthy voice use that includes lifestyle adjustments. This is especially true for patients with Reinke's edema who often have a history of excessive cigarette smoking, loud voice use, and episodes of vocal misuse. Preoperative voice therapy programs should involve a course of vocal hygiene.

A comprehensive voice therapy program includes exercises for muscle relaxation, posture and alignment, and breathing, as well as preparation for recovery after surgery if surgery is planned. The preoperative time is important because it provides the voice care team with an indication of the patient's level of compliance. If a patient is not compliant with the preoperative voice therapy, then phonosurgery may be best delayed or cancelled.

Muscle relaxation exercises are useful to scale down the force of voice onset and perhaps the overall loudness of the voice as well. A program of general body relaxation provided by a physical therapist may be helpful, along with specific exercises for the head and neck muscles. Specific exercises for the lips, tongue, jaw, and neck selected by the SLP should also be included in the program.[12-14] Direct laryngeal massage also has been shown to have a positive benefit in relaxing muscles of the neck area and altering laryngeal posture. With a relaxed laryngeal posture, the onset of phonation may be less forceful.[15]

Postoperative Voice Rest

Patients undergoing surgery for vocal fold cyst and granuloma are routinely placed on complete voice rest for 3 to 7 days following surgery, as are patients having surgery for vocal polyps or Reinke's edema. Although there are a number of opposing thoughts regarding complete voice rest, it is generally a good idea to plan several days of complete voice rest following surgery. The surgical treatments for vocal fold paresis and paralysis may involve some voice rest, but it need not be as extensive as it is following the removal of benign vocal fold lesions. Of specific importance in the voice rest period is the avoidance of whispering and coughing. Patients should be asked not to whisper but rather to use a pencil and paper during complete voice rest. Voice rest should always be used judiciously, as it does involve a significant hardship on most patients. Voice rest should be monitored, because the psychological strain of not talking sometimes is more difficult to tolerate than attempting to talk in a soft, breathy voice. It should be remembered that voice rest alone does not help a person return to healthy voice use if the person has not been treated for excessive traumatic vocal behavior or poor vocal habits that led to the disorder in the first place.

Postoperative Rehabilitation

The role of the speech-language pathologist immediately after surgery is to make sure the patient understands the reason for the voice rest period and to begin vocal exercises once the voice rest is completed. The acute voice rest period should end with the laryngologist and speech pathologist starting the patient on easy vocalization. Exercises may include using the consonants /n/, /w/, /y/, and /h/. With easy voice onsets using these consonants connected to vowels, the patient begins to sense the notion of easy voice onset and reduction of force. For patients with longstanding Reinke's edema, these exercises should be initiated above the patient's preoperative speaking pitch. At the outset of the therapy, it is important to refocus the voice to proper pitch range with low-effort level.

The acute postoperative period is also an excellent time to initiate voiceless muscle relaxation exercises or review the muscle relaxation and breathing exercises that were taught in the preoperative voice therapy sessions. Exercises for the lips, tongue, jaw, neck, and shoulders are appropriate at this time. Specifically, in a standing as well as a sitting position, the patient should be asked to take the pressure away from the upper part of the chest near the top of the sternum by using slow exhalations followed by inhalations. These may be accompanied by breathy vowels during the end of the voice rest. Once voice rest is complete, the patient should focus the vowels forward in the oral cavity and concentrate on ease of onset and the auditory perception of voice quality. Clearly, the acute postoperative period offers the patient a time to tune into his support systems for phonation and to prepare for easy voicing.

The first postoperative visit to the speech-language pathologist is extremely important. If the plan of treatment is not explained well, and if its rationale is not sound, patients may be reluctant to return for therapy, feeling that surgery corrected the problem. It is often a good idea to tell the patient to think of his voice much like a football player thinks of his knee or shoulder, that recovery is slow and requires limited and controlled use. As recovery of the voice improves, the voice use increases. In the first days of recovery, it is important for the patient not to overdo voice use or voice practice. Slow and controlled reacquisition of voice, especially pitch range and voice quality, helps patients develop confidence in voice use and prevents the opportunity for overuse and strain to recur.

Specific Voice Therapy Techniques

Confidential Voice

Casper and Murry described some of the more frequently used therapeutic techniques for voice therapy.[11] One technique is the use of the confidential voice. Confidential voice is used most often to reduce or eliminate excessive vocal fold contact, thereby decreasing the force of vocal fold collision. It also helps to reduce hyperfunctional behaviors such as false vocal fold adduction. The treatment is described as confidential voice, because it typically sounds like the voice that one uses to describe things in a quiet setting and almost in a breathy voice. It is produced with the vocal folds slightly abducted, which results in increased airflow and reduced loudness.[16] When produced correctly, the confidential voice results in reduction of excessive muscle tension and reduction of supraglottal constriction. The addition of tension to increase loudness may result in a vocal harshness that is readily identifiable to the patient.

Reduced vocal intensity is one positive feature of the confidential voice. Although it may be difficult for patients to use this voice throughout the day, it often can be employed at least part of the day. The intent of this technique is to eliminate hyperfunctional or traumatic behaviors to allow lesions, such as vocal nodules, to heal as a result of reduced excessive vocal contact in the area of the nodules and to help reduce muscle tension and vocal fatigue.[17] The patient should be aware that use of the confidential voice is not the endpoint of therapy and that

it is only a temporary means of promoting healing, especially when there are bilateral midfold lesions.

The confidential voice technique is useful for treating muscle tension dysphonias, hyperfunctional dysphonia, and vocal fatigue. It is also useful, as an early postoperative voice therapy technique, to reduce strong glottal attack. If the patient continues to report excessive fatigue during this phase of the treatment, further examination should be done; and the patient should be observed using the technique in conversational speech to verify that he or she is using it appropriately. It is important for both the SLP and the patient to understand that whispering is not acceptable, because it puts excessive tension on the vocal folds and is not a long-term solution to communication.

Resonant Voice Therapy

Resonant voice therapy, or a voice with a frontal focus, usually refers to a voice disorder associated with vibratory sensations felt in the facial area.[17] The focus in resonant therapy is on the production of the voice primarily through feeling and hearing. The feeling is specific, in terms of both vibratory sensation, and in terms of the use of onset of phonation. The patient is required to listen to changes in voice quality to achieve maximum ease of voice with the least amount of effort. This treatment method historically derives from the work of Lessac,[18] who used this approach to improve the voices of students in theatrical training. The goal is to place the voice high in the head so that resonance is achieved easily through all the resonators from the supraglottic area up through the face. Once placement is obtained, a variety of flexibility exercises related to pitch and intonation should be used. Initially, placement of the voice is obtained by humming the /m/ phoneme. It should be noted that patients often reject the more forward placement as it often leads to a higher pitch, and they do not sound like themselves.

Vocal Function Exercises

Vocal function exercises date back to the middle of the twentieth century when Briess described a series of specific muscle dysfunctions that could be alleviated by "rebalancing" various laryngeal postures. Recently, Stemple formalized this series of exercises.[19] No significant research supports the value of these exercises. However, there is some evidence that singers, as well as normal speakers, produce improved voice after the exercises are completed.

The exercises are centered on four distinct phases. These include muscle warm-up, muscle stretching, muscle contracting, and muscle power building. The exercises are recommended for many types of dyspho-

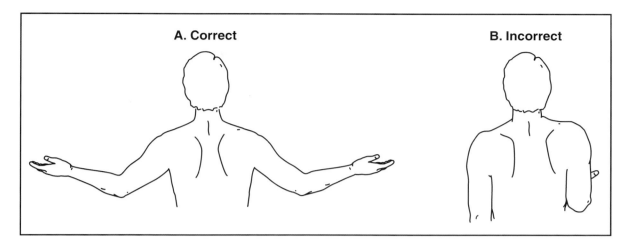

Figure 37–1. A. Alignment of the shoulder blades; shoulder blades are relaxed but in close proximity, with the upper chest remaining expanded. **B.** Incorrect alignment. Tensions of expressivity may pull the shoulders upward and/or forward, compromising breath efficiency.

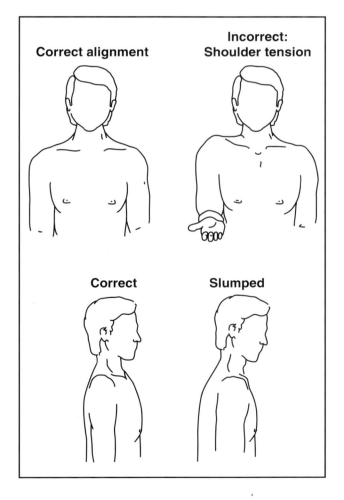

Figure 37–2. Correct and incorrect alignment of the upper torso. Excessive physical expressivity may result in lifted shoulders or slumped chest positions.

place them behind the fullest part of the back of the head. The elbows should be brought forward. The patient should then isometrically push the head back into the clasped hands and pull the head forward with the hands/arms, feeling the pull against the back and sides of the neck. The patient should breathe comfortably while maintaining this isometric exercise for approximately 20 to 30 seconds. Then he or she should suddenly release the clasped hands, allowing the head to move freely on the now-loosened neck. The patient should feel a reduction in neck/shoulder tensions, which may lead to improved access of lower breathing patterns (caused by reduced muscle tension of the upper torso).

Exercise 4:   "Figure 8s": With the patient standing, have him or her bring the hands to each shoulder, and raise the elbows (parallel to shoulder). Using the elbows as "paintbrushes," he or she is asked to attempt to paint the number 8 from the ceiling to the floor, bending the knees and moving the torso as necessary, maintaining a regular breathing pattern as the torso contorts to form the figure 8s. (*Note:* This is hard to do.) Repeat, with elbows facing the back. (*Note:* This is even harder to do!)

General Coordination

Trunk stability and general coordination are traditionally assessed in young children with a speech or language issue. Because the professional voice user with a vocal disorder is typically an adult, it is easy to overlook general coordination and stability of physical function. It is important to note carefully and bring to the patient's attention any observed episodes of slight hip swaying (while standing), particularly if it occurs during phonation. Instability of the lower trunk impairs respiratory control. Upon identification, many patients have difficulty controlling swaying movements of the torso. Many performers incorrectly add tension to avoid body swaying (which has significant ramifications for respiratory control). This may be redirected easily into energized, intention movement found in tai chi, for example. Many performers have also found this form of exercise helpful for stress management, in addition to the improved support and trunk stability.

Other issues of general coordination include eye movements/blinking (which are often associated with the swallow reflex, which would entrap the larynx during phonation) at the beginning of high notes, and arm or hand tension during speech and singing. Video documentation and analysis are usually sufficient to reinforce verbal comment by the voice specialist.

One standard vocal exercise that assesses respiratory-laryngeal-resonance coordination is a /β/ lip flutter (vibration therapy). This phoneme (a voiced bilabial fricative) tests the ability of the patient to balance the power, source, and filter subsystems during pitch change (see Figure 37–3).

It is, in effect, a test of the patient's general tendency to cheat in vocal technique. If the patient locks his or her support or fails to use adequate support, the lip flutter (a "raspberry" sound) will stop or fade away. If the patient uses hyperfunction at the source, the sound will stop. If the patient uses excess tension in the filter subsystem (usually at the lips), the sound will stop. If the lip flutter is tested in a *messa di voce* (crescendo-diminuendo) task (see Figures 37–4A, 37–4B), more detailed analysis is possible of the singer's strategy for use of hypofunction and hyperfunction. Initially, some patients may need to reduce lip tension by placing their hands gently on the corners of the mouth. Other patients may need to use a tongue flutter (with tongue extended over the lower lip) or a rolled "r" (/ɾ/) to achieve balanced coordination.

A more difficult vocal exercise to test coordination of the subsystems is a panting exercise. The DEVT panting exercise examines the patient's ability to coordinate the alternation between a delicate vocal task (*messa di voce* on vowels) and a dynamic respiratory task (panting) (see Figures 37–5A, B, C, and D).

This exercise may be done throughout the entire vocal range, and should begin on a medium low note for the patient, and at a moderately slow tempo. After each short *messa di voce*, the patient exhales and inhales three times. After completing the given vowels, the patient then executes a staccato (short, bouncy singing), legato (smooth, fluid singing) and then marcato (detached but still connected singing), diatonic scale. Most singers can accomplish the diatonic scales on one breath. Many singers typically view panting exercises as a repeated exhalatory exercise. It should be viewed as a *quiet inhalatory exercise* first and foremost. The

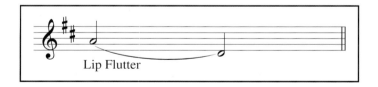

Figure 37–3. Descending lip flutter (vibration therapy exercise) to coordinate the subsystems.

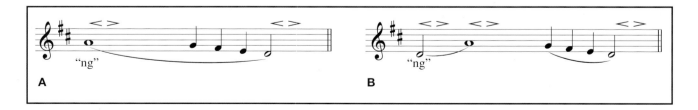

Figure 37–4 A. Descending slide on lip flutter (vibration therapy) with *messa di voce*. **B.** Lip flutter (vibration therapy) with messa di voce and change in fundamental frequency and descending scale.

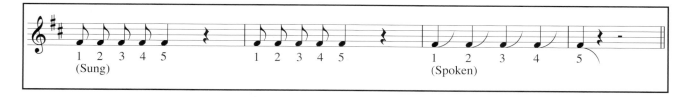

Figure 37–14. "Counting exercise" using rote speech task with transition from singing mode to speech mode with pitch inflections for speech mode.

They are identified as "Judy, the singer" or "Mark, the tenor" or "John, the great actor." When a vocal problem arises, they may not be able to function in part (or whole) as the professional vocal athlete they perceive as their identity. This is particularly true if the vocal athlete requires phonosurgery. They fear temporary or permanent loss of range, quality, flexibility, sensation, or laryngeal appearance. In essence, they have lost their trust of the voice. The voice care team must recognize these concerns.[33] Referral to a psychotherapist who specializes in performers may be necessary.

PSYCHOLOGIC AND PHYSIOLOGIC ISSUES OF STRESS

Performance anxiety is commonplace among performers and public speakers and is considered normal behavior in high-level performance. Performers with voice disorders can benefit from a team that includes professions for counseling, hypnotherapy, and other professional psychologic services. The voice specialist must handle referrals to other professionals through the referring physician in order to maintain integrity in the chain of referrals, avoid interfering inadvertently with medical care, and continue the successful team management process.

From the voice trainer's perspective, perhaps the most important strategy in stress reduction is attention to the interaction between the physiology of respiration and the psychology of stress. Public speakers tend to hold the breath while listening to a questioning reporter and then reply without refreshing the breath. Singers and actors may also fall into this trap, which can also increase laryngeal tension. The habit of holding one's breath is often seen prior to musical entrances or stage dialogue. Three deep breaths can make a significant difference in calming the nervous body and voice and preparing for efficient phonations physically and psychologically.

Physical exercise is a second important strategy in reducing overall stress. The choice of exercise should be carefully considered as the activity should reduce body tension and effort, rather than overindulgence in "strength training." Swimming, cross-country skiing, fencing, racquetball, and basketball are all good choices, depending on the needs and likes of the patient.

Meditative and hypnotic exercises are practiced regularly, either intentionally or unintentionally, by most great performers. Mesmerizing the audience with one's level of self occurs when techniques similar to those of meditation and self-hypnosis are implemented. Collecting energies and focusing concentration on the ultimate goal allow confidence in performance. Just as an Olympic athlete practices visualization of success, these strategies, both physical and mental, can be valuable to the vocal athlete.

The excitement of performance releases adrenaline in the body. This sudden surge of adrenaline may be unnerving to the performer, but should be channeled into "directed energy" rather than masked with medications or alcohol. Although many performers request beta-blockers, this practice is usually not recommended. These medications usually lead to dull lackluster performances. The voice trainer must help the voice user learn to perform with confidence.

DESIGNING AN EXERCISE PROGRAM

Vocal exercises should be prescribed in an organized manner, with rationales and expected results (or gains) for each exercise. If the patient does not understand the specific need for an exercise, he or she may misjudge when to use the exercise, or may misjudge the production found during the exercise.

All patients should be able to demonstrate good posture and be able to execute a *messa di voce* that is based on filter contributions rather than overt source or power supply contributions. Exercises should be designed to bring the higher registers (falsetto, loft register) down to the lower register (modal/chest). Register integration and balanced resonance are essential for all voices and vocal styles.

Perhaps the single most important education for the patient with a voice disorder is vocal warm-up prior to heavy voice use (such as a rehearsal, conference meeting, social meeting, or concert), followed by a vocal cool-down immediately after the heavy voice use. Much of the work on exercise physiology as applied to voice is contained in a text by Saxon and Schneider *Vocal Exercise Physiology*,[34] and it is worth reading to understand the basics of exercise physiology (although they are not well tested on voice). Essentially, the vocalist must adequately prepare and readjust the body and the voice for marathon vocal control, quality, and endurance. Marathon runners would develop muscle spasms if they suddenly stopped at the finish line, but with continuation of ever gentler activity, eventually slow walk, and finishing with stretches, the runner may avoid or reduce the possibility of injuries. The vocal warm-up consists of physical stretches, followed by specific exercises designed to optimize control and finesse of respiration, phonation, resonance, and articulation. Vocal exercises begin in midrange and gradually encompass the entire physiologic range. Exercises should be selected based on the needs of the voice that day, rather than a mechanical series of exercises.

A simple cool-down is the opposite of a warm-up and should proceed from the middle-high voice into the lower-middle voice. Descending scales, long, expressive tones, or a soulful expressive melody (humming "Amazing Grace," "Mary had a little lamb" or the Brahms "Lullaby") acts as a massage, encouraging blood circulation to the muscle of heavy use, evacuating lactic acid, and restoring oxygen debt incurred in anaerobic activity. After a strenuous performance or a difficult rehearsal, many performers instinctively want to be quiet or want to desist immediately from any vocal activity. Cool-down exercises are preferable. With use of vocal cool-down, the vocal muscles begin to recover and many vocalists report that their voice is more readily available the next day.

Many performers feel a sense of elation following a successful performance, and they often segue too soon into a party environment, carrying their elated and boisterous vocal tones with them. A few moments of descending hums (which can begin with the audience applause) to readjust the voice into a comfortably normal speech mode moderate the potential for injury at a noisy party or smoky restaurant.

In the development of an appropriate vocal exercise routine, simplicity is an important element. An exercise routine should take the typical injured voice user between 5 and 15 minutes and should not be excessively complex. In fact, a 5-minute routine of three simple exercises is often sufficient initially. This exercise routine should be accomplished in a program of 4 to 5 brief exercise sessions per day for optimal benefit.

It is vitally important that the issue of proper hydration during exercise be addressed simultaneously to avoid the effects of excessive friction on the vocal folds. Sipping room temperature water is recommended. Gulping large quantities of water (ie, a large glass) may exacerbate gastroesophageal reflux disease, especially when one is engaging in breathing and singing exercises. Moderation is recommended.

Physical Exercise

Overall body conditioning plays an important role in the rehabilitation of the voice. A healthy voice is usually accompanied by a healthy body. Aerobic exercise that is geared toward efficient use and coordination of muscles, without forceful or abrupt movements that could induce laryngeal tension (ie, avoiding a strenuous Valsalva maneuver) is recommended. Although some well-known singers are overweight, their success is from their efficiency of vocal production, despite the adverse effects their weight may have had on the body. Although an impressive masculine physique has launched more than a few careers, strenuous bodybuilding that includes serious weight-lifting is discouraged. Exercises such as basketball, rowing, tennis, fencing, and swimming, which require upper body coordination without excess tension, are advocated.

Patients should be cautioned on their use of strenuously aerobic exercise when experiencing a cold or upper respiratory infection. Rapid, full inhalations which occur with physical exercise (and with the "panting exercise" above) increase exacerbation of infection, including increased risk for myocarditis.[35]

Issues of Chronologic Age

The effects of age and general body conditioning on the voice have been researched in depth by Chodzko-Zajko and Ringel[36] and Hollien[37], and more recently reviewed by Linville.[38] A body maintained in good physical condition facilitates a younger-sounding voice. Likewise, vocal muscles that are abused or misused for a long period of time tend to maintain those behavior patterns and make voices sound "old" prematurely. It was once felt that older voices wobble naturally. However, any voice, young or old, may wobble (or weaken) when there is inefficient connection of the respiratory, phonatory, resonatory, and articulatory subsystems. The majority of "wobbly old voices" respond with new youthful capabilities when effective coordination of the voice is re-established.

Training of the voice can be undertaken at an early age with the understanding that the goals of training are to optimize the efficiency of the changing voice and reduce the vocal patterns of abuse and misuse often found in young speakers and singers. Many children enjoy the community involvement that participation in the theater affords. The projection of the young voice, however, may overdevelop the heavy (modal voice) mechanism to the detriment or total exclusion of the light (loft register) mechanism. Maintaining flexibility in vocal color, range, and dynamics has long been the goal of high-quality children's choral programs. It is strongly recommended that children who wish to excel in theater concurrently maintain their skills in choral ensemble singing. This helps avoid the habit of always singing too loudly (provided that the choral direction is appropriate). Likewise, extending the vocal fundamental frequency range should not be a primary goal with prepubescent or pubescent voices. If extension of the range of frequency and power is desired, it is best to wait until the effects of puberty have subsided. Efficient use of the entire vocal range is desirable for all ages.

HYDRATION

Dryness is an important issue in the continuing care of the voice. Simply drinking more water may be an important strategy in recovering from a voice disorder. The voice trainer may be helpful in educating the patient about issues which may adversely affect lubrication and, if necessary, bring them to the attention of the physician. Salivary flow is important: stimulating salivary flow with nonmedicated lozenges, lemon drops, and so forth, is prudent. Drinking lemon juice or vinegar, however, may not be prudent especially in patients with GERD or LPR. Foods and drugs that induce dryness should be avoided when possible. The voice trainer should encourage the professional voice user to ask his or her laryngologist about medications, whether over-the-counter or prescription. Alcohol is a vasodilator; its consumption causes drying and reduces fine motor control and sensations of tension or pain from inappropriate or potentially damaging vocal behaviors. (For the same reason, any lozenge that anesthetizes the pain of a sore throat should be avoided.) Alcohol dulls the sensorium and should be avoided if professional voice use is scheduled. Many commercial (alcohol-based) mouthwashes also induce dryness. Another drying agent may be silica–based toothpaste, which can leave behind a microscopic silica gel (used as an abrasive to clean teeth). On days of performances, it may be more prudent for some singers or actors to brush with commercially available isotonic baking soda toothpaste. Microscopic food par-

ticles will continue to stimulate salivary flow, contributing to "moister" voice use. The voice trainer helps ensure that the patient is aware of the importance of these and other vocal hygiene and lifestyle issues.

On the topic of baking soda and salt, the author would be remiss not to mention Dr. Wilbur James Gould's nonmedicated gargle recipe:

1/2 teaspoon sea salt

1/2 teaspoon baking soda

1/2 teaspoon corn syrup (Karo) (or honey or other syrup)

6 ounces of warm water

Gargle quietly and gently for 2 long, boring minutes. Do not rinse.

Although there has been some discussion on the remotely abusive effects of gargling, if it is done quietly and conservatively, or if the mouth is simple rinsed thoroughly (without swallowing), this folk remedy is generally recommended as an adjunct for preserving (or reacquiring) the sensation of a moist, fresh voice.

To maintain the proper level of laryngeal lubrication, the voice user should remember the old adages of Van Lawrence.[39] "Keep moist," and "mucus is our friend." The kidneys are the body's "computers" for adjusting the level of systemic hydration. If more fluid is needed, the kidneys conserve water, causing urine to be darker. Pale-colored urine generally indicates adequate levels of hydration. The amount of water necessary varies by the individual and environmental conditions. Drinking 1 ounce for every 2 pounds of body weight is recommended by some, while others recommend 8 to 10 glasses of water per day for adequate hydration. To avoid systemic dehydration, the voice user should drink enough water to "pee pale." Medications to assist in maintaining desirable lubrication may be helpful in some cases, as discussed elsewhere in this book.

The blanket of thin, runny mucus covering the entire mucous membrane is swept along by cilia (microscopic cytoplasmic hairs). Maintaining a high level of moist blanket keeps the mucus thin and runny. Failure of the mucus glands to secrete enough serous fluid results in a thicker blanket of mucus; secretions and foreign matter accumulate, and phlegm thickens. Further, in a performance situation, adrenaline attenuates the salivary flow in the mouth, thickening and decreasing the total fluid available in the vocal tract, and results in a failure to lubricate the vocal folds. The voice trainer helps ensure that the patient is aware of these normal phenomena and has effective coping strategies. In a performance the voice user can simply bite the tip of the tongue just to the point of pain, allowing an instantaneous flow of saliva in the oral cavity.

LIFESTYLE ISSUES FOR THE VOICE PATIENT

Being a professional voice user is comparable to being a violinist who carries a Stradivarius at all times. Everywhere a voice user goes, the instrument goes too. It is logical that voice conservation should be observed. The voice user should obviously avoid certain activities such as yelling at noisy sports events, speaking over noise at raucous nightclubs, and being in irritating, smoky environments. There are many other behaviors that a professional voice user may need to regard with care, including use of ingested substances.

LIFESTYLES AND LIFELONG VOCAL PREPAREDNESS

Poor technique is often blamed for vocal failures. Although poor technique is possible, especially when combined with other difficulties such as infection or injury, it is important not to discount the level of technique attained by many self-trained performers. Sound vocal training may be learned through formal or informal study. Although many acquire their muscle memory through formal training, others have stronger influence from performing experiences and mentors, and some are naturally good technicians. Singers such as Ella Fitzgerald and Mabel Mercer have developed incredibly complex and predictable vocal techniques based on years of experience and hard-learned lessons. Good vocal habits should be established early in the career, but when the voice continues to develop, a voice specialist can be a valuable helper for the predominantly self-trained voice. Although it is possible to develop a sound, reliable technique later in life, many patients fear that they will lose their vocal identity. They often do not understand that they will, instead, be expanding vocal skill while maintaining the critical personality aspects of their vocal style. Patient motivation is a key issue in adapting motor patterns and behavioral decisions. The assistance of an experienced voice specialist can be invaluable in dealing with the issues of compensation especially in light of moderate or major injuries. There is no substitute for someone else's experienced ears and eyes.

Each style of performance has its own demands. Technique is technique, however. Style is primarily an issue of interpretation. Although cross-specialization is possible among various vocal performance styles, it is not commonplace. A solid vocal technique and acting technique, however, can utilize the same sets of muscular strategies in the coordination of resonance, articulation, and respiration while reducing the risk to the phonatory mechanism. Healthy, efficient use of the voice is possible with all styles of voice use. People with certain vocal styles and occupations have traditionally had shorter careers. It is rare to see a commodities trader "in the pit" for more than a few years, primarily because of the extreme level of vocal misuse that pervades that industry. It may be rare to have the lead singer of a heavy metal band continue to heavily abuse the voice for more than a few years without noticeable vocal changes. It is not unusual for classical singers and classic actors to have significantly longer careers. This may be caused in part by the consistent reliance on skilled voice teachers, acting teachers, and coaches in that segment of the industry. Well-trained voice users usually take only well-calculated risks. They do not take extraordinary risks daily, and they tend to pamper their voices more than the untrained or nonprofessional voice user.

CANCELLATION OF APPEARANCES

When should a performance be canceled? If the voice user is technically strong enough to sing by sensation, not sound, it is generally safe to perform with those instructions after medical evaluation and clearance. The voice trainer can be invaluable in reconfirming vocal hygiene and ensuring good vocal technique. It is wise to note the admonition by Punt that performers should not "say an unnecessary word unless they are paid for it."[40] If there is a sudden and dramatic voice change, the performer should cancel, even if the voice change happens in the middle of the concert. Sudden voice change may indicate a hemorrhage or mucosal tear, and continued use of the voice may permanently impair normal healing of the membranes. The performer should seek an examination by a physician as soon as possible. Vocal trainers can help patients understand the importance of such precautions, and their professional acceptability.

If the performer's abdominal strength is compromised by illness or muscle cramping, the performer should not risk the voice. Inaccessibility of reliable, well-supported breath management imposes risks for vocal injury as support may be inadequate, and this may result in compensation by inappropriate muscles. When the performance is not critical, the performer should not risk the career. Judgment calls are never easy to make, however, and decisions should be made jointly by the patient, voice teacher/trainer, physician, and the performer's management. Officials who insist that the indisposed performer continue a performance obligation at the risk of permanent vocal injury should be advised that they must take responsibility for lifelong damage incurred because of their insistence.

AUDITORY FEEDBACK IN PERFORMANCE

Performing conditions and performance spaces vary considerably among the vocal arts forms. If microphones are used (which for singers—and ideally also for professional speakers—should always be a microphone designed for singing amplification rather than speech), the performer should be skilled in the proper use of the amplification system. Separate monitor speakers for the voice user are essential when amplification is used, particularly for singers. There are new in-the-ear monitors that are being used by nonclassical and classical performers in large theaters. They are individually molded and require supervision by an audiologist or otologist. They often require numerous readjustments to optimize function and preserve the hearing of the user. These monitors avoid the pitfalls of the monitor feedback squeal encountered in public address systems, but they are not foolproof. A backup monitor system must be available in the event of failure of the ear mold monitors.

Good hearing is as important as a good voice for the voice professional. The preservation of hearing is an important issue, especially with the commonplace use of portable stereos with headphones. Headphones allow a very high level of sound to be transmitted directly to the ear. Users typically listen to stereos, especially portable stereos and radios, at significantly higher levels of intensity than they realize. These higher levels may cause permanent hearing threshold changes. The Occupational Safety and Health Administration regulations state that prolonged exposure to noise (8 hours at 90 dBA) is unsafe and hearing protection is necessary.[41] The risk of temporary (and potentially permanent) hearing loss increases as intensity and duration increase. Hearing loss in singers and actors creates a special problem and may be the root of some inappropriate technical adjustments.

PARTNERSHIP OF THE VOICE SPECIALIST WITH THE SPEECH-LANGUAGE PATHOLOGIST

The voice specialist and speech-language pathologist share the common goal of optimizing vocal production but do so using different techniques. The experienced voice specialist has invaluable practical voice skills, as well as personal experience in professional voice use. The speech-language pathologist has stronger scientific and medically related training for speech and language development and disorders, but typically has only rudimentary to intermediate training in voice. Speech therapy focuses on maximizing efficiency of the colloquial speaking voice. Specialized voice training maintains a higher level of overall skill of vocal efficiency throughout the entire physiologic fundamental frequency range of phonation and critically examines the choices for transmitting that phonation in a variety of acoustic environments. Terminology may differ between the two specialties. Training methods to achieve vocal efficiency may differ. Although some voice specialists tend to stay "married" to one intervention method, the more successful approach is generally eclectic in nature, designed specifically for the individual patient. This is important because of the muscle memory patterns for each individual.

Traditional speech therapy addresses adjustments in behavior (such as yelling, level of hydration), then breath management, easy vocal onset, awareness of resonance, and connected speech patterns. Optimizing oral-nasal resonance is typically done by the voice specialist. Attention to habitual, abusive speech patterns (including excessive throat clearing and harsh glottal onsets) and language disorders is the primary province of a speech-language pathologist. In behavior modification, any addictive trait is given a substitute rather than an admonition of restraint. Whereas much of the literature in speech-language pathology recommends telling the patient, "Don't yell," the voice specialist teaches the voice user to substitute a rather high energy sound production that is based on elongation of the sound (gentle "calling"). Although earlier speech-language pathology texts reported singing (and acting) as "abusive," efficient vocalization is not abusive. The voice specialist and speech-language pathologist can work together very effectively as a team.

Locating a voice specialist can sometimes be problematic. In the past, many voice teachers and theater coaches were reluctant to collaborate with a medical team on the care of injured voices. Excellent voice teachers and theater coaches are highly skillful in detecting inefficient breath patterns, poor resonance choices, and instances of vocal strain. These professionals are excellent candidates for clinical training as voice specialists and, if they can afford the time for completing additional graduate education in speech-language pathology, to become vocologists. Advanced study in speech-language pathology and the resulting certification (CCC/SLP) are advocated and would enable those individuals to practice privately in the area of voice therapy as well as maintain their private voice training studios. Voice specialists who do not hold licensure (and in most states the Certificate of Clinical Competence from the American Speech-Language-Hearing Association) can participate in the rehabilitation process (generally as a speech aide) under the direct supervision of a physician or licensed speech-language pathologist, but cannot legally provide voice therapy independently.

Voice trainers who specialize in singing may be found in the community, or through local and national singing teacher associations (such as the National Association of Teachers of Singing). The New York Singing Teachers Association (which was a parent organization for the National Association of Teachers of Singing) has developed a Professional Development Program with curriculum for their Voice Professional Certificate for Teachers, testing their knowledge base in a variety of areas, including medical/therapeutic management. Voice trainers who specialize in acting voice may be located through local colleges, community theaters, or through the national organization Voice and Speech Trainers Association (VASTA). Speech-language pathologists who specialize in voice disorders may be found by contacting the American Speech, Language and Hearing Association (ASHA). ASHA has a variety of subspecialty divisions members may join, with voice (Special Interest Division 3) as one of the specialty areas.

Perhaps the most compelling rationale for use of specialized voice exercises as adjuncts to more traditional voice therapy exercises is access to a mode of phonation (singing or elocutionary speech) which may not have as many compensatory behaviors established, and the development of higher skill level (singing and elocutionary voice/acting voice) for lesser demanding tasks (colloquial speech).

CONCLUSION

Vocal rehabilitation is a simple yet complex process. It is simple in that it requires basic coordination of three main subsystems: respiration, source, and filter. Yet it is complex because of the many factors influencing the efficiency of each of those subsystems, particularly in the voice professional. A vocal disorder rarely emerges or resolves because of one facet of vocal production. The many nuances of phonatory control and compensation are best addressed through a combination of traditional and specialized therapy. Because singing and professional speaking require greater

control of the nuances of vocal quality and coordination across subsystems, it is logical to use select vocal exercises to improve vocal control and assist in resolution of the pathology. The voice specialist, with his or her additional training and experience in vocal production, is an invaluable asset to the voice care team.

FOR FURTHER INFORMATION, CONTACT:

The Voice Foundation:
www.voicefoundation.org

The New York Singing Teachers Association:
www.nyst.org

The National Association of Teachers of Singing: www.nats.org

Voice and Speech Trainers Association:
www.vasta.org

National Center for Voice and Speech:
www.ncvs.org

American Speech-Language-Hearing Association: www.asha.org

REFERENCES

1. Carroll LM: Application of singing techniques for the treatment of dysphonia. In: Rosen C, Murray T, eds. *Otolaryngologic Clinics of North America: Voice Disorders and Phonosurgery II.* Philadelphia, PA: WB Saunders Co; 2000.
2. Benninger MS, Jacobson BH, Johnson AF. *Vocal Arts Medicine: The Care and Prevention of Professional Voice Disorders.* New York, NY: Thieme Medical Publishers; 1994.
3. Peacher G. *How to Improve Your Speaking Voice.* New York, NY: Fell Publishers; 1966.
4. Riley WD, Carroll LM. The role of the singing-voice specialist in non-medical management of benign voice disorders. In: Rubin JS, Sataloff RT, Korovin GS, Gould WJ, eds. *Diagnosis and Treatment of Voice Disorders.* New York, NY: Igaku-Shoin; 1995:405–423.
5. Sataloff RT. *Professional Voice: The Science and Art of Clinical Care.* New York, NY: Raven Press; 1991.
6. Sataloff RT. Training teachers to work with injured voices. *NATS J.* 1992;49(1):2–26.
7. Sataloff RT. *Professional Voice: The Science and Art of Clinical Care.* 2nd ed. San Diego, CA: Singular Publishing Group; 1997.
8. Sataloff RT. *Vocal Health and Pedagogy.* San Diego, CA: Singular Publishing Group; 1998.
9. Brodnitz FS. *Vocal Rehabilitation: A Manual.* Rochester, MN: American Academy of Ophthalmology and Otolaryngology;1971.

10. Gould WJ, Sataloff RT, Spiegel JR. *Voice Surgery*. St. Louis, MO: Mosby; 1993.

11. Lawrence V. Singers and surgery. Part II; Vocal tract surgery. *NATS Bull*. 1982;38(5):20–21.

12. Spiegel JR, Sataloff RT, Hawkshaw MJ. Surgery for the voice. *NATS J*. 1990;46(5):28–30.

13. Riley WD, Korovin GS, Gould WJ. *Directed energy in vocal technique: a preliminary study of clinical application*. Presented at: The Voice Foundation Symposium: Care of the Professional Voice; 1990; Philadelphia, PA.

14. Hirano M. *Clinical Examination of Voice*. New York, NY: Springer-Verlag; 1981.

15. Prater RJ, Swift RW. *Manual of Voice Therapy*. Boston, MA: Little, Brown & Co; 1984.

16. Culver CA. *Musical Acoustics*. New York, NY: Blakiston; 1951.

17. Titze IR. *Principles of Voice Production*. Englewood Cliffs, NJ: Prentice-Hall; 1994.

18. Hollien H, Dew D, Philips P. Phonational frequency range of adults. *J Speech Hear Res*. 1971;14:755–760.

19. Coleman RF. Sources of variation in phonetograms. *J Voice*. 1993;7(1):1–14.

20. Schute HK, Seidner W. Recommendations by the Union of European Phoniatricians (UEP): standardizing voice area measurement/phonetography. *Folia Phoniatr*. 1983;35:286–288.

21. Kent RD. *Reference Manual for Communicative Sciences and Disorders*. Austin, TX: Pro-Ed; 1994.

22. Winholtz WS, Ramig LO. Vocal tremor analysis with the vocal demodulator. *J Speech Hear Res*. 1992;35(3):562–573.

23. Feldenkrais M. *Body and Mature Behavior*. New York, NY: International University; 1949.

24. Alexander FM. *The Use of Self*. London, England: Methuen; 1932.

25. Reed CM, Rabinowitz WM, Durlach NI, et al. Research on the Tadoma method of speech communication. *J Acoust Soc*. 1985;77:247–257.

26. Leanderson R, Sundberg J, von Euler C. Role of diaphragmatic activity during singing: a study of transdiaphragmatic pressures. *J App Physiol*. 1987;62:259–270.

27. Sundberg J. Breathing behavior during singing. *NATS J*. 1993;January/February:49–51.

28. Titze IR, Solomon NP, Luschei ES, et al. Interference between normal vibrato and artificial stimulation of laryngeal muscles at near-vibrato rates. *J Voice*. 1994;8(3):215–223,.

29. Lessac A. *The Use and Training of the Human Voice*. 3rd ed. Mountain View, CA: Mayfield Publishing Co; 1977:122–159.

30. Carroll LM. Interaction of laryngeal and velopharyngeal mechanics: a look at resonance in singers. Presented at: American Speech-Language-Hearing Association Annual Convention; 1999; San Francisco, CA.

31. Skinner E. *Speak with Distinction*. New York, NY: Applause Theatre Book Publishers; 1990.

32. Linklater K. *Freeing the Natural Voice*. New York, NY: Drama Book Publishers; 1976.

33. Rosen DC, Sataloff RT. *Psychology of Voice Disorders*. San Diego, CA: Singular Publishing Group; 1997.

34. Saxon KG, Schneider CM. *Vocal Exercise Physiology*. San Diego, CA: Singular Publishing Group; 1995.

35. Friman G, Ilback NG. Acute infection: metabolic responses, effects on performance, interaction with exercise, and myocarditis. *Int J Sports Med*. 1998;19(suppl 3):S172–S182.

36. Chodzko-Zajko WJ, Ringel RL. Physiological aspects of aging. *J Voice*. 1987;1(1):18–26.

37. Hollien H. "Old voice": what do we really know about them? *J Voice*. 1987;1(1):2–17.

38. Linville SE. The sound of senescence. *J Voice*. 1996;10(2):190–200.

39. Sataloff RT, Titze IR. *Vocal Health and Science: A Compilation of Articles for the NATS Bulletin and the NATS Journal*. Jacksonville, FL: The National Association of Teachers of Singing; 1991.

40. Punt NA. Applied laryngology—singers and actors. *Proc R Soc Med*. 1968;61:1152–1156.

41. Sataloff RT, Sataloff J. *Occupational Hearing Loss*. New York, NY: Marcel Dekker, Inc; 1987.

38

Laryngeal Manipulation

Jacob Lieberman, DO, MA
John S. Rubin, MD, FACS, FRCS
Thomas M. Harris, FRCS
Adrian J. Fourcin, PhD

This chapter, written by an osteopath, two laryngologists, and a speech scientist, is on manipulation of the larynx and the perilaryngeal structures. This is a young science, perhaps still more of an art than a science, but which takes as its predecessors, principles from anatomy, physiology, osteopathy, and physical therapy. We present a synopsis of the role that laryngeal manipulation plays in our clinical practice. Concepts presented in this chapter are fresh and still undergoing change. Many come out of an ongoing collaboration with the Sidcup Voice Unit.

Certain aspects of manipulation, for example, side-to-side movement of the larynx, have been used by physicians as part of the routine clinical examination for well over a century and by performers for centuries. One or two quick side-to-side movements of the larynx to help relax it are part of many performers' routine preparations.

Manipulation of the larynx has been reported on by practitioners as one form of treatment in patients presenting with functional voice disorders,[1-7] and more generally in patients with muscular tension dysphonia (Murray Morrison, Instructional Course, Annual

Meeting of the American Academy of Otolaryngology Head and Neck Surgery, September 1999; Murray Morrison, Laryngology Research meeting, AAOHNS annual meeting, San Antonio, 1998; John Rubin, Laryngology Research meeting, AAOHNS annual meeting, San Antonio, 1998).

Currently, the core team of the voice clinic at Sidcup consists of laryngologist(s), speech and language pathologist(s), an osteopath, and a singing teacher. The osteopath is also a certified child, family, and adolescent psychodynamic psychotherapist; similarly, the speech and language pathologist has taken extra training in counseling. There is also immediate access to a psychiatrist, other singing teachers, and coaches.

The role of the osteopath is to examine the relationship of posture, breathing mechanics, and the function of the larynx to voice production. In the Sidcup clinic the osteopath is frequently called on to assist in the diagnosis, as well as to assist at an early stage in the rehabilitative management (Table 38–1).

In this chapter we discuss laryngeal manipulation from an osteopathic perspective. Anatomy and physiology, indications for manipulation, the osteopathic

Table 38–1. Lieberman's Protocol (Revised)(Reproduced with permission from Lieberman J. Principles and techniques of manual therapy. In: Harris T, Harris S, Rubin JS, Howard DM, eds. *The Voice Clinic Handbook*. Whurr Medical Publishers, London, 1998, appendices 6.1 and 6.2: 132–137.)

Assessment of Posture and Laryngeal Apparatus (Joints and Muscles) in Hyperfunctional Dysphonia

This protocol is a nonexhaustive reference for the assessment of posture and the laryngeal apparatus. It is designed to accompany the instructional course on the detailed anatomy of the larynx, its palpatory assessment, and the assessment of posture-related aspects of voice dysfunction. It can be used in multidisciplinary voice clinics as part of the overall assessment of voice patients to provide a framework for practitioner agreement and research.

1. POSTURE and LARYNGEAL ACTIVITY

1.1 OBSERVATIONS:

Sitting: (while patient is providing history): — (tick as appropriate)

Anterior neck compartment:

Observation	Detail				
Signs of increased muscular activity:	Smooth		Conspicuous Rt	Conspicuous Lt	
Level and position of thyroid lamina	Static (patient is silent)	Normal	High	Low	Deviated
Bulging omohoid muscle activity in speech	Dynamic (talking)		Absent	Present Rt	Present Lt
Skin crease asymmetry			Absent	Present Rt	Present Lt
Head position in the sagittal plane	Tilt		Absent	Present Rt	Present Lt
Head gestures (head nodding in speech/swallowing)			Absent	Present Rt	Present Lt
Jaw movement (vertical and lateral plane)*	Asymmetric		Absent	Present Rt	Present Lt

1.1.2 Standing: (lateral view): — (tick as appropriate)

Observation	Detail			
Weight bearing (sagittal plane, observed from the side):		Normal	Anterior sway	Posterior sway
Spinal curve (exaggerated: hyperhypolordosis):	Lumbar	Normal lordosis	Decreased lordosis	Increased lordosis
	Thoracic	Normal kyphosis	Decreased kyphosis	Increased kyphosis
	Cervical	Normal lordosis	Decreased lordosis	Increased lordosis
Rib cage:	Flexibility	Normal	Decreased	Held
	Function	Normal	Raised	
Breathing patterns:	Diaphragmatic	Normal	Decreased	Paradoxical
	Upper chest	Absent	Present	Increased
	Clavicular	Absent	Present	Increased
Head position (cervical translation):	Anterior	Absent	Present	
	Cervical thoracic hump	Absent	Present	Cervical level

1.1.3 Spinal Curves

Standing: (anterior/posterior view):

Lumbar-thoracic (including scoliosis)	Normal	Asymmetry Rt	Asymmetry Lt
Scapular level	Normal	Raised Rt	Raised Lt
Head level	Normal	Tilt Rt	Tilt Lt

1.1.4 Spinal Curves

Standing: (vertical axis):

NOTE: the normal larynx moves with the torso

Torso rotation	Normal	Clockwise	Counterclockwise
Pelvis rotation	Normal	Clockwise	Counterclockwise
Head rotation	Normal	Clockwise	Counterclockwise

2.1 PALPATION:

(tick as appropriate)

Cervical spinous processes: Palpable	No	Yes	Cervical level
Suboccipital musculature (above C2): Tonus	Normal	Increased Rt	Increased Lt
Symmetry	Normal	Increased Rt	Increased Lt
Tenderness	No	Increased Rt	Increased Lt
Cervical musculature (other): Tonus	Normal	Increased Rt	Increased Lt
Symmetry	Normal	Increased Rt	Increased Lt
Tenderness	No	Increased Rt	Increased Lt
TMJ: Movement	Normal	Asymmetry Rt	Asymmetry Lt
Opening	Normal	Asymmetry Rt	Asymmetry Lt
Tenderness	No	Increased Rt	Increased Lt
Sternocleidomastoid muscle: Tonus	Normal	Increased Rt	Increased Lt
Symmetry	Normal	Increased Rt	Increased Lt
Tenderness	No	Increased Rt	Increased Lt

3.1 The LARYNGEAL APPARATUS:

OBSERVATION:

(tick as appropriate)

Superior suspensory muscles: Tone	Normal	Low	High
Laryngeal range of movement (in speech and swallowing):	Normal	Increased	Decreased
Inferior suspensory muscles: Tone	Normal	Asymmetric Rt	Asymmetric Lt

(continues)

Table 77–1. (continued)

4.1 The LARYNGEAL APPARATUS: PALPATION (tick as appropriate)

Palpate for position, tone, symmetry, tenderness both in static (passive) and dynamic (swallowing, speech singing):

Hyoid:				
Geniohyoid: static	Tone	Normal	High	Low
	Tenderness:	None		Present
Geniohyoid: dynamic		Normal	Asymmetric	
Superior suspensory muscles: static	Tone	Normal	Asymmetric Rt	Asymmetric Lt
	Tenderness:	None	Rt	Lt
Superior suspensory muscles: dynamic	Tone	Normal	Asymmetric Rt	Asymmetric Lt
Inferior suspensory muscles: static	Tone	Normal	Asymmetric Rt	Asymmetric Lt
	Tenderness:	None	Rt	Lt
Inferior suspensory muscles: dynamic		Normal	Asymmetric Rt	Asymmetric Lt
Thyrohyoid apparatus: static	Coronal: attitude hyoid to thyroid	Parallel	Tilt Lt	Tilt Rt
	Size of gap:	None	Diminished Rt	Diminished Lt
	Tenderness:	None	Rt	Lt
	Symmetry:	Normal	Asymmetric Rt	Asymmetric Lt
Thyrohyoid apparatus: dynamic (movement)		Normal	Rotation Rt	Rotation Lt
Cricothyroid muscles: static	Tone	Normal	Asymmetric Rt	Asymmetric Lt
	Tenderness:	None	Rt	Lt
Cricothyroid visor (joint)(head neutral): static	Resting state:	Closed	Mid position open	Open
	Anterior arch:	None	Present	
Cricothyroid joint: dynamic	Changes with siren:	No change	Closes	
	Changes with yawn:	No change	Opens	
	Posterior glide of arch with pitch rise:	No change	Diminishes	
Constrictor muscles: (perform lateral shift test):	Mobility:	Absent	Present Rt	Present Lt
	Tenderness:	None	Asymmetric Rt	Asymmetric Lt
	Accessible:	No	Rt	Lt
Internal laryngeal structures (for experienced therapists only):	Tenderness:	None	Rt	Lt
	Movement:	None	Rt	Lt

OSTEOPATHIC ASSESSMENT

The osteopathic assessment (see Table 38–1) begins with visual observation and then proceeds to palpation. Palpation is performed to assess the resting muscle tone, contracted muscle tone, resting joint position, range of motion, and ease of mobility.

If failure to relax a muscle following activity leads to hyperfunctional muscular behavior, and voice and swallow require repetitive, complex muscular activity, then it is hardly surprising that both the laryngeal and perilaryngeal musculature are at risk for hyperfunctional patterns. These patterns are identifiable by tight, tender, and contracted muscles. This results in loss of full joint range of movement and loss of movement pattern. It is experienced as stiffness.[43]

It should be recalled that, although the patient presents with a hoarse voice, the osteopath is interested in far more than the larynx; he or she needs to evaluate the entire vocal tract. Specifically, he or she will need to assess (1) general posture; (2) head position; (3) integrity of the deep and more superficial muscles of the neck; (4) integrity of the muscles, joints, and ligaments supporting breathing; (5) integrity of the muscles, joints, and ligaments of the pharynx and larynx; (6) position of the laryngeal cartilages and hyoid bone.

General Posture

The general posture of an individual plays a significant role in the development or perpetuation of voice problems. As noted above, there is a steady state between the extensors and the flexors of the body. In our society this balance is frequently abrogated. There is often peer pressure leading children to assume a "slumped" position. Adults spend much of their working day and evening seated in front of computer screens or televisions, often in unhealthy postural positions. Unfortunately, the media has paid much attention to bulging abdominal muscles (the "six pack" appearance) in individuals with flat stomachs. This has led to an emphasis in adults' sports time, on exercises designed to pull the lower rib cage down toward the pelvis. Thus, even during exercise, some adults tend to develop muscles that promote abnormal postural patterns.

These postural patterns lead to a cascade of compensatory postural changes with a resultant hyperlordotic neck. This in turn places the suprahyoid suspensory muscles at significant risk for the development of chronic spasm, and can lead to inefficient muscular patterns of voicing.

There are many other causes of general postural problems relating to spinal curvatures and asymmetries, injuries, or congenital problems affecting the pelvis, hips, legs, and feet, all of which can ultimately affect voice production.

Head Position

Head position has a direct effect on voice production. The adult head weighs 14 to 16 pounds. Position of the head can affect the resting length of the suspensory muscles. Hyperlordosis has already been discussed above. Head tilt or anterior-posterior displacement can affect voice. Examples of individuals with head tilt might include: teachers who work from a piano, with their students always singing from the same side of the piano; many instrumentalists (for example, some woodwind players, guitarists, violinists), and so forth.

Integrity of the Deep Muscles of the Neck

These muscles have been reviewed above briefly. All are involved in head, neck, or upper spine positioning or stability. Abnormalities in any of these muscles ultimately can lead to voice problems.

Integrity of the Muscles, Joints, and Ligaments Supporting Breathing

The mechanisms inherent to the "bellows" are crucial to voice production.[44] Limitation of motion, caused by injury, inflammation, infection, aging, and so forth, can decrease efficiency of these mechanisms. Examples might include: limitation of rib cage movement, for example, as caused by ankylosing spondylitis; reduction of efficiency of the muscles and ligaments supporting expiration, for example, stretching of the rectus abdominis muscles during pregnancy. Of note, at times the emotional state of the patient may also influence abdominal support or pattern of breathing.

Integrity of the Muscles, Joints, and Ligaments of the Pharynx and Larynx

These have been reviewed in some depth above. Palpation of these structures gives the osteopath insights into the voicing mechanism at the level of the sound source. Examples might include: (1) increased tension, tenderness, or guarding in the suspensory musculature; (2) a held cricothyroid visor with decreased range of motion of the cricothyroid joint, both changes often being found in prolonged voice misuse patterns.[22]

Much emphasis recently has been placed on the Morrison muscular tension dysphonia patterns, type 1 through 4[45,46]; however, they primarily have been identified by the patterns of visualized vocal fold closure. Harris has attempted to go one step further and characterize the specific muscular misuse patterns that have led to the observed vocal fold closure patterns.[47]

The relative size of the thyrohyoid space (and the thyrohyoid muscles) should be assessed. Lieberman notes that in individuals with hyperfunctional voicing disorders, the space is much reduced in surface area.[22]

Position and Mobility of the Laryngeal Cartilages and Hyoid Bone

1. Thyroid cartilage position. This can be observed readily as well as palpated. Deviation of the thyroid cartilage from center is frequently accompanied by major underlying postural changes. Examples might include rotation of the torso to one side, scoliosis, abnormal unilateral hypertrophy of the superficial muscles of the neck (for example, unilateral torticollis), surgery (for example, following a unilateral radical neck dissection), unilateral hyperostosis of the cervical spine, and so forth.

2. Limitation of movement of the thyroid cartilage on side-to-side movement (rotation). This finding may be associated with aging, hyperostosis of the cervical spine, or a tumor of the larynx or neck. In young, otherwise healthy performers, the most common cause of this limitation of movement, however, is increased resting muscular tone in the "strap" muscles. This is generally indicative of a musculoskeletal pattern associated with increased "holding" or "guarding" of these muscles. It is often associated with voice changes, including lowering of the fundamental frequency of the speaking voice and a gravelly quality to the voice. This muscular pattern is readily amenable to laryngeal manipulation.

3. Hyoid position. The hyoid bone is the principal structure below which the remainder of the larynx is suspended. It should lie in a horizontal plane, and be located just below the mandible. Typically it lies approximately 1/2 inch caudal to the body of the mandible. Angulation of either side toward the mandible suggests unilateral tight posterior hyoglossus or stylohyoid muscles or anterior thyrohyoid ligaments.[22] Such angulation may also be associated with inflammatory lymphadenopathy in zone two (the jugulodigastric region) of the neck (J. Rubin, personal observation, 2002). Lateral tilting of the hyoid bone may be associated with unilateral tightness of the superior suspensory muscles or to the unilateral pull of a tight thyrohyoid muscle. When the hyoid bone appears to be pulled forward anteriorly, a tight geniohyoid muscle should be suspected.[22] The reverse may occur should the middle constrictor muscle be hypertonic (J. Lieberman, personal observation, 2002).

In patients with a "held" larynx, or a posteriorly backed larynx, consideration should be given to the possibility of unresolved emotional issues. Aronson has noted that one common denominator of psychogenic voice disorders is a hypercontractile state of the intrinsic and extrinsic laryngeal musculature.[6] These considerations are very important to successful long-term intervention, but are outside the scope of this chapter (see chapter 33, Psychologic Aspects of Voice Disorders, for further insights).

The superior suspensory muscles consist of the stylohyoid, geniohyoid, hyoglossus, mylohyoid, and anterior and posterior bellies of the digastric muscles. As noted, excessively tight suprahyoid musculature in association with a high-held larynx signifies marked muscular hyperactivity often in association with unresolved emotional issues.[22] One example of such a clinical scenario is that not uncommonly found in mutational dysphonias.

The inferior suspensory muscles should be palpated. These include the sternothyroid, sternohyoid, and omohyoid muscles. These muscles are long, with thin bellies and are thus difficult to assess by direct palpation. Their quality can be inferred by assessing the resting level of the larynx and by stretching it upward and laterally (see below). An extremely low-held, or "anchored" larynx should be checked for. Koufman has classified one type of speaking-voice abuse pattern as the "Bogart-Bacall" syndrome, in which the patient speaks with a very low-pitched fundamental frequency. This is associated with a low-held larynx.[48,49]

ENDOLARYNGEAL EXAMINATION

Prior to laryngeal manipulation by an osteopath, the larynx should be examined by an otolaryngologist with a flexible or rigid endoscope, preferably with an attached stroboscope, and the results relayed to the osteopath. Particular attention should be paid to the characteristic appearance of any known patterns of dysphonia. Typically these include muscular tension dysphonia, as described by authors such as Morrison, Koufman, or Harris,[44-46,48] or bowing. There may also be evidence of asymmetry of vocal fold movement or of arytenoid position (see below).

The otolaryngologic examination should include evaluation for evidence of extraesophageal reflux (posterior interarytenoid "heaping," piriform pooling, posterior laryngeal edema or redness, and so forth), and for subtle laryngeal mucosal pathology that may be the source of the abnormal muscular behavior. The stroboscope will be of critical importance here, as subtle asynchrony of the mucosal wave, areas of adynamism, and so forth may lead the examiner to infer the possibility of such pathologies as a partially resolved vocal fold palsy, a small cyst, sulcus, or scar, all of which could be the source of the muscular dyskinesia.

The arytenoid cartilages and the cricoarytenoid joints are accessible to palpation by the osteopathic practitioner with adequate experience, particularly in long, thin-necked individuals. Similarly, the posterior cricoarytenoid muscles and interarytenoid muscles can be palpated and compared for tenderness and hypertonicity. These maneuvers require considerable skill and can be very uncomfortable to the patient, however. Thus, they should be considered to be outside the scope of this chapter. It is worth noting that the patient's response to such an examination can assist in the diagnosis, one example being the irritable larynx (Murray Morrison, Instructional Course, Annual Meeting of the American Academy of Otolaryngology Head and Neck Surgery, September 1999).

BASIC LARYNGEAL MANIPULATION

Generally speaking, common sense needs to be used when considering performance of laryngeal manipulation. For example, laryngeal manipulation is not advisable in patients with laryngeal or thyroid malignancies, or in instances of Graves' disease. In the presence of other anterior neck pathologies, the techniques should be modified appropriately to avoid unnecessary discomfort. Prior to manipulation, a thorough explanation of the proposed procedure, its risks and benefits, should be given to the patient, and his or her permission sought.

Particular care must be exercised when working in the area overlying the carotid artery and especially around the carotid body and sinus.

Prior to any manipulation, the osteopath gently palpates for any deviation from "normal" anatomic structures, for example, an unusually enlarged or prominent carotid sinus in relation to the hyoid bone and its attachments. Imaging has not been found to be necessary, as direct hands-on palpation is very sensitive to such abnormalities. While laryngeal manipulation proves to be a highly safe treatment in experienced hands, we teach that energetic or inadvertent manipulation should not be performed near the carotid; it can lead to rapid changes in blood pressure and/or pulse rate; it can also lead to loosening of atheromatous plaques in elderly patients.

Similarly, care should be exercised in instances of previous laryngeal trauma, surgery, or radiation where normal anatomy may be altered.

General

In cases of soft tissue damage caused by repetitive strain injury, similar to certain orthopedic problems, the muscles will be chronically shortened, fibrotic or scarred, and tender to touch. By working on the muscles, the osteopath is able to stretch scar contractures, lengthen the muscle belly, increase blood flow, and improve lymphatic drainage. The osteopath probably also affects the neuromuscular pattern of outflow locally and centrally, although this requires further clarification through research.[22]

Limitation of joint movement can also be addressed by direct joint manipulation, as well as by soft tissue techniques to surrounding musculature. In addition to reducing muscle spasm, the practitioner also attempts to alter head position, reduce hyperlordotic spinal curve, and improve mobility in the thoracic spine.

Treatment aims include restoration of joint mobility and muscle function. Perhaps as important is bringing to the conscious level the unconscious and habitual abnormal postural patterns that need to be corrected.[43]

General concepts of manipulation to attain these goals include those of:

1. Identification of the indicated muscle or structure to work on.
2. Stabilization of indicated muscle against a known, more fixed structure (for example, the cricoid cartilage).
3. Passive stretch where two structures (for example, hyoid bone and mandible) are held apart under gentle stretch for a period of time.
4. Dynamic stretch (the patient activates a muscle that the osteopath wishes to manipulate, and the osteopath works with or against the patient's own force).
5. Muscle kneading.
6. Working beyond guarding (the osteopath maintains stretch beyond the point at which the patient holds back).

BASIC MANIPULATION: GENERAL TECHNIQUE

Much of basic manipulation involves general soft tissue work on the posterior neck, shoulders, and upper back. The patient is treated while lying supine on a firm table or gurney with a movable head support.

First the cervical and upper thoracic spinous processes are carefully assessed for evidence of abnormal alignment, tenderness, and integrity or laxity of interspinous ligaments. The cervical and upper thoracic spine is gently investigated for range of motion. This will give the osteopath information as to what can be safely accomplished.

The posterior extensor muscles are then palpated and gently placed under stretch, during which time the osteopath checks for focal or point tenderness or guarding. Focal areas of spasm are identified and stretched to relax the hypertonic muscle, increase blood flow, and break the spasm.[22]

Not uncommonly the superficial neck muscles are addressed next. The levator scapulae and splenius are frequent sources of neck pain and often require specific work. The trapezius is another muscle frequently found to be tight or in spasm. Often certain fibers of the trapezius may be found to be contracted and others stretched, given the size of this muscle and its broad insertions.

Frequently the anterior neck, larynx, and laryngeal and pharyngeal muscles are next addressed. Areas particularly relevant to voice problems include: suprahyoid suspensory muscles, cricothyroid visor, scalenes, sternocleidomastoids, and lower strap muscles.

Suprahyoid Suspensory Muscles

As previously noted these muscles are at particular risk for chronic shortening, thereby causing the laryngeal complex to be elevated and effecting a change in resonatory pattern.

These are large powerful muscles and can be addressed individually. When using soft tissue techniques it is best to stabilize the hand against the mandible or the hyoid bone and work from this solid base.

The patient can actively assist by attempting to initiate a swallow (but not a full swallow) while the osteopath gently presses down against the hyoid. This type of combined patient/practitioner activity is termed "dynamic stretch."

Cricothyroid Visor

This "keystone" area has been anatomically characterized above. The osteopath can relax both cricothyroid muscles individually, applying soft tissue stretch techniques, working against the cricoid cartilage as his solid base. He can also work directly on each cricothyroid joint. Dynamic stretch, in this instance would involve the patient "sirening" the pitch up from low to high, thereby actively placing the cricothyroid muscle into contraction, while the osteopath stretches this muscle.

Scalenes, Sternocleidomastoids, and Lower Strap Muscles

The larynx frequently is found to be held in an abnormally low position, a typical correlate being tightly held and tender lower bellies of the SCM, scalenes, and lower strap muscles.

This is a common problem noted in 26% of Koufman's patients with "functional" voice problems,[49] but must be differentiated from a chronically high-held rib cage (as seen in some patients with severe emphysema).

These muscles can be stretched against the solid base of the upper sternum and medial clavicles, and are readily accessible to manipulation.

SUCCESSFUL OUTCOME AFTER LARNGEAL MANIPULATION

In our clinical experience, albeit anecdotal, the following are comments frequently made by patients immediately following laryngeal manipulation: immediate change in pitch, audible to patient and practitioner; increased resonance; increased ease of swallowing associated with a sense of "openness"; decreased hoarseness; decreased "wobble"; decreased pain and discomfort.

In the longer term, it is not uncommon for there to be reported an increase in stamina, vocal flexibility, and range, better negotiation of the passaggio, and shorter duration of recovery time following laryngeal exertions. Research to confirm these anecdotal impressions is needed, as discussed below.

There is often resolution of the laryngeal "click" (that is caused by anterior movement of the hyoid bone over the thyroid cartilage and is frequently associated with chronically shortened and tightly held thyrohyoid muscles) and a decreased need to clear the throat. Finally, JL finds in many of his patients acknowledgment of underlying emotional issues related to the laryngeal pathology (Jacob Lieberman, unpublished data, 1999).

Because of the relaxed laryngeal musculature and the small alteration in laryngeal position, professional voice users occasionally experience what they call a "wild voice," momentarily. Warming-up type exercises are required to allow the performer to get used to the changes.

In the pilot study assessing the efficiency of manipulation versus conventional speech therapy, the two modalities were found to be dissimilar but complementary.[7] Manipulation was found to excel at rapidly reducing tension in muscles that were tightly held in the "unaware" patient. With manipulation, early vocal fatigue was found to be reduced as was laryngeal discomfort. While conventional speech therapy was found to address these problems as well, the progress was slower. Speech therapy, however, was found to be better at substituting more efficient voicing patterns over the pretreatment dysphonic patterns.

ADVANCED MANIPULATION

Advanced manipulation is designed for instances in which the laryngeal intrinsic muscles require direct address. This might include times when the laryngeal "set" needs to be altered. For example, Lieberman has directly manipulated the intrinsic muscles of certain patients with granulomas who have failed traditional therapy, the aim being to reduce the hard prephonatory gesture and resultant impact of the arytenoid cartilages. In Lieberman's practice, advanced manipulation is not uncommonly combined with elements of psychotherapy that focus on unresolved emotional issues.

It must be remembered that manipulation of the intrinsic muscles of the larynx involves working on the posterior aspect of the larynx on muscles that are designed for mainly reflexogenic activities. Such manipulation requires considerable palpatory skill, as well as great sensitivity in working with patients.

ONGOING RESEARCH

Laryngeal manipulation has been developed, and practiced in Queen Mary's Hospital Sidcup, Kent, for the last 14 years. Initially the team looked at the relationship of head position, shoulder girdle, and hyperfunctional voice disorders.[7]

The clinic has developed a research protocol with Professor A. Fourcin using the laryngograph to record vocal parameters prior to and immediately following manipulation, in an attempt to validate the anecdotal findings described above. Preliminary laryngographic data have often confirmed clinical findings, including: immediate change in fundamental frequency of the speaking voice, better control, and wider vocal range. As an example, a patient with spasmodic dysphonia treated with manipulation is presented (Fig 38–1). The project is ongoing.

Other research projects in planning involve assessing cricothyroid joint activity, diaphragmatic breathing, and the function of the thyrohyoid mechanism.

CONCLUSION

We have presented a synopsis of the role that laryngeal manipulation plays in our practice. Certainly in our voice clinics, the more we have considered the possibility of musculoskeletal issues in patients with voice disorders, the more reasons we have found for referring such patients for diagnostic investigation and treatment by a physical therapist, osteopath, or by practitioners with similar skills. The critical issue is for the therapist to participate actively in the voice clinic so that he or she will develop sensitivity to the needs of the patient.

That said, muscles do not work in isolation. The musculoskeletal system is driven by thoughts and affects. The effects of physical therapy, passive and active manipulation in particular, are immediate and frequently effective in (at least temporarily) breaking through unconscious neuromuscular pathways (habits). To be long lasting, the "new" musculoskeletal behavior must be internalized by the patient. Many or most of our patients require refresher sessions to reinforce the beneficial behavior patterns.

Manipulation is a potent treatment modality, but it does not resolve underlying emotional conflicts. Hence, a small proportion of our patients will benefit from a short course of supportive counseling, or from more formal psychotherapy.

REFERENCES

1. Mathieson L. Vocal tract discomfort in hyperfunctional dysphonia. *Voice.* 1993;2:40–48.
2. Mathieson L. *Greene and Mathieson's The Voice and Its Disorders.* 6th ed. London, England: Whurr Publishers Limited; 2001.
3. Roy N, Leeper HA. Effects of the manual laryngeal musculoskeletal tension reduction technique as a treatment for functional voice disorders: perceptual and acoustic measures. *J Voice.* 1993;7:242–249.
4. Roy N, Bless DM, Heisey D, Ford CN. Manual circumlaryngeal therapy for functional dysphonia: an evaluation of short- and long-term treatment outcomes. *J Voice.* 1997;11:321–331.
5. Aronson AE. *Clinical Voice Disorders: An Interdisciplinary Approach.* 2nd ed. New York, NY: Georg Thieme Verlag; 1985.
6. Aronson A. *Clinical Voice Disorders.* 3rd ed. New York, NY: Thieme Medical Publishers; 1991:117–145.
7. Harris S, Harris T, Lieberman J, Harris D. The multidisciplinary voice clinic. In: Freeman M, Fawcus M, eds. *Voice Disorders and Their Management.* London, England: Whurr Publishers; 2000:313–332.
8. Harris T, Laryngeal mechanisms in normal function and dysfunction. In: Harris T, Harris S, Rubin JS, Howard DM, eds. *The Voice Clinic Handbook.* London, England: Whurr Publishers; 1998:64–90.
9. Rubin JS. The structural anatomy of the larynx and supraglottic vocal tract: a review. In: Harris T, Harris S, Rubin JS, Howard DM, eds. *The Voice Clinic Handbook.* London, England: Whurr Publishers; 1998:15–33.

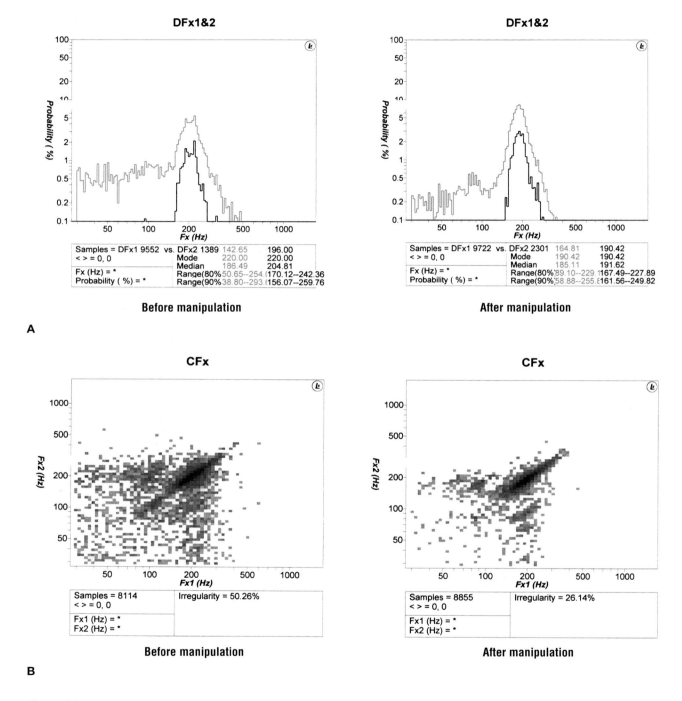

Figure 38–1. A. Laryngographic data taken from a patient with spasmodic dysphonia before and after one treatment with laryngeal manipulation. (Courtesy of Professor Adrian Fourcin). Plots show range, before and after one manipulation. Range as defined herein refers to the range of frequencies contained within the speaking voice, while reading from a standard text. Note the reduction in spread of the first order distribution *(in red)*, and the slight improvement in range definition shown by the second order distribution *(in black)*, both following manipulation. **B.** Plots shows regularity, before and after one manipulation. Regularity as defined herein refers to the extent to which successive vocal fold periods are comparable, while reading from a standard text. Note the reduction in irregularity in the postmanipulation distribution. *(continues)*

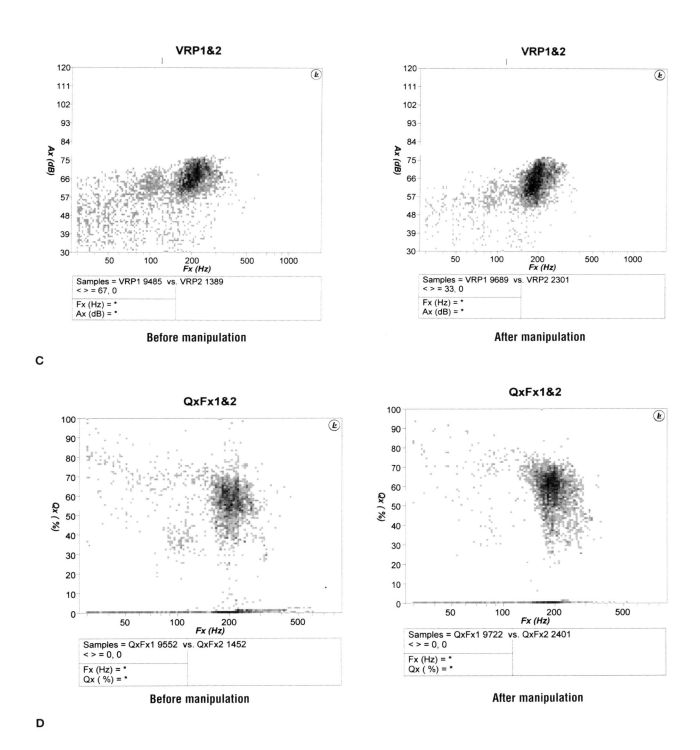

Figure 38–1. *(continued)* **C.** Plots show a phonetogram before and after one manipulation. The phonetogram as defined herein refers to the distribution of loudness against pitch, while reading from a standard text. Note that the postmanipulation plot demonstrates a more compact control of loudness (less dispersion) **D.** Plots show "quality" before and after one manipulation. "Quality" as defined herein refers to the extent to which the closed phase percentage of the total period is well defined in the speaking voice, while reading from a standard text. Note that there is a (somewhat) better definition of the closed phase in the postmanipulation plot.

10. Laitman JT, Noden DM, Van de Water TR. Formation of the larynx: from homeobox genes to critical periods. In: Rubin JS, Sataloff RT, Korovin GS, Gould WJ, eds. *Diagnosis and Treatment of Voice Disorders*. New York, NY: Igaku-Shoin Medical Publishers; 1995:9–23.

11. Scherer RC. Laryngeal function during phonation. In: Rubin JS, Sataloff RT, Korovin G, Gould WJ, eds. *Diagnosis and Treatment of Voice Disorders*. New York, NY: Igaku-Shoin Publishers; 1995:86–104.

12. Hast MH. Mechanical properties of the cricothyroid muscle. *Laryngoscope*. 1966;76:537–548.

13. Cooper DS, Partridge LD, Alipour-Haghighi F. Muscle energetics, vocal efficiency, and laryngeal biomechanics. In: Titze IR, ed. *Vocal Fold Physiology: Frontiers in Basic Science*. San Diego, CA: Singular Publishing Group; 1993:37–92.

14. Harris T, Lieberman J. The cricothyroid mechanism, its relationship to vocal fatigue and vocal dysfunction. *Voice*. 1993;2:89–96.

15. Rubin JS, Sataloff RT. Voice: new horizons. In: Sataloff RT, ed. *Professional Voice: The Science and Art of Clinical Care*. 2nd ed. San Diego, CA: Singular Publishing Group; 1997.

16. Fisher K. Early experience of a multidisciplinary pain management programme. *Hol Med*. 1988;3:47–56.

17. Robinson L, Fisher H, Knox J, Thomson G. *The Official Body Control Pilates Manual*. London, England: Macmillan Publishers; 2000.

18. Feldenkrais M. *Awareness Through Movement*. New York, NY: Harper & Row; 1972.

19. Rolf IP. *Rolfing: Reestablishing the Natural Alignment and Structural Integration of the Human Body for Vitality and Well-Being*. Rochester, VT: Healing Arts Press; 1989.

20. Dickson D, Dickson W. Functional anatomy of the human larynx. *Proc Penn Acad Ophthalmol*. 1971;29.

21. Boileau Grant JC. *Grant's Atlas of Anatomy*. 6th ed. Baltimore, MD: Williams & Wilkins; 1972.

22. Lieberman J. Principles and techniques of manual therapy: application in the management of dysphonia. In: Harris T, Harris S, Rubin JS, Howard DM, eds. *The Voice Clinical Handbook*. London, England: Whurr Publishers; 1998:91–138.

23. Dickson DR, Maue-Dickson W. *Anatomical and Physiological Basis of Speech*. Boston, MA: Little, Brown & Co; 1982.

24. Letson JA Jr, Tatchell R. Arytenoid movement. In: Sataloff RT, 2nd ed. *Professional Voice: The Science and Art of Clinical Care*. San Diego, CA: Singular Publishing Group; 1997:131–145.

25. Baken RJ, Isshiki N. Arytenoid displacement by simulated intrinsic muscle contraction. *Folia Phoniatr*. 1977; 29:206–216.

26. von Leden H. The mechanics of the cricoarytenoid joint. *Arch Otolaryngol*. 1961;73:63–72.

27. Arnold GE. Physiology and pathology of the cricothyroid muscle. *Laryngoscope*. 1961;71:687–753.

28. Choi HS, Berke GS, Ye M, Kreiman J. Function of the thyroarytenoid muscle in a canine laryngeal model. *Ann Otol Rhinol Laryngol*. 1993;102:769–776.

29. Fujimura O. Body-cover theory of the vocal fold and its phonetic implications. In: Stevens KN, Hirano M, eds. *Vocal Fold Physiology*. Tokyo, Japan: University of Tokyo Press; 1981:271–288.

30. Titze IR, Jiang J, Drucker DG. Preliminaries to the body-cover theory of pitch control. *J Voice*. 1988;1(4):314–319.

31. Vilkman E, Alku P, Laukkanen A. Vocal-fold collision mass as a differentiator between registers in the low-pitch range. *J Voice*. 1995;9:66–73.

32. Alipour-Haghighi F, Perlman Al, Titze IR. Tetanic response of the cricothyroid muscle. *Ann Otol Rhinol Laryngol*. 1991;100:626–631.

33. Alipour-Haghighi F, Titze IR, Perlman AL. Tetanic contraction in vocal fold muscle. *J Speech Hear Res*. 1989;32: 226–231.

34. Titze IR, Durham PL. Passive mechanisms influencing fundamental frequency control. In: Baer T, Sasaki C, Harris KS, eds. *Laryngeal Function in Phonation and Respiration*. San Diego, CA: College-Hill Press; 1987:304–319.

35. Broniatowski M, Sonies BC, Rubin JS, et al. Current evaluation and treatment of patients with swallowing disorders. *Otolaryngol Head Neck Surg*. 1999;120:464–473.

36. Hellemans J, Agg HO, Pelemans W, et al. Pharyngoesophageal swallowing disorders and the pharyngoesophageal sphincter. *Med Clin North Am*. 1981;65:1149–1171.

37. Estill J. *Voicecraft: A User's Guide to Voice Quality. Vol 2, Some Basic Voice Qualities*. Santa Rosa, CA: Estill Voice Training Systems; 1995.

38. Angsuwarangsee T, Morrison-Murray M. Extrinsic laryngeal muscular tension in patients with voice disorders. *J Voice*. 2002;16(3):333–343.

39. Rubin JS. The physiologic anatomy of swallowing. In: Rubin JS, Broniatowski M, Kelly J, eds. *The Swallowing Handbook*. San Diego, CA: Singular Publishing Group; 2000:1–20.

40. Sonninen A. The role of the external laryngeal muscles in the length-adjustment of the vocal cords in singing. *Acta Otolaryngol*. 1956;118:218–231.

41. Vilkman E, Sonninen A, Hurme P, Korkko P. External laryngeal frame function in voice production revisited: a review. *J Voice*. 1996;10:78–92.

42. Lumley JSP, Craven JL, Aitken JT. *Essential Anatomy*. Edinburgh, Scotland: Churchill Livingstone; 1973.

43. Rubin JS, Lieberman J, Harris TM. Laryngeal manipulation. *Otolaryngol Clin North Am*. 2000;33:1017–1034.

44. Rubin JS. Mechanisms of respiration (the bellows). In: Harris T, Harris S, Rubin JS, Howard DM, eds. *The Voice Clinic Handbook*. London, England: Whurr Publishers; 1998:49–63.

45. Morrison MD, Rammage LA, Gilles M, et al. Muscular tension dysphonia. *J Otolaryngol*. 1983;12:302–306.

46. Morrison M, Rammage L, Nichol H, et al. *The Management of Voice Disorders*. San Diego, CA: Singular Publishing Group; 1994.

47. Harris S. Speech therapy for dysphonia. In: Harris T, Harris S, Rubin JS, Howard DM, eds. *The Voice Clinic Handbook*. London, England: Whurr Publishers; 1998: 186–195.

48. Gould WJ, Rubin JS. Special considerations for the professional voice user. In: Rubin JS, Sataloff RT, Korovin G, Gould WJ, eds. *Diagnosis and Treatment of Voice Disorders*. New York, NY: Igako-Shoin Press; 1995:424–435.

49. Koufman J, Blalock O. Functional voice disorders. *Otolaryngol Clin North Am*. 1991;24:1059–1073.

39

The Effects of Posture on Voice

John S. Rubin, MD, FACS, FRCS
Ed Blake, MSc (Phty), MCST, SRP
Lesley Mathieson, DipCST, FRCSLT

This chapter looks at the potential adverse effects of abnormal posture on the vocal tract. Although it has been known for centuries that poor posture can have an adverse effect on voicing, there has been relatively little research into the subject. Recently, however, the importance of posture to well-being has become popularized through the works of authors such as Alexander,[1] Pilates,[2] Feldenkrais,[3] and others. Physiotherapy and osteopathy have become integral to the field of Sports Medicine and to rehabilitation of musculoskeletal injuries. Only very recently has consideration of these sciences been applied to voice research and rehabilitation.

Posture could, in one sense, be considered to be a constant battleground between the deep extensor and flexor groups of muscles. The long bones and pelvis, the skull, and the spine are the obvious targets and (in many cases) the origins and/or insertions of these muscle groups.

The larynx is suspended from the basicranium, not by direct bony attachment, but by a series of muscles and ligaments. It could be viewed as a victim in this struggle, in part due to its location in the anterior neck, in part to its dense muscular attachments to the pre-vertebral fascia, and in part due to its attachments to the basicranium above and the trachea below.

Rolf has described the ideal state of posture (what she calls "equipoise") in which the individual stands upright.[4] The head is held vertically over the perpendicularly oriented shoulder girdle, vertically over the hip joints and the pelvis, and vertically over the forward-facing feet. A plumb line through the coronal plane formed by the ears would pass directly over the plane of the shoulders and hip joints. The eye plane is horizontal, the rib cage is neutral. The spine "rests in the pelvis much as a person sits in a rocking chair."[4(p175)] It has four curves. The sacral and thoracic are concave ventrally, the lumbar and cervical are convex.

POSTERIOR EXTENSORS

In a free erect spine, the extensor system of the back (the "erector spinae" muscles) supply support and span the vertebrae (Figure 39–1). The erector spinae consist of three groups of superficial vertical fibers, which interweave, and numerous deeper oblique fibers.[5] The ac-

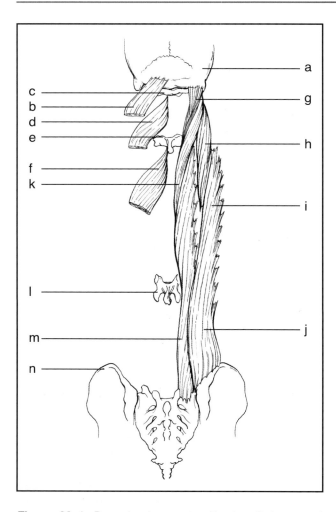

Figure 39–1. Deep back muscles Erector, Spinae, and Transversus Spinalis (**a.** Occiput, **b.** Semispinalis capitis, **c.** Atlas, **d.** Semispinals cervicis, **e.** C7, **f.** Semispinalis thoracis, **g.** Longissimus capitis, **h.** Iliocostalis cervicis, **i.** Iliocostalis thoracis, **j.** Iliocostalis luborum, **k.** Longissimus cervicis, **l.** T12, **m.** Longissimus thoracis, **n.** Pelvis).

tion of the erector spinae is to establish and maintain appropriate extension of the vertebral column. It contains three superficial muscles, the iliocostalis, longissimus, and spinalis. The iliocostalis is placed laterally. It extends from the iliac crest and angles of the ribs and inserts into the transverse processes of the cervical vertebrae. It has a lumbar, thoracic, and cervical portion.

The longissimus is intermediate in position, attached inferiorly to the transverse processes of the thoracic and cervical vertebrae. Its uppermost fibers, the longissimus capitis, reach the lateral surface of the mastoid bone. The medially placed spinalis passes alongside and is attached to the vertical spines.

Deeper muscles include the semispinalis and the deep short muscles (the levator costae, multifidis, rotatores, interspinus, and intertransversus muscles). Of the

several parts of the semispinalis that run from the lower (tenth) thoracic vertebrae, upwards and medially to the occiput, the massive semispinalis capitis, supporting the head, is almost vertical. It is attached to the occiput between the superior and the inferior nuchal lines.

The multifidis, arising from the dorsal sacrum, runs from the transverse processes and inserts into the lower border of the third cervical vertebra. It also has some role in neck extension.

The splenius capitis and cervicis also support the spine. The splenius will be discussed again later as a superficial anterior muscle, because of its lateral location and action. The splenius capitis attaches inferiorly to the ligamentum nuchae and spinous processes of the upper three or four thoracic vertebrae and the seventh cervical vertebra. Superiorly, it attaches to the mastoid process and lateral part of the superior nuchal line deep to the sternocleidomastoid. The splenius cervicis has a similar inferior attachment but passes to the transverse processes of the upper cervical vertebrae.

The major action of the erector spinae is to maintain the upright position of the body. When standing at rest, the center of gravity lies just in front of the second sacral vertebrae. Body movement, however, frequently carries the center of gravity forward. This mass of muscle is then required to restore the upright position.

The muscles attached to the skull produce extension, lateral flexion, and rotation of the head.[5]

SUBOCCIPITAL MUSCLE GROUP

The suboccipital muscles (Figure 39–2). are important because they permit accurate head positioning and thus stereoscopic vision. They extend the skull at the atlanto-occipital joints and rotate it at the atlanto-axial joints. Muscles in this group include the rectus capitis posterior (RCP) major and minor and the obliquus capitis (OC) superior and inferior. The RCP major arises from the spine of the axis and inserts into the occiput below the inferior nuchal line. The RCP minor is anteromedial to the RCP major and passes from the posterior tubercle of the atlas to insert into the occiput behind the foramen magnum. The OC superior arises at the tip of the transverse process of the atlas and inserts into the occiput between the superior and inferior nuchal lines, lateral to the semispinalis. The OC inferior originates at the tip of the transverse process of the atlas and inserts into the spine of the axis.[5]

DEEP ANTERIOR NECK FLEXORS

The three scalenes together with the prevertebral muscles make up the deep muscles of the anterior neck.

Muscular Imbalance and Voice

Upper and middle cervical extension results in a positional change of the styloid process of the mastoid, moving it anteriorly. This, we believe (E Blake, personal observation, 2003), allows for adaptive shortening of the stylohyoid muscle, as its origin and insertion have moved closer together as a consequence of head position. The stylohyoid muscle functions with improved force output in this position. It therefore elevates the larynx into a position that changes the shape of the vocal tract, altering resonance and pitch.

A muscular imbalance similar to that described earlier can now occur between the stylohyoid and sternohyoid muscles. The adaptive shortening that will occur in the stylohyoid will resist the forward translation of the hyoid bone and thyroid cartilage during singing. In turn, this may alter vocal fold length and tension (E Blake, personal observation, 2001). Consequently, there is potential loss of the singer's top range, in addition to the presence of breathy phonation. This is still postulation but fits with the clinical patterns seen in many of our patients.

Lieberman et al believe further that shortening (chronic contraction) of the cricothyroid muscle may occur.[10] This could be postulated to occur in response to the above-described laryngeal elevation or even to the forward translation of the larynx in relation to the hyperlordotic cervical spine. In this clinical scenario, the anterior cricoid ring often is positioned in a plane anterior to the inferior thyroid cartilage (J Rubin, personal observation, 2001).

As a correlate, Lieberman et al often note the resting anatomical relationship of the anterior cricoid ring/inferior rim of thryoid cartilage complex (which they designate the "cricothyroid visor") to be narrowed with little discernable space.[10] In this clinical scenario, they often identify a decreased range of motion of the cricothyroid visor as the individual changes vocal pitch from vocal fry to falsetto,[10] presumably in association with diminished cricothyroid muscle activity or efficiency. We have noted that some affected individuals recruit external muscles, particularly the suprahyoid muscles but also the strap muscles, and even at times other muscles of first and second branchial arch origin, to assist in pitch elevation. The physical consequence is an elevated larynx and tightened suprahyoid and perilaryngeal muscles.[12]

The issue of pain or discomfort in relation to muscular imbalance is relevant to this discussion, as well. A sense of discomfort commonly arises when muscles are not used appropriately. Further discomfort may occur as phonation is attempted while the anatomically related muscles are unduly tense. This can result in a cycle of muscle tension and pain, which further reinforces the behavioral muscular 'holding' pattern.[14]

TREATMENT

Various physical techniques have been developed to help alleviate the problems described above. Many are outside the purview of this chapter and can be found in texts on Alexander technique, in Pilates manuals, and so on. In essence, if we limit ourselves to the neck, physical techniques of use to our patients might include those that deal with:

1. release of tension/contraction of the suprahyoid musculature. Such techniques have been championed by workers such as Lesley Mathieson[14] and Nelson Roy[15];
2. release/stretch of the cricothyroid mechanism and release of tight strap muscles. Such techniques have been championed by Jacob Lieberman[10];
3. repositioning of the forward (hyperlordotic) cervical spine, including release of restriction of the cervical facet joints, release of contractions of the sternocleidomastoid and trapezius, stretch of the upper fibers of the erector spinae. These techniques are commonly used in physiotherapy, osteopathy, and to a lesser degree in massage. For voice patients, they have been championed by Ed Blake (E Blake, personal communication, 2001).

Lieberman et al[10] have described techniques for working directly on the cricothyroid joint and muscle and on the ligamentous and muscular attachments of the hyoid in such scenarios. They have identified rapid improvement of voicing in certain individuals. We have noted this as well but should note that laryngeal manipulation therapy may become possible only when other fundamental issues of posture have been addressed.

In her extensive work combining speech therapy with laryngeal manipulation, Mathieson has often found vocal improvement to occur immediately upon working on the muscular and tendinous attachments to the hyoid bone.[14] Roy has had similar experience.[15] Mathieson suggests that vocal improvement may occur when a muscle status is achieved that allows the larynx to respond easily to lateral digital pressure. This passive lateral laryngeal movement may well be an indicator that excessive tension has been eliminated or substantially reduced. As a result, vocal strategies can then be introduced in therapy, whereas previously they would have been counterproductive (L

Mathieson, personal observation, 2001). Teachers and performers, through the ages, have reported that lateral movement of the laryngeal cartilages is associated with a sense of freedom of the voice.[9]

Case Report

A case report (fictitious but based on our clinical experience) will help elucidate our current management approach. A 45-year-old professional female singer and dancer presented to the author (JR) on the day of an evening performance with a 2- to 3-week history of throat pain and increasing difficulty with the top register of the voice. Some months earlier she had suffered from a back injury for which she received intermittent physical therapy. On laryngeal examination, there was a satisfactory mucosal wave on stroboscopy with no definitive mucosal pathology; but the neck was found to be held in extension, and the anterior neck musculature was tight and tender to palpation.

An urgent referral was made to a physiotherapist (EB) who identified several musculoskeletal abnormalities, including resting extension of the upper cervical spine, deficits in force production of the deep neck flexor stability mechanism, and stiffness in the upper and midthoracic spine. Palpation of the second and third cervical vertebral facet joints demonstrated restriction of movement and duplicated the discomfort noted by the patient. There were also trigger points in the upper trapezius and levator scapulae and spasm of the sternocleidomastoid; and the lower trapezius was found to be inefficient, with difficulty initiating contraction.

Initial therapy focused on altering the resting position the larynx. Specific technical aspects are outside the scope of this chapter, but it was accomplished through direct manipulation and mobilization of the upper cervical and thoracic vertebrae and through soft tissue work on the affected muscles. The performer was able to perform that evening.

Intermediate therapy was designed to continue releasing the restricted muscular and arthrogenic structures. An exercise plan was also developed to strengthen the deep neck flexors and lower fibers of the trapezius. Following three or four additional sessions, the performer felt that she was back to normal voicing.

FURTHER THOUGHTS ON POSTURE AND VOICING

In discussing aspects of therapeutic intervention, one key issue is that changes in the resting position of the larynx often appear to be secondary to changes in the resting position of the cervical spine. These, in turn, may well be secondary to fundamental postural changes elsewhere in the body. Such postural issues require attention if local treatment of laryngeal position is to provide more than temporary relief of vocal symptoms.

Because this is a chapter on the effects of posture on voice, a final note should perhaps be referenced to posture with regard to breathing for speaking and or singing. Inappropriate posture frequently affects lung volume and subglottal air pressure; and inappropriate breathing patterns (eg, upper chest breathing) can affect posture, which in turn affects laryngeal position and phonation. Perhaps there will be a further chapter on this aspect of voicing in the fourth edition of this book as further clinical experience and research are accumulated.

CONCLUSIONS

Many types of musculoskeletal programs, including Alexander, Pilates, Feldenkrais, Rolf, and others, have emphasized the overall importance of posture to body "wellness." We believe that a clinical correlate to this is a balance of the deep flexor and extensor muscular systems of the body. An imbalance therein, even in the lower extremities or pelvis, can have far-reaching postural effects that ultimately affect the voice. We must emphasize that these are still, for us, early days in our interpretation and management of such complex musculoskeletal problems and the laryngeal manifestations thereof; but we believe these issues are important in the management of voice disorders and that further study is warranted.

REFERENCES

1. Fisher K. Early experience of a multidisciplinary pain management programme. *Holistic Med.* 1988;3:7–56.
2. Robinson L, Fisher H, Knox J, Thomson. *The Official Body Control Pilates Manual.* London, England: Macmillan Publishers Ltd; 2000.
3. Feldenkrais M. *Awareness Through Movement.* New York, NY: Harper and Row; 1972.
4. Rolf IP. *Rolfing: Reestablishing the Natural Alignment and Structural Integration of the Human Body for Vitality and Well-being.* Rochester, VT: Healing Arts Press; 1989.
5. Lumley JSP, Craven JL, Aitken JT. *Essential Anatomy.* Edinburgh, Scotland: Churchill Livingstone; 1973.
6. Ger R, Abrahams P, Olson TR. *Essentials of Clinical Anatomy.* 2nd ed. New York, NY: Parthenon Publishing Group; 1996.
7. *Stedman's Medical Dictionary.* 22nd ed. Baltimore, MD: Williams and Wilkins; 1972.

8. Boileu Grant JC, Basmajian JV. *Grant's Method of Anatomy.* 7th ed. Baltimore, MD: Williams and Wilkins; 1965.

9 Rubin JS, Korovin G, Epstein R. Care for the professional voice. In: Rubin JS, Sataloff RT, Korovin G., eds. *Diagnosis and Treatment of Voice Disorders.* 2nd ed. Clifton Park, NY: Thomson Delmar Learning; 2003.

10. Lieberman J. Principles and techniques of manual therapy. In: Harris T, Harris S, Rubin JS, Howard D, eds. *The Voice Clinic Handbook.* London, England: Whurr Publishers; 1998:91–138.

11. Koufman J, Blalock O. Functional voice disorders. *Otolaryngol Clin North Am.* 1991;24:1059–1073.

12. Rubin JS, Lieberman J, Harris TM. Laryngeal manipulation. *Otolaryngol Clin North Am.* 2000;33(5):1017–1034.

13. Aronson A. *Clinical Voice Disorders.* 3rd ed. New York, NY: Thieme Medical Publishers; 1991:117–145.

14. Mathieson L. *Greene and Mathieson's The Voice and Its Disorders.* 6th ed. London, England: Whurr Publishers Ltd; 2001.

15. Roy N, Leeper HA. Effects of the manual laryngeal musculoskeletal tension reduction technique as a treatment for functional voice disorders: perceptual and acoustic measures. *J Voice.* 1993;7:242–249.

40

Special Considerations for the Professional Voice User

John S. Rubin, MD, FACS, FRCS
Gwen Korovin, MD, FACS
Ruth Epstein, Ph.D., MRCSLT

OVERVIEW

A professional voice user may be defined as someone who uses the voice as a primary means of occupational communication. The crucial aspects of the definition revolve around: (1) a requirement of communication by means of the voice and (2) the production of a desirable and dependable vocal sound which carries its own message and which is, in many cases, compelling. Under this umbrella falls a large portion of the working population. Singers, actors, broadcasters and announcers, public speakers, politicians, and talk show hosts are immediately evident. Other important groups for whom the voice is critical include barristers and trial lawyers, lay preachers, clergy, teachers and coaches, telephone operators, receptionists, salespeople, stock and bond traders, exercise instructors; the list is almost indeterminable.

Within these groups, the voice is used in many differing ways: The salesperson uses the voice to convince others, and, frequently, to be "earnest" or "sincere." The trial lawyer's voice can cajole, soothe, or threaten, often within the same time frame. On radio and at sporting events, the "vocal signature" of the broadcaster assumes great importance, in many instances allowing for immediate recognition by the public. Many broadcasters' and performers' voices are so well known to the public that even the slightest vocal change due to illness or emotion is immediately apparent.[1] The voices of politicians and statesmen have probably effected significant changes in history as we know it. Franklin Delano Roosevelt's fireside chats gave the United States a collective will to carry on during the Depression. Winston Spencer Churchill's vocal presentation powerfully reinforced the image of the battling bulldog keeping all foes at bay. John Fitzgerald Kennedy's voice quite possibly won the presidential debate of 1960 and, hence, the presidency.

With some exceptions, a professional singer generally specializes in a particular musical style, be it classical, popular, rock, musical theatre, or rap; each style has its own requirements. For the classical singer, clarity of sound is necessary; harshness or hoarseness is immediately perceptible and undesirable. The rock singer may purposefully "color" the voice with harshness or graininess. Unlike the classical performer, who is generally comfortably balanced while performing, the rock singer may have developed a reputation for singing on the move. Problems associated therein include maintenance of sufficient breath control to sustain the required power and pitch of the voice. Problems may be exacerbated in musical theater where singing requirements may include a harness or trapeze or skates, a weighty head costume, or a constricting belt or sheath. This places a range of potential challenges in the path of satisfactory voice production.

Professional voice users as a group have the highest of work ethics and an unusually good appreciation of their state of health. They generally will not seek out the help of a laryngologist unless they are certain that something specific is wrong with their vocal tract; their level of anxiety as to its ramifications on their career will be great, and they will likely downplay the extent of the ailment and its duration.

THE LARYNGOLOGIST'S ROLE

What then is the laryngologist's role? As with all patients, when seeing a professional voice user, the laryngologist must assess the general medical condition of the patient as well as the specific vocal complaint. A holistic approach is necessary. A comprehensive, detailed patient history is essential, or else the laryngologist may well miss a vital clue.

The laryngologist must differentiate professional voice users from all of his or her other patients; voice is crucial to the professional's career and in many instances the career is the driving force and top priority of the professional's life. Some may even have difficulty in differentiating their voices from themselves as individuals. Although the health of the patient and his or her vocal apparatus is the laryngologist's foremost responsibility, the laryngologist always needs to consider the professional voice user's unique immediate and career requirements.

This chapter focuses on care of the singer, actor, and public speaker; however, principles discussed also apply to the other groups of individuals who fall within our definition of a professional voice user. For the sake of simplicity the text uses the male gender throughout; however, it applies equally to women.

ANATOMY: THE DRIVING FORCE OF THE VOICE

To care successfully for someone who relies on his voice, a critical understanding of how the voice is generated is necessary. Voice is produced through the function of three main mechanisms, which, together, encompass a large portion of the body: the breathing apparatus or "bellows," the true vocal folds or "oscillator," and the upper airway and oral cavity or "resonator." Mention should also be made of neural control both on a brainstem/cerebellar level, interrelating the respiratory apparatus and laryngeal musculature, and on a cortical level, with complex interrelationships allowing minor changes in emotional state to affect vocal quality. In addition, the body's musculature as it affects posture has an impact on the vocal mechanism and voice production. Effectively, therefore, one should consider the entire body as the vocal organ.

PRODUCTION OF VOICE

To producte voice, there must be a power source. This source, or "bellows," consists of the rib cage and pleurae, the diaphragm and intercostal muscles, the abdominal and back musculature, and the lungs. The back and thoracic musculature lifts and stabilizes the rib cage. The lungs expand and contract in association with the movements of the rib cage and pleurae. The diaphragm (and to a lesser extent the external intercostal muscles) is the major muscle involved in inspiration. The abdominal muscles and intercostals assume a greater and greater role as the demands on the expiratory system increase from simple reflexive expulsion to prolonged and controlled release of breath for phonation. The orientation of the ribs determines the range through which they can move, the upper ribs permitting more of a "pump-handle" type of motion and the lower ribs a "bucket-handle" movement.

Many problems therein can deleteriously affect the efficiency of the system. These might include intrinsic problems of the lungs and pleura, for example, asthma, chronic obstructive pulmonary disease, tuberculosis, or pleurisy. Musculoskeletal problems also can cause difficulties with the power source. Examples might include diastasis recti secondary to multiple parity, umbilical or inguinal hernia, muscle spasm of the shoulder girdle or paraspinous musculature, or age-induced calcifications of the costal cartilages.[2-5]

At the level of the glottis (the "oscillator"), expiration causes alternative buildup and release of air pressure at the vocal folds, which mechanically open and close in a caudad to cephalad direction. The pressure differential created by virtue of a large volume of compressed air streaming through the small glottal space initiates vocal fold vibration, partially through the Bernoulli effect (but only when the vocal folds are within the neartest 14% of their adductory range).[6] This effect is activated when an object prevents a flowing substance (such as air) from streaming freely, thus creating layers of stream. In the glottis, the middle layer of stream goes through undisturbed, whereas the lateral layers are deflected by the vocal folds; the negative pressure thus created draws the folds together.

This pulsatile stream is translated into sound, the fundamental frequency (F_0) being dependent on the number of oscillations per second. The sound wave can vibrate at a wide frequency range. Modal register in untrained speakers has been demonstrated to vary from 75 to 450 Hz in men and 130 to 520 Hz in women.[7,8] In primary school teachers, it has been postulated that the vocal folds may vibrate up to 1 million times per day (Erkki Vilkman, unpublished observation, 1999).

Pitch correlates nonlinearly with the physical measure of fundamental frequency.[6] It depends on vocal fold length and tension. In a string model, pitch is directly related to tension and inversely related to mass (or thickness) and length of the string. Researchers have attempted to apply this model to the vocal folds, with varying degrees of success, recognizing that the vocal folds do not function like vibrating strings.[9] Tension changes, both lateral and longitudinal, have been related to pitch variation. Increasing vocal fold length in modal register has been found to correlate to increased F_0; in falsetto, however, the vibrating length shortens as frequency increases. Vocal fold thickness or mass has been found to be of particular importance in modal range; an increase in length correlates with a decrease in mass and higher vibrating frequencies.[9-14] Colton relates this to the stretch of a rubberband; after certain stretch, the thickness remains the same.[9] Stretch is caused by contraction of the intrinsic laryngeal muscles.

The sound created at the level of the vocal folds is a buzz tone and contains a complete set of harmonic partials. It is then damped, amplified, and shaped by the "resonators," which consist of the soft tissues of the supraglottic larynx, pharynx, vault of the nasopharynx, and oral cavity, finally to be shaped into recognizable sound and language by the articulators, particularly the tongue, palate, and lips.[15-17] Certain frequencies are amplified. These are the formants. The adult male vocal tract is approximately 17 to 20 cm in length with formants at roughly 500 Hz, 1500 Hz, 2500 Hz, and 3500 Hz. The adult female formants are about 15% higher. The second formant is particularly sensitive to the tongue shape and the third to the position of its tip.[17]

To summarize, voice is produced by a power source causing the oscillator to vibrate, thereby producing a sound that is subsequently shaped by the resonators and articulators.

HISTORY

Detailed history taking is essential. It must incorporate ailments affecting the entire body, as well as those specific to the vocal tract. The history should be unrushed and detailed. Most professional voice users, when faced with what they perceive as a potentially career-ending vocal illness, will be extremely fearful when they come into the office.[18] A gentle and sympathetic approach will go a long way in obtaining an accurate history, which is essential to adequate treatment.

In many centers, the voice professional completes a questionnaire while in the waiting room. Some centers also incorporate questions that provide a psychological profile. This allows the patient to focus on the problem, makes him more receptive to questioning and, in a sense, begins the relaxation or unburdening process.

The taking of the history has already been elegantly described in chapter 11. In this chapter, we relate further information on history-taking in the singer/professional voice user on the basis that it is critical to formulation of any treatment strategy. Even if a cyst or other discrete vocal fold pathology is found during the examination, the question that the laryngologist needs to ascertain is what has caused the performer to fall from his performance plateau.

We present history-taking in terms of: (1) the current voice problem; (2) nonmedical events or stressors that may have caused or led to the voice problems; (3) medical problems that may have caused or led to the voice problems. Recall that a general medical history must evaluate overall health. Many problems including asthma, emphysema, chronic bronchitis, endocrinopathies, many central nervous system disorders, and so on can affect the vocal mechanisms directly. Although important to the professional voice user, it is outside the scope of this chapter.

The Current Voice Problem

This includes an overview by the patient as to what he or she perceives the problem to be and what has led to the problem. Vocal and career goals are investigated. Then a detailed vocal history is taken. This should include any history of vocal training both for the speaking and singing voice. The number and type of rehearsals or performances over the previous several months are important.

It is useful to know exactly when the performer noted the problem and in what context. For example, one performer described having intermittent voice problems in between a successful rehearsal and the actual performance, often with just hours between them. We discovered that he was regularly eating copious amounts of "junk" food in between. When he stopped this activity, the problems ceased.

Information regarding length and timing of warm-up and of rehearsals is important. Singers and actors frequently overrehearse, especially in the period just before a major performance.

The date of the next performance is an essential piece of information. Management may well vary depending on the timing therein. Usually, however, the laryngologist does not have the luxury of prolonged investigations, as the performer may seek care within hours or days of an important performance.[19]

The laryngologist needs to clarify exactly what the performer feels is wrong with his or her voice. This often gives the vital clue as to the etiology. A well-trained singer can generally sing for well over an hour without developing vocal fatigue. Fatigue suggests musculoskeletal issues and may point to oversinging or overuse of the voice, although serious neurologic problems may also present with this complaint. Prolonged warm-up time is frequently associated with reflux.[19] Pain while singing is often the result of vocal abuse, as are choking or coughing in rarer situations.

A harsh voice with loss of dynamic range may be associated with vocal polyps, Reinke's edema, or other mass lesions.[20,21] Difficulty with the passaggio and loss of the upper range could well indicate prenodular edema. Breathiness may be indicative of vocal fold palsy or other problems preventing closure of the vocal folds.[22] Postviral partial paresis is probably much more common than previously appreciated.[23] A voice weakening with use, especially in association with increased nasality and ptosis, could be indicative of myasthenia gravis.[24] Although other pathologies often are associated with these symptoms, the ones mentioned here must be included in the differential diagnosis.

Nonmedical Issues

These might include any of the following:

- Troubles in the family, home, or with friends
- Difficulties with the singing teacher/voice coach

- Difficulties in the production with the producer or members of the cast
- Difficulties with the acoustics, including the actual space or venue, difficulty with the microphones or with feedback, and so forth
- Difficulties with the role or activity. Part of which may be inappropriate for the performer's range. Furthermore, the role/part may require intensive learning and rehearsing or may have the potential to be abusive to the voice. Examples might include occupations such as aerobics instruction or primary school teaching; performances such as cartoon character voiceovers or a staged scream; operatic death scenes sung while lying down, and so forth Also, nonoccupational activities may be abusive, such as yelling at sporting events, cheerleading, and so forth.

Medical Problems or Issues

These are extremely diverse and are well covered elsewhere in this book. In synopsis, they may include (among others):

Infection—upper respiratory infection, laryngitis, bronchitis, sinusitis, and so forth

Inflammation/irritation—cigarette or passive smoke, reflux, pollution, stage effects, bulimia, cough, and so forth

Allergy and asthma

Hormonal issues

Neurologic issues

Physical injuries and or musculoskeletal issues

Medications and recreational drugs

Stress and anxiety

PHYSICAL EXAMINATION

The physical examination is well presented in chapter 12. We shall limit ourselves to what we see as critical issues in the examination for the performer. These include (1) the examination philosophy, (2) musculoskeletal and postural issues, (3) the general ear, nose, and throat (ENT) examination, and (4) the laryngeal examination.

The Examination Philosophy

In general, every effort should be made to allow the patient to feel at ease. Unlike many busy general ENT

ommend the use of these agents on the basis that: (1) they have many potential complications including hypotension, thrombocytopenic purpura, depression, exacerbation of certain pulmonary conditions, and so forth; (2) they can be dangerous, causing rebound hypertension if stopped precipitously; and (3) many performers use their anxiety/stress to produce a world-class performance, whereas with beta-blockers they would have a steady but lackluster performance.

Antacids taken about half an hour prior to performance may prevent some of the concomitant hyperacidity associated with preperformance anxiety. They may, however, also cause a slight dryness of the mouth, which could be deleterious.

In some individuals, there is a tendency toward shallow or decreased respirations as part of preperformance anxiety/stress. In these instances, two or three voiced yawn-sighs can prove beneficial. Not only will they (slightly) raise oxygen saturation and lower CO_2 levels, the act of yawning will also help release tightened and held muscles in the neck and lower the level of the larynx. (However it must be emphasized that repetitive deep breathing could bring about hyperventilation and carry with it its own side effects. Again, common sense is required.)

Overall, regular coaching, adequate preparation, and appropriate warm-up exercises remain the cornerstone to manage this problem.

The laryngologist must determine how much of a problem the anxiety is. Crescendoing anxiety or inability to perform in public without the benefit of medications, in a professional who spends most of his life in the public eye, could be a sign of an underlying psychologic disturbance which requires professional guidance.[29]

REFLUX PHARYNGOLARYNGITIS

Reflux is another problem commonplace among professional voice users. The reader is referred to chapter 28 for detailed information. In 1991, Sataloff reported reflux laryngitis in 45% of consecutive professional voice users.[40] Generalized symptoms include chronic cough, belching, throat clearing, throat pain, catarrh, and intermittent hoarseness, often improving as the day progresses. Frequently in the performer the condition is so chronic that he is totally unaware of the symptoms. It is also not uncommon for the performer to suffer from reflux only while singing and particularly while performing.

Symptoms may be brought on or exacerbated by weight lifting or abdominal workouts, or by a change in diet.

Should the laryngologist have his or her suspicions aroused to the possibility of reflux during the examination (arytenoid edema, etc), a course of H2 blockers, or proton pump inhibitors could be commenced without definitive proof. Apples, red wine, caffeine, chocolate, and highly spiced food should be stopped and an antireflux regimen begun. Modified barium swallow, cine-esophagram, or endoscopy may be useful to identify reflux and/or related pathology. The gold standard in quantification of laryngopharyngeal reflux is pH monitoring, but its sensitivity and specificity are not 100%.[41] Patient education in relation to diet and lifestyle and participation in the management of this disorder is of particular importance.

VOCAL ABUSE/MISUSE

Vocal abuse, either of the singing or the speaking voice, is not uncommon in the performer.

Vocal Abuse/Misuse When Singing

Vocal abuse/misuse in professional singers can occur in many forms. Singers in the two extremes of their careers have a tendency to try to overextend their vocal limits. There is a particular problem in choral masters asking children to perform work too difficult for their vocal ages.[42,43] The older performer is susceptible to the risk of accepting roles no longer suited for his or her voice. In all performers, there is always the possibility of inadequate time for preparation for a particular role. To make up for this, the performer is likely to overrehearse just before the performance.

Professional performers generally have a very high work ethic. This can lead to the unwise decision by the performer to perform when not at peak, when suffering from an upper respiratory ailment, and so forth. Among popular music singers, there is a tendency to color the voice. This vocal coloration may become a part of the performer's signature and be necessary for vocal recognition by the public, but may well lead to chronic irritation of the vocal folds. Musical theater has become the mainstay of Broadway and the West End in New York. Belting is perhaps more effortful than operatic style, and performers may be required to sing while on skates, leaping in the air, and during other athletic endeavors. Performing in eight shows a week can represent a significant stressor for the performer's larynx, particularly if the performer is not at his peak.

Cancellation of Performance

The role of the laryngologist is to diagnose the underlying problem and determine how serious it is with relation not only to any upcoming performance but also to the performer's career. The laryngologist must make up his or her mind on a case-by-case basis as to whether the performer can perform as is, or needs to cancel. He or she must also make certain that the performer is working closely with an appropriate singing and/or voice teacher. A close working relationship with a speech-language pathologist with a special interest in voice may be of great benefit to the performer.

Regarding general guidelines, the laryngologist should have a relatively low index for suggesting cancellation for an established performer. That said, the established performer will frequently have a very clear idea as to whether or not it is "safe" for him or her to undertake the performance. The laryngologist's role is one of support and gentle guidance.

It is the crucial or critical performance, especially in the young or not-yet-established performer, that requires the greatest deliberation. If there is sufficient time (several days) prior to the performance, voice rest in association with aggressive humidification and medical management may save the performance. It is not sufficient to let the performer state that he will "mark" the rehearsals, as what "marking" means can vary extensively from performer to performer; and some forms of "marking" (eg, whispering) may actually be detrimental. It must be recalled that it is the overall health of the performer and his or her future professional life that must be considered first and foremost.

Vocal Abuse/Misuse When Speaking

It is not uncommon for a professional trained in singing to have no training in speaking. Similarly, it is the rule rather than the exception for public speakers to have little or no formal training in speaking. Often an actor or public speaker will assume that he can project his voice or change the vocal pitch without proper training. Such performers may get away with the abuse for a time, but eventually it will catch up with them. For an actor, however, the most common cause of voice abuse is too much rehearsal, frequently in a dry environment.

Koufman classified one type of speaking-voice abuse seen among professional voice users as the "Bogart-Bacall" syndrome; he found it in 26% of his patients with functional voice disorders.[44] The patient speaks with a very low fundamental frequency, frequently at the lowest note of his pitch range. The use of an unnaturally low fundamental frequency for too long or at high intensities can lead to the formation of vocal fold nodules. Similarly, prolonged use of too high a speaking voice, a problem not infrequently encountered in the United Kingdom, can lead to vocal edema (Sara Harris, personal observation, 1997).

The laryngologist needs to have close interaction with a singing voice teacher or speech-language pathologist in these conditions. Refer to chapter 37 by Carroll in this book for further information.

Musculoskeletal Pathologies

Musculoskeletal and postural issues are frequently part of the process leading to voice disorders. A neck held in a hyperextended hyperlordotic position, a cervicodorsal shelf, or head tilt are commonplace among the general population. Limitation of motion of the cricothyroid joints with contraction of the cricothyroid muscle or tenderness of the muscles that attach to the lateral body of the hyoid bone may also be found during the examination. These conditions are amenable to intervention by an osteopath or physical therapist. We recently reviewed a series of patients in the voice clinic with musculoskeletal pathology and identified certain patterns. These included: high-held larynx; shortening, contraction of the suprahyoid and sternocleidomastoid muscles; and weak deep flexor mechanism.[45]

Tension Fatigue

This is one type of musculoskeletal voice disorder that is seen particularly in the hard-driving vocal professional. The patient presents with dysphonia, vocal fatigue, and pain on phonation. This was the most common finding among patients with functional voice disorders in Koufman's series.[44] It is somewhat less common among trained singers and actors, but more common among other professional voice users.

The condition is characterized by poor breath control and excessive muscular tension in the neck and base of tongue musculature.[44] The jaw is frequently held in a rigid position, the sternocleidomastoid and trapezius muscles are tight, and the base of tongue musculature is contracted and frequently in spasm. These patients also suffer from other musculoskeletal tension syndromes (eg, tension headache, temporal mandibular joint syndrome, bruxism, etc). Vocal quality is often strained and harsh and pitch range is limited. There are frequently hard glottal attacks.

Because most of these patients do not have voice coaches, a speaking-voice teacher will need to be consulted and relaxation techniques instituted (see chapter 37).

DISCRETE VOCAL FOLD PATHOLOGY

These pathological conditions are well covered elsewhere in this book and we will not belabor them. From the standpoint of the professional voice user, the key issues surrounding management of these vocal-abuse pathologies include:

1. The etiology of the pathology
2. Its effect on the voice
3. The risks versus benefits of the treatment plan chosen (particularly from the standpoint of time off work and upcoming commitments)
4. The effects on the professional voice user's career

Etiology of the Pathology

If prenodular edema or early nodules have been related to the performer working in 8 shows per week over the last 6 months, and the performer anticipates being in the production for the forseeable future, the treatment plan may well need to differ from a performer who has been overrehearsing for a single upcoming performance.

An example of the latter is a young professional voice user who was preparing for a singing competition. This individual presented to one of the authors 6 days prior to the competition, with the ultimate diagnosis of prenodular edema, secondary to overrehearsing and reflux. The treatment plan included relative voice rest and an antireflux program. The performer went on to perform credibly in the competition.

Effect of the Pathology on the Voice

The effects of prenodular edema or early Reinke's edema may well be devastating to the voice of a performer specializing in early music. In a performer specializing in Country and Western, R&B, or rap music, the pathology may actually be contributing to that performer's vocal signature.

An example of the latter is a self-trained "rap" singer. He was currently preparing a recording and the recording company was concerned about an increase in the gravelly quality of his voice. A previous recording confirmed the characteristics of his vocal signature. Laryngeal examination demonstrated Reinke's edema, supraglottic hyperfunction, and reflux. The laryngologist referred him to a speech-language pathologist and commenced an antireflux program. The performer felt that his voice returned to its previous state, without change in his underlying vocal signature, enabling him to fulfill his contractual obligations and finish the recording.

Risks Versus Benefits of the Treatment Plan Chosen (particularly from the standpoint of time off work and upcoming commitments)

As an example, one of the authors treated a performer in a musical theater production who was found to have a vocal polyp that was causing some difficulty with his upper range, but which he was more or less able to "sing around." At the time of assessment he only had a few more weeks in his current role, but was to start a in a new production 2 months thereafter. The treatment plan, after considerable discussion with him, was for the performer to start working with a speech- language pathologist immediately, and once the production was completed, to schedule surgical removal of the polyp. His larynx was stabilized and his voice was fine by the beginning of the next production.

Effect of the Pathology and Its Management on the Professional Voice User's Career

This is, of course, the ultimate consideration and is not always straightforward to answer.

One of the authors saw a professional voice user who presented with a granuloma of the arytenoid process, which had recurred following surgery. It affected his vocal stamina, and thus placed the patient's career in jeopardy. Reflux management in combination with work with a speech- language pathologist was initiated, but did not bring about significant improvement. The performer was referred for physical therapy of the larynx, as well as continuing to work with the other members of the team. The granuloma responded to this therapeutic intervention, but only over a course of several months.

VOCAL FOLD HEMORRHAGE

Vocal fold hemorrhage occurs in the submucosal layer, causing severe hoarseness and swelling. It is frequently precipitated by a cough, shout, or scream, especially in a patient on aspirin or nonsteroidal analgesics. Management is usually medical; it should be considered a laryngologic emergency. Management requires strict voice rest, for up to 2 weeks (or until it resolves), generally with total resorption of the hemorrhage. However, there are exceptions, and early surgical evacuation may be appropriate in rare cases.[46] It is not infrequent for the patient to be left with a prominent vessel on the vocal fold, which could rebleed at a later time, especially during times of vessel fragility. An example of this is at the beginning of the menstrual cycle. If necessary, a decision can be made to treat the vessel surgically if it continues to rebleed.

From the standpoint of the performer, the key issue is to get him to understand the potential risks of continuing to perform with the hemorrhage, and thus to get him to accept the relatively prolonged period of voice rest followed by vocal restriction that is usually necessary.

NONLARYNGEAL SURGERY

Certain issues that are particularly important in non-laryngeal surgery on performers shall be presented here. First and foremost, the surgeon and anesthesiologist must be aware that the patient is a performer. This information will generally heighten their level of care for the airway and soft tissues.

Following surgery, the performer should refrain from performing too soon, particularly after any surgery that may affect the production of the voice. This includes abdominal, pelvic, back, and thoracic surgeries.

There may well be a role for the performer to seek rehabilitation from a physiotherapist or voice teacher following such surgery to make certain that he is recovering properly.

Surgery on the neck frequently involves manipulation of the strap muscles. The surgeon should make an effort not to divide or denervate the strap muscles in this patient population because of their importance in controlling vertical laryngeal position and stabilizing the larynx. When operating on the thyroid, he should be aware of the needs of the patient and be particularly careful regarding the superior laryngeal as well as the recurrent laryngeal nerves. When operating on the upper neck, particular caution must be taken with the marginal mandibular nerve and the platysma muscle. Division of the former or imprecise resuture of the latter could affect the ability of the performer to use the depressors of the lower lip with a negative impact on voice production.

Indications for tonsillectomy or uvulopalatopharyngoplasty are the same as for the general public. However, the performer must be aware that both procedures can cause scarring and will change the shape of the pharynx. These changes may affect resonation, with resultant changes of tone. Both of these procedures must be considered carefully and thoughtfully by all parties prior to surgery.

Indications for nasal surgery do not differ in the professional voice user from other people. Nasal obstruction due to a deviated nasal septum leading to recurrent episodes of acute sinusitis is such an indication. The voice professional should not expect improvement in the singing voice. An awareness of a possible change in the voice is necessary.

VOICE REST

Voice rest is reserved for cases exhibiting severe mucosal redness and swelling, hemorrhage, or mucosal breaks. It is also prescribed at times for instances of aggravation of previously present vocal pathology. It is rarely necessary to prescribe absolute voice rest for more then 3 days. Acute vocal hemorrhage is the one instance where it should be extended for up to 2 weeks. Complete voice rest means, as it suggests, no use of the voice for communication. Whispering may be more traumatic to the larynx than speaking. This differs from restrictive voice use, which may be recommended by certain laryngologists following laryngeal surgery. Others recommend complete voice rest after laryngeal surgery, for up to 2 weeks.

CONCLUSION

Professional voice users as a group have special needs, the foremost being that their voice is crucial to their career. They should be referred to the subspecialist who has been trained in management of the particular ailments from which this group suffers. The laryngologist caring for these patients must be prepared to put aside the requisite time necessary to obtain an adequate history and physical examination. He or she should also have access to a large interdisciplinary body of specialists including a speech-language pathologist, voice coach, singing voice specialist, osteopath or physiotherapist, gastroenterologist, pulmonologist, neurologist, psychiatrist or psychologist, endocrinologist, and so forth to help in management of the frequently complex problems presented.

The role of the laryngologist is a demanding one. He or she must be able to make the correct diagnosis and initiate an appropriate treatment plan. The laryngologist must also be sensitive to the career needs of this group, but be able to put their patients' health over any immediate performance problem.

REFERENCES

1. Mitchell SA. The professional speaking voice. In Benninger MS, Jacobson BH, Johnson AF, eds. *Vocal Arts Medicine: The Care and Prevention of Professional Voice Disorders.* New York, NY: Thieme Medical Publishers, Inc; 1994:167–176.
2. Rubin JS. Treatment of voice disorders. *Cortlandt Forum.* 1993;6(7):123–126.
3. Dickson DR, Maue-Dickson W. *Anatomical and Physiological Bases of Speech.* Boston, MA: Little, Brown and Co; 1982.
4. Bunch MA. *Dynamics of the Singing Voice.* 3rd ed. Wien: Springer-Verlag; 1995.
5. Rubin JS. Mechanisms of respiration (the bellows). In: Harris T, Harris S, Rubin JS, Howard DM, eds. *The Voice Clinic Handbook.* London: Whurr Publishers Ltd; 1998: 49–63.

6. Scherer RC. Laryngeal function during phonation. In: Rubin JS, Sataloff RT, Korovin GK, Gould WJ, eds. *Diagnosis and treatment of Voice Disorders.* New York, NY: Igaku-Shoin; 1995:86–104.

7. Baken RJ. An overview of laryngeal function for voice production. In: Sataloff RT. *Professional Voice, The Science and Art of Clinical Care.* 2nd ed. San Diego, CA: Singular Publishing Group Inc; 1997:147–166.

8. Gould WJ. Caring for the vocal professional. In: Paparella MM, Shumrick DA, Gluckman JL, et al, eds. *Otolaryngology.* 3rd ed. Philadelphia, PA: WB Saunders Co; 1991:2273–2288.

9. Colton RH. Physiology of phonation. In: Benninger MS, Jacobson BH, Johnson AF, eds. *Vocal Arts Medicine: The Care and Prevention of Professional Voice Disorders.* New York, NY: Thieme Medical Publishers, Inc; 1994:30–60.

10. Perlman AL, Titze IR, Cooper DS. Elasticity of canine vocal fold tissue. *J Speech Hear Res.* 1984;27:212–219.

11. Titze I, Durham P. Passive mechanisms influencing fundamental frequency control. In: Baer T, Sasaki C, Harris K, eds. *Laryngeal Function in Phonation and Respiration.* San Diego, CA: College-Hill Press; 1986:304–319.

12. Hollien H, Colton R. Four laminagraphic studies of vocal fold thickness. *Folia Phoniatr.* 1969;21:179–198.

13. Hollien H. Vocal fold thickness and fundamental frequency of phonation. *J Speech Hear Res.* 1962;5:237–243.

14. Hollien H, Coleman RF. Laryngeal correlates of frequency change: a STROL study. *J Speech Hear Res.* 1970; 12:272–278.

15. Titze I. On the mechanics of vocal fold vibration. *J Acoustic Soc Am.* 1976;60:1366–1380.

16. Titze I. Comments on the myoelastic-aerodynamic theory of phonation. *J Speech Hear Res.* 1980;23:495–510.

17. Sundberg J. Vocal tract resonance. In: Sataloff RT. *Professional Voice: The Science and Art of Clinical Care.* 2nd ed. San Diego, CA: Singular Publishing Group Inc; 1997; 167–184.

18. Carpenter B. Psychological aspects of vocal fold surgery. In: Gould WJ, Sataloff RT, Spiegel JR, eds. *Voice Surgery.* St. Louis, Mo: Mosby; 1993:339–343.

19. Sataloff RT, Spiegel JR. Care of the profesional voice. *Otolaryngol Clin North Am.* 1991;24:1093–1124.

20. Sanada T, Tanaka S, Hibi S, et al. Relationship between the degree of lesion and that of vocal dysfunction in vocal fold polyp. *Nippon Jibiinkoka Gakkai Kaiho.* 1990;93: 388–392.

21. Bennett S, Bishop S, Lumpkin SMM. Phonatory characteristics associated with bilateral diffuse polypoid degeneration. *Laryngoscope,* 1987;97:446–450.

22. Tucker HM, Lavertu P. Paralysis and paresis of the vocal folds. In: Blitzer A, Brin MF, Sasaki CT, et al. *Neurologic Disorders of the Larynx.* New York, NY: Thieme Medical Publishers, Inc; 1992:182–189.

23. Sataloff RT, Mandel S, Rosen DC. Neurologic disorders affecting the voice in performance. In: Sataloff RT. *Professional Voice: The Science and Art of Clinical Care.* 2nd ed. San Diego, CA: Singular Publishing Group, Inc; 1997: 479–498.

24. Colton RH, Casper JK. Voice problems associated with nervous system involvement. In: *Understanding Voice Problems: A Physiological Perspective for Diagnosis and Treatment.* Baltimore, MD: Williams & Wilkins; 1990: 107–150.

25. Jahn AF, Davies, DG. A clincial approach to the professional voice. In: Blitzer A, Brin MF, Sasaki CT, et al, eds. *Neurologic Disorders of the Larynx.* New York, NY: Thieme Medical Publishers, Inc; 1992:149–162.

26. Sataloff RT, Spiegel JR, Hawkshaw M. The history. In: Gould WJ, Sataloff RT, Spiegel JR, eds. *Voice Surgery.* St. Louis, MO: Mosby; 1993:173–188.

27. Sataloff RT. Physical examination. In: Sataloff RT. *Professional Voice: The Science and Art of Clinical Care.* New York, NY: Raven Press; 1991:91–100.

28. Rubin JS, Lieberman J, Harris TM. Laryngeal manipulation. *Otolaryngol Clin North Am.* 2000;33:1017–1034.

29. Sataloff RT. Stress, anxiety, and psychogenic dysphonia. In: Sataloff RT. *Professional Voice: The Science and Art of Clinical Care.* New York, NY: Raven Press; 1991:195–200.

30. Jacobson BH, Johnson A, Grywalski C, et al. The Voice Handicap Index (VHI): development and validation. *J Speech-Lang Pathol.* 1997;6:66–70

31. Ma EPM, Yiu EML. Voice activity and participation profile: assessing the impact of voice disorders on daily activities. *J Speech Lang Hear Res.* 2001;44:511–524

32. Epstein R, Stewart L, Rubin JS. Who's reality is it anyways? The interrelationships of objective and perceptual evaluations and the patient's own perspective in a sequential series of voice patients seen in one voice center. In preparation.

33. Finkelhor BK, Titze IR, Durham PL. The effect of viscosity changes in the vocal folds on the range of oscultation. *J Voice.* 1988;1:320–325.

34. Cohn JR, Spiegel JR, Hawkshaw M, Sataloff RT. Allergy. In: Sataloff RT. *Professional Voice: The Science and Art of Clinical Care.* 2nd ed. San Diego, Calif: Singular Publishing Group, Inc; 1997:369–373.

35. Hocevar-Boltezar I, Radsel Z, Zargi M. The role of allergy in the etiogenesis of laryngeal mucosal lesions. *Acta Otolaryngol (Stockh).* 1997(527, suppl):134–137.

36. Lavy JA, Wood G, Rubin JS, Harries M. Dysphonia associated with inhaled steroids. *J Voice.* 2000;14:581–588.

37. Surow JB, Lovetri J. "Alternative medical therapy" use among singers: prevalence and implications for the medical care of the singer. *J Voice.* 2000;14(3):398–409

38. Rosen DC, Sataloff RT. Psychological aspects of voice disorders. In: Sataloff RT. *Professional Voice: The Science and Art of Clinical Care.* 2nd ed. San Diego, CA: Singular Publishing Group, Inc; 1997:305–318.

39. Aronson A. *Clinical Voice Disorders.* 3rd ed. New York, NY: Thieme Medical Publishers; 1990:117–145.

40. Sataloff RT, Spiegel JR, Hawkshaw MJ. Strobovideolaryngoscopy: results and clinical value. *Ann Otol Rhinol Laryngol.* 1991;100:725–727.

41. Sataloff RT, Castell DO, Katz PO, Sataloff DM. *Reflux Laryngitis and Related Disorders.* San Diego, CA: Singular Publishing Group, Inc; 1999:55–67.

42. Sataloff RT. The effects of age on the voice. In: Sataloff RT. *Professional Voice : The Science and Art of Clinical Care.* New York, NY: Raven Press; 1991:141–151.

43. Sataloff RT, Spiegel J, Rosen DC. The effects of age on the voice. In: Sataloff RT. *Professional Voice: The Science and Art of Clinical Care*. 2nd ed. San Diego, CA: Singular Publishing Group, Inc; 1997:259–268.

44. Koufman J, Blalock O. Functional voice disorders. *Otolaryngol Clin North Am*. 1991;24:1059–1073.

45. Rubin JS, Blake E, Mathieson LM. Postural patterns in voice patients. *J Voice*: in press.

46. Spiegel JR, Sataloff RT, Hawkshaw M, Rosen DC. Vocal fold hemorrhage. In: Sataloff RT. *Professional Voice: The Science and Art of Clinical Care*. 2nd ed. San Diego, CA: Singular Publishing Group, Inc; 1997:541–554.

41

Laryngotracheal Trauma

Yolanda D. Heman-Ackah, MD
Vijay Rao, MD
George S. Goding, Jr., MD

The incidence of laryngotracheal trauma is estimated to be 1 in 14,000 to 30,000 emergency department visits in the United States.[1,2] Trauma to the laryngotracheal complex can be classified as blunt, penetrating, caustic, thermal, and iatrogenic injuries. The morbidity associated with these injuries ranges from chronic airway obstruction to voice compromise, with complication rates as high as 15 to25%.[3-5] Because of their potential for airway compromise, these injuries can be lethal, with mortality rates of 2 to 15%.[3,5] Injuries to the larynx and trachea often accompany other severe injuries, and the neck can appear to be deceptively normal even in cases of serious laryngotracheal disruption.

BLUNT INJURY

Blunt injury to the larynx and trachea is the most common cause of laryngotracheal injury in the United States today, accounting for 60% of all injuries to the laryngotracheal complex.[2,4] These injuries result from motor vehicle collisions in the adult population and from accidents involving all-terrain vehicles, bicycles, contact sports, and hanging type injuries in the young adult, adolescent, and pediatric populations. Adults and children differ not only in the mechanisms of injury, but also in the types of injuries experienced. These differences can be accounted for, at least in part, by differences in the relative size, position, and degree of calcification of the larynx and trachea.

Adult Framework Injuries from Blunt Trauma

In the adult, the inferior border of the cricoid cartilage sits at the level of the 6th and 7th cervical vertebrae.[6] Thus, in the normal upright position, the larynx is relatively protected from trauma by the overhang of the mandible superiorly, the bony prominence of the clavicles and sternal manubrium inferiorly, and by the mass of the sternocleidomastoid muscles laterally. Laryngeal injuries are relatively rare except when there is a direct blow to the neck. The usual victim of laryngotracheal trauma in a motor vehicle collision is an unbelted front seat passenger or driver in a vehicle without protective airbags. Upon collision, the front seat passenger or driver is propelled forward with the neck in extension, eliminating the mandible as a protective shield. The laryngotracheal complex hits the dashboard or steering wheel with a posterior-superiorly based vector of force, and the thyroid and cricoid cartilages are crushed against the cervical vertebrae (Figure 41–1).[7,8] Direct blows to the larynx can also occur during athletic competition, while falling forward onto a blunt object, or with hanging of the neck from a suspended rope or wire.

A wide spectrum of predictable injuries occurs. The thyroid and cricoid cartilages interact dynamically to protect the airway from blunt injury.[8] Forces to the anterior larynx often are encountered first by the thyroid prominence, which bends against the cervical vertebrae on impact. The thyroid cartilage eventually reaches a point of maximal flexibility, and a single median or paramedian fracture occurs (Figure 41–2).

The force then impacts the cricoid ring, which was previously shielded by the anterior projection of the thyroid cartilage. In a patient with a marked laryngeal prominence, multiple fractures of the thyroid cartilage in both the vertical and horizontal planes may occur prior to the distribution of force onto the cricoid cartilage (Figure 41–3).[8] The cricoid has a relatively thin anterior arch that blends laterally into rigidly buttressed tubercles. Lower level impacts result in a single median fracture or multiple paramedian vertical fractures. The airway is maintained by the lateral buttresses (Figure 41–4). With higher impact forces, secondary lateral arch fractures can occur in the cricoid cartilage, resulting in airway collapse and possible injury to the recurrent laryngeal nerve caused by impingement at the level of the cricothyroid joint (Figures 41–5 and 41–6).

If the force is severe or low in the neck, complete laryngotracheal separation may occur.[9] Separation usually occurs between the cricoid cartilage and the first tracheal ring. The results is displacement of the trachea

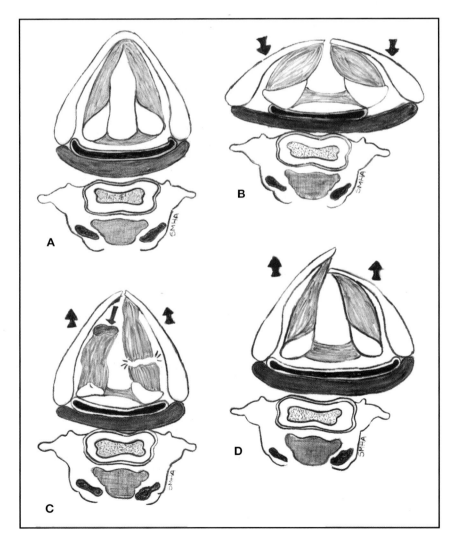

Figure 41–1. Mechanism of blunt laryngeal trauma. **A.** Normal laryngeal position; **B.** Posteriorly directed force crushing thyroid ala against cervical vertebrae, resulting in a midline fracture; **C.** Recovery of larynx from force resulting in detachment of the vocal ligament on the left, tear in the right thyroarytenoid muscle, and bilateral arytenoid dislocation; **D.** Recovery of larynx from force resulting in overlapping, displaced thyroid lamina fracture and malposition of the vocal fold. (Courtesy of Sabrina M. Heman-Ackah)

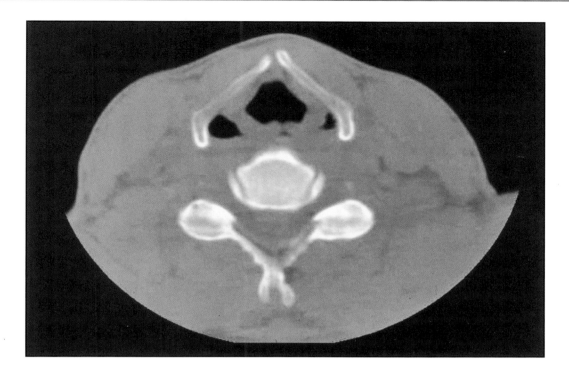

Figure 41–2. Axial CT scan of the thyroid ala. There is a midline thyroid ala fracture with diastasis of fracture segments.

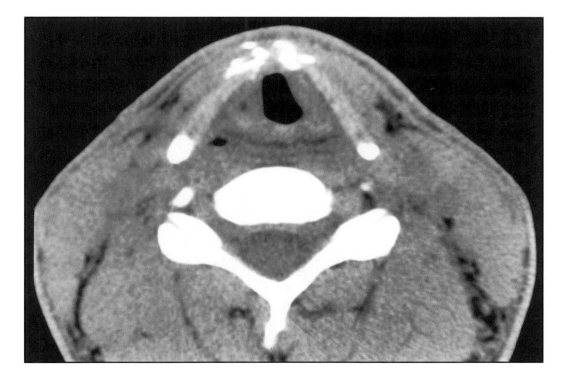

Figure 41–3. Axial CT scan of the thyroid ala demonstrating an anterior comminuted thyroid ala fracture sustained by the patient in a motor vehicle collision.

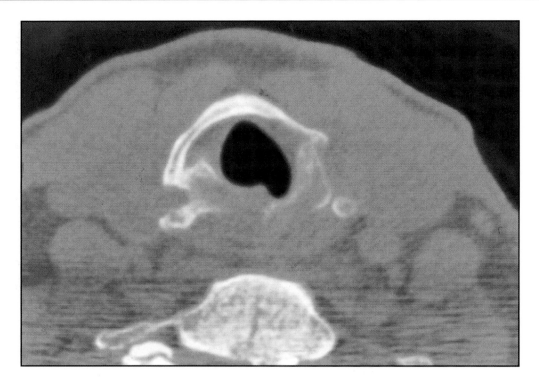

Figure 41-4. Axial CT scan at the level of the thyroid and cricoid cartilages. There is a vertically, displaced posterior cricoid lamina fracture with fusion of the right cricothyroid joint. The airway is maintained by the lateral buttresses.

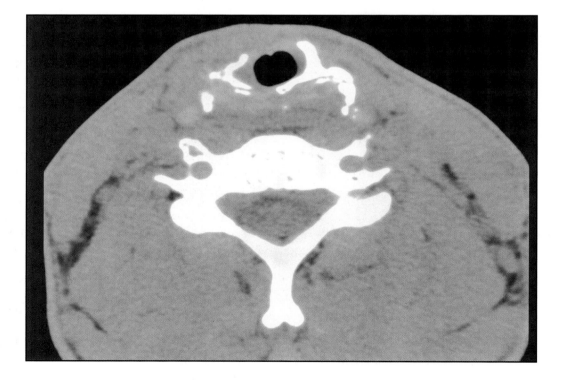

Figure 41–5. Axial CT scan of the cricoid cartilage. The airway is narrowed secondary to anterior and posterior vertically, displaced cricoid lamina fractures.

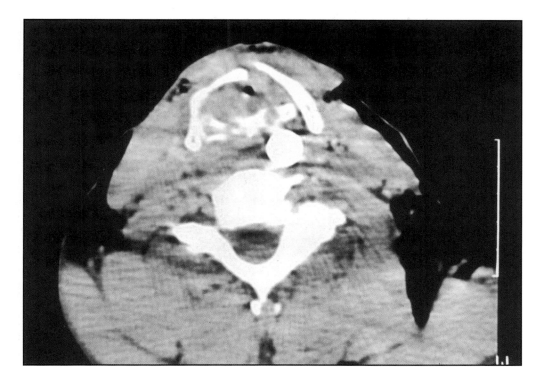

Figure 41–6. Axial CT scan at the level of the thyroid and cricoid cartilages. There are midline and left lateral fractures of the thyroid ala and comminuted fractures of the posterior cricoid lamina with loss of the airway space. The airway was secured below the fracture segments with tracheotomy.

inferiorly and soft tissue collapse into the airway, with consequent airway obstruction.[9-12] The strap musculature and surrounding cervical fascia can serve as a temporary conduit for air until edema and hematoma formation result in obstruction of this temporary airway.

Pediatric Framework Injuries from Blunt Trauma

Fractures of the thyroid and cricoid cartilage from blunt trauma are uncommon in the pediatric population. The pediatric larynx sits higher in the neck than in the adult, and depending upon the age, can lie between the 2nd and 7th cervical vertebrae. The mandible serves more as a protective shield in the child than it does in the adult.[13] The greater elasticity of the pediatric cartilaginous framework makes it more resilient to external stresses, and the mobility of the supporting tissues tends to protect the laryngotracheal complex more effectively. Children, however, are likely to sustain soft tissue injuries resulting in edema and hematoma formation.[12,13] This is of particular concern in a child because of the relatively smaller diameter of the pediatric airway.

The pediatric patient is more likely than the adult to sustain transection and telescoping injuries. An indi-

vidual who falls onto the handlebar of the bicycle may suffer a telescoping injury in which the cricoid cartilage is dislocated superiorly underneath the thyroid lamina (Figure 41–7).[12-15] With more forceful blows, complete laryngotracheal separation may occur. The adolescent and young adult riding a snowmobile or an all-terrain vehicle may sustain a "clothes-line" type injury to the neck. Upon collision with the cable or wire, a horizontal, linear force is applied low in the neck, compressing the cricotracheal complex against the anterior cervical vertebrae and resulting in cricotracheal separation.[15] The elasticity of the intercartilaginous ligaments contributes to substernal retraction of the trachea. These are often fatal injuries, but occasionally there is enough fascial stenting to maintain an adequate airway until an artificial airway can be established. There may be an associated injury, and possibly transection of both recurrent laryngeal nerves, which are also compressed against the cervical vertebrae during the injury.[12,15]

Young children may accidentally hang themselves while playing, and adolescents may do so intentionally in suicide attempts. In these instances, the fall to hanging position is usually less than 1 to 2 feet. The rope around the neck tightens usually in the region of

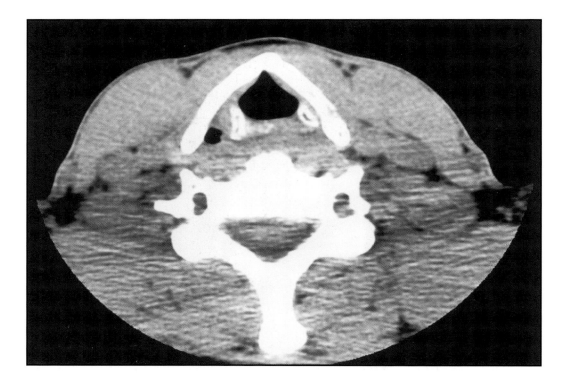

Figure 41–7. Axial CT scan at the level of the thyroid and cricoid cartilages. There is subluxation of the cricoid cartilage under the thyroid ala after the patient sustained an elbow injury to the neck while playing basketball.

the thyrohyoid membrane, resulting in airway obstruction as the epiglottis closes over the glottis. The distinction between this and the injury that results from hanging inflicted by a second party is that in accidental or self-inflicted injuries, death is not necessarily imminent; and, in those who survive, there is usually injury, possibly avulsion, at the level of the thyrohyoid membrane. In homicidal hanging, the person is usually dropped a distance of several feet, resulting in death secondary to tracheal transection or spinal cord injury from C_1-C_2 dislocation.[15]

Soft Tissue Injuries from Blunt Trauma

Blunt trauma to the larynx may result in soft tissue injuries with or without associated framework injuries. Rupture of the thyroepiglottic ligament can be associated with either horizontal or vertical fractures of the thyroid cartilage. Narrowing of the laryngeal lumen can occur secondary to herniation of pre-epiglottic tissue or posterior displacement of the epiglottic petiole.[7,11]

Vocal fold injuries result from vertical fractures of the thyroid ala (Figure 41–1). As the thyroid cartilage snaps back from its compression against the cervical vertebrae, the thyroarytenoid muscle and ligament may tear, resulting in a separation at any point along its length. This may be evident as mucosal lacerations or hemorrhage of one or both vocal folds. The mucosa on the arytenoids may be denuded or avulsed. Because of the traction on the arytenoids from this spring-like motion of the thyroid cartilage, the arytenoid cartilages may also become displaced from the cricoarytenoid joint into a more posterior and lateral or anterior position (Figure 41–8). If one segment of the thyroid cartilage fails to return back to its normal position, an overlapping fracture may occur, resulting in malposition of the vocal fold (Figures 41–9 and 41–10). Lacerations of the piriform sinus and upper esophagus may occur as the thyroid cartilage rubs against the cervical vertebrae.[7,11]

Soft tissue injuries associated with cricoid, tracheal, and cricotracheal separation injuries within the cartilaginous framework usually involve crushed or lacerated mucosa. Both recurrent laryngeal nerves are frequently injured and can be severed by blunt trauma that results in cricoid fractures and/or cricotracheal separation. The phrenic nerve can also be injured, especially in cases of cricotracheal separation.[7,9,11,12,15]

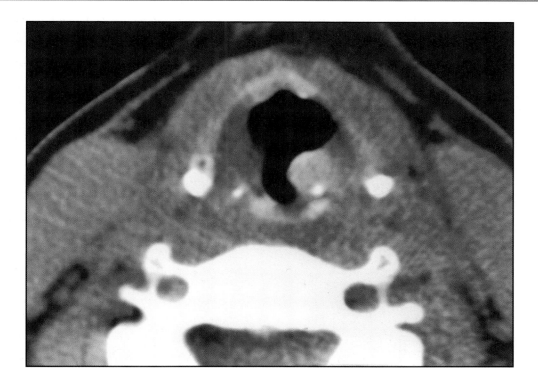

Figure 41–8. Axial CT scan of the larynx at the level of the arytenoids demonstrating anterior dislocation of the right arytenoid cartilage.

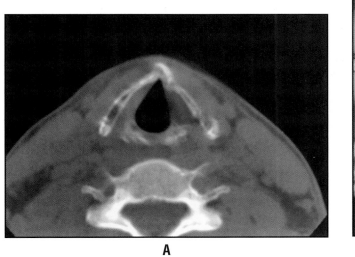

A

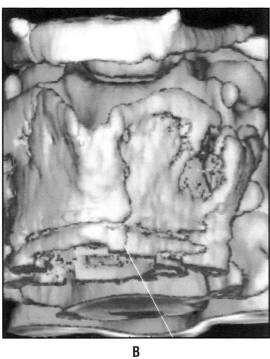

B

Figure 41–9. **A.** Axial CT scan of the subglottic larynx demonstrating a displaced, paramedian fracture of the left thyroid ala. **B.** 3-dimensional CT reconstruction of the left paramedian thyroid ala fracture demonstrating overlapping of the fracture segments.

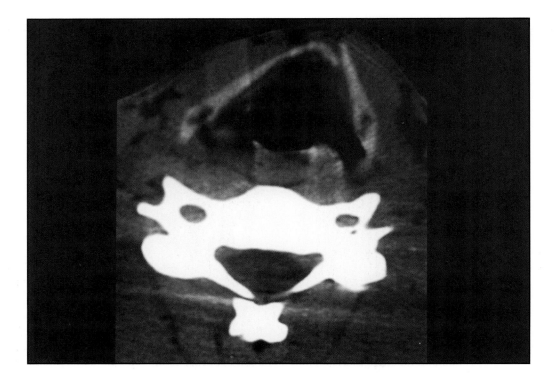

Figure 41–10. Axial CT of the supraglottic larynx. There is a displaced paramedian fracture of the right thyroid ala.

Associated esophageal lacerations and perforations are common.

Assessment of Blunt Injuries

Initial evaluation and assessment of the blunt trauma patient is similar for adults and children. It is important to obtain an understanding of the mechanism of injury. A high index of suspicion for blunt neck injury should be maintained in motor vehicle collisions, even without obvious external signs. Knowledge of the speed of the vehicle at the time of collision, the use of seatbelts by the trauma victim, and the presence and deployment of airbags can also be helpful in estimating the amount of force involved. In the patient with short stature, the force of deceleration against a locking "shoulder" strap that is draped over the neck may also produce significant injury. Assessment of the patient ́begins with evaluation and stabilization of the airway, paying particular attention to the status of the cervical spine. Assessment then proceeds with evaluation and stabilization of neurologic, cervical spine, cardiovascular, and other emergency organ system injuries. Management of aerodigestive tract injuries varies depending upon the presence of acute airway distress (Figure 41–11).

Evaluation of the Blunt Trauma Patient Without Airway Distress

In the patient without immediate signs of upper airway compromise, the evaluation can proceed with a complete examination, including palpation of the neck, assessment of voice quality, and flexible fiberoptic evaluation of the larynx and upper airway. Fiberoptic laryngoscopy allows assessment of the mobility of the vocal folds, patency of the upper airway, and integrity of the mucosa. If there is an adequate airway, intubation is not necessary. Because of the potential for the development of worsening laryngeal edema and airway compromise, serial examinations of the airway should be performed during the first 24 to 48 hours after injury if intubation is initially deemed unnecessary.

Management is based on the severity of the initial signs and symptoms.[16]

Patients with any sign of endolaryngeal injury (Table 41–1) should have a thin-cut (1 mm) computed tomography (CT) scan of the larynx with bone/cartilage windows to evaluate for possible laryngeal framework injury.[14,16,17] Minimally displaced fractures of the thyroid cartilage can be present with very mild endolaryngeal signs and should be evaluated to

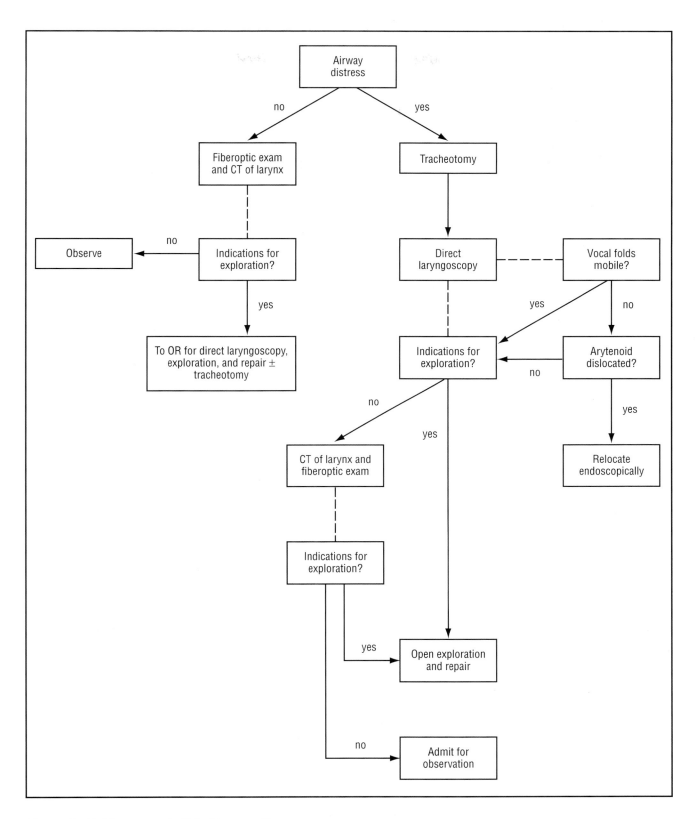

Figure 41–11. Management of blunt laryngeal trauma.

Table 41–1. Signs and Symptoms of Laryngeal Injury

Hoarseness/dysphonia	Dyspnea
Stridor	Endolaryngeal edema
Endolaryngeal hematoma	Subcutaneous emphysema
Endolaryngeal laceration	Neck pain/point tenderness
Dysphagia	Loss of laryngeal landmarks
Odynophagia	Impaired vocal fold mobility
Hemoptysis	Arytenoid dislocation
Ecchymosis/abrasions of anterior neck	Exposed endolaryngeal cartilage

determine the likelihood of fracture stability. Table 41–2 lists CT findings that suggest fracture stability and instability.

Fractures that appear to have the potential for instability should be evaluated further with direct laryngoscopy and open exploration for repair. Patients with minimally displaced fractures that are associated with significant endolaryngeal injuries also require direct laryngoscopy, open exploration, and repair of the soft tissue injuries (Table 41–3). Because of the high potential for concomitant cervical spine injuries, assessment of the cervical spine is always performed prior to operative intervention of the laryngeal injuries. The presence of a cervical spine injury may preclude the ability to perform a direct laryngoscopy, and repair is begun based on findings on CT scan and flexible endoscopic examination.

Patients without fractures on CT scanning and those with minimally displaced, stable fractures can be observed closely. Soft tissue injuries that consist of isolated mucosal lacerations of the supraglottic larynx, superficial lacerations of the nonvibrating edge of the true vocal fold, small hematomas of the true vocal fold, and/or mild mucosal edema may also be observed. Management of these patients includes the use of antibiotics, antireflux medications, reflux precautions, elevation of the head of bed, voice rest, and humidity. The use of antireflux medications and reflux precautions, including elevation of the head of the bed, help to limit additional inflammation and delays in wound healing caused by laryngopharyngeal reflux. Humidity helps to maintain lubrication of the vocal folds lubricated, which aids in the re-epithelialization process. The benefit of steroids in this scenario is controversial. The disadvantage of corticosteroids is that their anti-inflammatory action may interfere with and prolong the natural process of wound healing, and resulting in a prolonged healing phase. The advantage of using steroids is that they may minimize

the formation of granulation tissue and decrease laryngeal edema.[2,7,10,16,18,19] In the patient with mild to moderate mucosal edema, high-dose steroids are given during the first 24 to 48 hours to minimize mucosal edema acutely.

Evaluation of the Blunt Trauma Patient with Airway Distress

Signs of upper airway distress include stridor, sternal retraction, and dyspnea. The patient should be examined for signs of upper aerodigestive tract injury. In the presence of immediate post-traumatic airway distress, significant laryngotracheal injury is likely. The neck is stabilized to prevent worsening of unrecognized cervical spine injuries, and the airway is secured with a tracheotomy fashioned at least 2 rings below the injured segments or through the distal transected segment under local anesthesia.[1,2,7,9,12,20-25] Tracheotomy prevents further laryngeal injury, and may expose an unnoticed laryngotracheal separation. Orotracheal and/or nasotracheal intubation in the presence of severe laryngotracheal trauma can lead to further laryngeal injury and airway compromise.

In the child with upper airway distress, the airway is secured in the operating room, if time permits. General anesthesia is induced using an inhalational agent that is unlikely to cause laryngospasm. During spontaneous respiration, a rigid bronchoscope is passed gently through the injured larynx and trachea to a point distal to the sites of injury. Tracheotomy is performed over the bronchoscope followed by repair of the injuries.[10,13]

Operative evaluation of the larynx with direct laryngoscopy is performed after securing the airway. If direct laryngoscopy reveals significant endolaryngeal injuries (Table 41–3), open exploration and repair are performed. The presence of palpable laryngeal fractures is also an indication for open exploration and

Table 41–2. CT Findings That Suggest Fracture Stability

Fracture Type	Displacement	Likely Stable	Management
Single Vertical, Unilateral	Nondisplaced	yes	Observe, fixate if symptoms or exam worsen
	Minimally displaced (<1 cartilage width)	yes	Fixate if immediate or delayed voice change, otherwise observe
	Displaced (>1 cartilage width)	no	Reduce and fixate
Single Horizontal, Unilateral	Nondisplaced	yes	Observe, fixate if symptoms or exam worsen
	Minimally displaced	yes	Observe, fixate if symptoms or exam worsen
	Displaced	no	Reduce and fixate
Multiple Unilateral	Nondisplaced	no	Reduce and fixate
	Displaced	no	Reduce and fixate
Multiple Bilateral	Nondisplaced	no	Reduce and fixate
	Displaced	no	Reduce and fixate

Table 41–3. Indications for Operative Evaluation After Blunt Laryngeal Trauma

Laceration of vibrating edge of true vocal fold

Laceration of anterior commissure

Deep laceration of thyroarytenoid muscle

Exposed cartilage

Impaired vocal fold mobility

Arytenoid dislocation

Epiglottis displacement

Herniation of pre-epiglottic contents

Unstable/displaced laryngeal fractures

Airway compromise

Extensive endolaryngeal edema

repair. If direct laryngoscopy does not reveal a need for open exploration, then a postoperative CT of the larynx is obtained to complete the evaluation.

Surgical Evaluation

Intraoperative evaluation begins with direct laryngoscopy to assess the extent of endolaryngeal injury, esophagoscopy to assess for esophageal lacerations, and bronchoscopy to assess for subglottic and tracheobronchial injuries. The arytenoid cartilages are palpat-

ed for possible dislocation. In the patient with isolated cricoarytenoid joint dislocation, reduction can usually be accomplished endoscopically, especially if the dislocation is noted early. With delays in diagnosis beyond even a week, joint ankylosis can begin, making reduction more difficult. Nonetheless, an attempt should be made to relocate the arytenoid cartilage back to its normal position on the cricoid regardless of the interval from the time of injury. In cases of posterior dislocation, this can be accomplished by inserting the anterior lip of an intubating laryngoscope into the posterior aspect of the cricoarytenoid joint while exerting a lifting motion in an anteromedial direction on the arytenoid cartilage. Anterior dislocations can be reduced by exerting a posteriorly directed force on the cricoarytenoid joint using the tip of a rigid laryngoscope.[26,27] If no other injuries that require repair are noted on CT scan or on direct laryngoscopy, then open exploration is not necessary.

Open Exploration and Repair

Open exploration is performed to repair mucosal lacerations involving the anterior commissure and/or the vibratory edge of the vocal fold, to repair deep lacerations of the thyroarytenoid muscle, to restore mucosal cover over exposed cartilage, to reposition the vocal ligament and anterior commissure, to reposition a displaced epiglottis or herniated pre-epiglottic contents, to reanastomose separated segments, and to reduce and fixate displaced and/or unstable fractures. If not previously done, tracheotomy is performed to allow intraoperative access to the larynx and postoperative airway management.

Principles of Repair

The basic principles of repair follow the primary principles of wound healing elsewhere in the body. Repair within the first 24 hours after injury is most desirable to prevent granulation tissue formation from occurring prior to closure.[9,16] An attempt should be made to repair all mucosal lacerations and defects in order to promote healing by primary intention. Healing by secondary intention predisposes to a greater deposition of collagen and an increased likelihood of granulation tissue and scar formation, which may result in vibratory dysfunction, stenosis, or webbing of the vocal folds. All de-epithelialized areas that cannot be closed primarily without tension should be covered with local mucosal flaps to minimize scar formation. Free mucosal grafts can be used to cover de-epithelialized areas when local flaps cannot be fashioned; however, these are rarely needed. Fine, absorbable suture on an atraumatic needle also seems to help minimize granulation tissue formation.

Exposure

For open exploration, a horizontal neck incision is made and subplatysmal skin flaps are elevated. To expose the thyroid and cricoid cartilages, the strap muscles may be divided in the midline and retracted laterally. When endolaryngeal repair of soft tissue injuries is necessary, entry into the larynx is gained through fractures of the thyroid cartilage that are median or those that are paramedian and less than 0.5 cm from the midline. In patients with lateral or horizontal fractures of the thyroid cartilage, a midline thyrotomy is performed. A midline cut is then made through the anterior commissure under direct visualization, with care not to further disrupt the architecture of the vocal fold. Above the level of the glottis, the endolaryngeal incision is curved laterally to the epiglottis on one side to avoid cutting through its cartilage or mucosa. Care is taken during the exposure to avoid further injury to the recurrent and superior laryngeal nerves.

Endolaryngeal Repair

The functional goal of repair is to realign glottic tissues to their premorbid anteroposterior and transverse planes, beginning posteriorly and proceeding in an anterior direction to maximize exposure (Figure 41–12). The arytenoid is repositioned with meticulous closure of overlying mucoperichondrial defects. If the arytenoid mucosa is damaged badly, local rotation flaps can be developed from the piriform sinus or postcricoid region. Regardless of the extent of the injuries, an attempt should be made to repair severe unilateral and bilateral arytenoid injuries. Consideration of arytenoidectomy as a secondary procedure can be made at a later date after healing has occurred and the wounds have matured.[7] This approach allows for the possibility of vocalization and respiration if at least one of the arytenoids retains some function.

Lacerations in the thyroarytenoid muscle or mucosa may be repaired with fine, absorbable suture. Avascular and crushed mucosal injuries are debrided prior to closure. If primary closure of mucosal disruptions is difficult, local advancement or rotational flaps should be performed. Local advancement or rotational flaps from the piriform sinus or postcricoid region usually provide adequate coverage of the arytenoid and its vocal process. Adequate mucosa for coverage of the anterior commissure region usually can be obtained from the epiglottis. If an extensive amount of mucosa is needed, the epiglottic mucosa can be elevated off the laryngeal and lingual surfaces of the epiglottis with removal of the cartilage to allow for a large superiorly based epiglottic flap.[28] It is important to ensure meticulous closure and re-epithelialization of the anterior commissure region, as this is the region most likely to develop a web or stenosis as a late complication.

Mucosal defects on the false vocal fold and epiglottis are less likely to pose significant problems with stenosis. If primary repair or a local flap cannot be accomplished, this area can be left open to granulate and mucosalize by secondary intention. A ruptured thyroepiglottic ligament should be reattached anteriorly to reposition the epiglottis to its anatomic position. Herniated contents of the pre-epiglottic space should be removed or replaced anterior to the epiglottis and the thyroepiglottic ligament.

The attachment of the vocal ligament at the anterior commissure is inspected. If torn, it is repaired by placing a slow-absorbing monofilament suture through the anterior aspect of the ligament and bringing it through a midline fracture to secure to the thyroid cartilage. If the fracture is paramedian, the suture is brought through the midline of the cartilage and secured. It is important to re-establish the appropriate height of the vocal fold as well as the appropriate midline placement for optimal postoperative voice results. Proper placement of the vocal ligament helps to ensure the proper position of the remainder of the vocal fold.

Table 41–4. Indications for Operative Evaluation of Penetrating Laryngeal Injury.

Endolaryngeal lacerations

Expanding neck hematoma

Subcutaneous emphysema

Audible air leak from neck wound

Hemoptysis

Laryngeal framework disruption

Impaired vocal fold mobility

Endolaryngeal edema

Dysphagia/odynophagia

Stridor/dyspnea

have been reported in as many as 20 to 50% of the patients with laryngeal injuries, esophagoscopy should also be performed at the time of rigid endoscopy.[5,38]

Repair of Penetrating Injuries

Repair of penetrating laryngeal injuries and postoperative management is accomplished in a similar fashion as would be done with the blunt trauma patient. In patients with combined esophageal and posterior tracheal wall injuries, consideration should be made for placing a muscle interposition flap between the trachea and esophagus to prevent the formation of a tracheo-esophageal fistula. This can be accomplished with the use of a nearby pedicled strap or sternocleidomastoid muscle flap.

CAUSTIC AND THERMAL INJURIES

Caustic and thermal injuries to the larynx can cause significant acute and chronic airway compromise as well as late vocal complications. Caustic injuries occur in both the adult and pediatric populations. Caustic injuries can result from ingestion of bases, acids, or bleaches. The most severe injuries are caused by bases which produce a liquefaction necrosis of muscle, collagen, and lipids with progressively worsening injury over time. Acids cause a coagulation necrosis that occurs more rapidly and tends to damage superficial structures only. In children under age 5, these tend to be accidental ingestions. Adolescent and adult ingestions usually are suicide attempts, and, thus, tend to produce the most severe injuries.[42,43]

Caustic ingestions most often affect the oral cavity, pharynx, and esophagus, but can occasionally contact the larynx and result in edema and mucosal disruption secondary to burn injury. Because the epiglottis and false vocal folds are the initial barriers in preventing aspiration, the laryngeal edema typically seen in caustic ingestions involves the epiglottis and supraglottic larynx, often sparing the true vocal folds.[42,44] The larynx is examined in all caustic ingestions. Of particular concern is the ingestion of low-phosphate or nonphosphate detergents. Ingestions of even small amounts of these may cause severe upper airway edema and airway compromise 1 to 5 hours after ingestion and warrant admission to the hospital for airway observation even in the absence of other significant injuries.[44] If significant edema or stridor is present, the airway should be stabilized with tracheotomy. Because of the potential for exacerbating the laryngeal injuries, nasotracheal and orotracheal intubation are avoided; tracheotomy is the preferred method of airway stabilization. The mouth, pharynx, and laryngeal inlet should be irrigated with water to remove any remnants of the offending agent. The use of steroids and antibiotics remains common but controversial. Further evaluation and management of esophageal injuries should then proceed. A discussion of the protocol for evaluation and treatment of esophageal injuries is beyond the scope of this chapter but can be found elsewhere.[42,43,45,46]

Thermal laryngeal injuries are usually encountered in patients who have experienced significant burn injuries from closed-space fires.[47] The laryngeal injuries most often result from thermal insult to the supraglottic and glottic larynx.[48] Because inhalational injuries may affect the larynx, tracheobronchial tree, or the lung parenchyma, all patients experiencing significant inhalational injuries should undergo flexible laryngoscopy and bronchoscopy. The diagnosis of laryngeal or tracheal injury is made by the presence of carbonized materials with inflammation, edema, or necrosis.[47] In patients with hypovolemic shock, as commonly occurs in patients with significant burn injuries, there may be severe injury to the larynx or trachea without signs of edema initially. The edema usually ensues with cardiovascular resuscitation.[49] The epiglottis, aryepiglottic folds, and hypopharynx are most prone to edema, which is usually progressive in the first few hours after injury.[49]

The primary concern is protection of the airway. The decision to perform tracheotomy versus endotracheal intubation is controversial. Orotracheal and nasotracheal intubation carry the risk of causing further mucosal injury. There have been several studies to suggest that tracheotomy in the burn patient places the patient at increased risk of long-term sequelae such as tracheal stenosis and sepsis.[48,50,51] In general, tracheotomy is recommended in patients who cannot be endotracheally intubated because of significant laryngeal injury, those who fail extubation, and/or those in whom prolonged respiratory support will be necessary.[47,49,52]

Late complications associated with thermal and caustic injuries include stenosis and webbing. Scar formation may continue for several months following the initial insult.[47] Thus, the larynx and trachea should be serially evaluated over the course of several months. Repair is delayed until scar formation has stabilized. This helps to minimize the incidence of recurrent scar formation and enhances the likelihood of successful repair.[47,49]

IATROGENIC INJURIES

Iatrogenic injuries to the larynx include radiation injuries and injuries that result from intubation. Doses of radiation used to treat head and neck cancer (6,000 cGy–7,000 cGy) can result in injury to the mucosa and cartilaginous framework of the larynx if it is included in the radiation field. These injuries are an expected outcome of radiation therapy and can include mucosal drying, soft tissue edema, and laryngeal radionecrosis. The treatment of mucosal drying is symptomatic, encouraging frequent water ingestion. Several preparations are available to minimize xerostomia in patients receiving radiation therapy to the head and neck. These work with variable success. Laryngeal edema from radiation can become problematic, resulting in narrowing of the airway. In some patients, this can be treated effectively with intermittent steroid use. In others, tracheotomy is necessary to help maintain an adequate airway.[53]

The incidence of radionecrosis of the larynx is approximately 1% of patients who receive doses in the range of 6,000 cGy to 7,000 cGy and increases with larger daily fractions.[54] Patients who continue to smoke or drink alcohol during and after radiation therapy are at increased risk. The presence of laryngopharyngeal reflux may contribute to the development and exacerbation of radionecrosis. Radionecrosis can pose a diagnostic dilemma to the clinician, as the symptoms are similar to the symptoms of recurrent cancer and there is often associated edema and/or ulceration overlying the devitalized tissue. It is often difficult to distinguish between recurrent or persistent tumor and radionecrosis. These patients should undergo direct laryngoscopy and biopsy. Biopsy of radiation-damaged tissue often shows necrotic debris. However, in an inadequately biopsied

area, a similar specimen can be obtained in the face of recurrent tumor. Although deep biopsies may exacerbate necrosis, tumor recurrence must be ruled out.[54] Hyperbaric oxygen treatments can be offered to patients with radionecrosis of the larynx, as the increased tissue oxygenation induced by such treatments may promote healing and prevent further damage to the laryngeal framework.[55,56] If the signs and symptoms worsen or are not improved with conservative treatment, partial or total laryngectomy should be considered because of the risk of a life-threatening infection with a retained necrotic larynx and because of the high risk of malignancy in this scenario.[54-56]

The most common iatrogenic injury to the larynx results from intubation trauma.[57] Because children are more often subjected to prolonged intubation as premature infants and neonates in the intensive care unit, they are more likely to experience complications as a result of being intubated.[58] The reported incidence of intubation injury in adults and children has decreased in the last 20 years from 18% to 3% because of improved equipment and methods of intubation.[11] The advent of low-pressure cuffed endotracheal tubes of uniform diameter has significantly decreased the incidence of subglottic stenosis. In addition, the development of ventilator adapters to prevent excessive movement of the endotracheal tube has also contributed to a decrease in the incidence of intubation trauma.[11,57]

In neonates, prolonged intubation often leads to circumferential granulation tissue, scarring, and eventual stenosis of the subglottis. This region is most often affected because the cricoid is the narrowest portion of the airway in the neonate and is, thus, most traumatized by the endotracheal tube. The posterior tilt of the cricoid cartilage in neonates likely helps to prevent damage to the interarytenoid region, which is the most common site of injury in the adult.

Subglottic stenosis in the infant from intubation injury can be managed similarly to congenital subglottic stenosis. For stenoses that are less than 50% obstructing, management can consist of observation, dilatation, or CO_2 laser excision. If CO_2 laser is used for a circumferential stenosis, it is done serially with no more than 30% of the circumference resected during any one procedure to prevent restenosis. If the stenosis is 50 to 70% obstructing, one may consider either endoscopic procedures or open procedures, depending on the location and potential ease of an endoscopic procedure. Stenotic regions that are more than 70% obstructing are best managed using open techniques. Lesions isolated to the subglottic region may be treated with an anterior cricoid split procedure. Longer stenotic regions may be treated with either cartilage grafting or resection with end-to-end anastomosis. Completely stenotic regions require resection and reanastomosis.[59]

In the adult, the glottis is the narrowest portion of the airway, and the posterior glottis often supports the endotracheal tube in the adult. Movement of the arytenoids against the endotracheal tube with respiration often contributes to ischemic necrosis of the thin mucosa overlying the vocal process. This can be followed by ulceration, chondritis, granulation, granuloma formation, and scarring. Often, removal of the endotracheal tube will allow for normal healing in the absence of gastroesophageal reflux, which should be treated presumptively during the healing process.

Scarring of the posterior glottis uncommonly causes problems with airway compromise. Attempts to release posterior glottic scar bands usually should be avoided to prevent worsening stenosis unless substantial symptoms justify the risks. In cases of significant airway compromise and minimal posterior scarring, treatment with microscopic direct laryngoscopy and carbon dioxide laser division of the scar band is usually successful.[60] Care should be taken during these divisions to protect the normal mucosa of the interarytenoid region.[61] Occasionally, repeat microscopic direct laryngoscopy with repeat laser division is needed. In cases with moderate to severe interarytenoid scarring, a laryngofissure with a mucosal advancement flap from the interarytenoid notch or from an aryepiglottic fold or a similar endoscopic procedure can be performed.[62] The value of adjunctive treatment with topical mitomycin-C to prevent restenosis is being studied currently, but preliminary results are encouraging.[63]

CONCLUSION

Injury to the laryngotracheal complex can result from blunt, penetrating, caustic, thermal, and iatrogenic insults. The primary concern in the initial management of these injuries is the establishment and maintenance of an adequate airway. Treatment can then address the reconstruction of the normal anatomic relationships of the larynx and trachea in an attempt to restore the normal phonatory, respiratory, and protective functions of the larynx.

REFERENCES

1. Bent JB, Silver JR, Porubsky ES. Acute laryngeal trauma: a review of 77 patients. Otolaryngol Head Neck Surg. 1993;109:441-449.
2. Schaefer SD. The treatment of acute external laryngeal injuries. Arch Otolaryngol Head Neck Surg. 1991;117:35-39.
3. Jewett BS, Shockley WW, Rutledge R. External laryngeal trauma analysis of 392 patients. Arch Otolaryngol Head Neck Surg. 1999;125:877-880.
4. Gussack GS, Jurkovich GJ, Luterman A. Laryngotracheal trauma: a protocol approach to a rare injury. Laryngoscope. 1986;96:660-665.
5. Minard G, Kudsk KA, Croce MA, Butts JA, Cicala RS, Fabian TC. Laryngotracheal trauma. Am Surg. 1992;58:181-187.
6. Holinger PH, Schild JA. Pharyngeal, laryngeal, and tracheal injuries in the pediatric age group. Ann Otol Rhinol Laryngol. 1972;81:538-545.
7. Pennington CL. External trauma of the larynx and trachea: immediate treatment and management. Ann Otol Rhinol Laryngol. 1972;81:546-554.
8. Travis LW, Olson NR, Melvin JW, Snyder JG. Static and dynamic impact trauma of the human larynx. Am Acad Ophthalmol Otolaryngol. 1975;80:382-390.
9. Ashbaugh DG, Gordon JG. Traumatic avulsion of the trachea associated with cricoid fracture. J Thorac Cardiovasc Surg. 1975;69:800-803.
10. Gold SM, Gerber ME, Shott SR, Myer CM 3rd. Blunt laryngotracheal trauma in children. Arch Otolaryngol Head Neck Surg. 1997;123:83-87.
11. Bryce DP. Current management of laryngotracheal injury. Adv Oto-Rhino-Laryngol. 1983;29:27-38.
12. Ford HR, Gardner MJ, Lynch JM. Laryngotracheal disruption from blunt pediatric neck injuries: impact of early recognition and intervention on outcome. J Pediatr Surg. 1995;30:331-334.
13. Myer CM 3rd, Orobello P, Cotton RT, Bratcher GO. Blunt laryngeal trauma in children. Laryngoscope. 1987;97:1043-1048.
14. Offia CJ, Endres D. Isolated laryngotracheal separation following blunt trauma to the neck. J Laryngol Otol. 1997;111:1079-1081.
15. Alonso WA, Caruso VG, Roncace EA. Minibikes, a new factor in laryngotracheal trauma. Ann Otol Rhinol Laryngol. 1973;82:800-804.
16. Schaefer SD, Close LG. Acute management of laryngeal trauma. Update. Ann Otol Rhinol Laryngol. 1989;98:98-104.
17. Schild JA, Denneny EC. Evaluation and treatment of acute laryngeal fractures. Head Neck 1989;11:491-496.
18. Olson NR. Surgical treatment of acute blunt laryngeal injuries. Ann Otol Rhinol Laryngol. 1978;87:716-721.
19. Lucente E, Mitrani M, Sacks SH, Biller HF. Penetrating injuries of the larynx. Ear Nose Throat J. 1985;64:406-415.
20. Reece CP, Shatney CH. Blunt injuries to the cervical trachea: review of 51 patients. South Med J. 1988;81:1542-1547.
21. Chodosh PL. Cricoid fracture with tracheal avulsion. Arch Otolaryngol. 1968;87:461-467.
22. Harris HH. Management of injuries to the larynx and trachea. Laryngoscope. 1972;82:1924-1929.
23. Ogura J. Management of traumatic injuries of the larynx and trachea including stenosis. J Laryngol Otol. 1971;85:1259-1261.

24. Trone TH, Schaefer SD, Carder HM. Blunt and penetrating laryngeal trauma: a 13 year review. *Otolaryngol Head Neck Surg.* 1980;88:257-261.

25. Fuhrman GM, Stieg FH, Buerk CA. Blunt laryngeal trauma: classification and management protocol. *J Trauma.* 1990;30:87-92.

26. Sataloff RT, Feldman M, Darby KS, Carroll LM, Spiegel JR. Arytenoid dislocation. *J Voice.* 1987;1:368-377.

27. Sataloff RT, Bough ID, Spiegel JR. Arytenoid dislocation: diagnosis and treatment. *Laryngoscope.* 1994;104:1353-1361.

28. Olson NR. Laryngeal suspension and epiglottic flap in laryngopharyngeal trauma. *Ann Otol Rhinol Laryngol.* 1976; 85:533-537.

29. Thomas GK, Stevens MH. Stenting in experimental laryngeal injuries. *Arch Otolaryngol.* 1975;101:217-221.

30. Woo P, Kellman R. Laryngeal framework reconstruction with miniplates: indications and extended indications in 27 cases. *Oper Tech Otolaryngol Head Neck Surg.* 1972;3:159-164.

31. Woo P. Laryngeal framework reconstruction with miniplates. *Ann Otol Rhinol Laryngol.* 1990;99:772-777.

32. Pou AM, Shoemaker DL, Carrau RL, Snyderman CH, Eibling DE. Repair of laryngeal fractures using adaptation plates. *Head Neck.* 1998;20:707-713.

33. Grillo HC, Donahue DM, Mathisen DJ, Wain JC, Wright CD. Postintubation tracheal stenosis: treatment and results. *J Thorac Cardiovasc Surg.* 1994;109:486-493.

34. Crumley RL. Teflon versus thyroplasty versus nerve transfer: a comparison. *Ann Otol Rhinol Laryngol.* 1990;99:759-763.

35. Crumley RL. Update: ansa cervicalis to recurrent laryngeal nerve anastomosis for unilateral laryngeal paralysis. *Laryngoscope.* 1991;101:384-388.

36. Little FB, Koufman JA, Kohut RI, Marshall RB. Effects of gastric acid on the pathogenesis of subglottic stenosis. *Ann Otol Rhinol Laryngol.* 1985;94:516-519.

37. Harrison DF. Bullet wounds of the larynx and trachea. *Arch Otolaryngol.* 1984;110:203-205.

38. Grewal H, Rao PM, Mukerji S, Ivatury RR. Management of penetrating laryngotracheal injuries. *Head Neck.* 1995;17:494-502.

39. Feliciano DV, Bitondo CG, Mattox KL, et al. Combined tracheoesophageal injuries. *Am J Surg.* 1985;150:710-715.

40. Defore WW, Mattox KL, Hansen HA, Garcia-Rinaldi R, Beall AC, DeBakey ME. Surgical management of penetrating injuries to the esophagus. *Am J Surg.* 1977;134:734-737.

41. Glatterer MS Jr, Toon RS, Ellestad C, et al. Management of blunt and penetrating external esophageal trauma. *J Trauma.* 1985;25:784-792.

42. Hawkins DB, Demefer MJ, Barnett TE. Caustic ingestion: controversies in management. A review of 214 cases. *Laryngoscope.* 1980;90:98-109.

43. Schild JA. Caustic ingestion in adult patients. *Laryngoscope.* 1985;95:1199-1201.

44. Einhorn A, Horton L, Altieri M, Ochsenschlager D, Klein B. Serious respiratory consequences of detergent ingestions in children. *Pediatrics.* 1989;84:472-474.

45. Holinger LD. Caustic ingestion, esophageal injury and stricture. In: Holinger LD, Lusk RP, Green CG, eds. *Pediatric Laryngology and Bronchoesophagology.* Philadelphia, PA: Lippincott-Raven Publishers; 1997:295-304.

46. Wijburg FA, Beukers MM, Heymans HS, Bartelsman JF, den Hartog Jager FC. Nasogastric intubation as sole treatment of caustic esophageal lesions. *Ann Otol Rhinol Laryngol.* 1985;94:337-341.

47. Jones JE, Rosenberg D. Management of laryngotracheal thermal trauma in children. *Laryngoscope.* 1995;105:540-542.

48. Moylan J. Smoke inhalation and burn injury. *Surg Clin North Am.* 1980;60:1533-1540.

49. Miller RP, Gray SD, Cotton RT, Myer CM 3rd. Airway reconstruction following laryngotracheal thermal trauma. *Laryngoscope.* 1988;98:826-829.

50. Lund T, Goodwin CW, McManus WF, et al. Upper airway sequelae in burn patient requiring endotracheal intubation or tracheostomy. *Ann Surg.* 1985;201:374-382.

51. Eckhauser FE, Billote J, Burke JF, Quinby WC. Tracheotomy complicating massive burn injury. *Am J Surg.* 1974;127:418-423.

52. Calhoun KH, Deskin RW, Gorza C, et al. Long-term airway sequelae in a pediatric burn population. *Laryngoscope.* 1988;98:721-725.

53. Calcaterra TC, Stern FS, Ward PH. Dilemma of delayed radiation injury of the larynx. *Ann Otol.* 1972;81:501-507.

54. Parsons JT. The effect of radiation on normal tissues of the head and neck. In: Million RR, Cassisi NJ, eds. *Management of Head and Neck Cancer: A Multidisciplinary Approach.* Philadelphia, PA: JB Lippincott Co; 1984:183-184.

55. Feldmeier JJ, Heimback RD, Davold DA, Brakora MJ. Hyperbaric oxygen as an adjunctive treatment for severe laryngeal necrosis: a report of nine consecutive cases. *Undersea Hyperbaric Med.* 1993;20:329-335.

56. Ferguson BJ, Hudson WR, Farmer JC Jr. Hyperbaric oxygen therapy for laryngeal radionecrosis. *Ann Otol Rhinol Laryngol.* 1987;9:1-6.

57. Richardson MA. Laryngeal anatomy and mechanisms of trauma. *Ear Nose Throat J.* 1981;60:346-351.

58. Cotton RT, Seid AB. Management of the extubation problem in the premature child. *Ann Otol Rhinol Laryngol.* 1980;89:508-511.

59. Lusk RP, Wooley AL, Holinger LD. Laryngotracheal stenosis. In: Holinger LD, Lusk RP, Green CG, eds. *Pediatric Laryngology and Bronchoesophagology.* Philadelphia, PA: Lippincott-Raven Publishers; 1997:172-184.

60. Dedo HH, Rowe LD. Laryngeal reconstruction in acute and chronic injuries. *Otolaryngol Clin North Am.* 1983;16:373-389.

61. Dedo HH, Sooy FA. Endoscopic laser repair of posterior glottic, subglottic, and tracheal stenosis by division or micro-trapdoor flap. *Laryngoscope.* 1984;94:445-450.

62. Dedo HH, Sooy FA. Surgical repair of late glottic stenosis. *Ann Otol Rhinol Laryngol.* 1968;77:435-441.

63. Correa AJ, Reinisch L, Sanders DL, et al. Inhibition of subglottic stenosis with mitomycin-C in the canine model. *Ann Otol Rhinol Laryngol.* 1999;108:1053-1060.

42

Surgical Management of Benign Voice Disorders

Mark S. Courey, MD
Robert H. Ossoff, DMD, MD

Surgical management of benign voice disorders is predicated on a sound understanding of laryngeal anatomy, histology, physiology, and pathophysiology. It makes no sense to treat an ankle fracture with a foot amputation. Similarly, it seems to make little sense to treat diseases that arise in the subepithelial tissue by stripping normal laryngeal epithelium and cover. This important aspect in the surgical management of benign voice disorders—the preservation of surrounding normal tissue with as little disruption as possible—is crucial to the return of normal laryngeal function postoperatively.[1] To achieve this goal, surgical precision is aided by magnification and delicate laryngeal instrumentation. Furthermore, the timing of surgical intervention to coincide with minimal-surrounding inflammation, whenever possible, needs to be manipulated to the patient's and surgeon's benefit. Patients must be informed of the risks and benefits of surgical intervention. They need to realize that good results from voice surgery rely on adequate preoperative preparation as well as postoperative rehabilitation.[2] Just as orthopedic surgeons

would not consider joint replacement until preoperative medical management and physical therapy have been exhausted, laryngologists should not consider vocal fold surgery for benign lesions until this same attention has been given to preoperative voice management. In addition, orthopedic surgeons have found that postoperative rehabilitation is crucial to the success of their surgical procedures, and they initiate therapy as soon as possible during recovery. This same attention to postoperative rehabilitation seems to serve us well when applied to the management of benign voice disorders.

Benign vocal fold abnormalities have been discussed in chapter 6. In review, they consist of vocal fold nodules or polyps, vocal fold cysts (mucus retention or epidermal inclusion), vascular malformations, sulcus vocalis, polypoid corditis, and others. Knowledge of the initiating site of these lesions is imperative for successful surgical management. Briefly, inflammation and trauma, most commonly from abusive phonation, lead to shearing stress and strain in the superficial portion of the lamina propria. The body's reaction to this repeated trauma leads to the development of lesions such as polypoid corditis, polyps, nodules, and possibly cysts.

The surgical management of these lesions, which arise in the subepithelial tissue is directed at the subepithelial tissue. Many of these lesions, with the exception of nodules and some polyps, arise deeply enough within the superficial layer of the lamina propria (SLLP), that the basement membrane zone (BMZ) of the epithelium and the overlying portion of the SLLP are normal. In these instances, this tissue can and should be preserved. On the other hand, the surgical management of lesions involving the BMZ will require excision of a portion of the BMZ with the overlying epithelium. It is not technically possible to separate the epithelium from the supportive structure of the BMZ,[3] nor would it be necessary as re-epithelialization occurs reliably and rapidly over remaining vocal fold structures.[4] In either case, surgical manipulation of the surrounding normal tissue should be kept to a minimum.

PREOPERATIVE MANAGEMENT

Preoperative management relies on obtaining an accurate history, performing a complete physical examination, and performing and interpreting the videoendostroboscopic examination. These factors aid in diagnosis.[5] Often the diagnosis is not apparent at the first office visit and requires multiple or serial examinations to identify the subtle physical and stroboscopic findings. In addition, because the disorders are benign, and are most commonly caused by inefficient vocal behaviors, the surgeon should allow time to accurately diagnose and assess the effect that the lesion has on both the speaking and the singing voice before the initiation of surgical therapy. For men, periodic interval examinations may take place in 1-, 2-, or 4-week intervals as necessary. In women of childbearing age, however, serial examinations should take place at odd-week intervals, 1, 3, or 5, to assess the effect that menstruation may have on the physical appearance and function of the larynx.

If the diagnosis cannot be established through the interval examination process alone, then therapeutic measures such as voice rest, modification of voice use through speech therapy, and/or voice training may help establish the diagnosis. These measures, which are designed to reduce the causative factors of vocal abuse and misuse, aid in diagnosis by reducing changes and edema in the surrounding tissue. This al-

ters either the initiating or the compensatory vocal behavior. Still, even after vocal modification and serial examination, establishing the diagnosis may not be possible. If the voice disorder is severe, and a suitable voice cannot be achieved and maintained through vocal behavior modification and elimination of other potential sources of trauma, then direct operative microlaryngoscopy with vocal fold palpation and possible exploration is indicated for accurate diagnosis and therapy.

Before surgical intervention, the voice disability must be evaluated in the light of modified vocal behavior. This is necessary to assess the lesion's absolute effect in the life of the patient.[1,6] Surgical therapy is not without risk. Though small, the chance of postoperative scarring from even simple palpation or intubation exists, and the patient should be made aware of this possibility. Therefore, any possible behavior modification that may improve the speaking or singing voice should be employed before surgical intervention.

Initial behavior modification steps are aimed at the identification and elimination of vocal abuse and misuse through vocal abuse reduction programs and the adaptation of methods of efficient voice production. These steps, along with the elimination of harmful substances such as tobacco products, caffeine and high-fat or dairy products, and hydration, improve vocal fold lubrication and promote vocal hygiene.[7] After the abuses have been eliminated, assessment of the vocal mechanism for both the speaking and the singing voice helps identify and correct misuses.

These behavior modification measures have several benefits. First, they aid in diagnosis. Second, proper vocal technique improves function. Third, behavior modification has been shown to reduce the recurrence rate of vocal nodules postoperatively.[8,9] Finally, these measures promote vocal health and may have the added benefit of allowing the patient to continue to function with the pathologic lesion in place.[10] With close observation the patients can then continue their work schedule. Surgery or definitive therapy can be postponed indefinitely or until timing is ideal.

Prior to choosing surgical intervention patients need to understand that postoperative rehabilitation from surgical therapy usually requires between 8 and 12 weeks and that their compliance with these recommendations will have a substantial effect on their overall outcome. This type of postoperative rehabilitation necessitates substantial freedom from work responsibilities and requires considerable effort by the patient and the patient's employer to allow adequate time.

Informed Consent

The risks and benefits of surgery need to be discussed at length with the patient prior to intervention. Surgery is not indicated solely by the presence of a benign-appearing laryngeal lesion, but rather by the troublesome dysphonia that results from the lesion's interference with the normal vibratory patterns. Behavioral and medical intervention may allow patients to develop improved functional capabilities and with these improvements some patients may no longer believe that they require a surgical intervention to fulfill their daily vocal activities. In addition, in spite of improved surgical techniques, healing can still be unpredictable and may lead to worsening of the speaking or singing voice. Patients need to be aware of these possibilities preoperatively and must be willing to accept rare but potentially devastating vocal risks before proceeding. Typically, features that prompt us to recommend surgery include: a failure of the vocal capabilities to improve with medical and/or behavioral management; worsening appearance or enlargement of the vocal fold lesion on interval examination despite medical and/or behavioral management; and the patient's perception and our objective documentation of continued unacceptable limitations in daily vocal activity despite improvement with medical and behavioral therapy. Under these circumstances, the potential benefits of surgery outweigh the possible risks.

The length of the postoperative recuperative period also needs to be discussed with patients preoperatively. Healing of the operative site and resolution of edema need to occur before the resumption of full vocal activity. Heavy use of the vocal mechanism before sufficient healing may result in the development of vocal hyperfunction as the patient uses excess tension to overcome a stiff or edematous vocal fold. The recuperative period may take 8 to 12 weeks or occasionally longer and needs to be tailored to the individual patient based on the physical appearance and characteristics of the healing vocal fold as determined by interval videoendostroboscopic examinations performed during the postoperative rehabilitation period. General guidelines, however, can be discussed with the patient, and the patient can be informed that failure to comply with these restrictions may affect the overall permanent result.

SURGICAL PRINCIPLES— EXPOSURE AND ENDOSCOPES

Endoscopic surgery, like other surgical techniques, relies first on exposure. The largest-caliber laryngoscope that can be comfortably placed in the patient is used. A large variety of laryngoscopes is available, and surgeons should identify several with which they are most comfortable. Preferably, these will permit binocular viewing and be of large enough caliber to allow working space for at least two microlaryngeal instruments simultaneously. For most glottic work, nonhinged microlaryngoscopes of the Holinger or Dedo variety with an upward flair at the distal tip are simple to use and provide adequate exposure of the vocal folds and anterior commissure. The traditional Dedo microlaryngoscope has been enlarged to improve binocular vision and allow greater room for instrumentation (Figure 42–1).[11] Similarly, modifications of the Holinger-type anterior commissure laryngoscope also allow binocular vision and provide enhanced space for instrumentation (Figure 42–2).[12] Other characteristics of useful laryngoscopes include improved lighting for better visualization and photographic documentation and built-in smoke evacuation channels for use with carbon dioxide laser. Finally, some surgeons prefer straight laryngoscopes without an upward flair at the distal tip. In their hands these laryngoscopes provide an unobstructed view of the anterior commissure and allow easier manipulation of this region.[13] The reader is encouraged to become familiar with several different types of laryngoscopes. Anatomic differences between patients will require dexterity on the part of the surgeon to achieve optimal exposure.

Once the laryngoscope is inserted, the application of a suspension device with complete patient relaxation provides a stable field for inspection, manipulation, and surgical intervention. In delicate microlaryngeal surgery, where precision is of the utmost importance, this is preferable to indirect methods or methods under local anesthesia in which patient movement may be disastrous.[14]

Inspection and documentation are performed with the aid of large-caliber 0°, 30°, and 70° telescopes. These provide excellent monocular optics for visualization and can be coupled with either a video, digital, or 35-mm camera for teaching or documentation purposes.[15] The medial surface of the vocal fold is inspected and the exact extent of the lesion from upper vocal fold lip to lower lip is determined.

Binocular vision is next obtained with the use of an operating microscope. Typically, the 400-mm focal length lens provides good visualization and allows adequate working space. Some surgeons, however, feel more comfortable with a 350-mm focal lens.[16] High magnification with binocular microscope enhances visualization. Typical microscope optics with 1.6 to 2.5 power magnification of the distal lens combined with the 10 or 12.5 magnification of the eyepiece

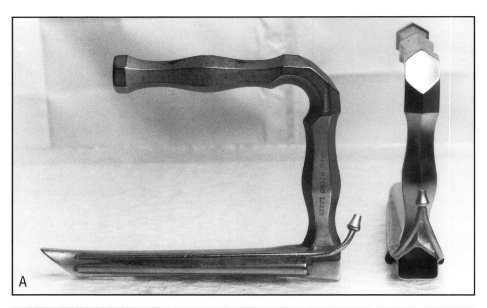

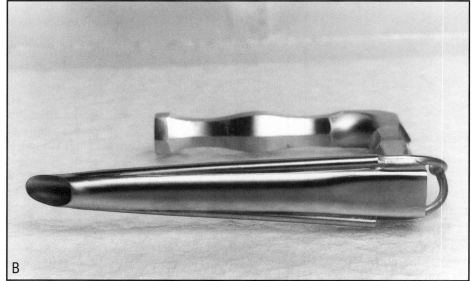

Figure 42–1. The Ossoff-Karlan modified Dedo laryngoscope. Important features include the upward flare at the distal tip to improve visualization at the anterior commissure, a built-in smoke evacuation port to facilitate use with the laser, and the expanded proximal port to improve visualization. **A.** Lateral view showing upward flair at the distal tip. **B.** View of the undersurface showing taper of laryngoscope and relative size of light channels.

and the focal length of the tube, allow overall magnification of the operative field by at least 6.8 to 12 times.

SURGICAL PRINCIPLES—INSTRUMENTATION

Newer microsurgical techniques are aimed at the preservation of surrounding normal structure. Knowledge of laryngeal anatomy, embryology, and physiology are essential for understanding laryngeal pathologic lesions and theories of their causes. This knowledge will then help direct the surgical approach. For most benign laryngeal lesions, standard cold knife excision techniques are preferable to laser excision techniques.[17] Surgical instrumentation has been improved to provide smaller equipment that is more appropriate for endolaryngeal use. New microscissors, knives, elevators, probes, cup forceps, and suction devices are available in 1- to 4-mm sizes.[18] Instrumentation of this size is essential for delicate and precise excision (Figure 42–3). Currently, several instrument companies produce this microlaryngeal instrumentation. The surgeon is encouraged to work with local representatives to find instruments with

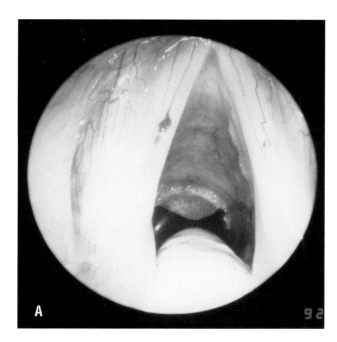

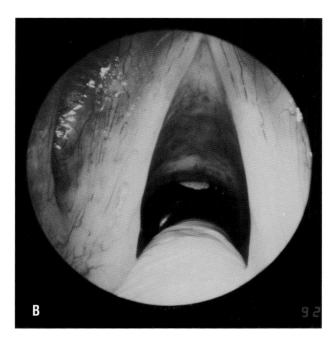

Figure 42–8. A patient with multiple vascular lesions that have been noted to hemorrhage repeatedly. **A.** Preoperative appearance. **B.** Postoperative appearance immediately following photocoagulation with the CO_2 laser at 1500 W/cm².

VOCAL FOLD CYSTS

The etiology of vocal fold cysts is uncertain. Vocal fold cysts are either mucosal retention cysts or epidermal inclusion cysts.[32] Mucosal retention cysts are presumed to arise secondary to obstruction of an excretory duct. The wall of the duct consists of cuboidal epithelium. How these excretory ducts come to lie in the true vocal fold, however, is uncertain, as the vocal fold itself normally has no salivary gland tissue. Presumably these mucosal retention cysts arise from ducts in the subglottis or supraglottis that then, secondary to pressure, migrate or expand into the area of the true glottis. If the cyst is of a presumed congenital nature, then the patient should have a lifelong history of dysphonia. Epidermal inclusion cysts, on the other hand, may be acquired secondary to recurrent vocal fold trauma. This trauma causes an infolding of the mucosa, which then breaks off and forms an inclusion cyst.

In either case the cysts are submucosal and are more frequently unilateral.[16] Their outline may be visualized with steady light examination. Videostroboscopy will enhance their outline and may show a significantly decreased or absent mucosal wave over the area of the cyst.[33] Surgical excision takes place after exposure is achieved. A sickle knife is used to make an incision on the superior surface of the vocal fold laterally, near the ventricle (Figure 42–9A). This place is chosen for the incision site for two reasons. First, the normal anatomy is relatively well-preserved, facilitating identification of the vocal ligament, and second, scarring and contracture on the lateral superior vocal fold have minimal effect on laryngeal vibratory patterns. The incision is finished with the up-cutting microscissors (Figure 42–9B). As in the case of submucosal scarring, a blunt elevator is inserted and used to separate superficial layers of the lamina propria and mucosal cover from the underlying intermediate and deep layers of the lamina propria (Figure 42–9C). Once the cyst is encountered, the dissection continues between the cyst and vocal fold ligament (Figure 42–9D). This may require either sharp or blunt dissection. Care is taken not to evacuate the contents of the cyst.

Once the lesion is free from the vocal fold ligament, blunt and sharp dissection are used to develop a plane between the lesion and the vocal fold cover (Figure 42–9E). Occasionally these steps can be reversed. The key to surgical success, however, is preservation of the vocal fold ligament and uninvolved SLLP. Thin epithelium may be sacrificed with acceptable results, while vocal ligament and excess SLLP sacrifice will lead to unacceptable voice results. Once the lesion is removed, the operative field is inspected for secondary lesions such as a second cyst. If none is found then corticosteroids are placed into the newly created pocket and the flap is redraped (Figure 42–9F).

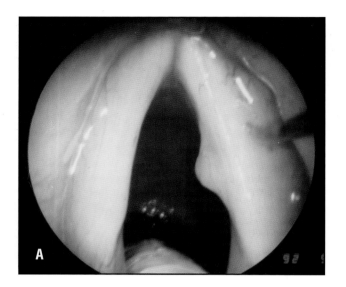

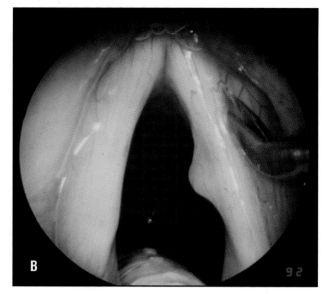

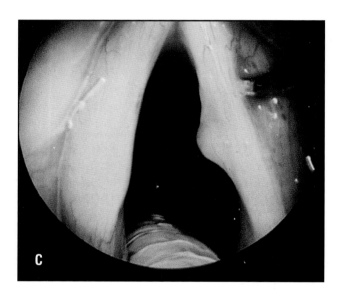

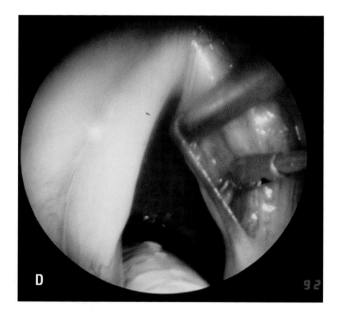

Figure 42–9. A patient with a vocal fold cyst. This was excised using a microflap technique to preserve the overlying, uninvolved mucosal cover. **A.** A sickle knife is used to make an incision laterally on the superior surface of the vocal fold. **B.** The incision is further defined with up-cutting scissors. **C.** A flap elevator is used to elevate the microflap. **D.** The lesion is dissected from the vocal ligament. (*continues*)

Well-circumscribed cysts may be approached through a medial microflap excisional technique if they appear to separate easily from the underlying vocal ligament. Some surgeons prefer this approach even for the more challenging cysts described previously.[25] On preoperative stroboscopy these lesions usually result in reduction or absence of mucosal wave. On palpation in the operating room, however, the surgeon can sometimes separate the lesion from the vocal ligament with gentle traction from a small suction. If the lesion appears to separate easily, then a medial microflap will usually allow adequate identification of the vocal ligament, particularly anteriorly and/or posteriorly to the lesion. The lesion can then be freed from the surrounding normal structures with minimal disruption. The surgeon needs to be confident in his or her abilities.

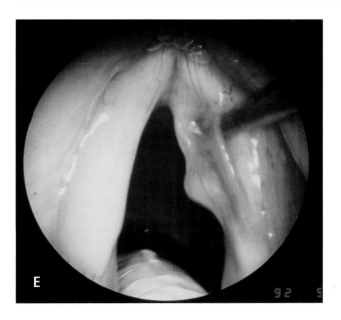

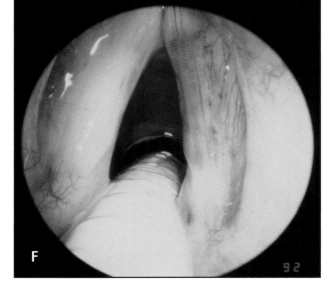

Figure 42–9. (*continued*) **E.** The lesion is dissected from the mucosal cover. **F.** The mucosal cover is redraped into position.

Mucosal retention cysts are often larger than they appear on initial observation. As the cysts expand they slowly lateralize the vocal ligament and can make dissection through a medial approach difficult. The cyst is more easily punctured through a medial approach. If the cyst is deflated too early in the procedure, then identification of appropriate dissection planes is difficult. If too much tissue is removed scarring will result and if cyst wall remnants are left, then the cyst will reoccur (Figure 42–10A and B).

SULCUS VOCALIS

Sulcus vocalis is a vocal fold lesion that appears as a furrow running the length of the vocal fold. It actually consists of a fold of mucosa running along the free surface of the vocal fold. The furrowed mucosa may be adherent to the vocal ligament. This adherence disrupts the mucosal wave and leads to increased vocal roughness and fatigue. The etiology of sulcus vocalis, acquired or congenital, is poorly understood. The lesions are, however, more commonly described in men and can be unilateral or bilateral. Sulcus vocalis lesions are occasionally associated with an epidermal inclusion cyst.[34]

Diagnosis relies on physical examination, stroboscopy, and microlaryngoscopy. Videostroboscopy usually shows an altered mucosal wave with incomplete glottal closure in the form of a slitlike or spindle-shaped deficiency between the vibratory portions of the vocal folds. The involved vocal fold may appear bowed on still-light examination. The furrow may or may not be visible on indirect examination. Operative palpation, therefore, is often necessary to confirm the diagnosis.

The treatment of choice when speech therapy does not produce sufficient improvement is surgical excision. One advocated technique involves precise excision of the involved mucosa. A sickle knife is used to incise the mucosa of the upper border. A blunt dissector is then used to dissect the furrow through Reinke's space and to separate it from the vocal ligament. The inferior mucosal border is then incised with either a knife or scissors. Advancement flaps are elevated on either side of the furrow and used to obtain coverage for the medial vibratory surface of the vocal fold. Suturing of the flaps to maintain their position has been advocated by some surgeons. Care must be exercised to avoid overaggressive mucosal resection, which will lead to a dehiscence on the vibratory surface and result in postoperative decreased voicing. Although experience with these lesions has been limited, initial results have been encouraging and have been reported as such by other authors.[35]

Other techniques advocated for surgical management of sulcus include mucosal slicing or fat implantation into the lamina propria. In the mucosal slicing technique originally described by Pontes et al, a surgical plane is created in the deeper layers of the lamina propria, deep to the base of the sulcus. Transverse incisions of variable length are then made in the flap

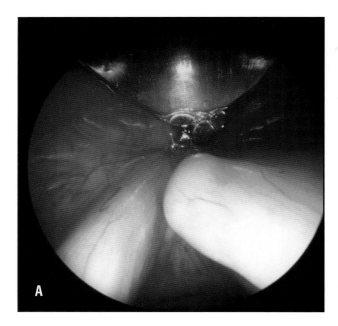

Figure 42–10. Well-circumscribed cysts can be excised with a medial microflap technique. The decision to perform medial versus lateral microflap is made intraoperatively. If the lesion, on palpation, appears to separate easily from the vocal ligament, then a medial approach will allow adequate identification of the appropriate plain within the superficial lamina propria. **A.** The 70° telescopic view demonstrates medial surface involvement preoperatively. **B.** Postoperatively the same 70° telescope shows a minimal disruption along the vibrating surface.

to break the tension created by the lesion. The flap is then redraped and re-epithelialization occurs. This technique has been reported with good results from two separate surgeons.[36,37]

Because of deficiency of normal superfical lamina propria deep to the sulcus, injection of substance into the SLLP to distend this region is difficult. Sataloff described surgically creating a pocket deep to the sulcus and placing a free-fat graft to help re-create a soft vibratory cushion.[25] Fat implantation techniques have been used successfully by other surgeons as well.[38]

VOCAL FOLD SCARRING

The treatment of vocal fold scarring from previous surgery is an arduous task for any laryngologist. It is often difficult to distinguish whether poor postoperative results are secondary to improper resection or continued vocal misuse. Therefore, before surgical re-exploration, exhaustive speech therapy should be conducted. If no functional improvement is apparent and examination reveals a persisting altered mucosal wave and impaired glottic closure, then surgical exploration may be indicated. The timing of re-exploration should be at least 18 month after the initial procedure. This allows stabilization of healing tissue and provides adequate time for exhaustive speech rehabilitation.

Surgical intervention usually takes the form of an exploratory cordotomy. An incision is made in the mucosal cover near the ventricle. Blunt and sharp dissection are used to find or create a surgical plane in the superficial lamina propria between the mucosal cover and the underlying vocal ligament (intermediate and deep layers of the lamina propria). Corticosteroids are then injected into this newly created pocket and the flap redraped.

Postoperative results with these types of lesions show some improvement in the appearance of the vibratory characteristics of the vocal fold on stroboscopy postoperatively. The main improvement in vocal capabilities, however, appears to result from a straighter vocal fold surface. This improves glottic closure and provides a straighter surface for the normal vocal fold to vibrate against. This improved glottic closure explains the decreased vocal strain, roughness, and vocal fatigue experienced by our patients.

If lysing of scar bands within the lamina propria is unsuccessful at relieving the vocal disorder, then other methods of reconstruction may be indicated. Again, the vibratory abnormality is usually secondary to a loss of normal lamina propria with re-epithelialization occurring directly over the vocal ligament or muscle. Currently, synthetic materials to reconstruct the LP do not exist. In addition, the injection of substances, such as collagen or fat, into this region is difficult if not impossible secondary to scarification and instrumentation. Injected materials will flow from the needle into less dense tissue. Therefore, the scar will remain undisrupted and the softer, more normal tissues, will be infiltrated by the injected material. With regard to the injection of fat into scar tissue, the large size of the needle, 18-gauge, required to transplant viable fat cells, limits placement. The bevel of most 18-gauge needles is 3 to 4 mm. The normal LP is at most 1 to 2 mm in width. Therefore, injection into adherent tissue with a large gauge needle is not possible. For these reasons, some surgeons have attempted LP reconstruction by surgically creating a pocket just deep to existing epithelium. A small piece of fat is then placed into this pocket and the epithelium repositioned over the top of the fat graft.[38] Alternatively, in animal models we have attempted to use synthetic materials of elastin and collagen with limited success.

If reconstruction of the LP is not possible, attempts at reducing the glottal closure defect by medializing the available soft tissue through framework surgery may be employed. Frequently, this can result in some reduction of effort required to phonate. However, because the vibratory structures are not restored, the vocal quality usually remains rough. In addition, if the vocal fold deficiency is in the form of a notch, it is difficult to medialize a small vocal fold segment without overcorrection in other regions.

POLYPOID CORDITIS

Polypoid corditis, also termed Reinke's edema or polypoid degeneration, is unlike other vocal fold polyps. It does not appear to be associated with vocal abuse but is intimately associated with cigarette smoking. Kleinsasser reports a 98% association.

Grossly, the vocal folds are sausage-shaped. As the polypoid changes progress, pedunculated lesions develop and involve the entire membranous vocal fold as their base. These lesions prolapse in and out of the glottis and inhibit phonation and, at times, respiration. Portions of the overlying epithelium may become keratotic, but the disease is not associated with an increased risk of cancer. Treatment is, therefore, aimed at excision of the polypoid changes of the superficial layer of the lamina propria with sparing enough mucosal membrane to cover the exposed, and carefully preserved, vocal ligament.

Surgical treatment, with mucosal preservation, allows simultaneous treatment of both vocal folds with minimal risk of web formation. In addition, the microflap excision technique facilitates proper identification of the vocal ligament and minimizes the risk of inadvertent injury. Comparison of surgical techniques indicates that excision via the microflap, or Hirano, technique results in the shortest duration of postoperative dysphonia.[35]

Regardless of the mode of treatment, the superficial layer of the lamina propria is diseased and must be removed. The term *edema* is a misnomer. The superficial layer of the lamina propria is not edematous but is replaced by a myxomatous-appearing stroma. Histologic examination of this stroma reveals relatively minimal increase in vascularity and minimal hyalinization, in contrast to the findings with polyps or nodules. Simple incision of the mucosa does not allow suction evacuation of the tissue, but rather, the tissue needs to be excised. Loss of the normal SLLP through the disease process, and then surgical excision, leads to a reduction in, or loss of, mucosal wave postoperatively. The SLLP does not appear to regenerate, and the mucosa attaches directly to the intermediate layer of the lamina propria. As such, patients need to be counseled with regard to postoperative voice quality. Voice will not return to normal. Reduction of vocal fold mass, however, usually results in an elevation of fundamental frequency and subjective increase in ease of phonation. In addition, patients usually report improved respiration, as the massive polypoid changes can lead to airway obstruction.

The surgical excision technique begins with adequate exposure through a binocular operating microlaryngoscope. A curved sickle knife is used to make an incision on the superior lateral surface of the vocal fold. The flap elevator is used to elevate a flap of mucosal membrane. The myxomatous stroma is then bluntly dissected from the underlying vocal ligament. The mucosa is trimmed with microscissors and redraped to cover the vocal ligament. Care should be taken not to leave excess mucosa as this will lead to an irregular vocal fold margin or increase the chance of recurrence.

POSTOPERATIVE MANAGEMENT

Postoperative management is divided into four phases. Phase 1 consists of 1 to 2 weeks of complete voice rest. Current recommendations regarding the use of voice rest among contemporary laryngologists show considerable variation. Recommendations range from zero to 14 days postoperatively.[1,2] Based on studies of vocal fold remucosalization and wound healing in general, 1 to 2 weeks seems most appropriate.[4] This allows adequate time for the majority of remucosalization to occur. In addition, collagen cross-linking for wound healing is at a point of steady incline. Laryngologists opposed to such lengthy periods of voice rest indicate potential vocal fold atrophy as their reason against use. No objective evidence, however, exists to support this view. In addition, examination of multiple patients after 2-week periods of complete voice rest does not show atrophy.

During phase 1, pharmacotherapy includes the use of antibiotics secondary to the presence of a contaminated surgical wound, pain medication, mucolytic agents, and control of hyperacidity if indicated.

Postoperative phase 2 includes postoperative weeks 2 through 4 and begins with an examination including videostroboscopy. If a microflap technique has been utilized, the operated vocal fold is edematous and stiff. Some evidence of return of the vertical phase difference and mucosal wave exists. The patient is allowed to phonate for 5 minutes the first day off voice rest. The time is then doubled to 10 minutes the second day, then 20 minutes, 40 minutes, 1.5 hours, 3 hours, and so forth. In this manner the patient is back to nearly full conversational speech by the midpoint of the fourth postoperative week.

Good vocal hygiene measures are continued. These include increased water uptake, mucolytic agents, and reflux control if appropriate.[39] The patient is instructed on easy-onset phonation and asked to observe frequent 10-minute periods of vocal rest. Vocal fatigue and strain are signs of overactivity, and the patient is asked to use biofeedback methods for regulating activity.

Postoperative phase 3 includes postoperative weeks 5 through 12 and consists of continued behavior modification and vocal hygiene. Physical examination should show continued resolution of edema with return of the vertical phase difference and the mucosal wave. Frequent examinations and videostroboscopy are performed to assess the effect of continued and increased function on the glottis. Vocal coaching for the singing voice is instituted during phase 3. The vertical phase difference, mucosal wave, and glottic closure should continue to improve with each examination. Should evidence of worsening of these factors develop, then vocal activity is decreased or halted.

Finally, phase 4 consists of weeks 13 and beyond and represents a return to full vocal activity with observation every 6 to 8 weeks. This is carried on for approximately 24 months from the time of surgery. Healing and changes in appearance of mucosal wave and glottic function will continue for up to 2 years postoperatively. Patients will continue to make improvement in their vocal technique and capability. Intermittent vocal re-education or rehabilitation enhances continued vocal hygiene and proper vocal function.

CONCLUSION

The surgical management of benign voice disorders relies on accurate history and examination. Videostroboscopy is essential for the examination of glottic vibratory behavior and vocal fold closure. With these tools the accuracy of diagnosis of vocal fold abnormalities is enhanced.[3] However, it is often still not possible to diagnose the exact nature of a vocal fold lesion on the initial examination. In this instance, serial or interval examination is helpful. In addition, behavior modification with vocal abuse reduction and correction of misuses may help to resolve surrounding vocal fold edema and further identify the true lesion. This principle of exhaustive behavioral and medical management before surgical intervention is essential for good surgical results. It is equivalent to the use of physical therapy by the orthopedic surgeon or neurosurgeon prior to definitive joint or disk surgery.

If surgical intervention is deemed necessary, then precise excision of the lesion with minimal disturbance to the surrounding normal tissue is crucial for the return of glottic function postoperatively. Patients who have had overaggressive resection of benign glottic lesions show altered mucosal wave formation and impaired glottic function on postoperative videostroboscopy. These patients have decreased vocal capabilities. To attain this goal of minimal disturbance to the surrounding normal tissues, the surgeon must time the surgical intervention with regard to treatment of the surrounding edema and use precise surgical techniques. Surgeons operating on benign vocal fold lesions should be well-versed in glottic anatomy, histology, and physiology. They should feel comfortable with the use of microlaryngeal instrumentation and in viewing the glottis under high magnification. Currently these techniques are not a standard practice in most residency programs.

After surgical intervention, postoperative rehabilitation with continued behavioral modification and improved vocal hygiene is important for adequate postoperative results. Preoperative physical or speech therapy is beneficial in establishing adequate vocal hygiene habits that can then be applied to the postoperative rehabilitation. Postoperatively patients should expect a 7- to 14-day period of complete voice rest followed by 2.5 months of rehabilitation. Overuse of edematous or stiff vocal fold(s) may result in the acquisition of functional disorders. Therefore, the patient's progress postoperatively needs to be monitored closely with repeat examination and videoendostroboscopy. Activity can be liberalized as the characteristics of vocal fold vibration improve.

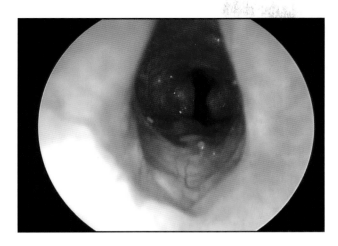

Figure 43–7. Tracheal injury seen at extubation.

ENDOTRACHEAL INTUBATION INJURY

Endotracheal intubation injury is the most common cause of acquired laryngotracheal stenosis in the developed world (Table 43–3). Prospective studies have shown some sort of intubation injury in up to 93% of patients who have been ventilated.[2] Although the risk of significant laryngeal injury correlates with duration of intubation, there does not appear to be a safe limit and significant injuries have been observed after only 8 hours of intubation in adults and 1 week in children.[3] The incidence of airway stenosis following prolonged ventilation is estimated at 6 to 10%.

The initial mucosal injury may be due to traumatic or repeated intubation. Trauma from the tube may also be related to the degree of agitation of the patient and movements produced through mechanical ventilation. Most commonly injury is seen at the mucosal contact points of the cuff or the tube. If a tube is too large the firm plastic material from which it is made can cause trauma. Too small a tube will require high cuff pressures, exceeding the capillary perfusion pressures of the mucosa. Mucosal ulceration leads to perichondritis, granulation, cartilage necrosis, and stenosis (Figure 43–7). In the majority of cases, these mucosal changes regress after the endotracheal tube has been removed. A chronic inflammatory process, with fibrous proliferation and healing by contracture, means the patient's symptoms may be delayed for up to a year. Injury from overinflated cuffs is less common since the widespread use of high-volume low-pressure cuffs. The sizing of an endotracheal tube in adults should be based on the patient's sex and height.

Endotracheal tubes and intubation trauma can also lead to injuries to the cartilaginous glottis and cricoid.

Table 43–3. One Hundred Consecutive Referrals to a Dedicated Adult Airway Reconstruction Unit

45%	Acquired tracheal or subglottic stenosis
	    43 secondary to endotracheal tubes
	    2 related to tracheostomy tube

20%	Bilateral impaired vocal cord immobility
	    thyroid/cardiovascular surgery
	    traumatic intubation
	    congenital
	    central nervous system deficit
	    rheumatoid arthritis

12%	Wegener's granulomatosis
11%	Idiopathic subglottic stenosis
7%	Previous treatment for papillomatosis
3%	Sarcoid
1%	Amyloidosis
1%	Relapsing polychondritis

They may produce granulomas, synechiae, or webbing (Figure 43–8). The cricoarytenoid joints may become fixed through scarring or hemarthrosis.

Patients ventilated on ICUs almost universally have gastroesophageal reflux. The vocal cords are held open by the endotracheal tube and the airway becomes bathed in a mixture of acid, enzymes, and microorganisms. Coexisting medical problems, reduced immunity, nutrition, and foreign body response to the tube are other exacerbating factors for laryngotracheal injury. Some of these problems can be addressed by appropriate medical therapies.

TRACHEOTOMY TUBE INJURY

In our series there have been virtually no cases of laryngotracheal stenosis secondary to a tracheotomy tube. Where it is anticipated that a patient may be ventilated beyond a week we recommend an early tracheotomy. Percutaneous tracheotomies should be performed under bronchoscopic control, surgical tracheotomies should be sited through the third and fourth tracheal rings and cricothyroidotomies should be avoided. This will reduce the incidence of cricoid cartilage necrosis and subglottic stenosis related to a tracheotomy. More than 90% of tracheotomy-related stenoses are suprastomal or stomal. The causative factors are poor sugery, inward buckling and collapse of the trachea from oversized tubes, and pooling of secretions and sepsis above the cuff. Cuff-related injuries and

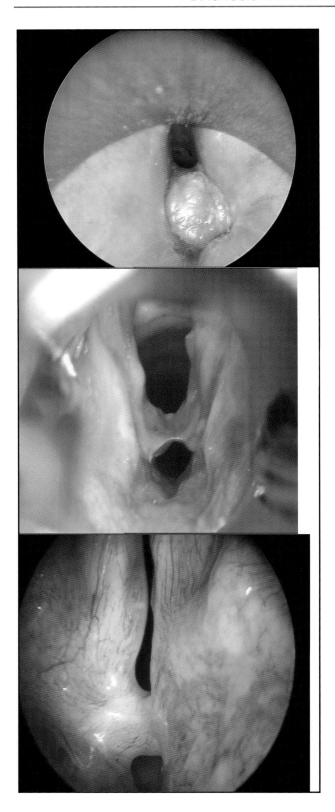

Figure 43–8. Glottic trauma from endotracheal tubes. Arytenoid granulation (*top*). Interarytenoid adhesion seen after extubation (*middle*) Synechiae (*bottom*)

tube-tip injuries are similar to those described with respect to endotracheal tubes.

GASTROESOPHAGEAL REFLUX DISEASE AND LARYNGOPHARYNGEAL REFLUX

Patients with gastroesophageal reflux disease (GERD) will usually have symptoms of heartburn or regurgitation. The larynx and trachea have little or no acid clearance mechanism and very little salivary bicarbonate comes into contact with the delicate epithelium of this part of the airway. The majority of our patients are therefore started prophylactically on proton pump inhibitor therapy prior to first endoscopy.

Laryngopharyngeal reflux (LPR), also referred to as "silent reflux," can be present even if there is no heartburn or esophagitis.[4] As well as acid, gastric refluxate also contains the proteolytic enzyme pepsin which has been shown to have activity up to pH 6.0. Pepsin can cause inflammation and edema of the larynx through this process of "nonacidic reflux" even in patients on definitive antacid medical therapy. In some cases of adult laryngotracheal stenosis, LPR may be an etiologic factor but, in many more cases, it is likely to be contributing to ongoing inflammation.

The "gold standard" for diagnosis of GERD is 24-hour esophageal pH monitoring. The diagnosis of LPR requires an esophageal probe combining intraluminal electrical impedance and pH monitoring. Patients with evidence of laryngotracheal inflammation, despite medical treatment for GERD, should be investigated for LPR and where appropriate a gastric fundiplication procedure is recommended.

ANESTHETICS

The surgeon and the anesthetist need to work closely and have experience in shared airway techniques for this type of surgery to be carried out safely. In our practice the majority of patients are paralyzed and ventilated using a laryngeal mask airway (LMA) to avoid further laryngotracheal trauma (Figures 43–9 and 43–10). During the procedure, supraglottic high-frequency jet ventilation techniques are employed so that there is no restriction to surgical access. The supraglottic jetting needle is mounted in the lumen of the laryngoscope. With severely restricted airways. subglottic jetting or transtracheal jetting may be used

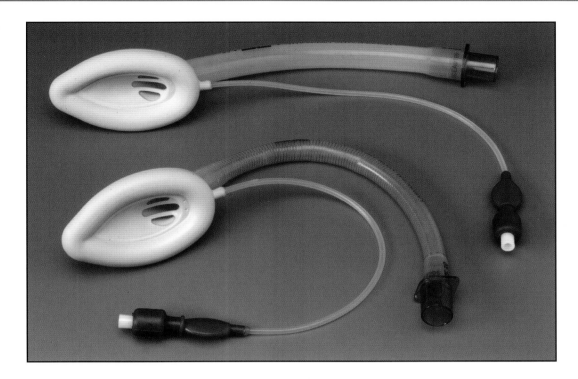

Figure 43–9. Laryngeal mask airways (LMA).

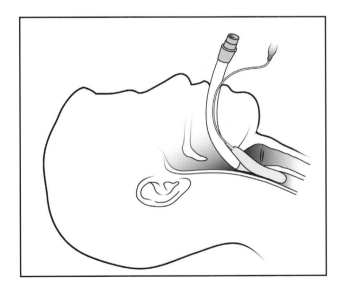

Figure 43–10. The laryngeal mask airway (LMA) in position.

(Figure 43–11) until the airway has been surgically enlarged. Use is also made of pre-existing tracheotomies. Following surgery the LMA is reinserted for ventilatory support until the recovery of reflexes.

MANAGEMENT OF SUBGLOTTIC AND TRACHEAL STENOSIS

At this stage, patients have been fully investigated and medical therapies have been optimized. Although the first endoscopy is a staging procedure, some form of surgery is usually possible. We have been able to decannulate 90% of patients at first endoscopy.

Thin stenoses (less than 5 mm in length) can be treated with radial cuts using a sickle knife or CO_2 laser mounted on a microscope. It is important to conserve strips of mucosa between these cuts to reduce the likelihood of restenosis (Figure 43–12). The stenosis can then be dilated using bougies of increasing size or by means of pulmonary balloon dilators. Topical mitomycin can also be applied to inhibit restenosis. This procedure is usually repeated every 1 to 2 months until the airway has stabilized.

Thick stenoses (greater than 5 mm length) can be managed in the same way as thin stenoses but these may require initial internal stenting (Figure 43–13). Soft silicone stents are preferable; however, firmer silicone stents are sometimes used (see stenting below). Even long lengths of complete airway stenosis can be managed in this way.

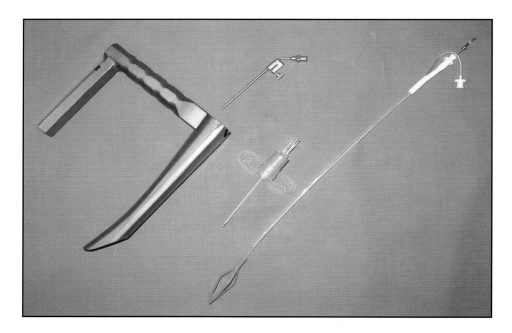

Figure 43–11. Jet ventilation devices: Supraglottic jetting needle (*left*). Transtracheal jetting needle (*middle*). Hunsaker subglottic jetting catheter (*right*).

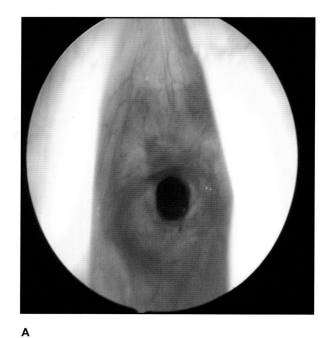

A

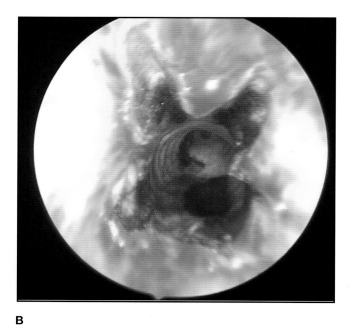

B

Figure 43–12. A. Subglottic stenosis. **B.** Subglottic steno-sis following radial CO$_2$ laser cuts and dilatation.

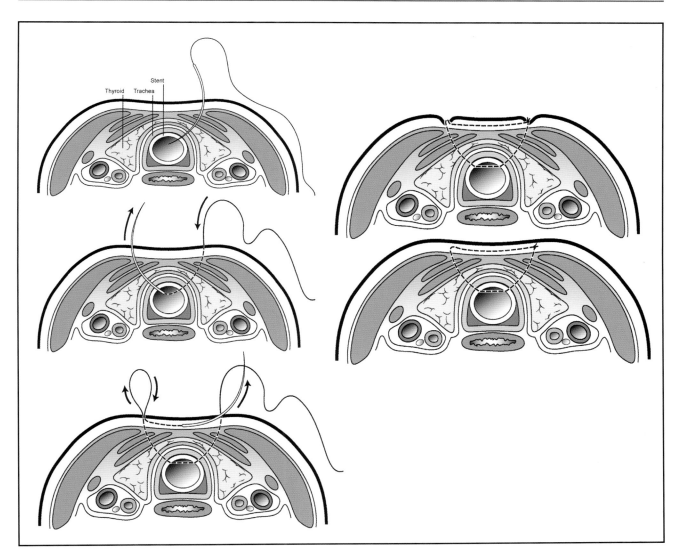

Figure 43–19. Securing an endoluminal Silastic stent.[14] The stent is held in the airway at laryngoscopy. A monofilament suture with a large needle is used to secure the stent as shown. The ends of the suture bury themselves within a few days. During stent removal the suture is divided endoscopically and removed through a small incision.

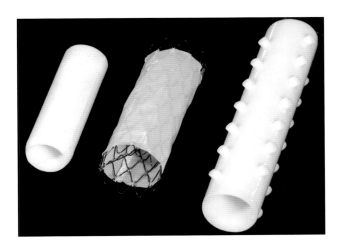

Figure 43–20. Soft Silastic stent fashioned from T-tube (*left*), Silastic-coated wire mesh stent (*middle*), Dumon Silastic stent (*right*).

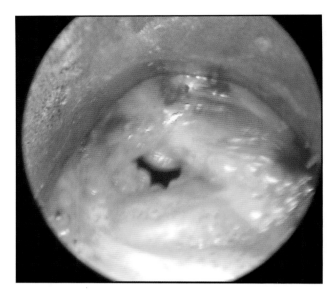

Figure 43–21. Glottic stenosis following multiple laser procedures for laryngeal papillomatosis.

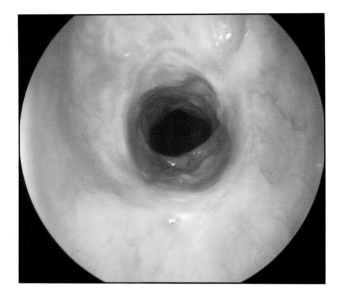

Figure 43–22. Idiopathic subglottic stenosis.

IDIOPATHIC SUBGLOTTIC STENOSIS

This is a slowly progressive, inflammatory, and fibrotic airway stenosis that is unremitting and affects almost exclusively women. There are only a few hundred cases in the world literature and the condition can occur at any age postmenarche. The diagnosis is one of exclusion and the patient must not have been intubated, received neck trauma, or had a significant respiratory tract infection in the preceding two years. Patients must also be investigated for GERD and autoimmune disorders including Wegener's granulomatosis. It is not unsual for these patients to be treated for asthma when the cause of their airflow restriction could simply be determined using flow-volume loop studies (see Figure 43–1).

The disease usually involves the subglottis and first two tracheal rings (Figure 43–22). The airway in these patients appears to have a heightened reactivity to any kind of trauma. Aggressive treatment with lasers or trauma from hard laryngeal stents can lead to more marked laryngotracheal stenosis (Figure 43–23). A conservative gentle approach is recommended. Most patients respond to radial laser incisions and dilatation with mitomycin application. Stenosis recurs usually over a period of 6 to 12 months at which time surgery can be repeated. Some surgeons recommend primary cricotracheal resection[11] but the high success rate has not always been

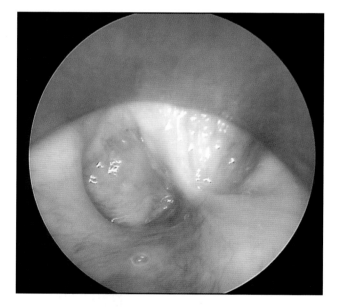

Figure 43–23. View of laryngeal glottis following overaggressive treatment of idiopathic subglottic stenosis.

repeated in other units. We manage most cases of idiopathic subglottic stenosis endoscopically. Often patients are referred with more significant stenosis following previous aggressive surgery and may require augmentation or resective surgery if endoscopic techniques fail.

BILATERAL VOCAL CORD IMMOBILITY

When vocal cord immobility is bilateral the patient may have good voice but experience dyspnea to such a degree that a tracheotomy is required. Many endoscopic and open procedures have been described to manage this problem, all with variable success. Vocal cord lateralization techniques have been used employing a suture or laser but they damage the membranous glottis and severely compromise voice. The interarytenoid region is normally the largest part of the glottic airway and surgery should therefore be aimed at improving this. We have had significant success with endoscopic partial posterior cordectomy and partial arytenoidectomy using the CO_2 laser (Figure 43–24). The resection is usually unilateral but can be bilateral. Mitomycin applied topically at the time of surgery will reduce the tendency for the resection to fill in with fibrosis and scar. The voice does become "breathier" but remains functional. If the cords have become fixed due to interarytenoid webbing then this can usually be corrected surgically (Figure 43–25). Reinnervation following recurrent laryngeal nerve injury has not been successful.

INFLAMMATORY AND IMMUNE DISEASES

There are several inflammatory diseases that may affect the mucosa or connective tissue of the airway resulting in stenosis. *Wegener's granulomatosis* is perhaps the most common. This is a condition of unknown etiology characterized by a necrotizing vasculitis involving the respiratory tract, kidneys, skin, eyes, and joints. About half will have laryngotracheal involvement (Figure 43–26) although the nose and ears may be involved in up to 75% of cases. Biopsies cannot always be differentiated from inflammation due to other causes. The most useful serologic test is cytoplasmic antinuclear cytoplasmic antibody (c-ANCA) which is positive in over 90% of patients with active disease. Corticosteroids are the mainstay of treatment in combination with other immune-modulating drugs. Subglottic and tracheal stenosis can be managed with intralesional steroid injections,[12] radial laser cuts, and dilatation. We have successfully extended this technique to the treatment of bronchial lesions. Even during periods of disease relapse we have managed to avoid tracheotomies in our patients.

Sarcoidosis is a noncaseating granulomatous condition of unknown etiology. Although there is no cure, corticosteroids may control the rate of disease pro-

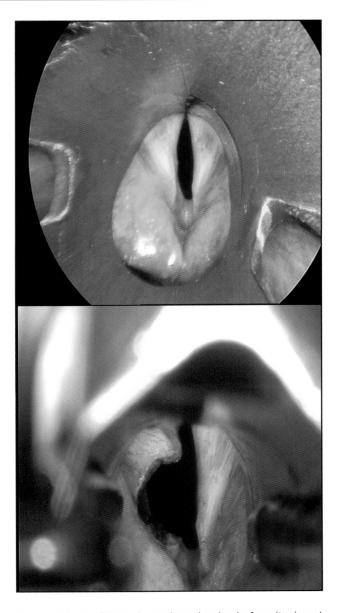

Figure 43–24. Bilateral vocal cord palsy before (*top*) and immediately after (*bottom*) partial laser cordectomy/arytenoidectomy.

gression. The larynx is involved in 1 to 5% of cases.[13] The supraglottic larynx tends to be affected more often than the subglottis (Figure 43–27). The laryngeal lesion is usually a pale pink, edematous swelling that can pedunculate into the airway and produce stridor. Intralesion steroids and CO_2 laser reduction of laryngeal lesions can be effective in restoring the airway.

Amyloidosis is a group of disorders characterized by acellular deposition of nonreactive proteinaceous material in one or many organs. Primary amyloid is not associated with other medical conditions and may be

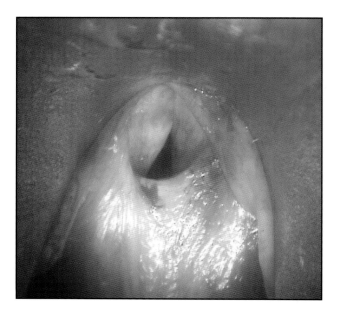

Figure 43–25. Interarytenoid web.

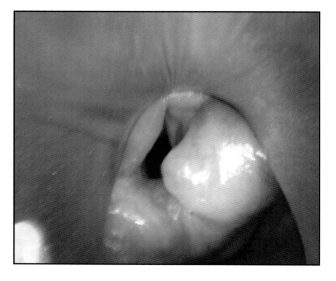

Figure 43–27. Laryngeal sarcoid involving the supraglottis and right arytenoid. Lesion appears as a pale pink swelling.

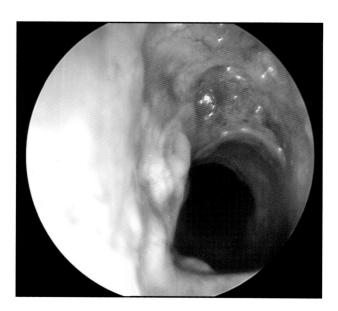

Figure 43–26. Subglottic stenosis due to Wegener's granulomatosis.

localized to one specific site or generalized throughout the body; however, multiple myeloma needs to be ruled out as a cause of the protein deposit. Secondary amyloidosis is associated with chronic inflammatory disorders such as tuberculosis or rheumatoid arthritis. Biopsy specimens stained with Congo red show the characteristic "apple green" birefringence under polarized light. Laryngeal involvement is extremely rare

and presents as a tumor mass or nodules, which can usually be removed endoscopically (Figure 43–28). These procedures can be repeated to maintain an airway and rarely is laryngeal or tracheal involvement fatal.

Relapsing polychondritis is an episodic inflammation of the cartilaginous structures of the body resulting in their destruction and replacement with scar tissue. The organs involved are principally the ears, nose, and peripheral joints and also the tracheobronchial tree. The pathogenesis is unknown but is likely to be autoimmune. Diagnosis is on clinical grounds and nearly half of the patients have layngeal involvement (Figure 43–29). Treatment is based on prolonged corticosteroid therapy, which is increased during disease flare-up. Prognosis is variable but a number of patients end up with a long-term tracheotomy. Death is usually due to airway collapse or pneumonia.

CONCLUSIONS

The most common cause of acquired laryngotracheal stenosis is prolonged ventilation on Intensive Care Units. Preventive measures should include careful sizing of endotracheal tubes based on height and sex, with close monitoring of cuff pressures and appropriate antireflux and antibiotic treatment. Where it is anticipated that a patient may be ventilated beyond a week, we recommend an early tracheotomy.

Voice and swallowing, as well as dyspnea, are important considerations in the management of estab-

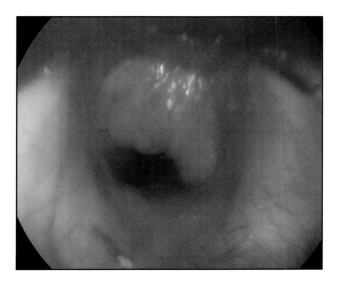

Figure 43–28. Primary laryngeal amyloid.

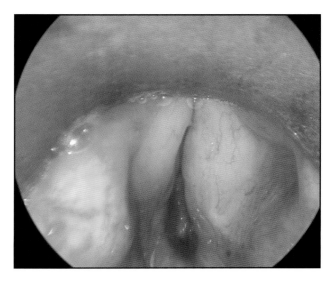

Figure 43–29. Relapsing polychondritis of the larynx showing results of loss of cartilage support.

lished airway stenosis. These patients need to be managed by a multidisciplinary team, which should include surgeons, anesthesiologists, speech and swallowing therapists, dieticians, and physicians. The majority of these patients can be managed by a staged endoscopic approach. Where this has failed, we prefer augmentation procedures using local vascularized flaps or tracheal homografts. Unlike the pediatric population, the results of rib graft augmentation of the airway in the adult have been disappointing. Tracheal and cricotracheal resection is used only as a last resort and usually in patients where there has been severe damage to laryngotracheal cartilaginous support.

The management of adult acquired laryngotracheal stenosis remains a challenge. There are multiple etiologic factors and the pathophysiology of many of these factors is poorly understood. Further basic science research is required for a better understanding of wound healing and new adjuvant therapies. The current hope is for tissue engineering to allow replacement of the damaged airway with laboratory-grown organs either from autologous tissues or stem cells.

REFERENCES

1. Schaefer SD. The acute management of external laryngeal trauma: a 27 year experience. *Arch Otolaryngol Head Neck Surg.*1992;118:598-604.
2. Colice GL, Stukel TA, Dain B. Laryngeal complications of prolonged intubation. *Chest.* 1989;96:877-884.
3. Whited RE. A prospective study of laryngotracheal sequelae in long-term intubation. *Laryngoscope.* 1984;9:367-377.
4. Koufman JA. The otolarygologic manifestations of gastroesophageal reflux disease (GERD): a clinical investigation of 225 patients using ambulatory 24-hour pH monitoring and an experimental investigation of the role of acid and pepsin in the development of laryngeal injury. *Laryngoscope.* 1991;101:1-78.
5. Papay FA, Eliachar I, Stein JM, Sebek BA, Ramirez HM, Tucker HM. Structural stability of the rotary door myocutaneous flap. *Laryngoscope.* 1998;108:385-392.
6. Duncavage JA, Ossoff RH, Toohill RJ. Laryngotracheal reconstruction with composite nasal septal cartilage grafts. *Ann Otol Rhinol Laryngol.* 1989;98:581-585.
7. Herberhold C, Stein M, Bierhoff E, Kost S. Tracheal reconstruction with preserved tracheal homograft —New aspects. *Laryngrhinootologie.* 1999;78(1):54-56.
8. Abdullah V, Yim AP, Wormald PJ, et al. Dumon silicone stents in obstructive tracheobronchial lesions: the Hong Kong experience. *Otolaryngol Head Neck Surg.* 1998;118:256-260.
9. Eliashar R, Eliachar I, Esclamado R, Gramlich T, Strome M. Can topical Mitomycin prevent laryngotracheal stenosis? *Laryngoscope.* 1999;109:1594-1600.
10. Mouney DF, Lyons GD. Fixation of laryngeal stents. *Laryngoscope.* 1985;95:905-907.
11. Ashiku SK, Kuzucu A, Grillo HC, Wright CD, Wain JC, Lo B, Mathisen DJ. Idiopathic laryngotracheal stenosis: effective definitive treatment with laryngotracheal resection. *J Thorac Cardiovasc Surg.* 2004;127:99-107.
12. Hoffman GS, Thomas-Golbanov CK, Chan J, Akst LM, Eliachar I. Treatment of subglottic stenosis, due to Wegener's granulomatosis, with intralesional corticosteroids and dilatation. *J Rheumatol.* 2003;30:1017-1021.
13. Krespi YP, Mitrani M, Husain S, Meltzer CJ. Treatment of laryngeal sarcoidosis with intralesional steroid injection. *Ann Otol Rhinol Laryngol.* 1987;96:713-715.

44

Vocal Fold Medialization: Injection and Laryngeal Framework Surgery

Steven M. Zeitels, MD, FACS

Restoration of vocal function with laryngeal framework surgery (laryngoplastic phonosurgery) was introduced at the beginning of the 20th century. Today, these procedures have emerged as the dominant surgical management approach for the treatment of the aerodynamic incompetence and acoustic deterioration associated with vocal fold paralysis/paresis. Other indications include cancer defects, vocal fold scar, sulcus vocalis, bowing associated with vocal fold atrophy, laryngeal trauma, and neuromuscular disorders including abductor spasmodic dysphonia and parkinsonism. Laryngeal framework surgery has also been employed to alter pitch for gender reassignment; however, this will not be detailed herein.

Although medialization of the musculomembranous vocal fold by means of rearranging the laryngeal cartilage framework was described by Payr[1] in 1915, and others in the mid-20th century,[2,3] Isshiki[4-6] championed the systematic analysis and laryngoplastic treatment of glottal incompetence in the 1970s. He designed his medialization procedure of the musculomembranous vocal fold with the use of a synthetic implant in 1974.[4] Gore-Tex has become the author's implant choice[7-10] for medialization laryngoplasty; the unique characteristics of this bioimplant are delineated below. In 1978, Isshiki designed the arytenoid-adduction[5] procedure to treat patients with large glottal gaps secondary to a malpositioned arytenoid. One of his outstanding contributions is that he taught surgeons that laryngeal framework procedures could be done with facility utilizing local anesthesia with sedation. The concept that the cricoarytenoid joint could be dissected and manipulated under local anesthesia to allow for phonatory feedback was revolutionary. Based on this seminal work, the adduction arytenopexy[2,7,8,11] and cricothyroid subluxation[7,8,12] procedures were introduced to further enhance phonatory reconstruction.

713

PRINCIPLES AND THEORY OF LARYNGEAL FRAMEWORK SURGERY

The ideal procedure(s) to treat aerodynamic glottal incompetence that is associated with paralytic/paretic dysphonia, should attempt to simulate the normal vocal fold position during phonation with regard to the following interdependent parameters:

1. Position of the musculomembranous region in the axial plane
2. Position of the arytenoid in the axial plane
3. Height of the vocal fold
4. Length of the vocal fold
5. Contour of the vocal fold edge in the musculomembranous region
6. Contour of the vocal fold edge in the arytenoid region
7. Mass and viscoelasticity of the vocal fold.

Furthermore, the procedure(s) should ideally be easy to perform, associated with few complications, be reliable, be reversible, and not be threatening to the airway.[13] Although not reversible, the adduction arytenopexy[2,7,8,11] procedure more closely models the synchronous agonist-antagonist function of the lateral cricoarytenoid, interarytenoid, lateral thyroarytenoid, and posterior cricoarytenoid muscles during phonatory adduction. Cricothyroid subluxation[7,8,12] is the first and only phonosurgical procedure designed exclusively to restore vocal fold tension in denervated soft-tissues associated with recurrent-nerve-induced paralytic/paretic dysphonia. This technique is designed to primarily increase unilateral length and tension of the vocal fold by simulating cricothyroid muscle function. Gore-Tex medialization[7,8,10] has a number of unique qualities but, like many prior innovations, is a modification of Isshiki's conventional implant approach.

TRADITIONAL APPROACHES

Surgical interventions for support or placement of the true vocal folds can be divided into injection thyroplasty techniques and laryngeal framework surgical techniques. A brief review of the traditional approaches serves to highlight the recent innovations in surgical technique. As this is an overview, the reader is referred to surgical atlases and surgical manuscripts to obtain detailed descriptions of these procedures.

Injection Medialization

Many materials have been used for injection medialization, each with its own indications, advantages, and disadvantages. These materials are typically injected deep within the paraglottic space to effect a change in the contour and medialize the edge of the paralyzed true vocal fold.

Teflon

Although popularized in the 1960s,[14] vocal fold augmentation with Teflon has fallen into disfavor due to its irreversibility, propensity to extrude, form granulomas, its imprecise placement, and stiffness, which can occur if it is injected superficially. Today, Teflon is best used in patients with terminal diseases who require a one-time, quick procedure that will decrease aspiration due to glottal incompetence. A disadvantage, which is common to all injected materials, is their inability to effect a change in the position of the arytenoid and height of the vocal fold. If there is not favorable synkinetic reinnervation, misalignment of the vocal folds remains with resultant air escape. In an effort to avoid the sequelae caused by Teflon, other materials have been used for medialization including autologous fat, collagen, and Gelfoam.

Autologous Fat Injection Thyroplasty

Autologous fat injection thyroplasty requires the harvesting of a small amount of fat (axillary or abdominal) and some preparation (washing, drying of excess moisture, and dicing into small pieces) prior to injection. A Brünings syringe is used to introduce the fat into the true vocal fold. As the Brünings injecting device was designed prior to the introduction of the surgical microscope, most surgeons do not perform the injections with microscopic control. Toward that end, Burns and Zeitels[15] designed an approach to facilitate microsteroscopic lipoinjection. Typically, the vocal fold is overinjected by up to 50% with fat as there is a variable loss of tissue during the first 6 weeks. Several studies have reported good long-term results with persistent glottal closure.[16,17] The obvious disadvantages include the imprecision of the final result due to limitations in quantifying the injection and unpredictable variable resorption.

Hyaluronic Acid and Collagen

When it is advantageous to volume-expand denervated paraglottic muscles, while awaiting potential reinnervation, we prefer office transoral injection.[18] That procedure is done with topical local anesthesia by means of laryngeal-telescopic guidance with phonatory gestures. Our temporary injectable of choice is hyaluronic acid preparations such as Restylane (Medicis Aesthetics, Inc). It does not require preparation or mixing (Cymetra: Lifecell), can be injected in the office through a long shaft and narrow-bore 25-guage needle, and is readily available. In large part, these substances have replaced collagen. Collagen's main disadvantages include variable resorption and relative high cost for the material. In an effort to decrease the resorption of collagen, autologous collagen has been introduced to eliminate the antigenicity associated with bovine collagen.[19] However, autologous collagen requires a donor site of resected skin from the patient.

Gelfoam

Gelfoam is still used by some surgeons as an intraoperative resorbable alternative to Teflon. It is injected into the paraglottic region in a fashion similar to Teflon. The procedure was introduced in 1978 by Schramm[20] and is easy to perform with a very low complication rate. Gelfoam is prepared prior to injection by mixing a gelatin powder with saline to form a Gelfoam paste, which is injected into the lateral paraglottic region. It is a very effective way to medialize the musculomembranous vocal fold in those who may have spontaneous return of activity for 2 to 3 months; other procedures, including medialization thyroplasty and arytenoid procedures can be performed subsequent to Gelfoam injections.

Laryngeal Framework Surgery

The foundation of laryngeal framework surgery was established by Isshiki et al during the early 1970s.[4-6] They demonstrated improvement in hoarseness by direct manipulation and rearrangement of the laryngeal framework to achieve closure of the glottal gap and restore competence to the glottal valve. Isshiki described four basic surgical procedures, which he termed thyroplasty types I–IV[6] for altering the conformation of the thyroid cartilage and the arytenoid adduction, which attempts to close the posterior (cartilaginous) glottis.

Thyroplasty Type I

Thyroplasty type I (Figure 44–1) is the most widely used of Isshiki's original thyroplasty techniques. It involves creating a rectangular cartilaginous window at the level of the true vocal fold and using cartilage, Silastic, Gore-Tex, or other implant materials to medialize the true vocal fold. This procedure achieves closure of the musculomembranous vocal fold only; arytenoid position is not appreciably altered by the implant. Thy-

roplasty type I is a relatively simple and reversible procedure, which is ideally performed with local anesthesia to facilitate fine-tuning of the voice with precise placement of the implant material. Many variations of the original procedure, primarily introducing different implant materials and their placement, have been described.. Because thyroplasty type I does not primarily influence arytenoid position, this procedure is often coupled with an arytenoid adduction or arytenopexy to close both the anterior (musculomembranous) and posterior (cartilaginous) glottis.

Isshiki's Other Thyroplasty Classifications

Thyroplasty type II is a procedure in which the posterolateral thyroid lamina is lateralized; there are few indications for its use. Thyroplasty type III is used to lower the vocal pitch by shortening the anteroposterior (A-P) dimension of the glottis. The primary function is to release vocal fold tension to lower pitch. Conversely, thyroplasty type IV increases the A-P dimension of the glottis, thereby increasing the tension on the vocal folds and raising the vocal pitch. Thyroplasty types III and IV have been used in gender reassignment surgery to bring the fundamental frequency into the normal range for the newly assigned sex.

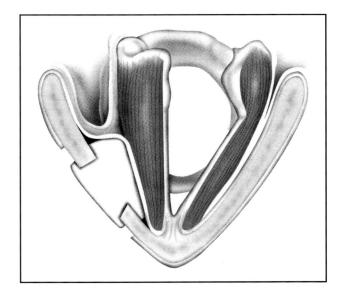

Figure 44–1. A small implant is placed lateral to the inner perichondrium of the thyroid lamina. (Reproduced with permission from Zeitels SM. Adduction arytenopexy with medialization laryngoplasty and cricothyroid subluxation: a new approach to paralytic dysphonia. *Op Techn Otolaryngol Head Neck Surg.* 1999;10:9–16.)

Arytenoid Adduction

Arytenoid adduction was described by Isshiki[5] as a way of mimicking the medializing effect of the lateral cricoarytenoid muscle on the vocal process. A paralyzed arytenoid will tend to fall forward and laterally on the cricoid facet, shortening the A-P length of the vocal fold and moving the arytenoid away from the midline. The classic arytenoid adduction procedure is performed under local anesthesia with sedation by exposing the posterior aspect of the thyroid lamina. The cricoarytenoid joint is identified, and a suture is placed through the muscular process of the arytenoid and passed anteriorly through the thyroid lamina, thereby rotating the vocal process medially to meet the opposite vocal process during phonation. Prior to the conclusion of the surgical procedure the position is visually verified by means of a flexible fiberoptic laryngoscope.

SURGICAL INNOVATIONS

Adduction Arytenopexy

Patients who require repositioning of the arytenoid secondary to paralysis-induced displacement typically have minimal or unfavorable synkinetic reinnervation of the intrinsic laryngeal musculature. Therefore, the arytenoid is malpositioned anteriorly, inferiorly, and laterally, resulting in a flaccid, foreshortened vocal fold. Isshiki's classical arytenoid adduction procedure mimics contraction of the lateral cricoarytenoid muscle and achieves rotation of the arytenoid by means of a suture that is placed through its muscular process and directed anteriorly through the thyroid lamina. However, the agonist-antagonistic adductor function of the other intrinsic muscles (lateral thyroarytenoid, interarytenoid, and posterior cricoarytenoid) is not simulated.

The adduction-arytenopexy procedure was designed to model the synchronous function of the aforementioned musculature.[2] In this technique, the arytenoid is positioned on the medial aspect of the cricoid facet, simulating normal adduction of the arytenoid during phonation. In addition, an implant (typically Gore-Tex) is placed lateral to the paraglottic muscles (inner thyroid perichondrium) to avoid wide excursion of the glottal tissues during entrained oscillation. The dennervated musculature of the paraglottic region is highly susceptible to the potential closing forces secondary to Bernoulli's effect. This fact is utilized to counterbalance the loss in normal elastic-recoil closing-forces from the denervation. Placing the arytenoid in appropriate position posteriorly, prior to the placement of an implant, achieves most of the medialization

that is necessary for the edge of the musculomembranous vocal fold.[2,7,8,11]

The adduction-arytenopexy procedure results in a slightly longer vocal fold, which is appropriately aligned in all three dimensions with a well-conformed medial edge of the glottal aperture. This clinical observation was confirmed in a cadaver study.[2,7,8,11] In contradistinction to the classical arytenoid adduction in which an anterolateral directed suture is used, the adduction-arytenopexy procedure achieves a longer vocal fold by posteromedially displacing the arytenoid and maintaining its position with a posteriorly based suture. In the same study, the adduction-arytenopexy procedure was more effective than the classical arytenoid adduction in closing interarytenoid gaps. Furthermore, the adduction arytenopexy does not result in excessive hyperrotation of the vocal process.

During adduction arytenopexy, the body of the arytenoid is medialized to the limit of the medial cricoarytenoid joint capsule in a normal gliding fashion along the cricoid facet. It is clear from the convex contour of the cricoid facet and the precisely accommodating concave contour of the arytenoid base that hyperrotation (simulating the lateral cricoarytenoid muscle) based on an axial plane does not simulate normal arytenoid adduction. Furthermore, pathological hyperrotation of the arytenoid and hyperfunction of the lateral cricoarytenoid are typically observed in patients who present with arytenoid granulomas.[21] Both Koufman's diagrammatic depiction of a typical arytenoid adduction[22] as well as cadaver studies by Neuman and Woodson et al[23] reveal an abnormally contoured medial arytenoid that results in an abnormal interarytenoid chink. In many patients, the clinical significance of this chink may be minimized by redundant interarytenoid and periarytenoid soft tissue.

The adduction-arytenopexy dissection method[2,7,8,11] of the cricoarytenoid joint can be performed without complication and is simpler than other techniques. Additionally, using the anatomic configuration of the cricoid facet to select the ideal position of the arytenoid has not been reported previously. These factors lead to placement of the arytenoid in a more normal adduction position, and, therefore, more effective glottal closure during laryngeal sound production.

Despite ideal positioning of the arytenoid from the arytenopexy procedure, intraoperative observations revealed that optimal vocal quality required an accompanying medialization laryngoplasty. This is due to the flaccidity of the dennervated glottis, which results in valvular incompetence. The dennervated glottal tissues have impaired elastic-recoil closing forces due to atrophy and fibrosis. On stroboscopy, this is revealed as an abnormally wide excursion of the vocal edge and as a long open-phase quotient during vibratory cycles.

A well-positioned arytenoid obviates the need for complex implant shapes that are intended to close the posterior glottis from an anteriorly positioned thyroid-lamina window. Additionally, there are a number of technical advantages to performing medialization laryngoplasty with adduction arytenopexy rather than with arytenoid adduction. As there is not an anterior thyroid-lamina suture, the implant is unencumbered by the adduction of the arytenoid. Furthermore, the adduction arytenopexy is done prior to the medialization so that the implant can be sized more accurately with the structural positioning of the posterior glottis already established. Finally, complex implant shapes that violate the thyroid-lamina inner perichondrium are unnecessary.

The adduction arytenopexy, which positions the arytenoid for normal phonation, can allow for a simple smaller implant shape to be placed lateral to the thyroid perichondrium because posterior glottic tissues are already aligned. *The primary goal of the implant with arytenopexy is to prevent lateral excursion of the flaccid paraglottic tissue during oscillatory cycles rather than to medialize the vocal edge, which is accomplished mostly by the adduction arytenopexy.* The technique for implant medialization becomes similar to what is required for patients with vocal muscle atrophy, which is easy to correct.

Observations made from the vocal outcome data in the patients who underwent adduction arytenopexy and medialization laryngoplasty revealed that fairly normal conversational-level phonation was achieved.[2,7,8,11] However, there were remarkable limitations of maximal range capabilities, especially frequency variation and maximal phonation time. This was thought to be secondary to suboptimal viscoelastic tension in the dennervated vocal fold soft tissues despite the aforementioned improvements in three-dimensional repositioning of the vocal edge. The need to increase viscoelastic tension in the dennervated vocal fold, and thereby improve aerodynamically efficient, entrained oscillation, catalyzed the development of the cricothyroid (C-T) subluxation procedure.[7,12]

In summary, repositioning the arytenoid should primarily be done when the malpositioned cartilage leads to phonatory aerodynamic glottal incompetence. Adduction arytenopexy[2] is the first modification of Isshiki's arytenoid-adduction procedure, which was designed over 20 years ago. The arytenoids-adduction procedure only simulates the lateral cricoarytenoid muscle, while the adduction arytenopexy models the synchronous adductor contraction of all the intrinsic musculature.

Gore-Tex Medialization Thyroplasty

The use of Gore-Tex as a medialization implant for the musculomembranous vocal fold was introduced by McCulloch and Hoffman[24] and has been employed by the author for 7 years.[7-10] The primary advantages of Gore-Tex are its ease of handling, placement, and adjustability, all of which enhance the speed and precision with which the operation can be performed. The position of the Gore-Tex can even be adjusted and fine-tuned extensively while the implant remains within the patient rather than removing it for modification as is done with Silastic. This is unlike virtually all other implant approaches. Furthermore, precise positioning of the thyroid-lamina window is less critical as Gore-Tex can be placed into appropriate position despite a slightly malpositioned window.

Because of these characteristics, Gore-Tex is also well-suited to restore aerodynamic glottal competence in scenarios in which there are complex anatomic defects such as those encountered with trauma and cancer resections. Even subtle contour changes from the loss of superficial lamina propria associated with sulcus vergeture can be reconformed to treat a small glottal gap. The versatility of Gore-Tex is evidenced by its ease of use in the treatment of these varied irregular tissue abnormalities. The clinical experience, in part reported in a recent review, revealed minimal complications in over 200 cases.[10]

To facilitate placement of the implant, an inferiorly based thyroid perichondrial flap is developed and a window is made in the thyroid lamina lateral to the musculomembranous vocal fold. The inner perichondrium of the thyroid lamina is preserved at the perimeter of the window. A small implant is then fashioned from a thin sheet of Gore-Tex so that it can be layered lateral to the inner perichondrium of the thyroid lamina. The Gore-Tex can be stabilized with a 4-0 Prolene suture. The thyroid lamina cartilage that was removed to make the window can be repositioned in its original site.

Cricothyroid Subluxation

Once the adduction arytenopexy and medialization laryngoplasty are completed, a cricothyroid subluxation is performed to further enhance vocal quality. The newly described cricothyroid subluxation is accomplished, by placing a 2-0 Prolene suture around the inferior cornu of the thyroid lamina on the dennervated side.[7,8,12] It is then passed in a submucosal fashion underneath the cricoid anteriorly. The suture is pulled taut, which increases the distance between the cricoid facet and the attachment of the anterior commissure ligament. This ultimately increases the tension and length of the musculomembranous vocal fold on the paralyzed side. The tension on this suture is adjusted by using a slip-knot while the patient performs phonatory tasks. These include maximal-range tasks such as use of pulse-register (vocal fry) through a falsetto register and glissando sliding scales.

This cricothyroid subluxation suture simulates cricothyroid muscle contraction for countertension on the thyroarytenoid muscle and for increasing length of the musculomembranous vocal fold.[7,8,12] Once this is completed, the strap muscles are reattached with 3-0 Vicryl suture in a running fashion. The wound is irrigated and a Penrose drain is placed. The platysma is approximated in a running fashion with Vicryl suture as well, and then the skin is closed with 4-0 nylon suture. A pressure dressing is applied and the drain is removed on the first postoperative morning. The patient is started on a liquid diet on the first postoperative morning and is advanced to a normal diet as tolerated. Fiberoptic laryngoscopy is performed prior to discharge to ensure that there is not an excessive amount of edema that would warrant further observation. Typically, patients can be discharged on the first postoperative day.

CLINICAL ELXPERIENCE WITH CRICOTHYROID SUBLUXATION

The cricothyroid-subluxation (C-T sub) procedure has further enhanced postoperative vocal quality as it is an easily adjustable method of increasing and varying tension and length of the paralyzed and dennervated musculomembranous vocal fold. This is unlike all prior operations, which were designed primarily to treat paralytic dysphonia by repositioning the vocal fold edge.[2,4-6,25] Procedures that alter tension and length of the vocal fold were conceived to modify pitch rather than to treat paralytic dysphonia.[6,25-27] The cricothyroid subluxation suture (1) models cricothyroid muscle contraction, (2) produces countertension on the thyroarytenoid muscle, and (3) increases the length of the musculomembranous vocal fold.[12] C-T subluxation is easy to perform, has been free from complications, and improves the acoustical outcome of other laryngoplastic phonosurgical procedures.

The modified biomechanical properties of vocal fold vibration that occurred subsequent to C-T sub resulted in improved vocal outcome in all patients[12] and was most remarkable in maximal range capabilities. C-T sub enhanced the postoperative voice of patients, regardless of whether they required medialization laryn-

goplasty alone or with adduction arytenopexy. Unlike stretching/lengthening procedures associated with gender reassignment, voice results in dennervated patients have not deteriorated with follow-up of a 1 year or more. *Due to the decreased elasticity of dennervated vocal folds, the optimal length (for vibration) is longer than that of normal vocal folds. Dennervated vocal fold tissue has a different resonant frequency than if it is innervated.*

Although the adduction arytenopexy had been shown to result in improvements in a number of objective measures of vocal function[2] by simulating normal glottal closure and reproducing the synchronous adductor contractile characteristics of all the intrinsic muscles, vocal outcome measures revealed limitations in maximal range tasks, especially dynamic frequency range.[2] This finding was most likely due to persistent flaccidity of the dennervated thyroarytenoid musculature. Both Isshiki's[5,6] and Zeitels'[2] adducting arytenoid techniques separate the cricothyroid joint to expose the cricoarytenoid joint. During a collaborative cadaver dissection, R. Sataloff (personal communication) observed that separation and destabilization of the ipsilateral cricothyroid joint impairs the function of the contralateral cricothyroid muscle. Based on a similar observation, other authors have exposed the cricoarytenoid joint during arytenoid adduction by removing a posterior window of the thyroid lamina and leaving the cricothyroid joint intact.[28]

Clinical observations revealed that, after the cricothyroid joint was opened, the inferior cornu of the thyroid lamina became retrodisplaced with relation to the cricoid. This meant that the previously fixed vocal fold length was shortened, and the tension of flaccid dennervated thyroarytenoid muscle was reduced further. Essentially, there was a decrease in the normal distance between the cricoarytenoid joint and the insertion of the anterior commissure tendon into the thyroid lamina.

Foreshortening of the paralyzed vocal fold, induced by separating the cricothyroid joint, probably led to compensatory hyperfunctional foreshortening of the normal vocal fold. This hyperfunctional adaptation occurs to align the vocal processes, which is a prerequisite for normal entrained oscillation during phonation. The decreased phonatory length of both vocal folds and the decreased viscoelastic tension of the paralyzed vocal fold resulted in limitations in acoustic maximal-range capabilities. Despite the fact that the paralyzed vocal fold was surgically placed under higher tension (than its preoperative state) after C-T subluxation,[7,8,12] almost all patients could reach a frequency lower than their preoperative state. This paradox is probably explained by the fact that the postsubluxation lengthened vocal fold results in reduced hyperfunction of the entire laryngeal complex.

The cricothyroid subluxation procedure was designed to rectify the mechanical impediments that were partially precipitated by disruption of the cricothyroid joint during cricoarytenoid joint dissection. However, C-T subluxation also improved the vocal outcome of those patients who did not require an arytenoid procedure (because of somewhat-favorable synkinesis). In both scenarios, the objective measures of vocal function reveal that C-T subluxation improved the aerodynamic efficiency of the glottal valve with a commensurate enhancement of the maximal-range acoustic characteristics of the voice. Subjective perceptions revealed that most patients demonstrated a register transition between modal and falsetto, an observation not previously reported.

OPERATIVE TECHNIQUE

Adduction Arytenopexy, Medialization Laryngoplasty, and Cricothyroid Subluxation

Unless contraindicated, most patients are started on a Medrol dosepak the day prior to surgery and are given 0.2 mg/kg of Decadron one hour prior to the procedure. This helps to minimize intraoperative swelling, which can alter judgment regarding the implant size, and reduces postoperative airway swelling. A hori-

zontal incision is made in a natural neck crease overlying the region of the cricothyroid space. Subplatysmal flaps are raised to expose the infrahyoid strap musculature and Gelpi retractors are placed to maintain the flaps. A transverse incision is made through the strap muscles to expose the thyroid lamina. A double-pronged skin hook is placed lateral to the edge of the thyroid lamina and it is rotated anteromedially. This defines the edge of the thyroid lamina and inferior cornu of the thyroid cartilage. A needle-tipped electrocautery knife is used to separate the inferior constrictor from the thyroid lamina (Figure 44–2). The inferior cornu is identified and isolated so that the cricothyroid joint can be separated with a Mayo scissors (Figure 44–3). Separating the cricothyroid joint and associated inferior constrictor muscle from the thyroid cartilage allows for further anteromedial rotation of the thyroid lamina (Figure 44–4). Blunt dissection is performed in a cephalad and slightly anterior direction from the cricothyroid facet along the cricoid cartilage until the superior rim of the cricoid is encountered (Figure 44–5). In performing these maneuvers, the lateral aspect of the piriform mucosa has been bluntly dissected from the inner aspect of the thyroid lamina and the medial aspect of the piriform mucosa has been separated from the posterolateral aspect of the cricoid (Figure 44–4). Posterior superior dissection along the top of the cricoid results in separation of the lateral cricoary-

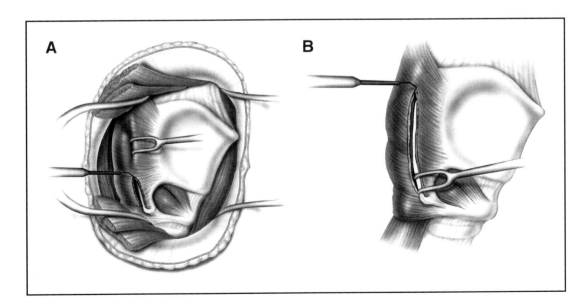

Figure 44–2. A needle-tipped electrocautery knife is used to separate the inferior constrictor from the thyroid lamina (**A** and **B**). (Reproduced with permission from Zeitels SM. Adduction arytenopexy with medialization laryngoplasty and crico-thyroid subluxation: a new approach to paralytic dysphonia. *Op Techn Otolaryngol Head Neck Surg.* 1999;10:9–16.)

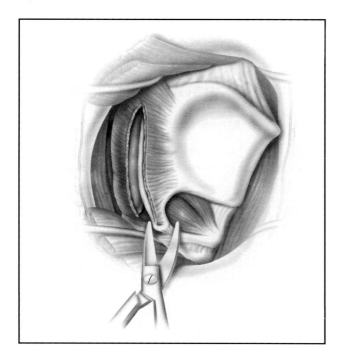

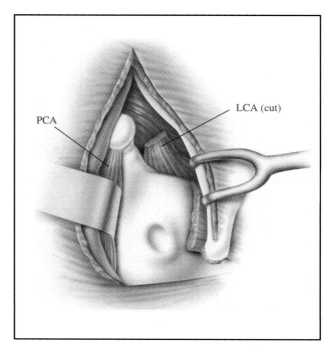

Figure 44–3. The inferior cornu is identified and isolated so that the cricothyroid joint can be separated with Mayo scissors. (Reproduced with permission from Zeitels SM. Adduction arytenopexy with medialization laryngoplasty and cricothyroid subluxation: a new approach to paralytic dysphonia. *Op Techn Otolaryngol Head Neck Surg.* 1999;10:9–16.)

Figure 44–5. Posterior-superior dissection along the top of the cricoid results in separation of the lateral cricoarytenoid muscle from the muscular process and ensures that the cricoarytenoid joint will be identified easily. (Reproduced with permission from Zeitels SM. Adduction arytenopexy with medialization laryngoplasty and cricothyroid subluxation: a new approach to paralytic dysphonia. *Op Techn Otolaryngol Head Neck Surg.* 1999;10:9–16.)

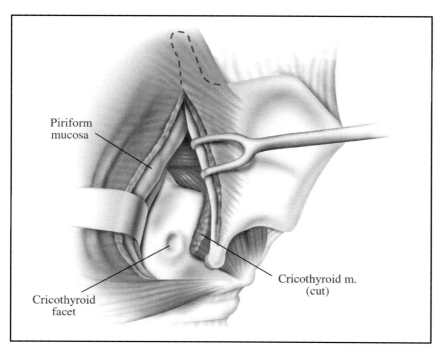

Figure 44–4. Separating the cricothyroid joint and associating the inferior constrictor muscle from the thyroid cartilage allows for further anteromedial rotation of the thyroid lamina. Blunt dissection is performed in a cephalad and slightly anterior direction from the cricothyroid facet along the cricoid cartilage until the superior rim of the cricoid is encountered. The lateral aspect of the piriform mucosa is bluntly dissected from the inner aspect of the thyroid lamina and the medial aspect of the piriform mucosa is separated from the posterolateral aspect of the cricoid. (Reproduced with permission from Zeitels SM. Adduction arytenopexy with medialization laryngoplasty and cricothyroid subluxation: a new approach to paralytic dysphonia. *Op Techn Otolaryngol Head Neck Surg.* 1999;10:9–16.)

tenoid muscle from the muscular process and ensures that the cricoarytenoid joint will be identified easily (Figure 44–5). The dissection along the superior rim of the cricoid leads to the muscular process of the arytenoid. The lateral cricoarytenoid muscle is severed from its attachment to the arytenoid. The posterior cricoarytenoid muscle is then separated from the muscular process of the arytenoids (Figure 44–5). The cricoarytenoid joint is opened widely with a Steven's scissors, and the curved, glistening white surface of the cricoid facet is identified (Figure 44–6). The posterior cricoarytenoid muscle is separated from the posterior plate of the cricoid so that the posterior aspect of the cricoarytenoid joint is seen well and so there is room to place a suture through this region (Figure 44–6). A 4-0 Prolene suture on a cutting needle is placed through the posterior plate of the cricoid just medial to the facet, and the needle is brought out through the medial aspect of the cricoarytenoid joint (Figure 44–7). The needle is then passed through the body of the arytenoid, followed by the inner aspect of the cricoid. The needle is then advanced under the cricoid facet and through the posterior plate of the cricoid, where a slipknot is placed (Figure 44–7). The arytenoid is positioned so that its body is subluxed medially, just off the facet, and so that it is rocked internally in the natural plane of the curved joint. Once the arytenoid is secured, the thyroid

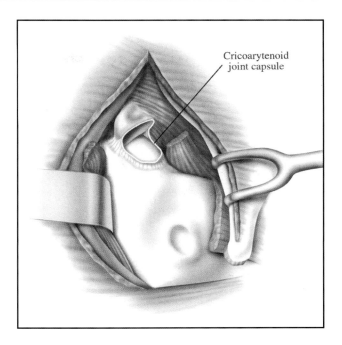

Figure 44–6. The cricoarytenoid joint is opened widely with Steven's scissors and the curved glistening white surface of the cricoid facet is identified. (Reproduced with permission from Zeitels SM. Adduction arytenopexy with medialization laryngoplasty and cricothyroid subluxation: a new approach to paralytic dysphonia. *Op Techn Otolaryngol Head Neck Surg.* 1999;10:9–16.)

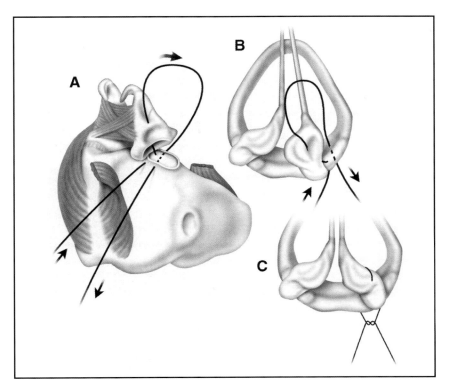

Figure 44–7. A 4–0 Prolene suture on a cutting needle is placed through the posterior plate of the cricoid just medial to the facet and the needle is brought out through the medial aspect of the cricoarytenoid joint (**A**). The need is passed through the body of the arytenoid and then through the inner aspect of the cricoid (**B**). The needle is advanced under the cricoid facet and through the posterior plate of the cricoid, where a slip knot is placed (**C**). (Reproduced with permission from Zeitels SM. Adduction arytenopexy with medialization laryngoplasty and cricothyroid subluxation: a new approach to paralytic dysphonia. *Op Techn Otolaryngol Head Neck Surg.* 1999;10:9–16.)

lamina is replaced into its natural anatomic position. The arytenoid is visualized by means of a flexible fiberoptic laryngoscope to check position during a number of phonatory tasks. If the arytenoid is in good position, the arytenoid suture is affixed permanently. The voice is typically still dysphonic until the implant is placed to support the paraglottic musculature.[2]

Subsequently, an inferiorly based thyroid perichondrial flap is developed and a standard window is made in the thyroid lamina lateral to the musculomembranous vocal fold as previously described by Isshiki (Figure 44–8). The inner perichondrium of the thyroid lamina is preserved as is appropriate at the perimeter of the window. A small implant is then fashioned from a thin sheet of Gore-Tex so that it can be layered lateral to the inner perichondrium of the thyroid lamina. The Gore-Tex can be stabilized with a 4-0 Prolene suture and the thyroid-lamina window can be repositioned. The external perichondrium (Figure 44–9) can be preserved and closed over the thyroid-lamina window.

Once the adduction arytenopexy and medialization laryngoplasty are completed, a cricothyroid subluxation is performed to further enhance vocal quality. The newly described cricothyroid subluxation is accom-

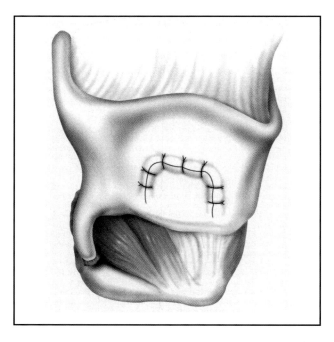

Figure 44–9. The thyroid lamina external perichondrium, is repositioned with 4-0 vicryl suture. (Reproduced with permission from Zeitels SM. Adduction arytenopexy with medialization laryngoplasty and cricothyroid subluxation: a new approach to paralytic dysphonia. *Op Techn Otolaryngol Head Neck Surg.* 1999;10:9–16.)

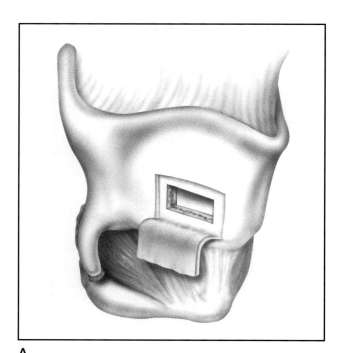

A

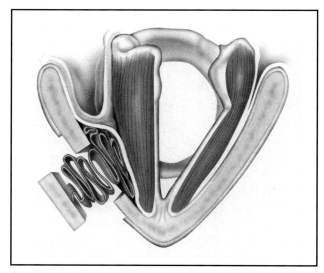

B

Figure 44–8. A. An inferiorly based thyroid perichondrial flap is developed, and a standard window is made in the thryroid lamina lateral to the musculomembranous vocal fold. **B.** A thin sheet of Gore-Tex is used and it is layered in position and can be stabilized with a 4–0 Prolene suture.

(Reproduced with permission from Zeitels SM. Adduction arytenopexy with medialization laryngoplasty and cricothyroid subluxation: a new approach to paralytic dysphonia. *Op Techn Otolaryngol Head Neck Surg.* 1999;10:9–16.)

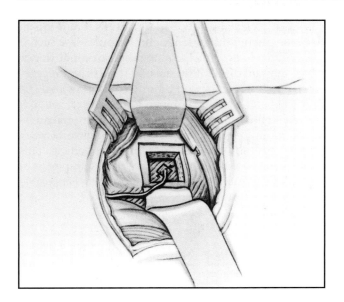

Figure 45–4. Nerve-muscle pedicle sutured to exposed surface of lateral thyroarytenoideus muscle.

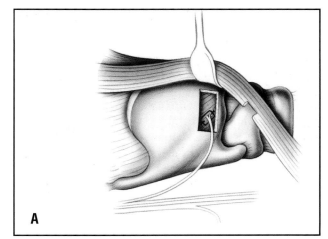

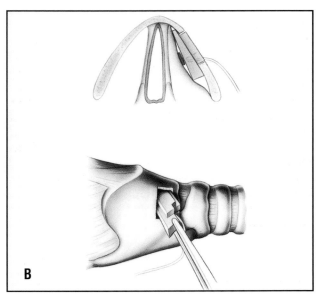

Figure 45–5. A. Nerve-muscle pedicle rotated and sutured to exposed muscle. **B.** Silastic prosthesis is inserted without disturbing pedicle. Note posterior-inferior corner has been removed to provide space for free passage of the nerve-muscle pedicle.

supply, and for reinnervation of a laryngeal transplant were already available. The one problem that remained to be solved at that time was the need for immunosuppression in a recipient who had recently been treated for a malignancy. It was felt that, unless the donor larynx could be rendered nonantigenic or that means of immunosuppression that would not potentiate malignancy could be found, the risks of laryngeal transplantation would not be justified.[29]

The first reported human laryngeal transplantation, and to date the only one, was accomplished[30] at the Cleveland Clinic on January 4th, 1998 in a patient whose larynx had been crushed and in whom reconstruction for voice and airway had been unsuccessful. Although the transplanted larynx has survived and the patient is now able to maintain nutrition by mouth, he still requires a "permanent" tracheostomy stoma for adequate airway. According to personal communications, the larynx transplant has not been successfully reinnervated.[30]

Any of several means of reinnervation could theoretically be applied in cases of laryngeal transplant. Nerve-muscle pedicle technique was reported to have been successful after reimplantation of totally excised canine larynges.[31] Any anastomotic technique should also succeed, but it will probably be necessary to selectively reinnervate only the abductor divisions, in order to restore adequate airway capability. Many studies have shown that, if both the adductor and abductor divisions are reinnervated, adduction usually overpowers any abductor function that may be restored, thus interfering in ability to eventually extubate the airway.

As the position assumed by bilaterally denervated vocal folds is usually appropriate for reasonable voice production, unopposed abductor function can be achieved more easily than when both divisions of the recurrent laryngeal nerve are reinnervated.

Which, if any of the currently available reinnervation techniques might be successful in restoring adequate voice and airway in a transplanted larynx will have to wait for further experience. Because the problem of immunosuppression is as yet unsolved, it seems unlikely that any such experience will be available in the near future.

ELECTRONIC PACING FOR VOCAL FOLD PARALYSIS

Several attempts to devise electronic pacemakers that could adduct or abduct paralyzed vocal folds have been reported.[32,33] Researchers who have reported direct implantation of wire electrodes into denervated laryngeal muscles have generally succeeded in an acute laboratory setting, but it seems unlikely that such an arrangement would be adequate in the long term. To begin with, laryngeal muscles denervated for several months are known to lose bulk, making direct implantation and the necessary fixation of the wires extremely difficult in an active person, whose laryngotracheal complex can be expected to move vigorously during swallowing, coughing, and even with necessary head and neck movements. Second, experience with direct implantation of wire electrodes into cardiac muscle shows that chemical changes and scarring around the tips eventually results in increasing electrical resistance. Finally, direct electrical stimulation does not seem to prevent deterioration and wasting of skeletal muscle, even though it may succeed in causing depolarization. Only restored neurohumoral depolarization appears to prevent further muscle deterioration.

Broniatowski et al have published several reports using perineural electrodes with a previously placed nerve-muscle pedicle.[34-39] This approach would appear more likely to succeed than direct implantation techniques in an actual clinical setting. The electrode contact with the nerve-muscle pedicle can be at some distance from the larynx itself, thus permitting more stable placement around the nerve (as opposed to implantation) and much less movement in an active patient. Moreover, this technique results in neurohumoral depolarization at the subtended motor end plate sites in the recipient muscle, thus preventing further deterioration of the reinnervated muscle. Finally, nerve-muscle pedicle electronic pacing lends itself to *selective* reinnervation so that the pacing efforts can be directed to those precise muscle groups that are needed, rather than gross reinnervation of all the muscles in the organ.

CONCLUSION

Loss of vocal capability because of immobility of one vocal fold can be corrected by any of several means, but only reinnervation can restore tensing capability and, thus, optimize voice quality. Anastomosis techniques have been successful, but require availability of sufficient length of donor nerve, as well as a distal nerve segment with patent neural tubules to which it can be attached. Direct implantation of a cut donor nerve may be difficult because of insufficient length. Nerve-muscle pedicle technique avoids most of these problems and can be combined with surgical medialization so that improvement in vocal strength can be achieved immediately, while the patient awaits onset of reinnervation from the nerve-muscle pedicle. This approach to voice rehabilitation offers the patient restoration of function as close to normal as is possible with existing techniques.

REFERENCES

1. Tucker HM. Vocal cord paralysis-1979: etiology and management. *Laryngoscope*. 1980;90:585–590.
2. Coleman SC, Netterville JL, Coury MS, Ossoff RH, Billante C. Etiology and outcome of vocal fold paralysis: unilateral and bilateral. *Trans Am Laryngol Assn*. 2004.
3. Evoy M. Experimental activation of paralyzed vocal cords. *Arch Otolaryngol*. 1968;87:155–161.
4. King BT, Gregg RL. An anatomical reason for the various behaviors of paralyzed vocal cords. *Ann Otol Rhinol Laryngol*. 1948;57:925.
5. Hogikyan ND, Johns MM, Kileny PR, Urbanchek M, Carroll WR, Kuzon Jr WM. Motion-specific laryngeal reinnervation using muscle-nerve-muscle neurotization. *Trans Am Laryngol Assn*. 2001.
6. Exner S. Notiz zu der Frage von der Faservertheilung mehrerer Nerven in einem Muskel. *Pflugers Arch Ges Physiol*. 1885;36:572.
7. Horsley JA. Suture of the recurrent laryngeal nerve with report of a case. *Trans Soc Surg Gynecol Assoc*. 1909;22:161.
8. Lahey FH. Suture of the recurrent laryngeal nerve for bilateral abductory paralysis. *Ann Surg*. 1928;87:481.
9. Colledge L. On the possibility of restoring movements to a paralyzed vocal cord by nerve anastomosis. *Br Med J*. 1925;2:547.
10. Frazier CH, Mosser WB. Treatment of recurrent laryngeal nerve injury. *Surg Gynecol Obstet*. 1926;43:134.
11. Ballance C. Some experiments on nerve anastomosis. *Mayo Clin Proc*. 1928;3:317.
12. Doyle PJ. Surgical treatment of bilateral adductor laryngeal paralysis. *Proc Can Otol Soc*. 1964:18.
13. Miglets AW. Functional laryngeal abduction following reimplantation of the recurrent laryngeal nerves. *Laryngoscope*. 1974;84:1996–2005.
14. Ballance C. Results obtained in some experiments in which the facial and recurrent laryngeal nerves were anastomosed with other nerves. *Br Med J*. 1924;2:349.
15. Taggart JP. Laryngeal reinnervation by phrenic nerve implantation in dogs. *Laryngoscope*. 1971;81:1330–1336.
16. Crumley RL. Experiments in laryngeal reinnervation. *Laryngoscope*. 1982;92(suppl 30):1–27.
17. Crumley RL. Update of laryngeal reinnervation concepts and options. In: Bailey R, Biller H, eds. *Surgery of the Larynx*. Philadelphia, PA: WB Saunders; 1988:135–147.

18. Crumley RL, Izdebski K, McMicken B: Nerve transfer versus Teflon injection for vocal cord paralysis: a comparison. *Laryngoscope.* 1988;98:1200–1204.

19. Crumley RL, Izdebski K. Voice quality following laryngeal reinnervation by ansa hypoglossi transfer. *Laryngoscope.* 1986;96:611–616.

20. Olsen DEL, Goding GS, Michael DD: Acoustic and perceptual evaluation of laryngeal reinnervation by ansa cervicalis transfer. *Laryngoscope.* 1998;108:1767–1772.

21. Paniello RC. Laryngeal reinnervation with the hypoglossal nerve: II. clinical evaluation and early patient experience. *Laryngoscope.* 2000;110:739–748.

22. Iwamura S. Functioning remobilization of the paralyzed vocal cord in dogs. *Arch Otolaryngol.* 1974;100:122.

23. Tucker HM. Reinnervation of the unilaterally paralyzed larynx. *Ann Otol Rhinol Laryngol.* 1977;86:789–794.

24. Applebaum EL, Allen GW, Sisson GA. Human laryngeal reinnervation: the Northwestern experience. *Laryngoscope,* 1979;89:1784–1787.

25. May M, Beery Q. Muscle-nerve pedicle laryngeal reinnervation. *Laryngoscope.* 1986;96:1196–2000.

26. Tucker HM. *Neurologic disorders. In: The Larynx.* New York, NY: Thieme Medical Publishers; 1987:chap 11.

27. Tucker HM. Combined laryngeal framework medialization and reinnervation for unilateral vocal fold paralysis. *Ann Otol Rhinol Laryngol.* 1990:99:778–781.

28. Tucker HM. Phonosurgery for voice disorders. In: *The Larynx.* 2nd ed. New York, NY: Thieme Medical Publishers; 1993.

29. Tucker HM. Laryngeal transplantation: current status. 1974. *Laryngoscope.* 1975;85:787–796.

30. Strome M, et al: Personal communication

31. Tucker HM. Selective reinnervation of paralyzed musculature in the head and neck: Functioning autotransplantation of the canine larynx. *Laryngoscope.* 1978;88:162–171.

32. Obert PM, Young KA, Tobey DN. Use of direct posterior cricoarytenoid stimulation in laryngeal paralysis. *Arch Otolaryngol.* 1984;110:88–92.

33. Bergman K, Wartzel H, Eckhardt HU, Gerhardt HJ. Respiratory rhythmically regulated electrical stimulation of paralyzed laryngeal muscles. *Laryngoscope,* 1984;94:1376–1380.

34. Broniatowski M, Tucker HM, Kaneko S, Jacobs GJ, Nose Y. *Entrainement electronique du larynx: etudes preliminaires—principes de base appliques aux muscles sous-hyoidiens reinnerves chez le chien.* Paper presented at the 81st meeting of the Congres Francais; September 25, 1984; Paris.

35. Broniatowski M, Kaneko S, Nose Y, Jacobs GJ, Tucker HM. Laryneal pacemaker, II. Electronic pacing of reinnervated posterior cricoarytenoid muscles in the canine. *Laryngoscope.* 1985;95(10):1194–1198.

36. Broniatowski M, Tucker HM, Kaneko S, Jacobs G, Nose Y. Laryngeal pacemaker. Part I. Electronic pacing of reinnervated strap muscles in the dog. *Otolaryngology-Head and Neck Surgery.* 1986;94(1):41–44.

37. Broniatowski M, Tucker HM, Nose Y. Laryngeal biostimulators: rational, clinical applications and future perspectives. *Otorhinolaryngol Head Neck Surg.* 1990.

38. Broniatowski M, Davies CR, Jacobs GB,, et al. Artificial restoration of voice. I: Experiments in phonatory control of the reinnervated canine larynx. *Laryngoscope.* 1990; 100(11):1219–1224.

39. Broniatowski M, Grundfest-Broniatowki S, Tyler DJ, et al. Dynamic laryngotracheal closure for aspiration: a preliminary report. *Laryngoscope.* 2001;111(11):2032–2040.

logic interpretation in 54% of the cases reviewed. However, the majority of cases differed by only one grade level (ie, mild vs moderate).

Although the rate of malignancy associated with a pathologic diagnosis of dysplasia varies widely, the pattern of increasing risk of malignancy with a worsening dysplasia grade is consistent. Fiorella et al[6] reported an incidence of 6% malignant transformation in keratosis without atypia and 17% when atypia was present. Kambivc et al[28] reported a rate of malignant change of 0.3% for keratosis and 9.5% for keratosis with atypia. Blackwell et al[31] retrospectively reviewed 65 patients with long-term follow-up after laryngeal biopsy and found the following cancer rates: 0% (0/6) for keratosis without atypia, 12% (3/26) for mild dysplasia, 33% (5/15) for moderate dysplasia, 44% (4/9) for severe dysplasia, and 11% (1/9) for carcinoma in situ.

While the presence and grade of dysplasia certainly have prognostic implications, the presence of keratosis has almost no predictive value. Frangeuz et al[29] reviewed 4,291 cases and reported that surface keratosis was present in simple and atypical hyperplasia in 68.8% and 85.5%, respectively. Follow-up of these patients showed malignant transformation to be 0.8% of cases with simple hyperplasia and 8.6% of those with atypical hyperplasia. Keratosis can mask epithelial changes and is not a predictor of underlying atypia. However, dyskeratosis is an important morphologic feature in the process of carcinogenesis[29] One study revealed a transformation rate of 50% (6/12) in patients with dyskeratosis.[7]

Blackwell et al[8,31] identified five histologic parameters that were found to be significantly different when comparing dysplastic lesions that resolved or remained stable to those that progressed to invasive carcinoma. These were abnormal mitotic figures, mitotic activity, stromal inflammation, maturation level, and nuclear pleomorphism. The five factors were not statistically different when comparing severe dysplasia and carcinoma in situ. Surface morphology, nuclear prominence, and koilocytosis were not significantly different in the two groups.

Histologic examination remains the basis of diagnosis in mucosal lesions of the larynx; however, the prognostic value of the morphologic criteria is limited. Quantification of histologic parameters may become an important supplement to the traditional grading of dysplasia. Proliferation associated changes such as a count of mitotic figures, or Ki67- or PCNA-labeling index gives additional hard data which are correlated to histologic grade.[9-11] DNA histograms are being utilized as an addition to microscopic evaluation. There is evidence that lesions with abnormal DNA content

are more likely to persist or progress to intraepithelial or invasive carcinoma. However, it is important to note that the same studies show that the lack of abnormal DNA content does not exclude malignant transformation and that some cancers have so few chromosomal abnormalities that they are below the threshold sensitivity of image analysis or flow cytometry.[12] The prognostic value of p53 immunohistochemistry is controversial and many studies have not found any significant association between p53 immunoreactivity and the evolution of carcinoma.[3,11,32-34]

All patients found to have dysplastic lesions of the laryngeal mucosa need to be followed closely for many years. Progression to invasive carcinoma often is a slow process allowing for early diagnosis, which should yield improved cure rates. Blackwell et al[31] reported that the average interval between the first biopsy and the diagnosis of invasive carcinoma was 3.9 years, suggesting that a 5- to 10-year follow-up plan is reasonable. Velasko et al[7] also suggested a more strict follow-up of patients with dyskeratosis as a result of a 50% (6/12) malignant transformation rate. Their report was based on a retrospective study in which all pathologies were reviewed by one pathologist. The period of follow-up ranged from one year to 130 months with a mean of 73 months follow-up. Their conclusion was that there is a longer interval between biopsy and malignant changes when you compare with patients having invasive carcinoma, the majority of whom will relapse within 2 years. The ability to provide dedicated long-term care for patients at risk for head and neck cancer is now limited by the financial constraints of managed care[30] in addition to all the other factors that have resulted in delayed diagnosis and treatment. The value of clinical examination, including strobovideolaryngoscopy, at regular intervals cannot be overstated. The senior author (RTS) follows his patients every 1 to 3 months for cancer surveillance with videostrobscopy performed at each office evaluation. Such practice allows for early diagnosis of small invasive carcinomas and use of surgical options that yield greater laryngeal preservation and better voice quality postoperatively.

The strategy of biopsy differs if there is a single area of suspicion versus broad or multifocal lesions. Single, small lesions should be excised with a small mucosal margin. This will be sufficient treatment for many dysplastic lesions and intraepithelial neoplasms. When excision requires the removal of a large area of the true vocal fold, or a critical site such as the anterior commissure or medial margin, a small incisional biopsy may be more appropriate to allow for treatment planning with optimal voice preservation. In patients with broad-based or multifocal lesions, accurate microscopic biopsy at multiple sites is required. While it is always possible for biopsy sampling to miss areas of invasive carcinomas, these techniques are usually sufficient. However, if invasion is suspected clinically and not confirmed pathologically, the surgeon and patient must be prepared to proceed with additional biopsies. The availability of high-resolution microscopic guidance with suspension laryngoscopy permits both aggressive diagnostic biopsy and mucosal preservation. Contact endoscopy may be helpful in guiding biopsy location. Vocal fold stripping is no longer indicated in the treatment of mucosal lesions of the vocal folds.

Carcinoma in Situ (CIS)

CIS is defined as cellular dysplasia involving the entire thickness of the mucosa without compromise of the basement membrane. The dysplasia may extend into adjacent mucous glands and is still considered an in situ lesion, as long as the lesion is confined to the duct and does not extend in the periductal lamina propia.[1,35] In other words, it is a malignant epithelial neoplasm which has all the characteristics of a true carcinoma except invasiveness and the ability to metastasize.[36] It may exist as an isolated lesion, but it is frequently associated with an invasive squamous cell carcinoma (SCCa), lying either adjacent to or remote from it.[1] Unlike cervical intraepithelial neoplasia, laryngeal CIS is not a required precursor to SCCa. Pathologically, the difference between CIS and severe dysplasia may be very difficult to determine with absolute certainty and is in many ways subjective, resulting in wide differences in the reported incidence and prevalence. However, in practice, the difference between these two lesions is not critical, as both indicate a significant risk for the future development of invasive cancer.

CIS must be evaluated carefully and invasive carcinoma must be ruled out. This is even more significant in the face of CIS of the supraglottis and subglottis than on the vocal folds,[1] as those two sites are considered the "silent area" that usually presents at a later stage of disease. Thus, CIS generally is present in association with an invasive carcinoma.[37] If a small biopsy reveals CIS, then there must be a high suspicion that an adjacent invasive cancer was missed, as reported by Ferlito.[36]

The incidence of CIS ranges from 1% to 15% of all malignant laryngeal tumors.[36] There is a distinct male predominance, and it is most frequently seen in the sixth and seventh decades of life.[1] Although it can occur anywhere in the larynx, it most often involves the anterior portion of one or both vocal folds.[1,36,38] It may

appear as leukoplakia, erythroplakia, or hyperkeratosis. CIS is a microscopic diagnosis, and its presenting signs, symptoms, and appearance are indistinguishable from other lesions of dysplasia or hyperkeratosis.[36]

The biologic behavior of this tumor is unknown. However, the main pathologic issue is whether or not all CIS will eventually develop into invasive carcinoma. Auerbach[15] presents indirect evidence that some cases of laryngeal CIS may be reversible in an autopsy study that showed lower rates of CIS in ex-smokers than in active smokers. Stenersen et al[4] observed 41 patients with the diagnosis of CIS or severe dysplasia, but who did not develop invasive carcinoma in the first year following their initial biopsy. The average observation time was 100 months. Forty-six percent (19/41) developed invasive SCCa after a mean interval of 50 months and 54% (22/41) returned to normal mucosa following biopsy. In a literature review, Bouquot and Gnepp[39] found that an average of 29% of cases of laryngeal CIS eventually resulted in invasive carcinoma with a reported range in the different studies of 3.5% to 90%. Untreated cases of CIS were associated with higher rates of transformation: 33.3% to 90%. When considering all these data, it appears that some cases of CIS are cured by excisional biopsy and some lesions are reversible if the patient controls tobacco use. Yet, despite close observation and treatment, many CIS lesions will progress to invasive carcinoma.

There are some prognostic factors that can be utilized to guide treatment of patients with CIS. Myssiorek et al[37] studied 41 patients with CIS retrospectively and found a much higher rate of transformation in lesions of the anterior commissure (92%) (11/12), than of lesions on the membranous vocal fold (17%) (5/29). This may reflect understaging caused by inadequate biopsy at the anterior commissure. This study also found no association of epidermal growth factor receptors (EGFR) in predicting lesions that will progress to invasive cancer. Epidermal growth factor (EGF) may play a role in the regulation of the growth of cancer of the larynx. Some in vitro studies have shown that cancer cells are stimulated by EGF/EGFR (immunohistochemical analysis of overexpression), while others evaluated if it had any prognostic value in determining which premalignant lesion or CIS would progress to invasive carcinoma. Results concerning its usefulness are inconsistent in the literature.[3,32] In another study, 37% (7/19) of patients with CIS who developed invasive laryngeal carcinoma were found to have had the carcinoma arise at a different anatomic site from the original CIS.[4] The authors concluded that there should be a high clinical suspicion of a lesion that arises separately from the site of known CIS.

47

Surgery for Laryngeal Cancer

Steven M. Zeitels, MD, FACS

GLOTTIC CARCINOMA; DISEASE PRESENTATION AND PHILOSOPHY OF MANAGEMENT

Although hoarseness is the most frequent symptom associated with glottic cancer, many patients have had this symptom for many years, while dysplastic mucosa undergoes malignant degeneration. Many patients describe frequent throat clearing; however, this is typically the result of reflux laryngopharyngitis, which is commonly observed in patients with laryngeal cancer. Advanced glottic cancer is associated with airway restriction and less commonly, hemoptysis and otalgia.

Tobacco smoking has been implicated as the primary risk factor associated with laryngeal cancer. In part, this was due to the fact that larynx cancer was a rare disease until the 20th century. Shortly after the introduction of mass-produced cigarettes, premalignant glottal epithelium is described along with escalating frequency of laryngeal cancer.[1] Large-scale studies typically report a 95% incidence of smoking in laryngeal cancer. However, in a recent report, Rosow and Zeitels (unpublished data: American Broncho-Esophagological Association, 2004) noted ~70% incidence of smoking in a small series of patients with doctoral degrees. This interesting observation is yet unexplainable and should heighten our awareness that there may be new carcinogenic risk factors, which may take decades to uncover. In fact, this pattern would mirror the acknowledgment of tobacco causing larynx cancer, which was not deemed to be a primary risk factor until well into the 1900s.

Squamous cell carcinoma comprises the overwhelming majority of laryngeal cancers.[2] Because of limited lymphatics in the glottis,[3,4] most patients presenting with glottic carcinoma have localized disease without regional or distant metastasis.[5] Glottic cancer presents almost exclusively in the musculomembranous region so that hoarseness occurs early, often facilitating identification of the disease at an earlier stage.[1] However, even advanced primary disease is adequately controlled with surgery and/or radiotherapy. Taken together, most patients will survive larynx cancer.

Similar to other tumor models, laryngeal cancer is staged using the standard TNM classification system (Table 47–1) The subsites are composed of the supraglottis, glottis, or subglottis and each geographic location has a discrete algorithm for stratifying T_1 to T_4. Understandably, the staging system has substantial limitations; however, it does provide broad language to communicate data to patients and physicians.

Surgery and radiotherapy (XRT) are the primary treatment modalities for laryngeal carcinoma. Solis

Table 47–1. TNM Staging of Laryngeal Cancer

Supraglottic

Tis:

T1: Tumor confined to site of origin with normal mobility

T2: Tumor involving adjacent supraglottic site(s) or glottis without fixation

T3: Tumor limited to larynx with fixation or extension or both to involve the postcricoid area, medial wall of piriform sinus, or pre-epiglottic space

T4: Massive tumor extending beyond larynx to involve oropharynx, soft tissues of neck, or destruction of thyroid cartilage

Glottis

Tis:

T1: confined to vocal cords with normal mobility (includes involvement of anterior or posterior commissure)

T1a: unilateral involvement

T1b: bilateral involvement

T2: supraglottic or subglottic extension of tumor or both with normal or impaired cord mobility

T3: tumor confined to larynx with cord fixation

T4: massive tumor with thyroid cartilage destruction or extension beyond confines of larynx or both

Subglottis

Tis:

T1: tumor confined to the subglottic region

T2: tumor extension to vocal cords with normal or impaired cord mobility

T3: tumor confined to larynx with cord fixation

T4: massive tumor with cartilage destruction or extension beyond confines of larynx or both

N0: no regional LN metastasis

N1: <3 cm, single ipsilateral LN

N2: 3 cm-6 cm

   N2a: single ipsilateral 3-6 cm

   N2b: multiple ipsilateral <6 cm

   N2c: bilateral or contralateral, all <6 cm

N3: >6 cm

Staging

Stage I: T1,N0,M0

Stage II: T2,N0,M0

Stage III: T3,N0,M0

     T1,T2 or T3, N1,M0

Stage IV: T4,Nx,Mx

     Tx,N2 or N3,M0

Tx,Nx,M1

Cohen[6] was probably the first individual to cure a larynx cancer by performing a transcervical vertical partial laryngectomy in 1869. Fraenkel[7] reported the first successful transoral (mirror guided) resection of laryngeal cancer in 1886. Radiotherapy was introduced in the late 19th century and gained progressive popularity through the 20th century. Despite the fact that endola-ryngeal surgery[1,8-15] and XRT[16,17] are equally successful in curing the early disease, radiotherapy became the dominant treatment modality due to many surgeons' concerns that their individual skills were not comparable to those reporting the endoscopic techniques, especially with regard to voice preservation. Many considered laryngoscopic treatment of glottic cancer too difficult and open surgery was deemed to be excessively morbid because of the associated vocal dysfunction and the frequent need for a temporary tracheotomy.

RADIOTHERAPY FOR GLOTTIC CANCER

Early Disease

Radiotherapy is the mainstay of treatment in untreated disease for surgeons who do not feel comfortable with microlaryngoscopic resection methods and associated reconstructive techniques. Patients who cannot be adequately exposed during staging endoscopy are ideal candidates for radiotherapy. The optimal clinical scenario for using XRT in early glottic cancer is diffuse superficial disease (T_{1b}, T_{2b}) in which surgical intervention would disrupt the basic architecture of both vocal folds; the anterior commissure tendon and/or the laminae propria.

The disadvantages of XRT include treatment of noncancerous vocal-fold tissue (T_{1a}, T_{2a}), which frequently results in scarring of the mucosa of the normal vocal fold with associated dysphonia.[18] Typically, the saccular glands are included in the treatment field, which can lead to further disruptions in glottal vibratory function and severe hoarseness. Atrophy of the saccular glands results in laryngitis sicca and the requirement of increased subglottal pressure for phonatory tasks. Administering radiotherapy to younger patients is a relative contraindication as it is a single-use treatment and there is a significant risk for metacronous lesions. In addition, there is the theoretic risk for radiation-induced cancer.[19] Finally, radiation is more expensive than endoscopic resection.[20]

More Advanced Disease (T_3, T_4)

Radiotherapy with or without chemotherapy is used when patients are not surgical candidates. Retrospective studies suggest that XRT as a single modality treatment for more advanced lesions results in diminished control rates as compared to surgery. Furthermore, morbid complications from XRT may include airway obstruction requiring a tracheotomy as well as acute odynophagia and dysphagia necessitating gastrostomy tube placement. Severe dysphonia and dryness may be permanent as is chondroradionecrosis.[21]

Radiation therapy is typically administered over 6 weeks to a total dosage of 5,600 to 7,600 rads. Investigations with neoadjuvant chemotherapy[22] (cisplatin and 5-fluorouracil) suggest that there is a subpopulation of individuals in whom this approach constitutes optimal management; however, this patient cohort has yet to be clearly delineated. Furthermore, it is difficult to determine whether induction chemotherapy provides a therapeutic advantage over advanced single-modality radiotherapy (ie, BID treatment).

SURGERY FOR GLOTTIC CANCER

Surgery has long been a mainstay of treatment for glottic cancer. If the correct procedure is selected and executed appropriately, local control is greater than 90% regardless of the disease stage. Effective management includes minimizing oncologically sound margins,[1,13,23-26] as well as creative reconstruction[25,26] to optimize the postoperative airway, voice, and deglutition. Surgery is typically less expensive than radiotherapy[20] and, unlike XRT, there is immediate oncologic eradication without intercurrent disease during the treatment course. Surgical resection of glottic cancer can be done transorally or transcervically.

Endoscopic Treatment of Early Glottic Cancer

The goal of endoscopic treatment of an isolated T_1 lesion of the musculomembranous vocal fold is eradication of the disease with maximal preservation of the normal layered microstructure (epithelium and laminae propria). This approach results in the optimal postoperative voice without compromising oncologic cure. The universal modular glottiscope was designed specifically to perform endolaryngeal resection of glottic cancer.[27] It has a number of advantages for exposing the tumor as well as for dissecting the tissue.

There are four basic procedures that are based on the depth of excision (Figure 47–1)[14,15,26,28]: (1) dissection just deep to the epithelial basement membrane and superficial to the superficial lamina propria for epithelial atypia and microinvasive cancer; (2) dissection within the superficial lamina propria microinvasive cancer that is not attached to the vocal ligament; (3) dissection between the deep lamina propria (vocal ligament) and the vocalis muscle for lesions that are attached to the ligament but not through it; (4) dissection within the thyroarytenoid muscle for lesions penetrating the vocal ligament and invading the vocalis. This approach can be fine-tuned further by performing partial resections of any of the layered microstructure. The specimen is always oriented for whole-mount histologic analysis and frozen-section margin assessment is employed selectively to verify a complete excision.

If dissection is performed in the SLP, cold instruments facilitate precise tangential dissection around the curving vocal fold (Figures 47–2, 47–3, and 47–4).[13,15,28,29] This allows for maximal preservation of

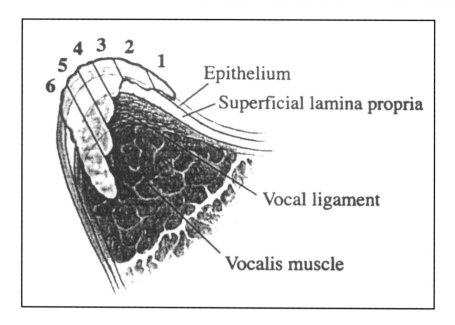

Figure 47–1. This diagram describes how a surface vocal fold lesion may harbor a variety of invasion patterns. (Courtesy of *Operative Techniques in Otolaryngology—Head and Neck Surgery*[26])

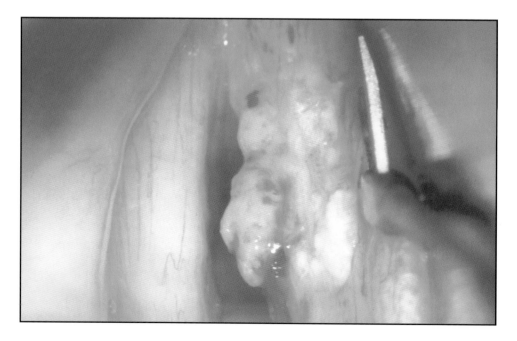

Figure 47–2. (7×) An upturned scissors is used to perform an epithelial cordotomy, which serves as a perimeter margin.

the superficial lamina propria and for pliability of the regenerating epithelium. Dissection between the vocal ligament and the vocalis muscle can be performed equally well with cold instruments alone or with assistance by the laser. Dissection within the muscle is performed most precisely with the CO_2 laser, which allows for improved visualization because of its hemostatic cutting properties.

through the underlying hyoepiglottic ligament until the pre-epiglottic fat is encountered. Once the dissection is done through the pre-epiglottic space anteriorly the laryngoscope is repositioned until the superior aspect of the thyroid cartilage can be palpated. In turn, the dissection is continued caudally just inside the thyroid lamina. Once this has been done, the laryngoscope is repositioned so that the upper blade is underneath the supraglottic tumor. The CO_2 laser is then used to incise the lateral aspects of the margin of the cancer. Optimally, a 7-mm margin is maintained. Once this is accomplished, the upper blade is repositioned back to its original position so that the supraglottic neoplasm is within the lumen of the bivalve laryngoscope. The specimen is gradually mobilized until it can be removed en bloc. Throughout the procedure, suction electric cautery is used as necessary to maintain hemostasis.

Endoscopic Resection for Cure

Transoral resection of supraglottic cancer as a single modality is successful when lesions are selected for small to medium size and endoscopic accessibility. Lesions that arise on the suprahyoid epiglottis, aryepiglottic fold, and vestibular fold are more amenable to endoscopic resection because they are more perpendicular to the distal lumen of the laryngoscope. Lesions arising on the infrahyoid epiglottis and upper false vocal fold are more difficult to resect transorally because they are visualized tangentially.[81]

Specimen margins are ideally established through multiple section analysis of the en bloc resected specimen rather than by means of frozen sections from the patient. Decisions about postoperative radiotherapy and treatment of "the necks" should be based on the pathologic assessment of the lesion. Consideration should be given to the volume of the cancer, the depth and location of its penetration, and the pattern of its invasion. Even small lesions of the aryepiglottic fold and vestibular fold will demonstrate early invasion of the paraglottic space. This places the neck at risk for occult metastasis. In contrast, early suprahyoid epiglottic carcinomas rarely invade the pre-epiglottic space and rarely metastasize to the neck if there is not occult tongue base invasion.[68]

Endoscopic Excisional Biopsy with Radiation Therapy

Transoral resection of larger supraglottic cancers followed by full-course radiotherapy to the primary site and both necks offers a more aggressive treatment approach for those individuals who otherwise would have undergone radiotherapy as a sole treatment. The endoscoscopic resection is a neoadjuvant therapy with a histopathologically controlled result. This approach stresses laryngeal function preservation (airway, swallowing, and voice) rather than organ preservation.[22] These patients become endoscopic resection candidates because they refuse to have an open laryngectomy or because they are medically unsuitable for an open partial laryngectomy.

These endoscopic supraglottic resections are considered excisional biopsies as margins are frequently close and the deep compartments (pre-epiglottic and paraglottic spaces) are not excised completely. The patients, however, have no clinical evidence of cancer when they commence radiotherapy. The success of obtaining clear margins on these excisional biopsies is based upon the typical pattern of invasion that is broad and pushing with a pseudocapsule. This pseudocapsule probably arises from the epiglottic perichondrium and the quadrangular membrane.[23,68,69]

Laryngeal Function After Endoscopic Supraglottic Laryngectomy

The airway is not typically impaired by an endoscopic supraglottic resection. Often however, the airway is improved when an exophytic lesion is excised. In approximately 3% of patients who are also irradiated, a late tracheotomy is required secondary to late stenosis from severe gastro-esophageal reflux. A fundoplication and open laryngeal reconstruction may facilitate decannulation.[23]

Laryngeal protective function may be impaired from several days to 6 weeks depending on the extent of the supraglottic tissues excised. There has not been permanent swallowing impairment in patients who have otherwise normal swallowing mechanisms. Previous impairment such as that sustained from a stroke or previous head and neck surgery is a relative contraindication to any partial laryngeal resection.

Limited resections of the suprahyoid epiglottis, aryepiglottic fold, or vestibular fold does not impair swallowing function because most of the sphincteric function of the supraglottis is unaffected. The epiglottis is a vestigial organ in man.[82] More extensive resections may predispose to aspiration from several days to 6 weeks depending upon the magnitude of the resection. Although patients may require nasogastric feeding during this time, none in our series have sustained an aspiration pneumonia during swallowing rehabilitation or from salivary soilage.

The favorable swallowing rehabilitation after the extensive transoral supraglottic resections occurs for several reasons. Most importantly, the superior laryngeal nerves are not disturbed proximal to the larynx. Therefore, the neosupraglottic region becomes fully sensate. Secondly, laryngeal elevation is not impaired either by disturbance of the suprahyoid musculature or by performing a tracheotomy. Finally, since the supraglottic defect heals completely by secondary fibrosis and epithelialization, there is favorable cicatrixation which functions as a new supraglottic valve. Hospitalization from this procedure is usually 1 to 3 days.

Open Supraglottic Laryngectomy: Background

Transcervical resection of an epiglottic neoplasm can be traced to Prat in 1859.[83] However, Alonso,[84] who presented his technique for excising supraglottic cancer in 1947, is responsible for inspiring the current approach to supraglottic laryngectomy. He described a two-staged procedure that was not widely adopted. Later, Ogura {1958} and Som[85] published their approaches with primary closure. The oncolgic justification for this procedure was based in part on the finding that the supraglottic structures are derived from the buccopharyngeal anlage and the glottic and subglottic regions are derived from the tracheopulmonary anlage.[86] However, the embryologic details of this concept have remained obscure.[87] Whole-organ sections have failed to demonstrate an anatomical structure that serves as a barrier between the supraglottis and glottis despite the fact that the sections document the typical confinement of supraglottic lesions to the supraglottis.[88] Bocca[65] furthered the concept of embryologic separation of the supraglottis and glottis in his landmark article in 1968. That work, which catalyzed current treatment paradigms, discussed the indications, technique, and results from 124 supraglottic laryngectomies.

Oncologic Results

In the 1970s and 1980s supraglottic laryngectomy became a mainstream approach for the treatment of early supraglottic cancer so that today, the concerns about the oncolgic safety of this procedure are resolved.[89] The extensive investigations of serially sectioned total-laryngectomy specimens helped differentiate which lesions were amenable to conservation laryngeal surgery. This information was utilized at numerous centers so that selection criteria were established for lesions that were oncologically appropriate. Local failure after appropriately selected lesions is unusual. In the Mayo and Pittsburgh series, less than 2% of patients failed locally after supraglottic laryngectomy.[89,90] Kirchner has noted that typically, local failure occurs in the cephalad margin (the pharynx), not in the laryngeal remnant, where there was concern about occult disease in the deep paraglottic space.[88] This lends further sup-

port to the oncologic effectiveness of this conservation procedure.

Early supraglottic cancer has been treated in a number of centers alternatively with supraglottic laryngectomy or radiation therapy. In recent years it has become evident that more voices and lives are preserved with the surgical option.[89] Recurrence in the larynx after failed radiation therapy can only rarely be managed with a conservation procedure. In an exhaustive literature review of 69 studies (1974–1993) and almost 15,000 patients, Staffieri et al[91] found that the 5-year survival of patients treated by supraglottic laryngectomy was 75% as compared to 64% for radiation.

Patient Selection

Through the 1970s, criteria were also established for selecting patients that could be successfully rehabilitated after supraglottic laryngectomy. As nearly all patients who undergo supraglottic laryngectomy have some degree of aspiration postoperatively, and as many have persistent low-grade chronic aspiration, care must be taken in choosing individuals who can withstand this pulmonary insult. Most patients who develop supraglottic cancer have a long-term smoking history and many surgeons have utilized pulmonary function tests in the selection of candidates for conservation laryngeal surgery. Obtaining an adequate history about a patient's aerobic activities and capabilities may suffice.

There are relative contraindications to performing supraglottic laryngectomy. Patients should be approached cautiously if they have cerebrovascular disease that has led to impaired mentation or deficits in function in cranial nerves IX to XII or if they have undergone previous head and neck surgery that has altered normal deglutition.

Functional Results

The primary functional goals of conservation laryngeal surgery are normal deglutition, an adequate tubeless airway, and a normal voice. The experienced surgeon can usually achieve these goals with minimal difficulty. Prompt resumption of a normal diet has been the most common problem for those undergoing supraglottic laryngectomy. This can be technically facilitated in a number of ways. Preservation of the hyoid bone has been demonstrated to be oncologically sound in most cases and facilitates laryngeal reconstruction by securing the neolarynx in an elevated position.[41] This consequently assists in swallowing rehabilitation. Often, one or part of one paraglottic space can be preserved.[57] This in turn facilitates preservation of one superior laryngeal nerve,[92,93] which improves sensation and proprioception in the neolarynx. Finally, decannulation of the tracheotomy tube allows for improved elevation of the laryngotracheal complex, which assists in effective protection of the airway and improved swallowing.

Removal of the tracheotomy tube is seldom a problem in patients who have not had previous irradiation. Some individuals may require the tube for direct access to the tracheobronchial tree for suctioning and pulmonary toilet. Occasionally, a difficult decision must be made about whether the tube is a greater liability toward laryngeal elevation and impaired swallowing as opposed to being an asset for direct access for removing secretions. The surgeon may wish to delay decannulation in those patients requiring postoperative radiation.

Voice should not be altered substantially after a supraglottic laryngectomy if Broyle's ligament is not disturbed. Voice changes that do occur relate to an increase in volume in the superficial lamina propria of the vocal fold secondary to altered venous and lymphatic drainage in the larynx. Consequently, there is mass loading of Reinke's space and a lower fundamental frequency (pitch). The other typical voice alteration relates to secretions that accumulate in the neolarynx. This may be improved in the immediate and latter postoperative periods by aggressive antireflux management.

Endoscopic Versus Open Transcervical Resection

There is an evolving controversy about whether early supraglottic cancer should be resected endoscopically or transcervically. The variables for consideration in this decision relate to the lesion, the patient, the surgeon, and available instrumentation. There is no discrete formula for this decision, which must be made based upon a critical understanding of all of the aforementioned variables.

The goals of endoscopic resection may be different than conventional transcervical supraglottic laryngectomy. Frequently (with the N_0 neck), open supraglottic laryngectomy is a single-treatment alternative to radiation.[94] This single-modality treatment philosophy is also employed for endoscopic excision of small, mostly T_1 lesions. However, for most T_2 and T_3 lesions (paraglottic and pre-epiglottic space invasion) that are confined to the supraglottis, endoscopic resection serves as a neo-adjuvant excisional biopsy prior to radiation therapy. Although Steiner[47] has used a single-modality endoscopic treatment for some T_2 and T_3 lesions, most investigators employ postoperative radiation. The endoscopic resection is considered to be a narrow-margin excisional biopsy that does not comprehensively remove the pre-epiglottic and paraglottic spaces.

Selection of lesions that are amenable to endoscopic resection is based on endoscopic accessibility to the lesion. Carbon dioxide laser excisional biopsy has been shown to be an effective single-modality treatment option for selected smaller lesions on the suprahyoid epiglottis, aryepiglottic fold, and vestibular fold.[23] These lesions are perpendicular to the distal lumen of the laryngoscope and angulated tissue retraction allows for minimal tangential cutting. This results in more precise surgical margins. In this minimally invasive approach, there is negligible morbidity and the staging endoscopy is therapeutic. Larger lesions and lesions that are located on the infrahyoid epiglottis or between the aryepiglottic and vestibular folds can be treated by endoscopic excisional biopsy. These procedures are technically more difficult and should be followed by full-course radiotherapy.

The pulmonary status and wishes of the patient are also important factors for consideration during the selection of an open or endoscopic procedure. Patients who were not considered viable candidates for an open supraglottic laryngectomy because of poor pulmonary reserve were ideal for transoral resection and comprised a large proportion of the individuals in the multi-institutional investigation reported by Zeitels et al.[23] None of these individuals sustained an aspiration pneumonia or any untoward postoperative pulmonary complications. It was not surprising to find that if a clear-margin resection was achieved endoscopically, no patient failed locally.[23] This is consistent with De-Santo's[94] data, which clearly demonstrated that there were no local failures after open supraglottic laryngectomy for early disease. Had these patients who were medically unfit for a supraglottic laryngectomy received single-modality radiation treatment, data in the literature indicates that approximately 20 to 35% of these individuals would have failed locally and have undergone a laryngectomy with loss of voice.[95,96]

Finally, successful endoscopic supraglottic laryngectomy requires a late generation CO_2 laser, a bivalve laryngoscope,[75] and appropriate hand instrumentation. Furthermore, the surgeon needs to select cases for transoral resection that are commensurate with his/her skills. Larger lesions on tangential surfaces such as the infrahyoid epiglottis and upper false cord should be approached by more experienced surgeons. In the treatment of T_2 and T_3 lesions that are confined to the supraglottis, open supraglottic laryngectomy remains as the standard by which other treatments should be measured. Endoscopic resection of these lesions can be difficult and available data remain preliminary due to the small number of cases.

Management of the Neck

Decisions to treat the neck with early supraglottic cancer should not be affected by the selection of open or endoscopic management of the primary. Unlike early glottic cancer, early supraglottic cancer has a clear predilection for cervical metastasis. This correlates to simultaneous invasion of the pre-epiglottic and/or paraglottic spaces that accompanies early supraglottic cancer. These deep compartments contain lymphatic channels that facilitate metastasis to the neck. Zeitels et al[68] demonstrated that 24 of 27 clinically staged T_1 and T_2 infrahyoid epiglottic cancers demonstrated invasion of the pre-epiglottic space and were therefore pathologically staged T_3. In this group, a 50% incidence of occult cervical metastasis was noted after elective neck dissection in clinically staged N_0 necks. Conversely, suprahyoid lesions that were confined to the epiglottis and did not invade the pre-epiglottic space, were unlikely to develop neck disease.[68]

There is little doubt that individuals who present with early supraglottic cancer and metastatic neck disease fare worse than those who are clinically staged N0.[90,94] Furthermore, the magnitude of the neck disease portends a worse prognosis.[89] Finally, a high percentage of patients who fail initial treatment, will fail in the neck and many these patients will die.[90,94]

It is clear that individuals who present with neck disease should be treated, and that most surgeons would perform a neck dissection. When there is documented ipsilateral disease, both necks should be treated because of frequent failure in the contralateral neck.[90,94] Management of the N_0 neck is more complex. The decision to perform a neck dissection would most logically be based on whether careful assessment of the primary suggested paraglottic or pre-epiglottic space invasion. If an open supraglottic laryngectomy is performed for such a lesion, an elective neck dissection is warranted on the more suspicious side. Because the incidence of contralateral failure is relatively low with a pathologically N_0 neck, DeSanto suggested dissecting the contralateral neck if intraoperative findings revealed metastatic disease.[94] This fits well with data reported by Zeitels et al[98] in which a trend was noted demonstrating that the surgeon's intraoperative assessment of the neck was more sensitive than radiographic imaging.

The decision to perform elective neck dissections for an individual that undergoes a transoral resection of a T_2 or T_3 lesion who is scheduled for postoperative radiotherapy is less clear than with open surgery without planned radiation. Each case should be individualized based on the intraoperative assessment of the primary lesion, the suspicion of occult neck disease clinically or radiographically, the difficulty of the clinical exam, and the wishes of the patient.

Transcervical Horizontal Supraglottic Laryngectomy: Technique

The procedure is begun by performing a tracheotomy. Unless the hyoid bone has been invaded, it is typically preserved. The strap musculature is separated in the midline with an electric cautery knife until the thyroid and cricoid cartilages are clearly identified. Then, the infrahyoid musculature is separated from the undersurface of the hyoid bone. The hyoid bone is then retracted anteriorly with a double-prong skin hook. Sharp dissection is done from the undersurface of the hyoid through the hyoepiglottic ligament to enter the vallecula superior to the lingual epiglottis (Figure 47–11). The infrahyoid pharyngotomy is then opened. The upper portion of the thyroid lamina is incised with a saw as is oncologically appropriate. Then, the supraglottis is withdrawn through the pharyngotomy so that the tumor can be well visualized. Incisions are made around the lateral aspects of the neoplasm under direct vision and in front of the arytenoid cartilages. In this way the entire deep compartments (paraglottic space, pre-epiglottic space) that are invaded by the tumor can be resected en bloc (Figure 47–12). Once the specimen has been removed, limited mucosal suturing is done anterior to the arytenoid by borrowing epithelium from the piriform sinus and suturing it to the lateral ventricular mucosa of the vocal fold. Complete anterior closure cannot be achieved. The most anterior portion of the neosupraglottis must close by secondary intention; 2-0 prolene sutures are placed around the hyoid bone superiorly and through the thyroid cartilage remnant. These sutures are placed to reposition the larynx anteriorly and superiorly, which facilitates postoperative deglutition. Anterior perichondrium of the thyroid lamina is typically preserved and this is utilized to oversew the defect (Figure 47–13). Subsequently, the residual strap musculature is used to do the same. Two quarter-inch Penrose drains are placed in the lateral aspect of the wound. The platysmal layer is closed with 3-0 vicryl sutures in a buried interrupted and/or running fashion. The skin is closed with 4-0 nylon suture in a running fashion and a pressure dressing is applied.

Supracricoid Laryngectomy with Cricohyoidopexy (SLCHP)

Supracricoid laryngectomy with cricohyoidopexy has been done for many years in Europe to treat T_1 and T_2 glottic cancer. Essentially, it is a form of horizontal subtotal laryngectomy in which the tracheotomy tube

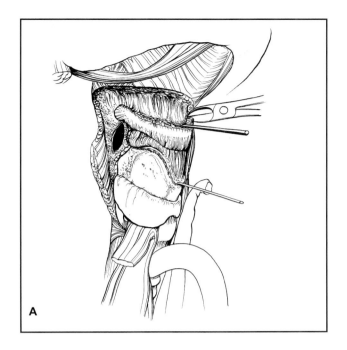

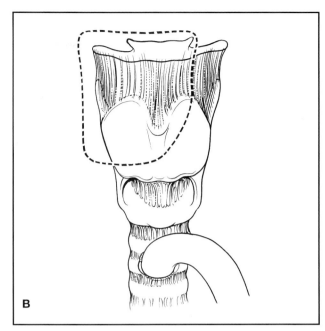

Figure 47–11. Supraglottic subtotal laryngectomy. **A.** The larynx has been skeletonized. The perichondrial flap is reflected, exposing the portion of thyroid cartilage to be resected. **B.** The bone and cartilage cuts are shown. Resection will include the body and right greater cornu of the hyoid bone, the upper half of the right thyroid ala, and an oblique portion of the left thyroid ala. From: Silver CE, Rubin JS. *Atlas of Head and Neck Surgery*. 2nd ed. New York, NY: Churchill Livingstone; 1999:210. Reproduced with permission.

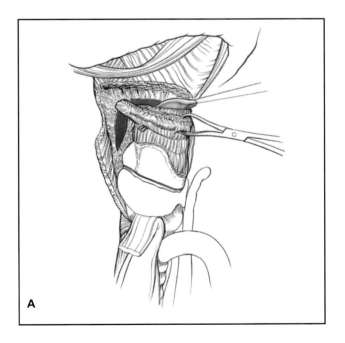

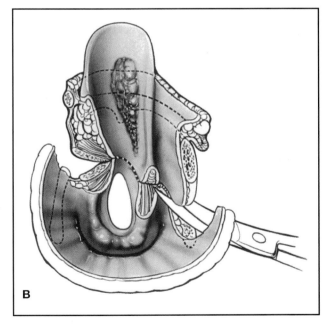

Figure 47–12. A. The hypopharynx is entered through the piriform sinus and the incision is extended through the valleculae. Careful inspection is required. The epiglottis is delivered through the mucosal incision. **B.** The incision has been carried through the posterior part of the false vocal fold into the ventricle and continued anteriorly through the ventricle to the anterior midline. As wide a margin of normal mucosa as possible is maintained, although inferiorly this may be no more than a few millimeters. From: Silver CE, Rubin JS. *Atlas of Head and Neck Surgery*. 2nd ed. New York, NY: Churchill Livingstone; 1999:210,211. Reproduced with permission.

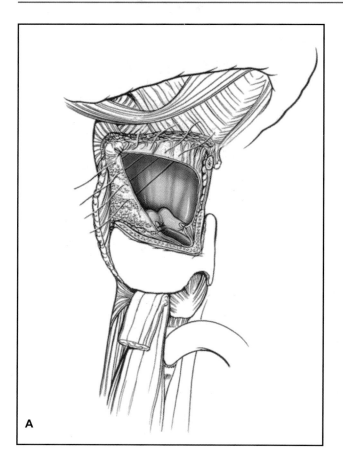

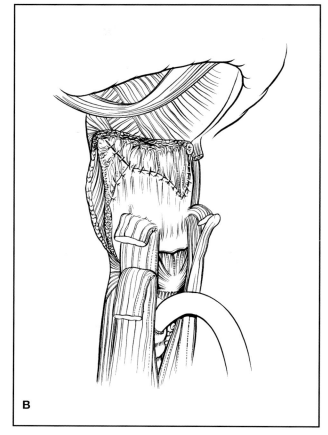

Figure 47–13. A. The mucosal defect is seen from the external aspect. Starting posteriorly, the hypopharyngeal mucosa is sutured directly as far as approximation without tension will allow. **B.** The remaining defect is closed by suturing the perichondrial flap to the base of the tongue. Resultant nonmucosal surfaces will re-epithelialize spontaneously. From: Silver CE, Rubin JS. *Atlas of Head and Neck Surgery*. 2nd ed. New York, NY: Churchill Livingstone; 1999:213,214. Reproduced with permission.

can usually be removed over time (Figure 47–14). Although SLCHP has been demonstrated to be oncologically efficacious, the procedure has never gained widespread popularity. Presumably most surgeons believe that endoscopic resection and/or radiotherapy provided similar oncologic success but with better functional results. Additionally, the procedure has been deemed by some to be difficult, although this probably is simply an issue of training. Because all the thyroid lamina along with the pre-epiglottic and paraglottic spaces are removed, extensive mesolaryngeal tumors are suitable for this technique. Invasion of the anterior commissure is not a contraindication. The reader is referred to detailed desciptions of this procedure to understand the technique as a cursory review is inadequate. Postoperative swallowing difficulty with aspiration is common initially but typically resolves over time. The corniculate-region mucosa typically becomes quite edematous

and becomes the laryngeal sound source by sphincteric closure medially and anteriorly. Arytenoid mobility is preserved and corniculate mucosa does remain sensate, which is why swallowing function recovers.

Near-Total Laryngectomy

Near-total laryngectomy as described by Pearson creates a narrow myomucosal shunt that has sphincteric function to prevent aspiration yet provide for a lung-powered laryngeal sound source (Figure 47–15). It is not intended to allow for an adequate airway so that the patient must live with a tracheotomy permanently. Large neoplasms can be resected by this approach; however, most surgeons believe that the procedure is difficult and that. functionally, the patients are fairly similar to those undergoing total laryngectomy with subsequent tracheoesophageal puncture. Detailed de-

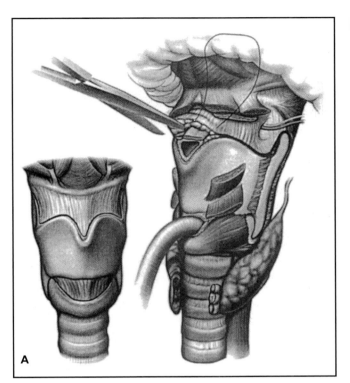

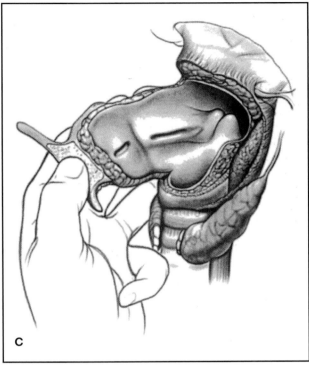

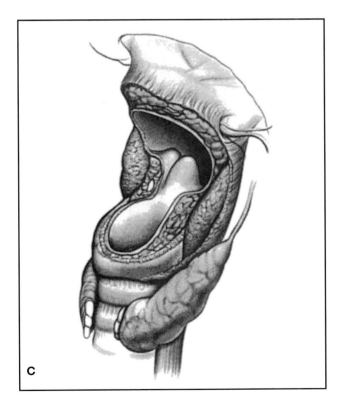

Figure 47–14. Supracricoid laryngectomy. **A.** The inferior constrictors have already been incised along the posterior border of the thyroid cartilage and the piriform sinus dissected from the internal aspect of the thyroid alae. The cricothyroid joint has been separated, being aware of the location of the recurrent laryngeal nerve. The larynx has been entered through the cricothyroid membrane and the incision extended posterolaterally. An incision has been made through the thyrohyoid membrane and the epiglottis sharply transected at the petiole, thereby allowing the larynx to be entered into. The incision is now extended posteriorly on either side. It follows the contour of the thyroid cartilage and will transect the aryepiglottic fold. **B.** The glottic structures are retracted posteriorly and the tumor visualized and assessed. A vertical incision is made through the aryepiglottic fold, anterior to the arytenoid on the contralateral side and carried forward. The surgeon now fractures the larynx along its midline, opening it "like a book" and now allowing for complete removal of the tumor under direct visualization. **C.** Remaining structures after resection include both arytenoids, cricoid, epiglottis above the petiole (in this case), and both piriform sinuses. (*continues*)

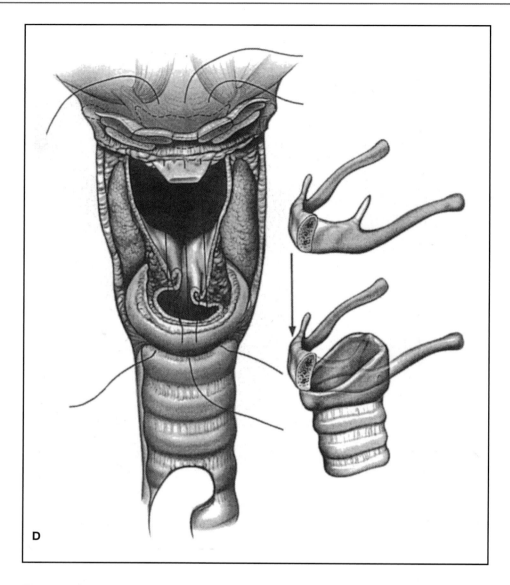

Figure 47–14. (*continued*) **D.** Reconstruction commences, with the hyoid bone and anterior cricoid brought together. From: Silver CE, Rubin JS. *Atlas of Head and Neck Surgery.* 2nd ed. New York, NY: Churchill Livingstone; 1999:218-220. Reproduced with permission.

scriptions of this procedure are also necessary to understand the subtleties of the reconstruction.

Total Laryngectomy

Total laryngectomy was first done to resect larynx cancer by Billroth in 1874. Although the resection was successful the first patients who underwent this procedure died of aspiration shortly thereafter. It was not until Solis-Cohen in United States and Gluck in Germany perfected separating the pharynx from the airway by creating a tracheostomy to the anterior skin of

the neck. This innovation led to the viability of total laryngectomy as a viable treatment to cure larynx cancer. For the most part, the procedure has changed very little since the nineteenth century. It is an outstanding procedure to resect large lesions of the larynx and the piriform sinus. Most patients heal extremely well and are typically eating a full diet within 7 to 10 days. Furthermore, there is seldom difficulty with the airway. Understandably, phonatory function is permanently impaired; however, there are a variety of ways to restore communication and most patients accommodate to one of these reasonably well.

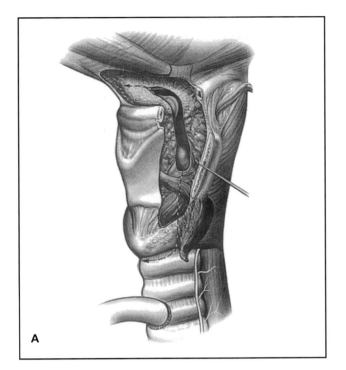

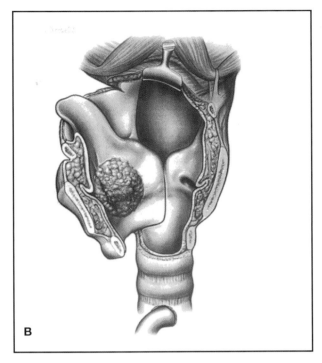

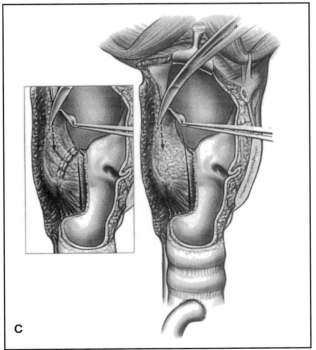

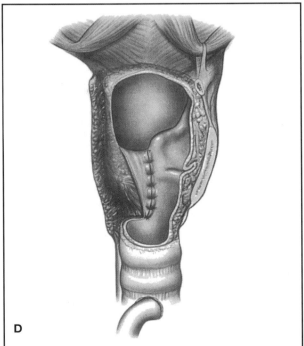

Figure 47–15. Near-total laryngectomy. **A.** Removal of a vertical portion of mid-lateral thyroid ala has exposed the soft tissues overlying the ventricle, through which the larynx is entered, at the level of the ventricle, the incision then being carried up into the vallecula. The larynx is inspected. **B.** The incision is carried down through the cricoid, around under the cricoid, and then vertically up between the ary- tenoids, posteriorly. The cricoid is fractured posteriorly in midline and deeper structures incised, care being taken to preserve the underlying hypopharyngeal mucosa. **C.** The specimen is then removed and the reconstructive phase begun. This consists of creating a phonatory shunt from myomucosal tissues, augmented by a rotation flap of piriform sinus mucosa. **D.** The flap is sewn to itself. (*continues*)

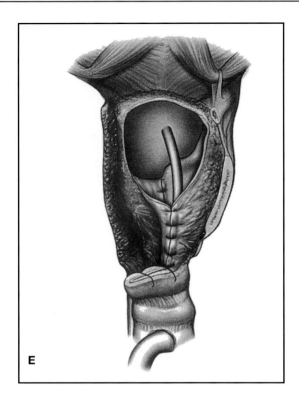

E

Figure 47–15. (*continued*) **E.** The myomucosal segment is now tubed, using a small catheter as a template. From Silver CE, Rubin JS. *Atlas of Head and Neck Surgery.* 2nd ed. New York, NY: Churchill Livingstone; 1999:241-245. Reproduced with permission.

Technique

A subplatysmal apron flap is developed to widely expose the laryngeal framework and overlying musculature. The flap is retracted with elastics and the strap muscles are separated in the midline to expose the thyroid isthmus. The thyroid isthmus is then cross-clamped, separated, and oversewn with 2-0 silk suture. This allows for an incision at approximately the second tracheal ring for replacement of the endotracheal tube. Once this is done, blunt dissection is performed lateral to the thyroid lamina to separate cartilage and associated inferior constrictor muscle from the structures of the carotid sheath. A double-prong skin hook is placed in the lateral aspect of the thyroid lamina and rotated medially. The inferior constrictor is separated from the thyroid lamina with a needle-tip electrocautery knife. Dissecting is done in the thyrohyoid space to identify the superior laryngeal neurovascular pedicle. The vein and artery are dissected, cross-clamped. and tied with 2-0 silk sutures. The same procedure is performed on the contralateral side (Figure 47–16).

Lateral dissection continues alongside the trachea. The thyroid gland is separated from the trachea until the recurrent laryngeal nerve is identified and severed. If there is extension of tumor extension through the cricothyroid space, a thyroidectomy can be performed as is appropriate given the extent of the laryngeal le-

sion. If the vallecula is free of cancer, attention is now focused on the superior aspect of the resection so that a suprahyoid pharyngotomy can be performed {Zeitels, 1991 #271}. The superior strap musculature is separated from the hyoid bone and the hyoid bone is retracted interiorly. Blunt dissection is done overlying the hyoepiglottic ligament so that the vallecula mucosa is separated from the lingual epiglottis. The median glossoepiglottic fold is easily seen as a condensation of fibers of the hyoepiglottic ligament and leads to the cephalad line aspect of the suprahyoid epiglottis. Further blunt retraction allows for a precise suprahyoid pharyngotomy. Once this is done, incisions are made along the aryepiglottic folds to visualize the neoplasm. The larynx is retracted through the pharyngotomy and the resection is continued by preserving mucosa of the piriform sinuses that is uninvolved with the cancer (Figure 47–17). Mucosal incisions continue on each side along the piriform aspect of each aryepiglottic fold until the incisions are joined in the postcricoid region. At this point, the initial incision through the trachea is extended. The trachea is transected in an oval fashion by incising the lateral trachea in a superior-posterior diagonal. The mucosa at the inferior aspect of the cricoid is incised and the dissection continues through the cricoid region until the postcricoid mucosal incision is encountered to release the larynx. The specimen is then removed and attention is paid to the closure. A

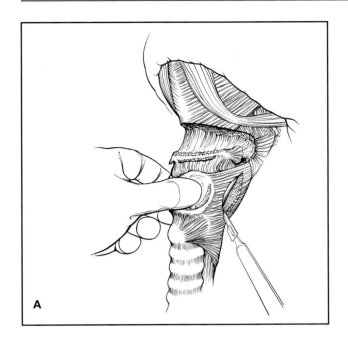

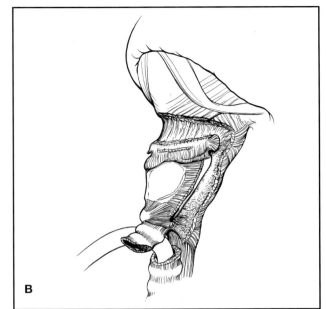

Figure 47–16. Total laryngectomy. **A.** The strap muscles have already been transected low in the neck, and the ipsilateral thyroid lobe mobilized to be included in the specimen. Paratracheal tissues have been mobilized and the surface of the trachea dissected free along the proposed line of resection. The mobilization has proceeded superiorly, the superior thyroid artery ligated, and the suprahyoid musculature freed along the body and greater cornu of the hyoid bone. On the contralateral side the thyroid gland is preserved, and separated from the trachea. The superior thy-roid artery is ligated on this side as well and the inferior constrictor fibers sharply freed off the posterior thyroid lamina. **B.** The larynx is now completely mobilized, the trachea transected and a cuffed endotracheal tube inserted. The trachea should be divided at least 2 cm below the tumor, and beveled upward, posteriorly, to increase the size of the tracheostoma. From: Silver CE, Rubin JS. *Atlas of Head and Neck Surgery.* 2nd ed. New York, NY: Churchill Livingstone; 1999:228,230. Reproduced with permission.

running Connell suture is typically done to perform the initial closure of the pharynx. With this type of mucosal-sparing resection, a straight closure is routine. A second reinforcing layer is done with 3-0 vicryl sutures in an interrupted fashion. Before closing the pharynx a nasogastric tube is placed. The wound is then copiously irrigated with Bacitracin solution. Bilateral Hemovac drains are placed and the platysma is closed with 3-0 vicryl in an interrupted varied fashion. Prior to this the trachea is sutured to the inferior and superior neck flaps in a similar fashion with 2-0 vicryl sutures. The skin is then closed with staples or 4-0 nylon sutures

REFERENCES

1. Zeitels SM. Premalignant epithelium and microinvasive cancer of the vocal fold: the evolution of phonomicrosurgical management. *Laryngoscope.* 1995;105(suppl 67):1–51.

2. Batsakis JG. *Tumors of the Head and Neck: Clinical and Pathological Considerations.* 2nd ed. Baltimore, MD: Williams & Wilkins; 1984.

3. Pressman J, Dowdy A, Libby R, Fields M., Further studies upon the submucosal lymphatics of the larynx by injection of dyes and isotopes. *Ann Otol, Rhinol Laryngol.* 1956;65:963–980.

4. Pressman JJ, Bertz MB, Monell C. Anatomic studies related to the dissemination of cancer of the larynx. *Trans Am Acad Ophthalmol Otolaryngol.* 1960;64:628–638.

5. Lindberg R. Distribution of cervical lymph node metastases from squamous cell carcinoma of the upper respiratory and digestive tracts. *Cancer.* 1972;29:1446–1449.

6. Solis-Cohen J. Clinical history of surgical affections of the larynx. *Med Rec.* 1869;4: 244–247.

7. Fraenkel B. First healing of a laryngeal cancer taken out through the natural passages. *Archiv fur Klinische Chirurgie.* 1886;12:283–286.

8. Lynch RC. Intrinsic carcinoma of the larynx, with a second report of the cases operated on by suspension and dissection. *Trans Am Laryngol Assoc.* 1920;40:119–126.

9. LeJeune FE. Intralaryngeal operation for cancer of the vocal cord. *Ann Otol Rhinol Laryngol.* 1946;55:531–536.

10. Lillie JC, DeSanto LW, Transoral surgery of early cordal carcinoma. *Trans Am Acad Ophthalmol Otolaryngol.* 1973; 77:92–96.

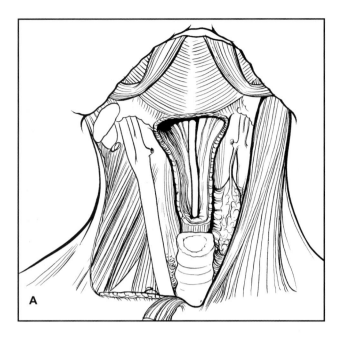

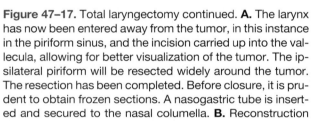

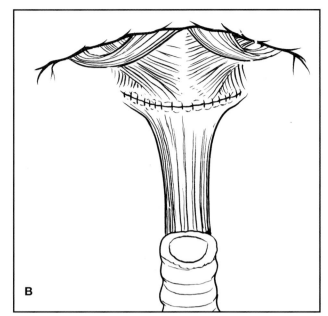

Figure 47–17. Total laryngectomy continued. **A.** The larynx has now been entered away from the tumor, in this instance in the piriform sinus, and the incision carried up into the valecula, allowing for better visualization of the tumor. The ipsilateral piriform will be resected widely around the tumor. The resection has been completed. Before closure, it is prudent to obtain frozen sections. A nasogastric tube is inserted and secured to the nasal columella. **B.** Reconstruction commences. Closure is frequently performed with interrupted sutures with the knots tied on the inside. Generally a transverse closure, without tension, can be attained; occasionally a "t" shape closure is required. The closure is reinforced by approximating the cut edges of the inferior constrictor muscles. From: Silver CE, Rubin JS, *Atlas of Head and Neck Surgery*. 2nd ed. New York, NY: Churchill Livingstone; 1999:231,232. Reproduced with permission.

11. Vaughan CW, Strong MS, Jako GJ. Laryngeal carcinoma: transoral treatment using the CO_2 laser. *Am J Surg.* 1978;136:490–493.

12. Blakeslee D, Vaughan CW, Shapshay SM, Simpson GT, Strong SM. Excisional biopsy in the selective management of T1 glottic cancer: a three year follow-up study. *Laryngoscope.* 1984;94:488–494.

13. Zeitels SM. Microflap excisional biopsy for atypia and microinvasive glottic *cancer. Op Techn Otolaryngol Head Neck Surg.* (Phonosurgery ed). 1993;4:218–222.

14. Zeitels SM. Phonomicrosurgical treatment of early glottic cancer and carcinoma in situ. *Am J Surg.* 1996;172:704–709.

15. Zeitels SM. Vocal fold atypia/dysplasia and carcinoma. In: Zeitels SM. *Atlas of Phonomicrosurgery and Other Endolaryngeal Procedures for Benign and Malignant Disease.* San Diego, CA: Singular Publishing Group; 2001:177–218.

16. Kanonier G, Rainer T, Fritsch E. Radiotherapy in early glottic carcinoma. *Ann Otol Rhinol Laryngol.* 1996;105:759–763.

17. Cragle SP, Brandenburg JH. Laser cordectomy or radiotherapy: cure rates, communication, and cost. *Otolaryngol Head Neck Surg.* 1993;108:648–653.

18. Lehman JJ, Bless DM, Brandenburg JH. An objective assessment of voice production after radiation therapy for stage I squamous cell carcinoma of the glottis. *Otolaryngol Head Neck Surg.* 1988;98:121–129.

19. DeSanto LW. Selection of treatment for in situ and early invasive carcinoma of the glottis. In: Alberti PW, Bryce DB, eds. *Workshops from the Centennial Conference on Laryngeal Cancer.* New York, NY: Appleton-Century-Crofts; 1976:146–150.

20. Myers EN, Wagner RL, Johnson JT. Microlaryngoscopic surgery for T1 glottic lesion: a cost-effective option. *Ann Otol Rhinol Laryngol.* 1994;103:28–30.

21. Mendenhall W, Parsons JT, Stringer SP, Cassissi NJ. Management of Tis, T1, T2 squamous cell carcinoma of the glottic larynx. *Am J Otolaryngol.* 1994;15:250–257.

22. Wolf GT, et al. Induction chemotherapy plus radiation compared with surgery plus radiation in patients with advanced laryngeal *cancer. New Engl J Med.* 1991;324:1685–1690.

23. Zeitels SM, Koufman JA, Davis RK, Vaughan CW. Endoscopic treatment of supraglottic and hypopharynx cancer. *Laryngoscope.* 1994;104:71–78.

24. Kass ES, Hillman RE, Zeitels SM, The submucosal infusion technique in phonomicrosurgery. *Ann Otol Rhinol Laryngol.* 1996;105:341–347.

25. Desloge RB, Zeitels SM. Endolaryngeal microsurgery at the anterior glottal commissure: controversies and observations. *Ann Otol Rhinol Laryngol.* 2000;109:385–392.

26. Hartig G, Zeitels SM. Optimizing voice in conservation surgery for glottic *cancer*. Op Techn *Otolaryngol Head Neck Surg.* (Phonosurgery, Part 1). 1998; 9: 214–223.

27. Zeitels SM. A universal modular glottiscope system: the evolution of a century of design and technique for direct laryngoscopy. *Ann Otol Rhinol Laryngol.* 1999;108(suppl 179):1–24.

28. Zeitels SM, Hillman RE, Franco RA, Bunting G. Voice and treatment outcome from phonosurgical management of early glottic *cancer. Ann Otol Rhinol Laryngol.* 2002; 111(suppl 190):1–20.

29. Zeitels SM. Laser versus cold instruments for microlaryngoscopic surgery. *Laryngoscope.* 1996;106:545–552.

30. Zeitels SM, Vaughan CW. A submucosal true vocal fold infusion needle. *Otolaryngol Head Neck Surg.* 1991;105: 478–479.

31. Zeitels SM, Dailey SH, Burns JA, Technique of en bloc endoscopic fronto-lateral laryngectomy for glottic *cancer. Laryngoscope.* 2004;114:175–180.

32. Killian G. Die Schwebelaryngoskopie. *Archiv fur Laryngologie und Rhinologie.* 1912;26:277–317.

33. Killian G. Suspension laryngoscopy and its practical use. *J Laryngol Otol.* 1914;24:337–360.

34. Lynch RC. Suspension laryngoscopy and its accomplishments. *Ann Otol Rhinol Laryngol.* 1915;24:429–446.

35. Lynch RC. A resume of my years work with suspension laryngoscopy. *Trans Am Laryngol Assoc.* 1916;38:158–175.

36. Grundfast KM, Vaughan CW, Strong MS, De Vos P. Suspension microlaryngoscopy in the Boyce position with a new suspension gallows. *Ann Otol Rhinol Laryngol.* 1978; 87:560–566.

37. Zeitels SM, Vaughan CW. "External counter-pressure" and "internal distension" for optimal laryngoscopic exposure of the anterior glottal commissure. *Ann Otol Rhinol Laryngol.* 1994;103:669–675.

38. Zeitels SM. Suspension laryngoscopy revisited. *Ann Otol Rhinol Laryngol.* 2004;113:16–22.

39. Zeitels SM. Infrapetiole exploration of the supraglottis for exposure of the anterior glottal commissure. *J Voice.* 1998;12:117–122.

40. Kirchner JA, Carter D. Intralaryngeal barriers to the spread of cancer. *Acta Otolaryngologica (Stockh).* 1987;103: 503–513.

41. Kirchner JA. What have whole organ sections contributed to the treatment of laryngeal cancer? *Ann Otol Rhinol Laryngol.* 1989;98:661–667.

42. Wolfensberger M, Dort JC. Endoscopic laser surgery for early glottic carcinoma: a clinical and experimental study. *Laryngoscope.* 1990;100:1100–1105.

43. Davis RK, Jako GJ, Hyams VJ, Shapshay SM. The anatomic limitations of CO2 laser cordectomy. *Laryngoscope.* 1982;92:980–984.

44. Wetmore SJ, Key M, Suen JY. Laser therapy for T1 glottic carcinoma of the larynx. *Arch Otolaryngol Head Neck Surg.* 1986;112: 853–855.

45. Krespi Y, Meltzer CJ. Laser surgery for vocal cord carcinoma involving the anterior commissure. *Ann Otol Rhinol Laryngol.* 1989;98:105–109.

46. Benninger M, Gillen J Thieme P, Jacobson B, Dragovich J. Factors associated with recurrence and voice quality following radiation therapy for T1 and T2 glottic carcinomas. *Laryngoscope.* 1994;104:294–298.

47. Steiner W. Results of curative laser microsurgery of laryngeal carcinomas. *Am J Otolaryngol.* 1993;14:116–121.

48. Eckel H, Thumfart WF. Laser surgery for the treatment of larynx carcinomas: indications, techniques, and preliminary results. *Ann Otol Rhinol Laryngol.* 1992;101:113–118.

49. Zeitels SM. Glottic reconstruction and voice rehabilitation. In: Zeitels SM: *Atlas of Phonomicrosurgery and Other Endolaryngeal Procedures for Benign and Malignant Disease.* San Diego, CA: Singular Publishing Group; 2001:219–221.

50. Zeitels SM, Dailey SH, Burns J.A. Microstereo-laryngoscopic lipoinjection: practical considerations. *Laryngoscope.* 2004;114:1864–1867.

51. Zeitels SM, Jarboe J, Franco RA. Phonosurgical reconstruction of early glottic *cancer. Laryngoscope.* 2001;111: 1862–1865.

52. Gray S, Titze IR, Alipour F, Hammond E. Biomechanical and histological observations of vocal fold fibrous proteins. *Ann Otol Rhinol Laryngol.* 2000;109:77–85.

53. Jia X, Burdick JA, Kobler J. et al. Synthesis and characterization of in situ crosslinkable hyaluronic acid-based hydrogels with potential application for vocal fold regeneration. *Macromolecules.* 2004;37:3239–3248.

54. Gussenbauer C. Ueber die erste durch Th. Billroth am Menschen, Ausgerfuhrte Kehlkopf Exstirpation und die Anwendungeines kunstlichen Kehlkopfes. *Archiv fur Klinische Chirurgie.* 1874;17:343–356.

55. Solis-Cohen J. Two cases of laryngectomy for adeno-carcinoma of the larynx. *Trans Am Laryngol Assoc.* 1892;14: 60–67.

56. Solis-Cohen J. Pharyngeal voice:iIllustrated by presentation of a patient who phonates without a larynx and without the use of the lungs. *Trans Am Laryngol Assoc.* 1893;15:114–116.

57. Silver CE. Supraglottic subtotal laryngectomy. In *Surgery for Cancer of the Larynx.* New York, NY: Churchill Livingstone; 1981:127–137.

58. Laccourreye O, Weinstein G. Supraglottic laryngectomy. In: Weinstein G, Laccourreye O, Brasnu D, Laccourreye H, eds. *Organ Preservation Surgery for Laryngeal Cancer.* San Diego, CA: Singular Publishing Group, 2000:107–125.

59. DeSanto LW. The "second" side of the neck in supraglottic *cancer. Otolaryngol Head Neck Surg.* 1990;102:351–361.

60. Kirchner JA. One hundred laryngeal cancers studied by serial section. *Ann Otol Rhinol Laryngol.* 1969;78: 689–709.

61. Tucker GF. Some clinical inferences from the study of serial laryngeal sections. *Laryngoscope.* 1963;73:728–748.

62. Kirchner JA, Som ML. Clinical and histological observations on supraglottic *cancer. Ann Otol Rhinol Laryngol.* 1971;80:638–645.

63. Olofsson J, Van Nostrand AWP. Growth and spread of laryngeal and hypopharyngeal carcinoma with reflections on the effect of preoperative radiation: 139 cases studied by whole organ serial sectioning. *Acta Otolaryngologica.* 1973;(supplement 308):1–84.

64. Pillsbury RC, Kirchner JA. Clinical vs histopathological staging in laryngeal cancer. Arch Otolaryngol. 1979;105:157–159.

65. Bocca E, Pignataro O, Mosciaro O. Supraglottic surgery of the larynx. Ann Otol Rhinol Laryngol. 1968;77:1005–1026.

66. Clerf LH. The preepiglottic space: its relation to carcinoma of the epiglottis. Arch Otolaryngol. 1944;40:177–179.

67. Ogura JH. Surgical pathology of cancer of the larynx. Laryngoscope. 1955;65:867–926.

68. Zeitels SM, Vaughan CW. Preepiglottic space invasion in "early" epiglottic cancer. Ann Otol Rhinol Laryngol. 1991;100:789–792.

69. Zeitels SM, Vaughan CW, Domanowski GF. Endoscopic management of early supraglottic cancer. Ann Otol Rhinol Laryngol. 1990l 99:951–956.

70. Zeitels SM, Kirchner JA. The hyoepiglottic ligament in supraglottic cancer. Ann Otol Rhinol Laryngol., 1995;104:770–775.

71. Vaughan CW. Transoral laryngeal surgery using the CO2 laser. Laboratory experiments and clinical experience. Laryngoscope. 1978;88:1399–1420.

72. Davis RK, Shapshay SM, Strong SM, Hyams V. Transoral partial supraglottic resection using the CO2 laser. Laryngoscope. 1983;93:429–432.

73. Steiner W, ed. Transoral microsurgical CO2 laser resection of laryngeal carcinoma. In: Wigand ME, Steiner W, Stell PM, eds. Functional Partial Laryngectomy. Berlin: Springer-Verlag; 1984:121–125.

74. Steiner, W. Experience in endoscopic laser surgery of malignant tumours of the upper aerodigestive tract. Adv Oto-Rhino-Laryngol. 1988;39:135–144.

75. Zeitels SM, Vaughan CW. The adjustable supraglottiscope. Otolaryngol Head Neck Surg. 1990;103:487–492.

76. Zeitels SM, Vaughan CW, Domanowski GF, Fuleihan NF, Simpson GT. Laser epiglottectomy: endoscopic technique and indications. Otolaryngol Head Neck Surg. 1990;103:337–343.

77. Davis RK, Kelley SM, Hayes J. Endoscopic CO2 laser excisional biopsy of early supraglottic cancer. Laryngoscope. 1991;100:680–683.

78. Boyce JW. Duties of the second assistant in endoscopy per os. In: Jackson C, ed. Tracheobronchoscopy, Esophagoscopy and Gastroscopy. St. Louis, MO: The Laryngoscope Co; 1907:145–147.

79. Jackson C. Position of the patient for peroral endoscopy. In: Peroral Endoscopy and Laryngeal Surgery. St. Louis, MO: The Laryngoscope Co; 1915:77–88.

80. Jackson C, Jackson CL. Direct Laryngoscopy, in Cancer of the Larynx. Philadelphia, PA: WB Saunders; 1939:10–29.

81. Shapiro J, Zeitels SM, Fried MF. Laser surgery for laryngeal cancer. Op Techn Otolaryngol Head Neck Surg. 1992;3:84–92.

82. Kirchner JA. Pressman and Kellman's Physiology of the Larynx. Vol. 78. [Monograph series]. Washington DC: American Academy of Otolaryngology-Head and Neck Surgery Foundation; 1986:689–709.

83. Mackenzie M. Removal of growths by division of the thyrohyoid membrane or suprathyroid laryngotomy. In: Diseases of the Pharynx, Larynx, and Trachea. New York, NY: William Wood & Co; 1880:241–243.

84. Alonso JM. Conservation surgery of cancer of the larynx. Trans Am Acad Ophthalmol Otolaryngol. 1947;51:633–642.

85. Som ML. Surgical treatment of carcinoma of the epiglottis by lateral pharyngotomy. Trans Am Acad Ophthalmol Otolaryngol. 1959;63:28–49.

86. Frazier EJ. The development of the larynx. J Anat Physiol. 1909;44:156.

87. Hast MH, ed. Applied embryology of the larynx. In: Alberti PW, Bryce DB, eds. Workshops from the Centennial Conference on Laryngeal Cancer. New York, NY: ppleton-Century-Crofts; 1976:6–9.

88. Kirchner JA. Spread and barriers to spread of cancer within the larynx. In: Silver CE, ed. Laryngeal Cancer. New York, NY: Thieme; 1991:6–13.

89. DeSanto LW. Cancer of the supraglottic larynx. Otolaryngol Head Neck Surg. 1985;93:705–711.

90. Lutz CK, Johnson JT, Wagner RL. Supraglottic cancer: patterns of recurrence. Ann Otol Rhinol Laryngol. 1990; 99:12–17.

91. Staffieri A, Miani C, Pedace E.. Supraglottic laryngectomy today. In: Smee R, Bridger P, eds. Laryngeal Cancer: Proceedings of the 2nd World Congress on Laryngeal Cancer. Amsterdam: Elsevier; 1994:471–475.

92. Tucker GF. Human Larynx Coronal Section Atlas. Washington, DC: Armed Forces Institute of Pathology; 1971.

93. Sato K, Kurita S, Hirano M. Location of the preepiglottic space and its relationship to the paraglottic space. Ann Otol Rhinol Laryngol. 1993;102:930–934.

94. DeSanto LW. Early supraglottic cancer. Ann Otol Rhinol Laryngol. 1990;99:593–597.

95. Mendenhall WM, Million RR, Cassisi NJ. Squamous cell carcinoma of the supraglottic larynx treated with radical radiation: analysis of treatment parameters and results. Int J Radiat Oncol Bio Phys. 1985;10:2223–2230.

96. Spaulding CA, Krochak RJ, Seung SH, Constable WC. Radiotherapeutic management of cancer of the supraglottis. Cancer. 1986;57:1292–1298.

97. Levendag P, Sessions R, Bhadrassin V, et al. The problem of neck relapse in early stage supraglottic larynx cancer. Cancer. 1989;63:345–348.

98. Zeitels SM, Domanowski GF, Vincent ME, Malhotra C, Vaughan CW. A model for multidisciplinary data collection for cervical metastasis. Laryngoscope. 1991;101:1313–1317.

48

Diagnosis and Management of Postoperative Dysphonia

Peak Woo, MD

Persistent dysphonia and recurrent dysphonia after endoscopic laryngeal surgery are clinical problems that have confronted all laryngologists. An unsatisfactory postoperative voice, as perceived by the patient, can be a particularly vexing problem. On the one hand, the patient's expectation of an improved and long-lasting postoperative voice may not have been met. On the other hand, the surgeon is faced with a new set of diagnostic and therapeutic dilemmas imposed by surgical trauma superimposed on existing impairments caused by the initial lesion.

The literature on this topic is sparse. As the problem of voice impairment is traditionally largely one of patient perception, residual dysphonia may be neglected by the clinician if no obvious masses are present. If the patient failed to improve in function, rehabilitation by referral to a speech-language pathologist is commonly the only recommendation. The impetus to "find" a better voice is a result of patient dissatisfaction; to satisfy the patient's request for a better voice. The laryngologist has several therapeutic options, which include further surgery,[1,2] evaluation and treatment by speech-language pathologists,[3-5] and patient counsel-

ing with therapeutic assurance. Brodnitz, in his large series of patients undergoing speech therapy for a variety of organic and functional disorders,[3] mentions several situations in which speech therapy resulted in a successful return of the voice following surgical treatment of laryngeal webs. He also cited the poor results with speech therapy in several patients with intubation-related injury to the larynx.

Spectrographic analysis and vocal measurements after surgical treatment show a variety of residual postoperative dysphonias ranging from mild to severe.[5] Baker et al[4] studied a small series of patients with persistent dysphonia after vocal fold surgery and correlated persistent dysphonias with other medical illnesses such as allergies, sinus infections, and chronic respiratory tract infections. Renowned endolaryngeal surgeons have noted variable voice results after microlaryngeal surgery for benign disease.[6-8] From their writings, one gathers that voice results may be variable depending on the size and type of lesion involved. More recently, vocal measurements after laser cordectomy, partial laryngectomy, and microlaryngeal surgery have provided evidence of residual disabilities in voice varying between slight dysphonia and aphonia.[9-12]

The optimal treatment of patients with postoperative dysphonia is not established; clearly, there is no consistently effective and corrective surgical treatment. Ford and Bless reported use of collagen for a variety of vocal fold defects.[1] Other autologous implants and thyroplastic phonosurgical treatments are being investigated, including autologous fat implanted in the vibratory margin of the vocal fold.[13]

At the Voice Clinic at SUNY Health Science Center at Syracuse, a multidisciplinary approach to the persistently dysphonic postsurgical patient gave us a perspective not easily obtained by one physician. By combining the referral base from otolaryngology, speech-language pathology, and speech and voice science, the medical, surgical, and speech rehabilitation needs of the persistently dysphonic patient can be better appreciated. Increasingly, patients who are persistently dysphonic after prior endolaryngeal microsurgery are being referred or are referring themselves for evaluation. This makes one suspect that the true incidence and scope of persistent dysphonia after laryngeal surgery are significant.

This chapter (1) highlights etiologic factors that contribute to persistent postoperative dysphonia, (2) discusses the differential diagnostic evaluations of patients with persistent dysphonia—as an accurate diagnosis is critical to the selection of patients who may benefit from medical, surgical, or speech therapy, the diagnostic aspects of the workup are emphasized—and (3) discusses medical, surgical, and speech therapy options for patients with postsurgical dysphonia.

DIAGNOSIS OF POSTSURGICAL DYSPHONIA

It is often not clear which component of persistent postoperative dysphonia is caused by which lesion: intrinsic disease, residual disease, or hyperfunctional voice disorder. Postoperative dysphonia is not one entity. It occurs in patients with recurrent contact granulomas shortly after removal, poor voice results after PTFE (Teflon) injection, poor voice results after vocal fold stripping for benign and neoplastic lesions, and poor voice results after endomicrolaryngeal surgery. One should also include patients with poor voice after hemilaryngectomy, subtotal laryngectomy, laryngeal fracture, and prolonged intubation; however, such inclusion would make this discussion overly expansive. Thus, although many of the diagnostic and therapeutic treatments may be applicable to these "more severe" problems, this discussion will be limited to patients with persistent dysphonia after endolaryngeal surgery. These surgical procedures include (1) microlaryngeal surgery with and without CO_2 laser for benign vocal fold lesions (polyps, webs, microangiomas, papillomas, cysts, nodules); (2) microlaryngeal surgery with and without CO_2 laser for dysplastic, hyperplastic, or neoplastic disorders of the vocal fold cover (eg, carcinoma in situ [CIS], sulcus vocalis, hyperplastic laryngitis, hyperkeratosis of the vocal folds); (3) endoscopic treatment of vocal fold paralysis (PTFE injection, PTFE granuloma); (4) endoscopic treatment of contact granuloma; and (5) diagnostic endoscopy and biopsy.

Scope of Problem

In a review of 1,380 stroboscopies performed in our clinic from 1987 to 1992, 62 patients sought consultation for improved vocal function after endolaryngoscopic surgery. The numbers would be larger if patients with dysphonia after surgical intubation and dysphonia after open laryngeal surgery were included. Prior surgical treatment included microlaryngoscopy with surgical excision (n = 44), direct laryngoscopy and excision (n = 13), and PTFE injection (n = 5). Women outnumbered men by a 2:1 margin. This may be related to sociocultural aspects of voice perception in women compared with those in men.

These patients present difficult management problems. The average number of otolaryngologists visited by these patients was 2.4. The actual number of visits to their otolaryngologists was far higher. Many had had their complaints dismissed or trivialized or were told the cause of their dysphonia was psychogenic or functional. Diagnostic examination carried out to reach these conclusions had consisted of mirror examination or flexible laryngoscope examination. Many patients had tried multiple courses of empirical therapy that included watchful waiting, antibiotic therapy, speech therapy, or a combination of these. The mean duration between the initial surgery and consultation with us was 3.4 months, with a range of 1 month to 18 years.

Clinical Presentation

One common situation at the voice clinic is the referral of a postsurgically dysphonic patient for speech therapy to reverse functional ventricular dysphonia. Figure 48–1 shows an example of ventricular phonation viewed by endoscopy.

In view of the clinical presentation, it is not surprising how many patients with persistent dysphonia are

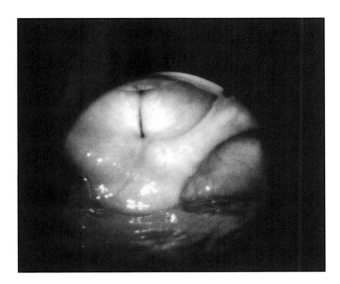

Figure 48–1. Ventricular phonation after prior laryngeal surgical intervention. The patient was referred for reversal of ventricular hyperfunction. The undiagnosed problem of poor vibratory fold function is the most common cause of this finding.

told by well-meaning physicians to seek psychological or speech therapy help. When viewed by indirect mirror or flexible laryngoscopy, the vocal folds often appear straight and free of organic disease. Yet when the patient is asked to phonate, the larynx takes on a tight, squeezed appearance. The ventricles adduct, the arytenoids may roll forward, and a raspy rough sound quality is produced (Figure 48–1). This has the appearance of ventricular dysphonia or dysphonia plica ventricularis (DPV). Ventricular dysphonia in the absence of vocal fold abnormality is often thought to have a functional or psychogenic cause, thus the reason for referral to speech therapy. What is not clear from observations using direct light is the vibratory function of the vocal folds. Vocal fold vibratory function is a dynamic process that cannot be evaluated adequately by mirror examination. The presentation of persistent dysphonia after microlaryngeal surgery is one indication for stroboscopic examination of vocal fold vibratory function as it is now known that DPV is often a compensatory effort (rather than psychogenic) to overcome vocal fold pathology.

A second pattern of failure occurs in the patient who undergoes microlaryngeal surgery with good initial restoration of vocal function. This good voice, unfortunately, lasts for only a brief period and is followed by progressive deterioration of function or renewal of symptoms.

A third pattern of failure occurs in the patient noted to have some improvement of vocal function, but the

degree of improvement does not meet the patient's expectations. This prompts revisits to the physician or self-referral for a second opinion.

Differential Diagnosis of Postoperative Dysphonia

The history and examination of clinical voice disorders have been covered in chapter 5, 12, and 13. In addition to a careful history, it is important for the laryngologist to review the clinical voice history after surgical treatment. With a good history, the clinician should be able to distinguish persistent dysphonia after surgery from recurrent dysphonia after surgery. The degree of clinical improvement and/or lack of improvement after surgery should be documented by specific examples. This helps the clinician to (1) gauge the extent of patient expectations, (2) assess the efficacy of the previous laryngeal surgery, and (3) direct the search for contributing causes of dysphonia. If the patient had a good voice after surgery followed by voice deterioration, one suspects a recurrent lesion (ie, recurrent vocal fold nodules, contact granuloma). If the patient always had a poor voice after surgery, the cause may be the results of healing (hypertrophic scarring) or the surgery (adynamic segment). If the voice remained the same or improved marginally, comorbid causes such as chronic laryngitis, reflux laryngitis, habitual hyperfunctional voice disorder, and residual disease should be considered. Table 48–1 lists the varieties of clinical failure and their possible causes. This should be considered only a partial list of likely causes, as a new unrelated vocal fold lesion could present with a similar history and symptomatology.

The severity of the patient's complaints may not be well-correlated with the examiner's perception of the severity of dysphonia. Some patients with severe to moderate dysphonia after surgery only want to be reassured that recurrent lesion or neoplasm is absent. Others have dysfunctional voices that interfere with activities of daily living. Still others have subtle dysphonia that affects only a small range of their phonation, and the patients seek help because of professional voice needs. True psychogenic dysphonia caused by conversion reaction and functional dysphonia for purposes of secondary gain are rare.

Without adequate preoperative documentation of the severity of dysphonia, the preoperative state cannot be appreciated. In almost all patients with postoperative complaints, vocal characteristics that can be readily identified by the examiner as a "hoarse" voice are generally present. The voice qualities are usually rough, husky, strident, or combinations thereof. Further questioning usually reveals a voice that is decreased in loudness and pitch range. The onset of phonation may require more effort. The duration of voicing per breath may be reduced. Speaking or singing effort is often increased. In some, a loss of clarity, brilliance, and timbre after surgery is the main complaint. For the experienced clinician, these are typical vocal characteristics of scarred vocal folds, of immobile vocal folds caused by inflammation, or of residual mass lesions. These vocal qualities should spur the clinician to examine the vibratory capabilities of vocal folds and reach a clearer diagnosis.

Physical Examination

Examination of the larynx should include videolaryngostroboscopy. Stroboscopy offers the clinician the most practical way to observe vibratory function of the vocal folds. Without direct observation of vibratory function, much of laryngoscopic diagnosis is guesswork. With direct observation, the interpretation of the pathophysiology of dysphonia can be made much clearer. For example, one common diagnosis made by referring physicians is hyperfunctional voice disorder with ventricular adduction. When laryngostroboscopy examination is carried out, a nonvibratory segment or diffuse edema with poor mucosal amplitude or mass differences between the vocal folds is often detected. When these factors are corrected medically or surgically, the ventricular hyperadduction often clears spontaneously. Thus, one can conclude that ventricular hyperadduction is very often a compensatory gesture of the larynx to attempt phonation at higher pressures. In our series of 62 postoperative dysphonic patients seen in the clinic, 33 were found on flexible laryngoscope to exhibit features of ventricular adduction. When stroboscopic examination was used to further examine vocal fold vibratory function in these 33 patients, 26 had poor vibration of the true vocal folds (TVFs). This suggests that ventricular adduction is a compensatory gesture in these patients. In this series, only 7 of 33 patients had the diagnosis of hyperfunctional voice disorder without vibratory anomaly.

Stroboscopy helps the clinician to distinguish between the various differential diagnoses. For the patients with persistent dysphonia, the differential diagnosis groupings can be separated into (1) scar and localized stiffness, (2) a residual mass lesion, (3) diffuse inflammation with bilaterally poor vibratory function, (4) lesion recurrence, and (5) hyperfunctional voice disorder. Table 48–2 lists the relative incidence in our series of 62 patients.

Scar and Stiffness

Localized scar with stiffness is the most common cause of persistent dysphonia after surgery (Table 48–2). This can be differentiated easily from the other causes as a diminution of mucosal amplitude and mucosal wave on stroboscopy. The site of involvement may be localized to a small area over the vocal fold or

Table 48–1. Possible Causes of Poor Voice After Surgery

1. Residual disease
   (ie, papilloma on the undersurface of the vocal fold, contralateral cyst or scar)

2. Unrecognized comorbidity
   Scar and prior vocal fold injury
   Inflammatory laryngitis

3. Recurrent disease
   Recurrent vocal nodules
   Recurrent polypoid degeneration
   Recurrent contact granuloma

4. Poor surgical result
   Hypertrophic scar
   Nonvibrating segment
   Overinjection of the vocal fold with PTFE (Teflon)
   PTFE granuloma

5. Surgical scar caused by repeated surgery or injury
   Repeated papilloma surgery
   Postradiation scarring
   Scarring after repeated vocal fold stripping

6. Patient expectations not met

7. Functional and hyperfunctional dysphonia

Table 48–2. Stroboscopic Diagnosis of 62 Patients with Persistent Postoperative Dysphonia

Diagnosis	No. of Patients
Scar and stiffness	27
Diffuse inflammation	13
Residual mass	8
Hyperfunction	7
Recurrent lesion	4
Unclear	3
Total	TT62

it may involve the entire fold. Grossly, the affected vocal fold is usually whiter or pinker than the uninvolved vocal fold. When viewed by magnifying laryngoscope, the translucent, clear Reinke's layer is often absent. Figure 48–2 shows some typical stroboscopic findings, including one vocal fold with a translucent layer that vibrates. The contralateral fold is white and stiff (*arrow*). If these patients were re-examined under anesthesia, palpation of the vocal folds would show them to be stiff and lacking resilience and pliability, although stroboscopy may be better at detecting such problems. Compared with the contralateral vocal fold, the affected vocal fold may seem atrophic and bowed. A vocal fold that is pink or rose-colored may also be increased in size and have prominent vascular ectasias. This appearance suggests the presence of a hypertrophic scar (Figure 48–3).

Diffuse Inflammation or Edema

Poor mucosal hygiene is often present in patients developing benign laryngeal lesions. Infectious laryngitis, chronic nonspecific laryngitis, hyperplastic laryngitis, chronic allergic laryngitis, and reflux laryngitis all contribute to make phonation more of an effort. The changed rheology of mucous membranes caused by poor mucosal hygiene contributes to the development of polypoid corditis and hyperplastic laryngitis. If these factors are not carefully corrected preoperatively and persist or recur after phonosurgery, they will contribute to persistent dysphonia that will disappoint both the surgeon and the patient. Inflammatory edema that affects vibration can be identified by

visual means. By mirror examination, the vocal folds appear thick and have increased mucus production or stranding. The arytenoids are often erythematous from chronic throat clearing. The superior surfaces of the vocal folds often have a salt-and-pepper appearance (Figure 48–4). The stroboscopic examination shows a symmetrically decreased amplitude and a decreased mucosal wave. Vocal characteristics of chronic laryngitis are characterized by a reduced dynamic range in both loudness and frequency. Many

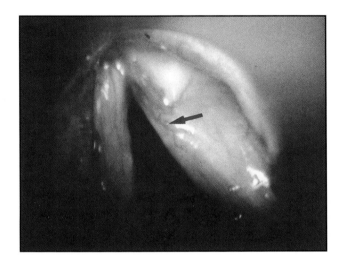

Figure 48–3. Hypertrophic scar of the right vocal folds with telangiectasia after previous microlaryngoscopy. Notice the neovascular changes originating from the center of the scar (*arrow*).

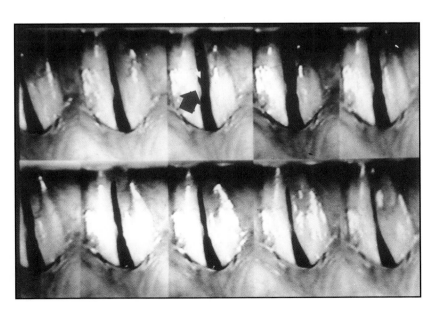

Figure 48–2. A series of stroboscopic images of a nonvibrating vocal fold after microsurgery. The vocal fold that vibrates is the one with the translucent jelly layer. The nonvibrating vocal fold is whiter and stiffer and has a residual nodule (*arrow*).

patients have a reduced ability to phonate a soft, easy low tone.

Mass Lesions

Residual mass lesions such as a small subglottic papilloma or intracordal cyst can be difficult to see (Figure 48–5). This is especially so if they are small enough to cause only intermittent dysphonia at certain frequen-

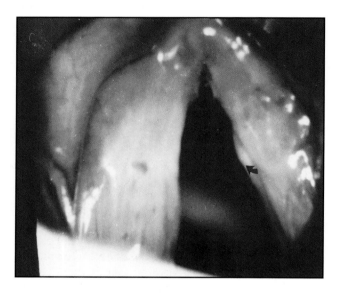

Figure 48–4. Hyperemia, edema, and salt-and-pepper appearance of the vocal folds in a patient with excessive inflammation and small right sulcus vocalis (*arrow*).

cies. By mirror examination, the vocal fold edge usually appears linear. Mirror examination may show a small area of mucus stranding that is confused with a nodule. Stroboscopy helps to isolate the effects caused by residual masses from other problems. One method to assist in the visualization of the vocal folds is to request loud phonation during stroboscopy. With loud phonation, the phase shift is accentuated and a subtle subglottic mass often becomes obvious. Another technique that is useful is to view the vocal folds at an angle using rigid or flexible laryngoscopy. When the videolaryngoscopy is being reviewed, particular attention should be paid to the abduction during deep inspiration. This maneuver helps to flatten the vocal folds laterally and accentuates any subglottic asymmetry. Figure 48–5 is an example of residual mass lesion after prior microlaryngeal surgery. Notice that the superior edge of the vocal fold is linear and shows good vibration, but the inferior lip is irregular and has small areas of papilloma.

In a small percentage of patients, recurrence of the original lesion can occur. Lesions prone to recurrence are (1) contact granulomas, (2) recurrent benign keratosis, and (3) recurrent vocal fold nodules. These lesions present with features similar to their original presentation.

Hyperfunctional Voice Disorder

In a select group of patients, postoperative healing occurs uneventfully, but residual dysphonia persists. Flexible examination and stroboscopic examination demonstrate good vibratory function of both vocal

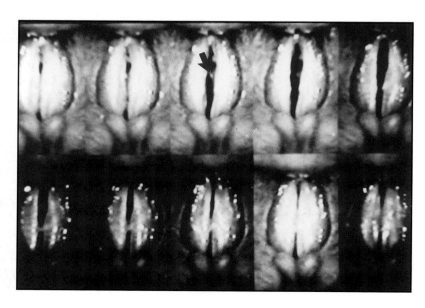

Figure 48–5. Residual subglottic papilloma (*arrow*) in a patient after recent microlaryngoscopy. The voice was improved but not perfect.

folds, yet the patient continues to be dysphonic. Flexible laryngoscopy of these patients may reveal the larynx to phonate in unusual supraglottic and glottic configurations. These patterns can be systematically evaluated by a review of the flexible laryngoscopy tape. In the absence of vibratory abnormalities of vocal folds, these patients are classified as having hyperfunctional or functional voice disorders. The possible causes of hyperfunctional dysphonia may be (1) poor vocal habits developed before surgery, (2) an intrinsic hyperfunctional voice disorder that predates the laryngeal lesion, or (3) psychogenic posturing of vocal folds.

Laryngoscopic findings in patients with functional dysphonia are best appreciated by flexible laryngoscopy using connected speech. The speech-language pathologist is particularly valuable during this portion of the examination. When hyperfunction is suspected, the speech-language pathologist should be present to help in the diagnosis and try therapeutic maneuvers while the flexible laryngoscope is in place.

On flexible laryngoscopy, the features that are relevant to the diagnosis of hyperfunction include the observation of pharyngeal and laryngeal squeeze during speech. Some features of hyperfunction are

1. Pharynx squeezing during speech
2. Inappropriate elevation of the larynx during phonation
3. Shortened anteroposterior diameter of the vocal folds

4. Ventricular hyperadduction (Figure 48–6)
5. Excessive arytenoid approximation and anterior displacement of the arytenoids
6. Myasthenia larynges with poor closure
7. Coup de glotte with harsh glottal attack during onset of phonation.

Stroboscopic features of hyperfunction are characteristic but are not critical to the diagnosis. These include

1. Abnormally shortened vocal folds suggestive of thyroarytenoid muscle (TA) hyperfunction (Figure 48–7)
2. A shortened or prolonged closed phase during the glottal cycle
3. A shortened closing time
4. A phase shift difference between vocal folds
5. Habitually too loud or too soft phonation during comfortable phonation

Figure 48–8 shows a patient with residual nodular diathesis after previous surgery. The vocal folds show preferential midfold contact. There is an hourglass appearance to the vocal folds, and there is only brief vocal fold contact with large posterior chink (Figure 48–8).

Interdisciplinary evaluation is often a critical part of the evaluation of postsurgical dysphonia. Our preference is to perform the history and examination together so that discussions of the pathophysiology can be

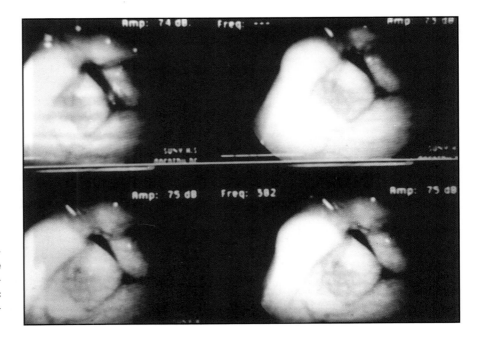

Figure 48–6. Ventricular hyperadduction in a patient with incomplete closure of the folds after lesion removal. The series of stroboscopic pictures shows the false folds to oscillate with an open glottis below.

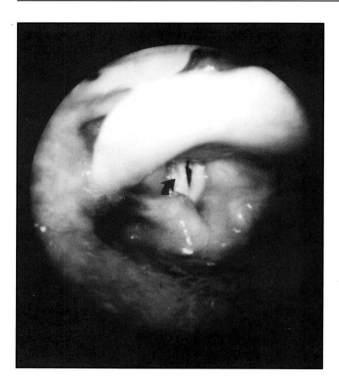

Figure 48–7. Excessive shortening of the posteroanterior diameter of the vocal folds during phonation in a patient with benign keratosis after prior resection. This gesture may be indicative of TA hyperfunction. Speech therapy is useful to correct this after lesion removal. However, if there is excessive scarring, the prognosis for voice is guarded.

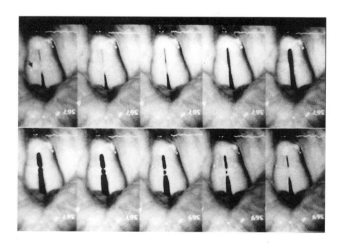

Figure 48–8. Nodular diathesis after previous laryngeal polypectomy. The patient had an excellent postoperative voice initially but returned to her previous vocal habits.

done immediately. When the speech-language pathologist is present, therapeutic speech therapy probes can be done at the same time as fiberoptic laryngoscopy.

This often provides clues about which interventional maneuvers to try during subsequent speech therapy sessions. The speech-language pathologist should, in most cases, independently verify the validity of the diagnosis prior to instituting a course of therapy. Because many patients may already have tried speech therapy, the validation of the diagnosis is a critical step before a recommendation for further speech therapy. Both the laryngologist and speech-language pathologist must have confidence in the accuracy of the diagnosis.

OBJECTIVE EVALUATIONS

The objective evaluation of vocal function is a useful adjunct to understanding changes in vocal function. As a research tool, it helps to identify specific acoustic, aerodynamic, and visual features that correlate with improved voice and vocal function. As a clinical tool, it helps to document the condition before and after treatment.

Of the various instruments, the recording of the voice and videostroboscopy appears to be the most useful. Aerodynamic measures, electroglottography (EGG), and acoustic waveforms help to identify relevant parameters that can be compared among treatment groups.

Measures such as glottal efficiency (AC/DC ratio), mean airflow, phonation time, and maximal loudness and pitch range give some objective "feel" for the patient's phonatory ability. Other acoustic measures such as jitter, shimmer, signal/noise ratio, and ratio of spectral energy of high frequency to low frequency energy help to simplify and document the complex acoustic signal.

TREATMENT

Avoidance of Complications

The best way to treat postoperative dysphonia is by prevention. This comes in the form of realistic patient counseling, accurate diagnosis, and careful preoperative, operative, and postoperative management. However, even in the best of hands, complications sometimes occur.

Preoperative Evaluation and Counseling

If a hyperfunctional voice disorder is present and surgery is unavoidable, speech therapy consultation before and after the surgery should be incorporated into the treatment plan. The patient should meet with the speech-language pathologist before surgery in an attempt to reverse the hyperfunctional habits before surgery. In these patients, the surgical treatment and speech rehabilitation of voice should be discussed as a unified treatment.

If there is significant inflammation of the laryngeal structures, reversal of the causative factors before surgery usually means a less turbulent postoperative course. This includes corrective measures for factors such as hydration, voice abuse, smoking, sinobronchial infections, and reflux laryngitis. If such factors cannot be reversed, their implication for return of "normal" vocal function should be honestly discussed and documented. Occasionally, preoperative treatment with systemic antibiotics and steroids for 72 hours before surgery and carried through the postoperative period may be useful to reduce postoperative inflammation.

Because the most common cause of postsurgical dysphonia is a nonvibratory segment, the surgeon should use the smallest microinstruments—laser or nonlaser—to achieve the most precise treatment of tissue lesions. Conservation of normal mucosa and preservation of the layered structure is the best insurance against a nonvibratory segment.

The scarred and immobile vocal fold that is free of residual mass lesions does not participate functionally in modulating airflow. All steps should be taken to avoid such results. In general, successful rehabilitation of voice by surgery or speech therapy is accompanied by the restoration of mucosal vibration and mucosal wave. This feature is often more important than a fine linear vocal edge. Failure to achieve good vibratory function may be related to a host of factors, including (1) the type and extent of the lesion, (2) the amount of fibrosis and scar involving Reinke's layer, (3) the amount of surgical dissection, and (4) the extent of epithelial resection and the resultant secondary healing. Several authors have stressed the importance of preserving the delicate layered structure of the vocal folds.[14,15] Loss of the layered structure of the vocal folds coupled with inflammation, fibrosis, and secondary re-epithelialization all contribute to produce a scarred, stiffened vocal fold. Such scarred vocal folds will not vibrate with ease, creating a crippled phonatory layer and a poor functional result.

The excision of large surface epithelial lesions contributes to the production of reduced amplitude of vibration. To avoid excessive injury, the dissection should be limited to within the layer of pathologic involvement. When the lesion is intraepithelial, the histologic specimen should stop at the basement membrane. The glistening gelatinous structures deep to the vocal fold epithelium should be left undisturbed. This helps ensure a vocal fold that is not tethered to the vocal ligament. When in doubt, it is often preferable to

leave an irregular vocal fold edge that vibrates rather than a vocal fold that is straight yet stiff. Likewise, when the lesion spares the epithelium, normal epithelium should be left and preserved. The cordotomy procedures, in which an incision is made on the superior surface followed by microdissection, spares the normal epithelium better than cup forceps and scissor excision. In the management of intracordal masses, cysts, and polypoid degeneration, cordotomy followed by careful gentle evacuation of the subepithelial lesion may give the best chance for the restoration of normal vibratory function. Figure 48–9 illustrates this concept

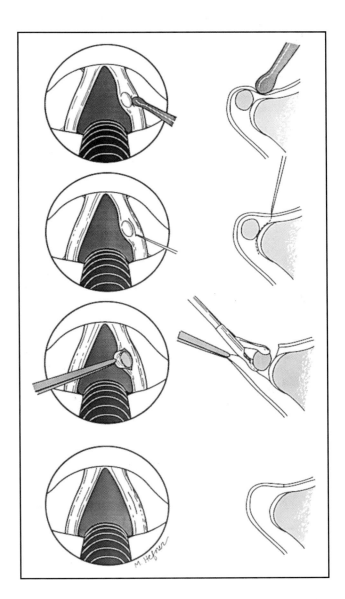

Figure 48–9. Schematic diagram of cordotomy incision and evacuation of a subepithelial lesion. The mucosa is spared using this approach.

diagrammatically. Figure 48–10 illustrates a typical lesion evacuated without excessive epithelial removal. To help reduce the size of the epithelial defect, a small 6-0 plain gut suture can be placed endoscopically to approximate the vocal fold edge. This seems to help reduce the amount of secondary healing.

One problem of postsurgical care that can result in poor function is excessive perioperative and postoperative inflammation. Patients at risk are smokers with polypoid corditis who have chronically thick mucus. Patients having a large amount of tissue resection are also at risk for prolonged inflammation after surgery as are patients who use their voices excessively in the immediate postoperative period. Evaluation of vocal fold vibration 1 week after surgery helps to assess the healing progress. If there is excessive edema and inflammation, aggressive retreatment by broad-spectrum antibiotics, mucolytics, and systemic steroids may be indicated as well as relative voice rest and voice therapy. Factors that contribute to laryngeal irritation should be considered and ruled out. These factors include smoking, excessive throat clearing, coughing, reflux laryngitis, allergic laryngitis, and voice abuse. Antitussives are used liberally in the postoperative patient to reduce chronic irritation and cough. Hydration, mucolytics, and antitussives coupled with careful monitoring of abusive behavior often can reverse the prolonged healing process and allow vibration to begin.

MANAGEMENT

Some patients with persistent dysphonia after laryngeal surgery do not need further treatment. Each patient has his or her own needs and motivations. Some are seeking to be reassured that there is no evidence of neoplasia, while others seek improvements in vocal function even at the expense of a great deal of time and money. The degree of motivation to follow treatment suggestions is a key factor in determining whether further treatment should be suggested. An accurate assessment of patient needs and whether these needs can be met by further treatment is the first step in treatment planning.

Appropriate pretreatment discussions should provide the patients with an in-depth review of their pathophysiology and of what can and cannot be done realistically to improve the situation. The surgeon and speech-language pathologist should not be overly optimistic about the hoped-for results. In deciding to undergo another treatment course, the patient may indeed risk being "disappointed" again. In general, the patients the laryngologist can reasonably expect to help are those with realistic expectations in whom the objective evidence of vibratory abnormality can be directly related to their dysphonic complaints. For example, the evacuation of a small residual intracordal cyst can be reasonably expected to improve vocal fold mass and symmetry and improve the voice if the mass is causing the dysphonia. A small subglottic papilloma that interferes with speaking can be removed by CO_2 laser bounced off a subglottic mirror. Other clinical problems are more challenging. For example, the patient with stiff vocal folds after PTFE injection is especially challenging. If there is no evidence of granuloma formation or airway obstruction, what is the role of speech therapy or surgery? Indeed, it is doubtful that repeat endolaryngeal surgery in the face of mas-

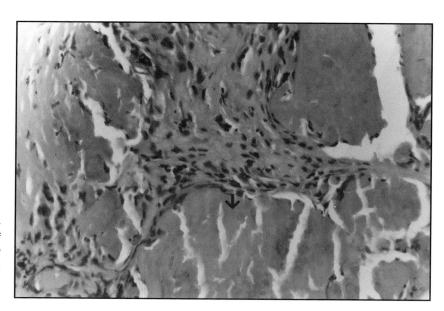

Figure 48–10. Histopathology of a subcordal mass lesion. Notice the absence of epithelium in the specimen evacuated by cordotomy. Arrow points to hyaline material seen in a pseudocyst of the subcordal space.

sively stiffened vocal folds will improve the voice. At worst, voice results may even suffer. One example of carefully limiting further surgery is in the patient with benign keratosis and a poor voice. If the diagnosis of benign keratosis is certain from prior biopsies, repeated stripping of an offending lesion that recurs can lead to worsening of vocal fold function. In these patients, selective biopsies based on supravital staining may be more appropriate than repeated strippings that leave the patient further disabled. In patients with benign keratosis, close follow-up is essential; selected biopsies may prolong vocal function with little increased risk.

In the absence of an obvious residual or recurrent mass lesion, a graduated approach of treatment planning seems appropriate. Generally, aggressive medical therapy and mucosal hygiene are instituted. This includes the restriction of caffeine and nicotine in the diet. Mucosal hygiene and hydration alone yield benefits in many patients. If such an approach fails, all drugs taken by the patient are reviewed with an eye toward side effects of mucositis and drying. If such drugs are identified, they are replaced by an alternative medication. The third step in medical management consists of careful environmental and dietary control and review. Avoidance of heavy coughing, throat clearing, and shouting is stressed and reviewed by the voice care team. Medications that have been found useful to restore vibratory function include steroidal and nonsteroidal anti-inflammatory agents, mucolytics, and broad-spectrum antibiotics. A steroid given in systemic form is much preferable to topical sprays. Longer-term steroid use can be managed with less endocrine suppression using an alternate-day dosing. If the introduction of mucolytics, anti-inflammatory medication, and antibiotics fails to bring about less erythema and edema, further treatment is instituted. This includes an antitussive and nonmedical antireflux regimen and nasal irrigations to remove offending thick secretions. The possibility of reflux laryngitis, sinobronchial infection, and allergic laryngitis should be considered, and, if tests are positive, medical treatment for these problems should begin.

Once maximal medical treatment has been achieved, a course of voice therapy is instituted to reverse hyperfunction and improve vocal fold flexibility. Despite moderate to severe functional loss of vocal fold vibration, many patients with isolated nonvibratory segments can have their vibratory function restored using a regimen of vocal fold exercises.

If the patient is motivated, the speech-language pathologist meets with the patient in six to eight 1-hour sessions. Instruction on proper vocal care and usage is given along with vocal fold exercises and a voice practice regimen designed to increase vocal fold flexibility. In our center, these therapeutic exercises include:

1. Lip and tongue trills at an ascending and descending scale and loudness
2. Vocal range and loudness exercises
3. Easy-onset phonation and tone focus exercises
4. The use of aspirate voice

Using such an approach, some patients show dramatic improvements in vocal fold vibratory function and better voice results in 6 to 8 weeks. If improvements are not present at the end of 8 weeks, further speech therapy is not advocated in most cases.

Surgical re-exploration is indicated for recurrent or residual masses that fail to respond to conservative measures. In the patient with poor closure and a nonlinear edge, reoperation to improve closure has a good chance of improving function. If the scarring is localized, surgical re-excision with lysis of the tethered scar band, followed by steroid injection, can lead to an improvement in voice. The number of patients undergoing such treatments is too small for any definitive conclusions regarding long-term efficacy.

Table 48–3 shows the initial diagnosis and the primary treatment rendered in our patient series. The equal distribution of patients undergoing primary treatments by medical, surgical, speech rehabilitation, and no therapy supports the equal role each treatment has in the management of these patients.

CASE HISTORIES

Some clinical case histories help to illustrate the management issues.

Table 48–3. Initial Diagnosis and Treatment Given in 59 Patients with Postsurgical Dysphonia

Initial Diagnosis	Primary Treatment[a]
Polyps, nodules, cysts (n = 22)	Surgery (n = 14)
Epithelial lesion (n = 15)	Speech therapy (n = 15)
Sulcus vocalis (n = 4)	Medical therapy (n = 17)
Contact granuloma (n = 3)	None (n = 16)
Cancer (n = 4)	
Paralysis (n = 5)	
Unknown (n = 6)	

[a]The treatment plan may include combinations of surgery, speech therapy, medical therapy, and therapeutic assurance.

Case A

Patient A was a 36-year-old male science teacher with intermittent voice breaks and easy vocal fatigue. He underwent a direct laryngoscopy and biopsy for a "polyp" at another hospital. Postoperatively, his voice failed to return to its preoperative function. He began to experience persistent and continuous dysphonia and pain with speaking. He was unable to return to his teaching. After 6 months of persistent dysphonia he presented to our voice clinic. His voice had a rough, breathy, and diplophonic quality with frequent voice breaks. Strobovideolaryngoscopy showed a stiff immobile segment on the left vocal fold with poor vibratory function (Figure 48–11). He was diagnosed to have a stiff vocal fold segment caused by surgical scarring. He underwent 6 weeks of voice therapy consisting of exercises designed specifically to increase vocal fold flexibility, such as trill exercises and vocal range exercises. Re-examination at the end of 8 weeks of voice therapy showed a remarkably improved voice. Repeat strobovideolaryngoscopy showed a mobile, less stiff vocal fold with excellent amplitude and mucosal wave (Figure 48–12).

This case demonstrates the value of speech therapy in restoring vibratory function in a stiffened vocal fold

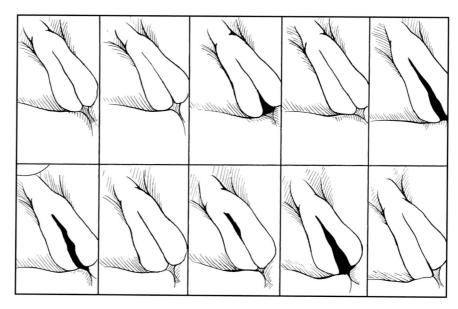

Figure 48–11. Case A, before speech therapy. This series of stroboscopic illustrations shows irregular vocal fold opening from aperiodic vocal fold oscillation caused by a scarred and stiff vocal fold. There is an irregular posterior chink and an absence of a discrete open and closed phase.

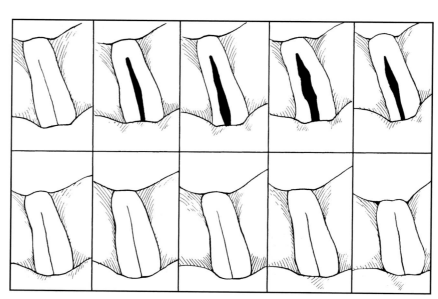

Figure 48–12. Case A, after speech therapy. With improved voice the videostroboscopy shows a regular opening and closing phase, good amplitude, and increased vibration of the side with the vocal fold scar.

caused by microlaryngoscopy. It is unlikely that the return of vocal vibratory function came about through continued spontaneous postoperative healing as the therapy was given 6 months after his surgery.

Case B

Patient B was a 45-year-old female smoker who had a "polyp" removed from the left vocal fold 1½ years ago. She stated that her voice never became normal after her surgery. Her voice was inappropriately low and continued to be mistaken for a man's. On examination, she was found to have a fundamental frequency of 180 Hz. Her voice was slightly rough with a veiled, husky quality. Strobovideolaryngoscopy revealed a mass differ-

ence between the right and the left vocal folds. Her previously operated side vibrated well with good amplitude and mucosal wave. On the right side there was evidence of Reinke's edema with polypoid degeneration. After a course of mucolytics and aggressive vocal hygiene failed, she was taken to the operating room, where a right subcordal evacuation of mucoid material was done by microdissection. Postoperatively, her voice was immediately improved. Her fundamental frequency was restored to 205 Hz with increased loudness and clarity of voice. Her laryngostroboscopy from the preoperative and postoperative examination is shown in Figures 48–13 and 48–14.

This case illustrates the added role of strobovideolaryngoscopy in detecting subtle mass differences be-

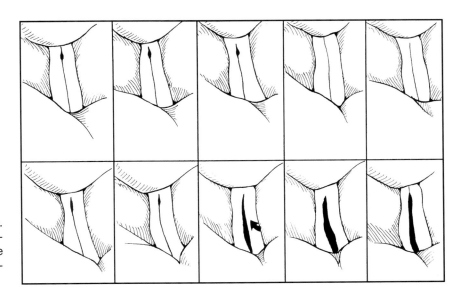

Figure 48–13. Case B, before surgery. A fullness of the right side is appreciated by stroboscopic examination. The fullness failed to oscillate (*arrow*), thereby indicating a residual mass lesion.

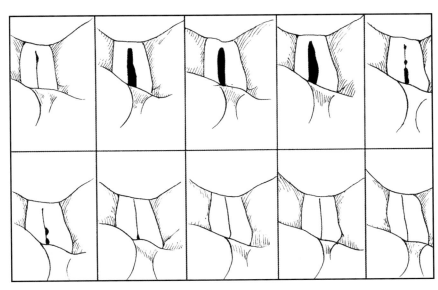

Figure 48–14. Case B, after surgery. Improved vocal fold oscillation of both vocal folds is apparent.

tween the vocal folds that could not be appreciated by nonstroboscopic means. The repeat operation restored vocal fold vibration and symmetry, resulting in a more normal vibratory pattern of vocal fold function. This correlated well with improved vocal function.

Case C

Patient C was a 58-year-old female smoker who worked in a noisy, smoky environment. She developed large bilateral laryngeal polyps with polypoid degeneration of the vocal folds. These were removed by microlaryngoscopy. She failed to experience voice improvement after surgery and brief voice rest. Examination 4 weeks after surgery revealed a diffusely reddened larynx with little vibratory amplitude or mucosal wave on either vocal fold. Further questioning revealed that the patient worked in a hot, noisy environment that required her to shout dietary orders. She also continued to smoke and cough. She was given a course of antibiotics, systemic steroids, and mucolytics and put on further voice rest for 2 weeks. Re-examination at the end of 2 weeks revealed an improved voice with good vocal function.

The diagnosis was inflammatory laryngitis exacerbated by her work environment and smoking. She was excused from her work environment and has continued to function well. Figure 48–15 shows vocal folds that are swollen and fail to vibrate. The ventricular folds are adducted with a posterior glottic chink. After medical therapy, the vocal folds show much less erythema with good vibratory function (Figure 48–16).

This case illustrates the impact of medical and environmental factors that prevented the return of vocal function. Optimizing her work environment, improv-

ing vocal hygiene, and medical treatment resulted in a more functional voice.

RESULTS

The results of treatment using such an approach can be good. In our experience, patients who are motivat-

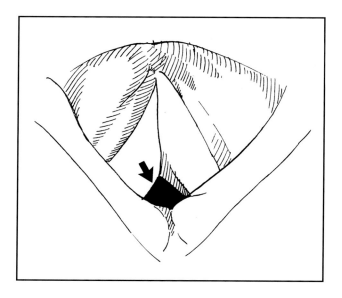

Figure 48–15. Case C, swollen and edematous vocal folds after microlaryngeal surgery. The patient's attempt at phonation results in a large posterior chink without vocal fold oscillation (*arrow on posterior chink*).

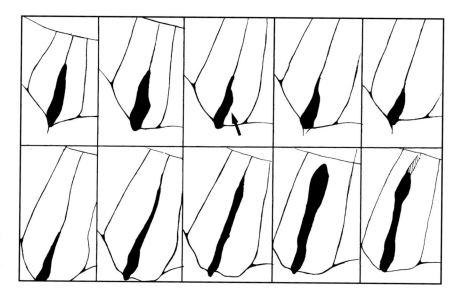

Figure 48–16. Case C, after medical therapy with steroids and antibiotics. Vocal folds now oscillate. There is still a sizable posterior chink (*arrow*).

ed and follow through on a diagnostic and treatment voice therapy program have a good chance of improved function using a combined approach. Table 48–3 shows the primary diagnosis and the various primary treatments rendered. Table 48–4 lists the results broken down by the types of problems. Patients with lesion recurrence, residual mass lesions, and hyperfunctional voice disorders did better than patients with localized scar with stiffness and inflammation. But despite the high rates of no improvement in the latter groups, improved vibratory function and voice were achieved in a significant percentage of patients.

The objective measures of vocal function help to lend support to stroboscopic observations of improved vibratory function. Table 48–5 lists some acoustic measures in 30 individuals undergoing treatment, while Table 48–6 lists the aerodynamic measures in 41 patients undergoing treatment. The acoustic measures show trends toward decreased perturbation, decreased shimmer, improved signal/noise ratio, and improved average SPL and pitch range. The mean flow was reduced from 160 ml/s to a more normal 120 ml/s, while glottal efficiency as defined by the AC/DC ratio has in-

creased. The maximum loudness was slightly decreased. This may be because of less stridency and fewer harsh glottal attacks noted in the majority of patients.

In summary, using a multidisciplinary approach to the diagnosis of postsurgical dysphonia, management issues in these difficult patients can be made easier. Moreover, treatment of these patients, utilizing the skills of the otolaryngologist, speech scientist, and speech-language pathologist, can be combined to improve vocal function in a large percentage of patients. Careful observation and understanding of vibratory function before and after phonosurgery should assist the phonosurgeon in avoiding pitfalls that result in persistent postoperative dysphonia.

REFERENCES

1. Ford C, Bless D. Collagen injection in the scarred vocal fold. *J Voice.* 1987;1:116–118.
2. Dedo HH. Injection and removal of Teflon for unilateral vocal cord paralysis. *Ann Otol Rhinol Laryngol.* 1992;101: 81–86.
3. Brodnitz FS. Results and limitations of vocal rehabilitation. *Arch Otol.* 1963;77:148–156.

Table 48–4. Results in the Series Treated by Combined Approach

	Diagnosis					
Results	Scar With Stiffness	Residual Mass	Inflammation	Hyperfunction	Recurrence	Unknown
Excellent	7	5	6	2	2	0
Improved	3	2	2	3	1	0
No improvement	8	1	3	0	0	0
No follow-up	4	0	2	2	1	3
Total	22	8	13	7	4	3

Table 48–5. Acoustic Measures in 30 Patients Undergoing Combined Treatment for Postsurgical Dysphonia

	Pre (n = 30)	Post (n = 30)
Mean speaking F_0 (Hz)	179	219
Dynamic range (dB)	25.7	25.2
Pitch range (semitones)	26.0	27.1
Average SPL (dB)	74.6	77.8
Signal/noise ratio (dB)	25.6	26.9
Shimmer (%)	1.7	0.25
Perturbation (ms)	0.015	0.01

Table 48–6. Selected Phonatory Function Measures in 41 Patients Before and 39 Patients After Combined Speech, Medical, and Surgical Treatment

	Pre (n = 41)	Post (n = 39)
Mean flow rate (ml/s)	160	120
AC/DC ratio	0.23	0.30
Maximum loudness (dB)	85	84

4. Baker et al. Persistent hoarseness after surgical removal of vocal cord lesions. *Arch Otol.* 1981;107:148–151.

5. Wolfe VI, Ratsunik DL. Vocal symptomatology of postoperative dysphonia. *Laryngoscope.* 1981;91:635–643.

6. Andrews AH. Surgery of benign tumors of the larynx. *Otolaryngol Clin North Am.* 1970;3:517–527.

7. Strong MS, Vaughn CW. Vocal cord nodule and polyps—the role of surgical treatment. *Laryngoscope.* 1971;81:911–923.

8. Kleinsasser O, Glanz H, Kimmich T. Endoscopic surgery of vocal cord cancers. *HNO.* 1988;26:412–416.

9. Leeper HA, Heeneman H, Reynolds C. Vocal function following vertical hemilaryngectomy. A preliminary investigation. *J Otolaryngol.* 1990;19:62–70.

10. Casiano RR, Cooper JD, Lundy DS, et al. Laser cordectomy for T_1 glottic carcinoma: a 10 year experience and videostroboscopic findings. *Otolaryngol Head Neck Surg.* 1991;104:831–837.

11. Watterson T, McFarlane SC, Menicacci AL. Vibratory characteristics of Teflon injected and noninjected paralyzed vocal folds. *J Speech Hear Dis.* 1990;55:61–66.

12. McGuirt WF, Blalock D, Koufman JA, et al. Voice analysis of patients with endoscopically treated early laryngeal carcinoma. *Ann Otol Rhinol Laryngol.* 1992;101:142–146.

13. Sataloff RT, Spiegel JR, Hawkshaw M, et al. Autologous fat implantation for vocal fold scar: a preliminary report. *J Voice.* 1996;11(2):238–246.

14. Bouchayer M, Cornut G, Witzig E. Microsurgery for benign lesions of the vocal folds. *Ear Nose Throat J.* 1988; 67:446.

15. Kleinsasser O. Restoration of the voice in benign lesions of the vocal folds by endolaryngeal microsurgery. *J Voice.* 1991;5:257–263.

Index